UNDERSTANDING & EVALUATING
COMMON LABORATORY TESTS

Gail Vaughn, MT, (ASCP), MSEd
Instructor and Network Coordinator
Central Kentucky Technical College,
Danville Campus
Danville, Kentucky

APPLETON & LANGE
Stamford, CT

Notice: The author and the publisher of this volume have taken care to make certain that the doses of drugs and schedules of treatment are correct and compatible with the standards generally accepted at the time of publication. Nevertheless, as new information becomes available, changes in treatment and in the use of drugs become necessary. The reader is advised to carefully consult the instruction and information material included in the package insert of each drug or therapeutic agent before administration. This advice is especially important when using, administering, or recommending new or infrequently used drugs. The author and publisher disclaim all responsibility for any liability, loss, injury, or damage incurred as a consequence, directly or indirectly, of the use and application of any of the contents of this volume.

Copyright ©1999 by Appleton & Lange

www.appletonlange.com

99 00 01 02 / 10 9 8 7 6 5 4 3 2 1

Prentice Hall International (UK) Limited, *London*
Prentice Hall of Australia Pty. Limited, *Sydney*
Prentice Hall Canada, Inc., *Toronto*
Prentice Hall Hispanoamericana, S.A., *Mexico*
Prentice Hall of India Private Limited, *New Delhi*
Prentice Hall of Japan, Inc., *Tokyo*
Simon & Schuster Asia Pte. Ltd., *Singapore*
Editora Prentice Hall do Brasil Ltda., *Rio de Janeiro*
Prentice Hall, Upper Saddle River, *New Jersey*

Vaughn, Gail.
    Understanding and evaluating common laboratory tests /
by Gail Vaughn.
        p.   cm.
    ISBN 0-8385-9273-2 (alk. paper)
    1. Diagnosis, Laboratory.   2. Nursing.   I. Title.
    [DNLM: 1. Laboratory Techniques and Procedures handbooks.
2. Laboratory Techniques and Procedures examination questions.   QY
39 V372u 1999]
RB37.V36   1999
616.07'56--DC21
DNLM/DLC
for Library of Congress   98-31573

ISBN 0-8385-9273-2

Acquisitions Editor: David P. Carroll
Production Service: Tage Publishing Service, Inc.
Interior Designer: Maryann Dube
Cover Designer: Mary Skudlarek

PRINTED IN THE UNITED STATES OF AMERICA

To my family. . . . . .
for your support, encouragement, and endurance!

CONTENTS

PREFACE

The field of laboratory medicine is a large and diverse one that does not readily lend itself to texts that are complete, concise, and instructional. Although many excellent text and reference books are available, those that are complete are generally either limited to one specialty area of laboratory medicine (such as hematology or chemistry) or present information related to all testing areas in a very abbreviated fashion for quick reference (such as those providing a brief test description and reference ranges). In addition, laboratory text and reference books are often written for a specific health care profession in order to best meet the needs of that discipline. Texts targeted primarily for clinical laboratory scientists must incorporate a great deal of technical and procedural testing information in addition to theoretical concepts, while those developed for other health care professionals must often sacrifice useful explanatory information for the sake of brevity. *Understanding and Evaluating Common Laboratory Tests* was developed to:

- appeal across disciplines to health care professionals who may have occasion to evaluate laboratory data.
- provide a basis for understanding test principles, factors affecting test results, and indications for the most common procedures as well as for applying these concepts to the evaluation of laboratory data in health and disease.
- present information in an instructional format and provide frequent opportunities to check understanding with review questions and self-tests.
- provide summary information throughout the text in table and chart form to facilitate use of the text for quick reference or review purposes.

The intent of the text is to present the technical aspects of laboratory testing along with pertinent clinical information. In addition to assessment of organ/system function, discussions typically include a review of anatomy and physiology; factors influencing test results; general test selection and usage considerations, including diagnostic and screening test results; general clinical findings; and signs, symptoms, and brief descriptions of related disease processes. Although treatment considerations are included in some discussions, the text is not intended to serve as the basis for determining patient treatment regimens nor to infer the indication for a particular treatment option. It is my hope that presenting laboratory test information in this context will facilitate understanding the principles of laboratory tests, the evaluation and application of laboratory data, and the role of laboratory medicine as it relates to other aspects of medicine.

This text is designed for use in both academic and clinical settings. It is appropriate for use in a variety of academic programs including those for practical nurses, registered nurses, nurse practitioners, and physician assistants. It is also beneficial for clinical laboratory technician/scientist programs as an adjunct text, for introducing laboratory medicine concepts to medical students, and as a reference for health care professionals seeking increased understanding of clinical laboratory data.

General information regarding the laboratory, test characteristics, evaluation of test performance, reference ranges, and related topics are presented in the first chapter to provide an overview of laboratory organization and basic concepts of laboratory medicine applicable throughout the rest of the text. Stressed here, and repeated in other sections, is the reminder that reference ranges provided in this or any other text cannot be universally or arbitrarily applied to the interpretation of laboratory data. Reference ranges specific to the test results under consideration must always be used. Appendices are included to provide additional information on topics covered in the body of the text and are generally presented in summary fashion. Answer keys for the self-tests at the end of each chapter are also found in the appendices.

The format of the text allows individual chapters to be used independently, though some closely related chapters may best be studied together or referred to as related chapters are studied. The text is not, however, intended to be all-inclusive with detailed information on all available laboratory analyses, to provide in-depth instruction for advanced students of laboratory medicine, nor to provide procedural steps for test performance. Other excellent materials, many of which are included in the list of references for this book, are available for these purposes.

Finally, an attempt has been made to find an acceptable balance that permits material to be offered with thorough coverage of the concepts presented, yet preserves a reasonable degree of brevity.

Advances in laboratory medicine and the development of new tests and test applications occur continually. As is the case in all aspects of medicine, continued study is necessary to maintain current knowledge in laboratory medicine. No individual author can be an expert in all areas of laboratory medicine. To develop a text based on the diverse and extensive body of knowledge encompassed by laboratory medicine, one must incorporate the knowledge, experience, and expertise of a variety of others in the field.

GAIL VAUGHN

ACKNOWLEDGMENTS

There are a number of individuals without whom this text would not have been possible and various others whose efforts have contributed to the quality, completeness, and accuracy of the material presented. Although any effort to acknowledge all those involved in this undertaking is certain to be incomplete, it is important that appreciation be expressed to a number of people. For the initial nudge toward publication, I am grateful to Jackie Lesperance, Laboratory Administrative Director at Ephraim McDowell Regional Medical Center as well as to JoAnn Rice, PharmD and Patricia Wynd, MT (ASCP), MSEd.

To David Carroll, Senior Editor at Appleton & Lange, I express not only appreciation for getting the "ball rolling" and for expert guidance, but also for encouragement and support along the way and for an unerring sense of humor. Dave was always available with appropriate and calming words of encouragement, whether my hysteria was related to an impending (or missed) deadline or to a personal crisis, and could invariably supply a humorous anecdote. Zöe Daniell, Editorial Assistant, was also an invaluable resource. Angela Dion, Tony Caruso, and many others at and associated with Appleton & Lange are also to be acknowledged for their dedication and professionalism.

To Doctors W. L. Pesci, MD, and Richard G. Jackson, Jr., MD, Medical Directors of Laboratory and Pathology Services at Ephraim McDowell Regional Medical Center, I offer my sincere gratitude for the encouragement, support, guidance, and mentoring provided over the years, along with appreciation for review of some of the text's subject matter.

Finally, tremendous gratitude goes to my family, especially my husband, for support and encouragement throughout the long and often difficult process of making this book a reality. Being blithely ignorant of the extraordinary amount of concentrated and continuous work required to bring such a project to fruition, I initiated this effort with excitement and delight. However, somewhere around the time the text came to be referred to as "that eternal book" and our children asked at least weekly if "she" was "*still* working on *that*," I came to rely heavily on his unwavering confidence and supportive encouragement.

1. ABOUT THE LABORATORY

Although many health care organizations are now promoting a more interdisciplinary approach to the delivery of services, professional groups within these organizations may be somewhat tribalistic and territorial. Stemming perhaps from the initial establishment of a professional identity, delineation of responsibility, organizational structure, and a sense of professional pride, this tribal mentality can result in the various "tribes" having only a vague and simplistic impression of the responsibilities, skill, and knowledge of their sister tribes (nurses take temperatures and give shots; laboratorians draw blood and send back reports; physical therapists walk patients and massage sore muscles ...). The information in this chapter is provided to familiarize you with the layout of the home territory of the laboratory tribe, the members of the tribe and their roles, and some of the elements of the tribal language.

DEPARTMENTS

Laboratories vary widely from large, fully automated and highly specialized regional reference laboratories to laboratories serving hospitals of various sizes and small laboratories with a limited test menu and little automation in physicians' offices and small clinics. A number of separate departments (or testing areas in smaller settings) make up the clinical laboratory. A general listing of these departments along with examples of the test procedures performed in each is provided below.

- **Hematology:** compute blood count; erythrocyte sedimentation rate; platelet count
- **Chemistry:** glucose; potassium; chemistry profiles/panels
- **Therapeutic Drug Monitoring (TDM):**[1] dilantin; valproic acid; theophylline
- **Toxicology:**[1] abused drug screens and individual drug levels

---

[1] TDM and Toxicology are sometimes combined and, in smaller settings, may be performed in Chemistry.

1

- **Coagulation:**[2] prothrombin time; activated partial thromboplastin time; fibrinogen; factor assays
- **Urinalysis:**[2] routine urine testing; semen analysis; urine pregnancy tests
- **Serology/Immunology:** mononucleosis; antistreptolysin O; immune function/autoimmune disorder tests; antibody levels
- **Transfusion Service (Blood Bank):** ABO/Rh typing; compatibility testing; antibody detection and identification
- **Microbiology:**[3] cultures; parasite detection and identification; virology tests; fungal tests; antibiotic sensitivities

THE LABORATORY STAFF

The laboratory operates under the medical oversight of a **Medical Director**. The Medical Director is a physician and is usually a pathologist, a medical doctor with additional training, experience, and board certification in clinical and/or anatomical pathology.

Administrative direction of the laboratory is usually provided by a Clinical Laboratory Scientist (CLS), also called a Medical Technologist (MT), with at least a bachelor's degree and often with a master's degree in a related field or in business administration. Laboratories of sufficient size have a supervisor for each of the departments within the laboratory and/or for various shifts who is also a bachelor's degree technologist. Larger facilities and laboratories at university teaching hospitals may also have a doctoral-level department head for each testing section.

Testing personnel include bachelor's degree technologists (sometimes with graduate degrees as well)and associate degree technicians who perform testing of moderate and high complexity classifications. A national examination administered by the American Society of Clinical Pathologists (ASCP) certifies technicians and technologists, and some states require a state administered examination for practice in that state. Each laboratory is required by regulatory and licensing agencies to ensure the ongoing competency and proficiency of personnel on at least an annual basis.

With the large and diverse body of knowledge included in laboratory medicine, laboratorians often specialize in a particular department through education, certification, or experience. Much as nursing personnel specialize in critical care, pediatrics, or obstetrics, a laboratorian's area of expertise may be in chemistry, microbiology, hematology, transfusion medicine, or other clinical testing areas. Specialization allows a more in-depth knowledge of test principles and procedures, as well as increased familiarity with and experience in detecting and identifying abnormalities and associated disease processes. Technologists may seek ASCP cer-

---

[2]Sometimes combined with Hematology; urinalysis may be in the department of Clinical Microscopy.

[3]In larger settings Bacteriology, Parasitology, Virology, and Mycobacteriology may each be a separate department.

tification in individual departments and, in some cases, specialist certification such as that offered for technologists with advanced education and experience in blood bank practice (SBB).

Phlebotomists and laboratory assistants are generally responsible for the collection of specimens for testing and may perform some basic laboratory procedures under the direction of qualified testing personnel. Preparation for these positions may be from an academic program or, in some cases, on-the-job training, and certification may be obtained by examination. Medical assistants with an associate degree may also fill these positions in the laboratory. Clerical staff support the laboratory's delivery of services by filing reports, retrieving results for clients, receiving specimens, and providing a variety of clerical support services.

REGULATORY AGENCIES

Laboratories are required to meet the standards of the Health Care Financing Administration (HCFA) as set forth by CLIA '88 (Clinical Laboratory Improvement Act of 1988). Compliance is ensured by state laboratory inspectors. Many hospital laboratories achieve voluntary accreditation by meeting the standards of the Joint Commission on Accreditation of Health Care Organizations (JCAHO) in addition to those mandated by CLIA. A further voluntary accreditation is provided through the College of American Pathologists (CAP), considered by some laboratorians to be the highest level of accreditation because of its stringent requirements.

Laboratories are under the regulation of a variety of health care oversight agencies and workplace regulatory agencies, including the Occupational Safety and Health Administration (OSHA) and often look to the Centers for Disease Control and Prevention (CDC) for recommendations and guidelines in specific areas of practice.

USING LABORATORY DATA

Data obtained from laboratory analysis may be used in a variety of ways:

1. to confirm a condition suspected based on clinical presentation.
2. to rule out certain conditions (pregnancy prior to surgical procedure; other causes of a positive test result).
3. to monitor the effectiveness of therapy (therapeutic drug levels; prothrombin time monitoring of warfarin [Coumadin] therapy).
4. to assess the severity of a disease or to provide prognostic information (T-cell counts in AIDS patients).
5. screening for disease (donor blood testing; newborn phenylketonuria testing).

Screening tests are best used when applied to a defined population (eg, blood donors, newborns) for specific indications or risk factors. Random screening without population selection and in the absence of clinical suspicion or other indication, raises questions of medical necessity and provides questionable benefit related to the resource expenditure. About twice as many tests are requested to follow patients who have been previously diagnosed as those requested to establish a diagnosis.

Laboratory data should always be used in conjunction with clinical findings, patient history, and information available from any other diagnostic procedures. Dr. John Bernard Henry, in the 19th edition of *Clinical Diagnosis and Management by Laboratory Methods* (1996), provides three fundamental principles to be followed in the interpretation of laboratory data:

1. Diagnosis should not be made based upon a single abnormal value.
2. In patients under the age of 60, an effort should be made to attribute all abnormal results to the same condition, with multiple diagnoses considered only if it is impossible to do so (Osler's Rule).
3. Significantly abnormal values, especially if inconsistent with clinical impression or other findings, should be verified by repeat analysis. It may be beneficial to confirm results by repeat analysis on the original sample as well as with analysis of a new specimen. This is true not only of abnormal values, but of any inconsistent results.

In addition to understanding the applications of a specific test, general knowledge of the performance characteristics of laboratory tests is beneficial in using the data obtained from laboratory analyses.

■ VALIDITY OF DATA

The final test result received from the laboratory is no better than the sample upon which the analysis was performed; therefore it is imperative not only that samples be completely and accurately identified and collected in appropriate containers, but that established collection and storage procedures for each sample be adhered to exactly. Some test procedures require a fasting sample for valid, useful data; some should be collected at specified time intervals or at a given time following administration of medication; others, because of diurnal variations, require morning collection only. Certain samples must be protected from light; others immediately chilled or frozen; and some require analysis within a very short time period after collection. Failure to adhere to collection and storage requirements can yield invalid results, usually due to the deterioration of the element or analyte in question. In such situations a falsely decreased value may be obtained. For example, bilirubin in a serum sample that is not adequately protected from light will be broken down and the sample will yield a bilirubin level that is lower than the actual serum level upon analysis. By the same token, a cerebrospinal fluid (CSF) sample not delivered promptly to the laboratory for immediate testing may result in a laboratory report indicating a lower than actual number of white cells since these cells deteriorate fairly rapidly in CSF.

A variety of medications, vitamins, and, in some cases, dietary intake can interfere with or alter test results. The manner in which results are affected may be either from interference with the chemical reaction that takes place in the test procedure or as a result of actual physiologic changes attributable to the medication or other substance.

The terms *false positive* and *false negative* are applied to invalid results obtained as a result of an interference of some sort or resulting from an improper specimen. **False negative** refers to a result that does not detect a substance or condition that is actually present. A negative urine pregnancy test on a woman who is actually pregnant might result from a failure to test a first morning specimen (most concentrated)—false negative. **False positive** refers to the detection of a substance or condition that is not present. A nonpregnant woman may have a positive pregnancy test as a result of a human chorionic gonadotropin (hCG) producing tumor—a false positive result.

Some false positive results may be caused by an interference with the actual test methodology, as in cases where certain drugs or other substances may interfere with a chemical reaction or cause a reaction producing a similar end product that will be detected by the method employed. In other cases false positives may result from physiologic causes, whether from a physiologic change produced by a medication or by the presence of an unrelated disease state that produces a positive result.

The rate of false positive results obtained by a particular test method is influenced by the **specificity** of the test. Specificity refers to how well the method performs in detecting *only* the desired substance or condition and is defined mathematically as

$$\frac{\text{\# negative test results}}{\text{\# normal individuals}} \times 100.$$

Although many test methods now approach a 100 % specificity level, no method is truly 100 % specific. The greater the likelihood that a particular method will detect substances or conditions other than those intended, the lower the specificity for that method. For example, a positive screening test for mononucleosis does not establish the presence of infectious mononucleosis (IM) with 100 % accuracy. Patients with some leukemias and lymphomas will also produce a positive result in this test. The Venereal Disease Research Laboratory (VDRL) test for syphilis is notorious for false positive results as it is not a highly specific test. Thus a notable number of patients may have a positive VDRL test in the absence of syphilis (any connective tissue disorder, such as rheumatoid arthritis, can produce positive results as can a variety of other diseases, including tuberculosis, IM, and chronic liver disease) and all positive VDRL tests require confirmation by a more specific test, the fluorescent treponemal antigen (FTA) test. Screening tests, used only as an initial indicator of the possible presence of the condition screened for, will have a lower level of specificity than do the confirmatory tests used to verify positive results obtained using the initial screening method.

Tests that do not have a high sensitivity will yield more false negative results than procedures that are very sensitive. The **sensitivity** of a test reflects the level or concentration of a substance that must be present in order for the methodology to detect its presence. Sensitivity is defined mathematically as

$$\frac{\text{\# positive results}}{\text{\# with disease}} \times 100.$$

A highly sensitive method will detect very small amounts of a substance, whereas a less sensitive method will require the substance to be present in greater concentrations for detection. A very highly sensitive test—detecting even minute amounts of a substance—may not have an acceptable level of specificity due, in part, to the high sensitivity (ie, the method is so sensitive that it detects virtually every similar substance resulting in a low specificity). The sensitivity of a test can determine at what point a condition will be detected. For example, the sensitivity level of a pregnancy test (the lowest concentration of hCG the method detects) determines, in part, how soon after conception pregnancy is detected. Just as it is not possible for a method to be 100 % specific, neither can a method be perfect in terms of sensitivity.

In choosing appropriate methodologies, laboratorians often must balance the specificity and sensitivity levels of methods. Ideally, the methods chosen for patient testing would be 100 % specific and 100 % sensitive. Since this is, of course, not possible in the real world in which clinical laboratory medicine is practiced, a degree of either sensitivity or specificity may be sacrificed depending upon the purposes for which the test value will be used. A maximum level of sensitivity is preferred for disease detection, while a higher level of specificity is desirable for confirmation of a suspected condition. Screening tests used to detect the possible presence of disease may be of low specificity, yet have a high degree of sensitivity. In addition to the examples provided in the preceding discussion of test specificity, excellent examples are provided by the methods employed to screen donated blood for the presence of infectious disease. Since the goal is to provide a safe blood supply that will not transmit infectious disease to transfusion recipients, it is better to exclude perfectly healthy donors (due to false positives—low specificity) than to miss the detection of true carriers (low sensitivity) of disease. The tests donor centers use to screen for the presence of hepatitis are highly sensitive, but may be "positive" in the absence of hepatitis, leading to the unnecessary exclusion of a donor without the disease. However, in terms of providing the safest blood supply possible, the negativity of unwarranted exclusion of healthy donors is greatly outweighed by the desire to ensure that no inappropriate donors are missed.

Confirming a condition that is suspected (based upon either clinical findings or other testing results) requires a more specific test even if the level of sensitivity is lower. Continuing with the blood donor testing example, donor blood that tests positive with an HIV antibody screening test is subjected to confirmatory testing by a more specific methodology such as the Western blot.

The performance of a test method is also described in terms of accuracy and precision levels. The **accuracy** of a method refers to how close the value obtained by this method is to the "true" value. It may be evaluated based upon the value yielded by an accepted standard and should be evaluated at low, normal, and high levels of the substance tested for.

Precision describes the *reproducibility* of the results obtained by a method. In other words, how close are repeated measurements of the same sample? Both precision and accuracy are evaluated by statistical analysis of an established number of measurements to determine the presence of statistically or medically significant differences. It is possible for a test method to be highly precise, but inaccurate, or to be accurate, but imprecise. A test method that yields glucose results of 100, 99, 101, 99, 100, 100, 101, 102, 100, 99, 98, 98, 100, 99, 100, 101, 101, 100, 102, and 100 on repeated measurement of the same sample has a high degree of precision (the differences in the measurements are neither statistically nor medically significant). However, if the "true" value for the glucose present in the sample is 300, the method has a low degree of accuracy. Good test methods should have a high degree of both precision and accuracy.

Good laboratory practice dictates that all test methods be evaluated in terms of sensitivity, specificity, precision, and accuracy prior to implementing the method for patient testing. If the method is being implemented to replace an existing method, a statistical comparison of the two methods is also necessary. Other performance characteristics of test methods are also evaluated by laboratorians prior to implementing new methodologies in addition to practical concerns regarding the cost per test, ease of performance, time required to produce results, chemicals and equipment required, and other considerations.

■ SOURCES OF ERROR

All laboratory analyses can be divided into three separate phases, with potential sources of error in each.

1. Pre-analytical: patient preparation; specimen collection, handling, and processing
2. Analytical: actual sample analysis
3. Post-analytical: calculations; transcribing results; charting report

Examples of errors in the **pre-analytical stage** include improper patient or specimen identification, patient not fasting when required, collection in the wrong preservative, collection at the wrong time, and storage at incorrect temperature.

An improperly maintained analyzer, expired or contaminated chemicals and reagents, improperly calibrated measuring devices, inaccuracies in the length or temperature of incubation phases, or poor laboratory technique would result in errors in the **analytical stage**. Errors may occur **post-analytically** when a calculation is made incorrectly, numbers are transposed when reports are written or read, results are stated or understood incorrectly in telephoned reports, or reports are placed on the wrong patient chart.

Fortunately, such errors are relatively rare as a result of a variety of "checks and balances" in place in all reputable laboratories, nursing units, physician offices, hospitals, and other health care facilities.

■ QUALITY CONTROL

A number of steps are taken to ensure the reliability of patient test results in addition to the evaluation of the performance characteristics of a test method. Samples of known concentrations are tested to ensure acceptable performance by the test system and testing personnel. A **quality control** protocol is established for each test method that establishes the frequency at which quality control (QC) samples are tested, the number and type of QC samples (low, normal, high), and an acceptable range for results.

Results are further evaluated to detect any shifts or trends that may occur even in QC results falling within acceptable ranges. To detect these more subtle changes or problems in QC data, a series of control rules called Westgard Rules are usually employed and are particularly beneficial to laboratorians lacking years of experience in evaluating Levy-Jennings plots of control data. Westgard Rules may initially appear confusing to those inexperienced in their use, but actually provide a logical, step-wise approach to the evaluation of QC data. Some of the rules are sensitive to **random error** (the variability resulting from imprecision inherent to some degree in all testing and affecting isolated or single values), while others are better at detecting **systematic error** (errors in the analytic process that can affect a series of results such as would be seen with an incorrectly calibrated pipette or an incorrect wavelength setting for endpoint detection).

Laboratory computer systems and many modern analyzers are capable of automatically applying selected Westgard Rules to control data and alerting the operator to any QC failures so that appropriate corrective actions can be immediately instituted. The rules will not be detailed here except for the following two examples of how their application could lead to rejected results.

- Reject when four consecutive QC results are 1 SD above the same mean or are 1 SD below the same mean.
- Reject when ten consecutive QC values fall on one side of the mean.

The examples of Levy-Jennings charts of QC provided (Figures 1–1, 1–2, and 1–3) may be beneficial to an understanding of basic QC principles.

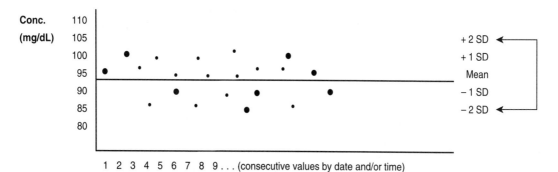

FIGURE 1–1. Graph of glucose control results. *All values acceptable; bracketed area denotes acceptable range.*

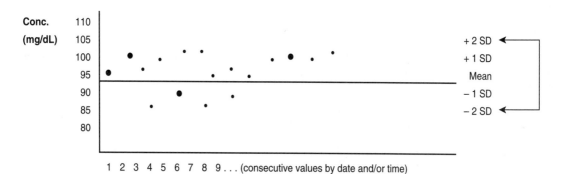

FIGURE 1–2. Control results depicting four consecutive values 1 SD above mean. *All values acceptable; bracketed area denotes acceptable range.*

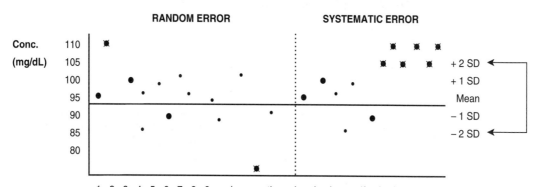

FIGURE 1–3. Control results representative of random and systematic error. *Bracketed area denotes acceptable range; values representative of random error—left of dotted line—and of systematic error—right of dotted line—are represented by ¤.*

Definitions of and formulas for the calculation of some **basic statistical parameters** used in the laboratory to evaluate control data, reference ranges, and instrument performance are provided below. Symbols and abbreviations used in these formulas are defined below.

Symbol or Abbreviation	Meaning
Σ	The sum of
$\bar{x}$	Mean or average
$\times$	Each measured value
x_d	Difference of a measured value from the mean
SD	Standard deviation
CV	Coefficient of variation
N	Total number of measurements

Mean: an average; calculated by adding results and dividing by the total number of measurements, or

$$\frac{\Sigma X}{N}$$

x_d: calculated by

$$x - \bar{x}$$

Standard deviation: an expression of variation from the mean calculated by determining the square root of

$$\frac{\Sigma(x - x_d)^2}{N - 1}$$

Coefficient of variation: another measure of variation; used to compare the performance of different test methods and to compare data from one laboratory to that of other laboratories; expressed as a percentage and calculated by determining the square root of

$$\frac{\Sigma(x - x_d)^2}{N - 1}$$

and dividing the result by the mean times 100.

■ DELTA CHECKS AND PROFICIENCY TESTING

Additional methods used in the laboratory to ensure the validity of patient data include delta checks and external quality control programs or proficiency testing. **Delta** (symbolized by "Δ" and meaning "change") **checks** involve a comparison of a test result to a previous result, if available, on the same patient. A time period for which results will be compared and the level at which a difference is considered clinically significant is defined for each parameter. Many analyzers have the capability to automatically perform delta checks and alert testing personnel of significant variations requiring follow-up. Laboratory information systems (LIS) also provide automatic delta checking as defined by the user on initial system setup. Some small laboratories may lack instrumentation capable of delta checks and may not have an LIS. In such situations, significant obstacles to effective delta checking are presented. Delta checks in these laboratories will likely be limited to a quick review of result logs over a very short time period (and then, most likely only when an abnormal result of significance is obtained or results are questioned by nursing or medical staff) or to testing personnel's memory of performing previous testing on the patient with a significantly different outcome.

Laboratories are required to participate in an approved **proficiency testing** program such as that provided by the College of American Pathologists. In such programs, the laboratory receives sets of samples (referred to as a "survey") at established intervals (four times per year for most analytes) for every regulated test the laboratory performs. The samples are analyzed by the same methods used for patient testing and results sent back for evaluation. A report is issued of the laboratory's performance that not only includes an evaluation of the accuracy of results, but also compares the laboratory's performance relative to all other reporting laboratories. Proficiency testing scores less than 80% are considered failures regardless of the cause of the error leading to the low score (eg, the laboratory obtained the correct test result, but a clerical error resulted in the value being recorded in the wrong column or associated with the wrong methodology on the report). Laboratories must have written policies and procedures in place detailing what actions will be taken in response to proficiency testing failures and how testing will be handled in the event proficiency testing failures require suspension of testing for a particular analyte and method (Is an alternate method available for testing? Will samples be referred to another laboratory and, if so, can results be provided within an acceptable time period?).

■ REFERENCE RANGES

Reference ranges, sometimes called normal ranges, are provided along with patient test results to assist the clinician in the interpretation of laboratory data. These ranges are established by testing a significant number of "normal," healthy subjects and statistically determining a range at a specified confidence level, usually 95% or 2 SD, based upon a Gaussian (normal) distribution curve (Fig. 1–4). Using this range (with the assumptions that persons exhibiting no signs of disease are normal and that test results from normal individuals have true random distribution) means that 95 % of clinically normal individuals can be expected to have values that fall within the established range. Note that this also means that 5 % of clinically normal individuals can be expected to have values outside this range (2.5 % above the upper limit of the range and 2.5 % below the lower limit of the range).

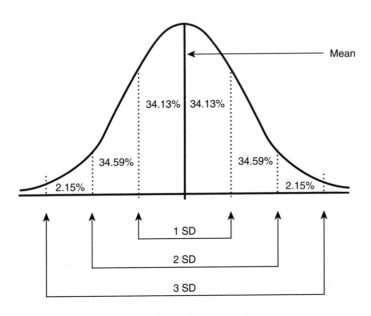

FIGURE 1-4. Normal (Gaussian) distribution.

Because of the number of variables that influence the establishment of a reference range, it is not possible to definitively establish one range that is applicable for an analyte across methods, location, and population. Reference ranges provided with the patient's report must be used in the evaluation of that particular laboratory value. Because of a lack of uniform standardization for all instruments, one test method may yield a glucose reference range of 90 to 110 while another methodology used in a different laboratory may have a reference range of 80 to 100, and home test meters may have yet another range.

Reference ranges are not only affected by the obvious differences in test methodology, but may also differ based upon age and gender. The alkaline phosphatase reference range for actively growing children will be higher than that for adults; newborns have a higher normal bilirubin level than adults; women generally have a lower hemoglobin level than men and pregnancy alters a variety of normal values. In some cases geographic location is an influencing factor, as can be seen in hemoglobin and red blood cell reference ranges for those living at high altitudes. Although racial and ethnic variations are generally not significant, there are some instances in which reference ranges may be impacted by these variations.

Each laboratory should evaluate the reference ranges used and establish ranges appropriate for their particular methodology and population. Patient data must be evaluated based upon the appropriate reference range, not upon "generic" ranges that may be found in test handbooks or other sources. *Reference ranges provided in this text should not be used to evaluate patient data unless the range is consistent with that provided by the testing laboratory.* It is also important to note the units of measure provided with both reference ranges and patient results. Are results reported in conventional units such as mg/dL or mEq/L or in mmol/L SI units (a standardized international system of measurement based on the metric system)? Values may be very different in some cases depending upon the units of measure.

■ CRITICAL VALUES

Each laboratory, ideally in conjunction with the medical staff of the facility, establishes a listing of test results that require immediate notification of the clinician. These values are typically called *critical values* or *panic values.* These values may differ somewhat from one institution to another, just as reference ranges do. Immediate notification is required for such results since they indicate the possible need for prompt intervention. Laboratories often verify critical values by repeat analysis, particularly when it is the first such result on a patient or is unexpected for other reasons. An example of a critical value list is included in the appendices.

■ ORDERING TERMINOLOGY

Many tests are available in a variety of panels or profiles. Laboratories may have different test combinations included in these panels and designate the panels by a variety of names. It is important that those with responsibility for requesting test procedures be familiar with the test menu of their laboratory. Further, an emphasis on the "medical necessity" of laboratory procedures by Medicare makes it imperative that tests be ordered in groups only when indicated. If a physician needs only glucose and potassium levels based upon the patient's medical condition and history, it would not be medically necessary to request a chemistry profile consisting of these two analytes along with another 10 or 20 other tests.

Designation of testing priority when a test is requested assists the laboratory in the effective management of workload and allows the clinician to receive those results needed for immediate patient care in a more timely manner. Most tests can be completed as a part of routine batch testing, but others are needed as quickly as possible and are designated "stat." It is important that only those tests required at once be designated as stat, in order that the completion of truly stat procedures is not compromised. Many laboratories have established stat lists containing those procedures that may be requested and performed on a stat basis. Tests not included in this listing would not be made available on a stat basis. For example, a lipid profile is not a procedure that would be needed on a stat basis for immediate medical intervention and would not be included on a laboratory's stat test list.

1. SELF TEST

Choose the best response by circling the appropriate letter. The answer key may be found in the appendices.

1. **A complete blood count (CBC) would be performed in which laboratory department?**
   A. chemistry
   B. serology
   C. hematology
   D. microbiology

2. **The medical director of the laboratory is a**
   A. bachelor's degree technologist
   B. physician
   C. master's degree technologist
   D. bachelor's degree RN

3. **A false negative test result would indicate that**
   A. the test detected a substance or condition that was not present
   B. the test had a low level of precision
   C. quality control results were not in the acceptable range
   D. a substance or condition that was present was not detected

4. **A test method with a low degree of specificity would be most likely to produce**
   A. false positive results
   B. false negative results
   C. highly precise values
   D. high levels of accuracy

5. **Reference ranges can be altered by**
   A. testing method
   B. age
   C. gender
   D. all of the above, as well as other variables

6. **Established sample collection and storage standards are**
   A. general suggestions for obtaining specimens
   B. requirements necessary to ensure appropriate testing samples
   C. an unnecessary addition to the workload of collection personnel
   D. the same regardless of the type of test ordered

7. **Tests should be designated as stat**
   A. when the physician is late for a scheduled meeting
   B. when needed before a nursing change of shift
   C. when results are needed for immediate medical intervention
   D. when the laboratory is notoriously slow in completing procedures

8. **With a normal distribution of values, the percentage of healthy individuals with results within a 2 SD range is**
   A. 85%
   B. 95%
   C. 100%
   D. 34.13%

9. **In a comparison of a screening test with a confirmatory procedure, the screening test would be likely to have**
   A. the same level of sensitivity and specificity
   B. lower sensitivity and higher specificity
   C. a higher degree of precision and accuracy
   D. higher sensitivity and lower specificity

2. ROUTINE URINALYSIS AND TESTS OF RENAL FUNCTION

Before undertaking a study of the tests of renal function and the clinical significance of test results, it is important to have a good understanding of the basic anatomy and physiology of the kidney and the urinary system. Although some of this information may be a review for you, this knowledge forms an important basis for understanding, and using the results from, renal function tests.

■ MAJOR FUNCTIONS

Looking at the functions of the urinary system demonstrates the importance of this system to our overall health and well-being and the necessity of a properly functioning renal system for a variety of bodily functions. The primary functions of the kidney and urinary system are as follows:

1. removal of metabolic wastes and toxic substances
2. regulation of volume and composition of body fluids by reabsorption and secretion
3. maintenance of acid-base balance
4. maintenance of blood pressure and erythropoiesis, producing substances important to the metabolism of other body tissues:
    - *renin:* a protein that acts as an enzyme converting an alpha-2-globulin of the blood into angiotensin I, which is rapidly transformed into angiotensin II, a powerful vasoconstrictor
    - *erythropoietin:* necessary for erythropoiesis (the formation of red blood cells)
    - *vitamin D and metabolites:* essential in calcium and phosphorous metabolism

■ BASIC ANATOMY

The two kidneys are embedded in fatty tissue known as the adipose capsule against the posterior wall of the abdomen under the lower ribs, one on either side of the vertebral column. The kidney is surrounded by the renal fascia, a sheath of fibrous tissue that helps to hold the kidney in place. It is interesting to note that the right kidney is slightly lower than the left one. The outer portion of the kidney is the cortex and the inner part is the medulla. These bean-shaped organs are greatly specialized and are highly vascular structures (Figs. 2–1 and 2–2).

From the pelvis of the kidney, a tube called a **ureter** carries urine from the kidney to the bladder where it empties into the base of the bladder. The **bladder**, a muscular, membranous, distensible reservoir for urine, is situated in the anterior part of the pelvic cavity—in females, in front of the anterior wall of the vagina and uterus; in males, in front of the rectum. The lower part of the bladder, the neck, is continuous with the urethra, a canal for the discharge of urine. It extends from the bladder to the outside. In the female, its orifice lies in the vestibule between vagina and clitoris. The male urethra transverses the penis and opens at the tip of the glans penis, serving as the passage for semen as well as urine.

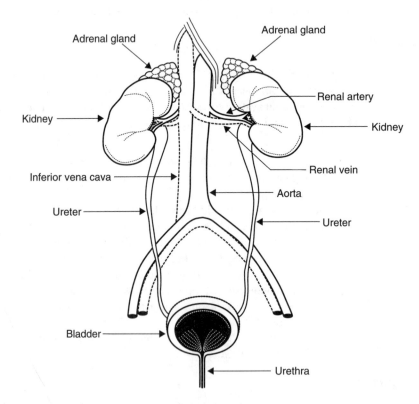

FIGURE 2–1. Organs of the urinary system.

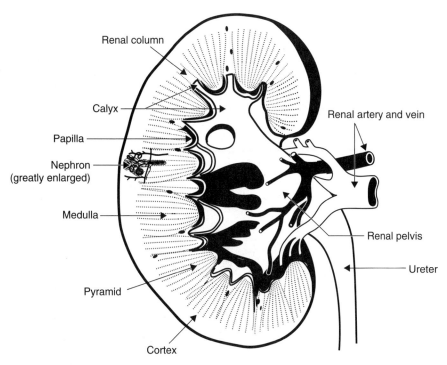

Renal column

Calyx

Papilla

Nephron
(greatly enlarged)

Medulla

Pyramid

Cortex

Renal artery and vein

Renal pelvis

Ureter

FIGURE 2-2. Internal structure of the kidney.

■ THE NEPHRON

Urine is formed in the basic structural and functional unit of the kidney, the **nephron**. Each kidney contains more than one million nephrons. The nephron consists of a renal corpuscle (which is a glomerulus enclosed in a membrane called **Bowman's capsule**) and its attached tubule. The **glomerulus** is a network of capillaries that serves as a filtering system. Blood enters the glomerulus through the afferent arteriole and leaves via the efferent arteriole. The tubular portion consists of the proximal convoluted tubule, the **loop of Henle**, and the distal convoluted tubule. The **proximal convoluted tubule** is the uppermost portion and is continuous with the glomerulus. It has finger-like projections that serve to increase the surface area used for resorption. The loop of Henle extends into the medulla, where the salt concentration is increased in the surrounding interstitium. Shorter than the proximal tubule, the **distal convoluted tubule** convolutes in the area of the afferent arteriole. It has numerous mitochondria which would indicate marked enzymatic activity. These tubular portions connect by arched and straight collecting tubules. Each nephron empties into a collecting tubule to which other nephrons are connected (Figs. 2–3 and 2–4).

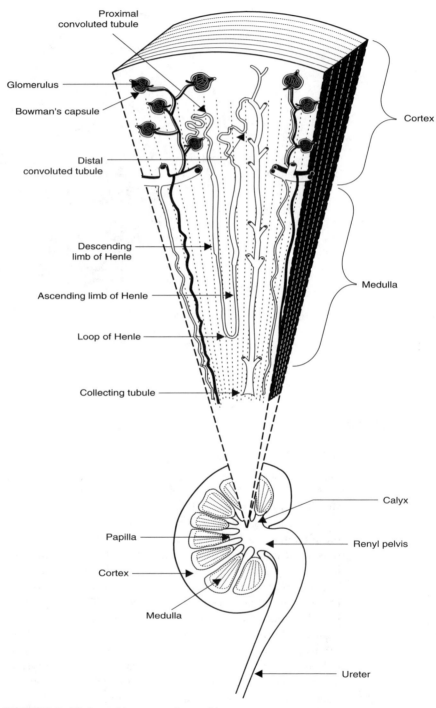

FIGURE 2–3. Wedge cut from a renal pyramid.

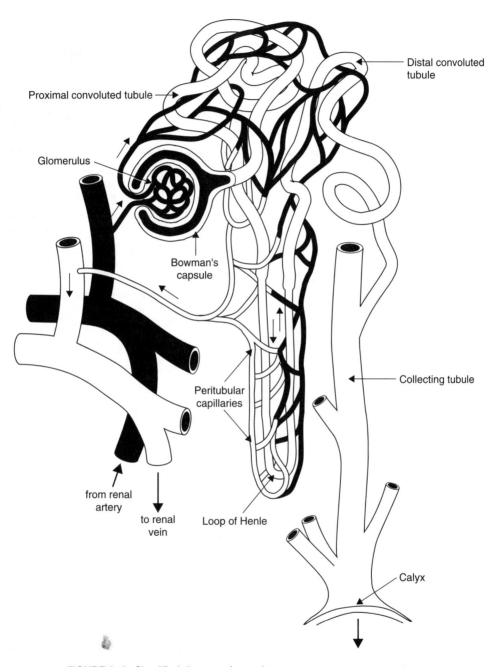

Distal convoluted
tubule

Proximal convoluted tubule

Glomerulus

Bowman's
capsule

Peritubular
capillaries

from renal
artery

to renal
vein

Loop of Henle

Collecting tubule

Calyx

FIGURE 2–4. Simplified diagram of a nephron.

■ FUNCTION OF NEPHRON COMPONENTS

Ultrafiltration and tubular reabsorption, secretion, and concentration are vital functions carried out by the components of the nephron that result in the formation of urine. **Ultrafiltration** is a function of the **glomerulus**, which acts as a nonselective filter of plasma substances with a molecular weight (MW) of less than 70,000. In other words, the only "selection criteria" for passage through the filtering mechanism is a MW < 70,000 regardless of the other characteristics of the substance in the plasma. This filtration process is influenced by the cellular structure of the capillary walls and Bowman's capsule, by hydrostatic (pressure of liquids in equilibrium and exerted on liquids) and oncotic (by "swelling") pressures, and by the feedback mechanism of renin-angiotensin and aldosterone. Substances that are *unable* to pass through the glomerulus include blood cells, high MW proteins, and large molecules; substances that *do* pass through the glomerulus include glucose, amino acids, urea, and water. (This distinction is important because the presence of substances normally unable to pass through the glomerulus can indicate renal damage.)

Tubular reabsorption, secretion, and concentration are responsible for the elimination of waste that is not filtered by the glomerulus and for the maintenance of acid-base balance by secretion of hydrogen ions. Before describing these processes, it is appropriate to define two terms:

- *reabsorption:* the process of removing substances from the filtrate and returning them to the blood
- *secretion:* passage of substances from the blood into the peritubular capillaries to the tubular filtrate

Over 80% of the filtrate is reabsorbed in the proximal convoluted tubule. **Reabsorption** may be **active** (requiring energy; substance must be combined with a "carrier" protein from the membrane of cells lining the tubules to create electrochemical energy) or **passive** (molecules move across the membrane due to differences in concentration or electrical potential on the opposite sides of the membrane). Sodium chloride, amino acids, glucose, phosphate, and bicarbonate are reabsorbed by active reabsorption, while water, uric acid, and urea are reabsorbed passively.

In the loop of Henle, the filtrate is exposed to the increased salt concentration of the medulla, changing the concentration gradient. Water is removed by osmosis in the descending loop of Henle and sodium and chloride are reabsorbed in the ascending loop. The ascending loop is not permeable to water, preventing excessive reabsorption of water.

Reabsorption amounts in the distal tubule are under the control of the hormones **aldosterone** and **antidiuretic hormone** (ADH, also called vasopressin), which have the ability to make the tubule walls permeable or impermeable to water. Under the control of aldosterone, sodium and water are reabsorbed; under the control of ADH, potassium, hydrogen and ammonia are secreted. Urine can be further modified in the collecting duct by the reabsorption of water, sodium, and potassium and the secretion of hydrogen. From this description of the formation of urine we can see that urine may be defined as an ultrafiltrate of plasma from which substances essential to the body's metabolism (such as glucose, amino acids, and water) have been reabsorbed.

 TIME FOR REVIEW. After studying the preceding sections, you should be able to respond correctly to the following:

■ List the four major functions of the urinary system.

■ Describe the location of the kidneys, ureters, bladder, and urethra.

■ Identify the basic structural and functional unit of the kidney and its components.

■ List the function of the glomerulus and the functions of the tubules.

■ List substances that are not able to pass through the glomerular membrane.

■ Define secretion, active reabsorption, and passive reabsorption.

■ Define urine.

Check your responses by reviewing the preceding pages.

THE ROUTINE URINALYSIS

■ HISTORY OF URINALYSIS

The study of urine in an effort to determine disease processes has been with us for a very long time. In fact, the study of urine was the beginning of laboratory medicine. Urine was perhaps the first body fluid studied in this manner because it is so readily available and easily collected. The initial tests were certainly less sophisticated and exact than those in use today, and in some cases, may seem rather offensive to modern health care practitioners. The early study of urine involved noting the appearance of the urine (cloudy, bloody, clear) and the odor of the sample (unpleasant, fruity). These pioneers were resourceful in the development of tests for what we now know as glucose, using the "ant test" (whether or not ants were attracted to the specimen) and the "taste" test (tasting a small aliquot of the urine). Fortunately, our methods have advanced from these initial efforts to study the urine!

■ IMPORTANCE AND USAGE OF URINALYSIS

Although the tests performed as a part of the routine urinalysis are relatively simple in comparison with some of the other laboratory tests, they can provide information about the major metabolic functions of the body, and about renal disease, and may provide the first clues to a disease process in asymptomatic (or when symptoms are not recognized or reported by the patient) diabetes mellitus and some liver diseases. The relative simplicity combined with the information that can be gained are probably the primary factors that lead to the majority of patients hospitalized in the United States having a urinalysis performed. Most types of medical practice use information about the changes that occur in urine characteristics when disease processes occur in the kidney or throughout the body.

However, we must not allow the relative simplicity of testing or the frequency of requests to diminish our understanding of the tests' importance, the clinical usage of the results obtained, or the testing standards applied to the testing processes.

■ SPECIMEN COLLECTION AND HANDLING

Since final test results are no better than the specimen used for testing, it is essential that all specimens, including urine, be properly collected. The method of urine collection is dependent upon the test(s) that are to be performed on the specimen, and in some cases, on the ease of collection. Use of the simply voided specimen should be avoided because of the large amount of contamination likely to be present. Such contamination can make it more difficult to detect and identify significant urinary constituents.

The **catheterized** specimen is the ideal specimen for most routine studies because it is collected under sterile conditions. However, collection of a catheterized specimen is not always practical because of cost and time considerations and particularly in young children or in other circumstances that may make the procedure difficult to perform. Catheterized specimens are, of course, best for bacterial cultures and should be collected for this purpose when possible.

The **clean-catch midstream** urine sample is a good alternative to the catheterized specimen in instances for which catheterization is not practical. A mild antiseptic solution is provided for cleansing and explicit instructions given to the patient. It is imperative that good instructions be provided to the patient and that the patient understands the collection instructions in order to provide an appropriate sample for testing. This specimen has the advantage of being easier to collect than the catheterized specimen and is superior to a voided sample in that it is more representative and less contaminated for microscopic analysis and bacterial cultures.

Pediatric patients are often not candidates for either of the previously described collection methods. Special pediatric collection containers are available for this purpose. These containers should be used exactly as described by the manufacturer and care taken to avoid contamination. It is important to note that squeezing urine out of a soaked diaper into a container is not an acceptable method of collection. A specimen collected in this manner is a filtered urine specimen with most of the important structures remaining in the diaper. Further, the specimen will contain numerous fibers that may mask any structures that do remain. Results obtained on such specimens are inaccurate and misleading, and should not be used.

In a much less common method of collection, the **suprapubic puncture**, a sterile needle and syringe are used to aspirate urine directly from the bladder, resulting in a specimen completely free of extraneous material. This method may be used for cytology examinations.

In addition to the different collection methods, there are **different types of urine specimens** based upon when the specimen is collected. For the purposes of routine urinalysis, specimens are usually random or first morning. A **first morning specimen** is the ideal specimen for screening purposes because of its increased concentration. A higher concentration increases the likelihood of detecting abnormalities that may not be evident in a dilute specimen. For urine pregnancy tests a first morning specimen should always be used. Otherwise, particularly in early pregnancy when the test is most likely to be performed, the urinary concentration of human chorionic gonadotropin (hCG) may not be sufficient for detection thus providing misleading results. The most common specimen is a randomly collected specimen because of the ease and convenience of this type of specimen. A **random specimen** is acceptable for obvious abnormalities, but will be affected by physical activity just prior to collection and to diet. **Fasting specimens** are sometimes used to avoid the interference of metabolites of food. Although generally not necessary for a routine screening specimen, this specimen may be used if indicated. It is collected as the second specimen after a period of fasting. **Timed specimens** are required for accurate quantitative analysis (of analytes such as creatinine or protein), but not for routine urinalysis. These specimens are collected according to explicit instructions over a designated period of time. The most common time periods are 24 hours and 12 hours. Specimens are sometimes, though not often, collected as 2 hour post-prandial (pp) specimens. The patient voids before the meal then collects a specimen 2 hours after the meal.

Since changes occur in the urine *in vitro* as well as *in vivo,* appropriate handling is essential to accurate results. Specimens should be delivered to the testing area as soon as possible after collection. Because of the changes taking place, *delayed delivery and testing can lead to inaccurate results.* Bacteria present in the urine will split urea to form ammonia. Ammonia combined with hydrogen ions forms ammonium, which will raise the pH (more alkaline) of the specimen. The increased pH will further hasten the decomposition of cellular elements and will destroy casts. If glucose is present, bacteria will use it as a source of energy. This can result in a false negative test for urine glucose. Bacteria present will also multiply, leading to a falsely elevated quantitation of the organisms present.

If a specimen is maintained at room temperature, analysis must be completed within a maximum of 2 hours. Cells and casts will deteriorate on standing (this process is accelerated in alkaline urines with a specific gravity < 1.015). This process would, of course, lead to misleading results. If there will be delay in delivery or testing, the specimen should be refrigerated. Refrigeration slows, but does not stop, the deterioration process and bacterial proliferation. Refrigeration does, however, sometimes cause an increased specific gravity and causes amorphous phosphates and urates to precipitate. The specimen should be returned to room temperature before testing. This will correct the specific gravity and may dissolve amorphous precipitates. Preservatives may be used in some cases, but must be compatible for the test to be performed as most preservatives interfere with some test procedures. Preservatives are not generally recommended for routine specimens, but are required for some specimens requiring a prolonged collection period for quantitation of analytes.

Containers for all urine specimens should be clean, dry, and well sealed. Sterile containers are required for bacterial culture specimens in order to avoid contaminating bacteria. The specimen container should be appropriately labeled with the patient's first and last name and hospital identification number to avoid sample mix-ups in the testing area. It is important that the container itself bear the label instead of the transport bag because the bag and the container will be separated prior to initiation of test procedures. Larger containers are provided for timed specimens collected over longer periods. These containers are labeled with the patient's identifying information and the preservative (if any) and any appropriate warning labels (ie, if acid has been added as a preservative, cautionary label would be required).

■ PHYSICAL EXAMINATION

The urinalysis begins with a physical examination. Urine **color** may range from colorless to black as a result of normal metabolic functions, physical activity, ingested materials, and pathologic conditions. Color is affected by the concentration of the urine, with concentrated urines being darker and dilute urines appearing more pale. Ingested substances, such as food or medications, may also affect urine color. Multivitamins can give a bright yellow color; pyridium, an orange color; and in patients with an inherited metabolic sensitivity, beets will produce a red color. Urine color may also be affected by certain chemicals and the color that many chemicals produce in urine is affected by the pH of the urine. For example, phenolsulfonphthalein, used in a kidney function test, will appear red in alkaline urine and will become more and more yellow as the acidity increases.

Another physical characteristic evaluated in the urinalysis is the **transparency** or **turbidity** of the sample. This is generally reported using terms such as clear, slightly hazy, or cloudy. Normal urine is generally clear, but can be hazy or cloudy because of the presence of amorphous phosphates or amorphous urates. (Amorphous phosphates can be dissolved in acid and urates with heat.) After amorphous phosphates and urates, the most common causes of hazy, cloudy, or turbid urines are white cells, red cells, epithelial cells, and bacteria. This can also be caused by mucus crystals, sperm, and extraneous material such as talcum powder. The presence of significant amounts of fat can give urine a milky appearance.

Volume is another important physical characteristic of urine, but its significance cannot be evaluated accurately without controlled circumstances (period of collection, hydration); therefore, the volume of a random specimen may or may not have clinical value. The volume of the specimen is not generally included as a standard part of the urinalysis report. It may, however, be noted on the report in instances in which the quantity is a significantly small amount. Urine volume is variable, with the daytime output about 2-3 times more than the nighttime output. Urinary volume is dependent upon the amount of water excreted by the kidneys, which is usually dependent on the body's state of hydration. There are several **factors that influence the urine volume**:

- fluid intake
- nonrenal fluid loss
- variations in the secretion of ADH
- the necessity to excrete large amounts of dissolved solids (salt, glucose)

Polyuria, an increased urine volume, is seen in diabetes mellitus and diabetes insipidus. The increased volume in diabetes mellitus results from the increased water necessary to excrete the higher levels of glucose, while in diabetes insipidus, the cause is impaired function or decreased production of ADH. A decreased urine volume, **oliguria**, is commonly seen in dehydration due to vomiting, diarrhea, or severe burns.

The **odor** of urine is seldom of clinical significance and is not a part of the urinalysis report. The characteristic ammonia odor is a result of the breakdown of urea. There are some disease processes associated with particular urine odors: diabetic ketones can produce a sweet, fruity odor; bacterial infections may produce a strong unpleasant odor; and an uncommon, serious metabolic disorder called maple syrup urine disease also produces a characteristic odor. Our sense of smell is not a standardized diagnostic tool, however, and although a particular odor may bring a particular disorder to mind it is, of course, not a reliable basis for diagnosis.

 TIME FOR REVIEW. After studying the preceding sections, you should be able to respond correctly to the following:

■ List and describe common collection methods and types of specimens.

■ Choose the best specimen for bacterial culture.

■ Describe at least two changes that occur in urine remaining at room temperature.

■ List two factors influencing urine color.

■ List three common causes of hazy or cloudy urine.

■ List three factors affecting urine volume.

■ Define and give an example of the causes of polyuria and oliguria.

Check your responses by reviewing the preceding pages.

■ CHEMICAL TESTING

Although in years past urine chemical tests required the use of various test tubes, chemicals, beakers, and other equipment, today a number of analytes in urine are commonly tested for using a reagent strip containing areas impregnated with various chemicals necessary for detection and semi-quantitation of these analytes. This reagent test strip is commonly known as the "dipstick" and has made chemical testing of urine a simplified and efficient process (as opposed to performing individual chemical analyses for each analyte). The reagent strip may be manually compared to a standardized color chart for determination of results, but instrumentation providing automated reading of results and standardization of color comparisons is now more commonly used. Such instruments are simple to use and to maintain. Daily calibration is required along with scheduled quality control specimens to ensure proper functioning of the instrument and the ability to detect both normal and abnormal results.

Specific Gravity
Specific gravity is a measurement that indicates the density of the urine. It is derived from the ratio of the weight of a given volume of urine to the weight of the same volume of water under standardized conditions:

$$\text{Specific gravity} = \frac{\text{weight of urine}}{\text{weight of water}}$$

Water has a specific gravity of 1.000 at the defined standard conditions. Specific gravity indicates the relative proportions of dissolved solid components to the total volume of the specimen and reflects the relative degree of concentration or dilution of the specimen. Knowledge of the specific gravity is needed in interpreting most tests performed on the routine urinalysis. Under the appropriate standardized conditions of fluid restriction or increased fluid intake, the specific gravity can provide a basic measure of the concentrating and diluting abilities of the kidney.

EXPECTED VALUES. Specific gravity varies widely, but usually remains between 1.010 and 1.025, with the highest reading found on the first morning specimen. The reference, or normal range, for specific gravity is **1.003 to 1.025**.

CLINICAL SIGNIFICANCE. The most severe and obvious, though uncommon, example of the **loss of effective concentrating ability of the kidney** (and thus a **low specific gravity**) is diabetes insipidus. Recall that the cause of diabetes insipidus is the impaired functioning or decreased production of ADH (which makes the walls of the distal tubule either permeable or impermeable to water, depending upon need). This disorder is characterized by large volumes of urine with low specific gravity—usually 1.001 to 1.003. Low specific gravity may also occur in patients with glomerulonephritis, pyelonephritis, and various renal anomalies in which the kidney has lost its ability to concentrate the urine because of tubular damage. Specific gravity is *elevated* whenever there has been excessive extra-renal loss of water, as with sweating, fever, vomiting, and diarrhea. Specific gravity is also high in patients with adrenal insufficiency, hepatic disease, and congestive heart failure. Abnormally high amounts of some urinary constituents, in particular glucose and protein, increase the specific gravity as measured by some methods such as the refractometer; x-ray contrast media will do the same. Reagent strip tests for specific gravity are not affected by these constituents. A urine with a *fixed* specific gravity (approximately 1.010) that varies very little from one specimen to another is known as isosthenuria and is indicative of severe renal damage with disturbance of both the concentrating and diluting abilities of the kidney.

METHODS OF MEASUREMENT. Although rarely used today, the **urinometer** was used for the measurement of specific gravity for many years. The urinometer is a weighted bulb-shaped instrument that has a cylindrical stem containing a scale calibrated in specific gravity readings. It is floated in a cylinder of urine and the depth to which it sinks indicates the specific gravity, which is read on the urinometer scale at the meniscus on the floating stem. The urinometer can be somewhat difficult to read and is probably the least accurate method of measurement available. Improved accuracy and readability are afforded by the **refractometer**, providing an indirect method of specific gravity measurement by measuring refractive index. Refractive index is the ratio of the velocity of light in air to the velocity of light in a solution. This measure is proportional to, but not identical to, specific gravity, so the scale readings have been calibrated in terms of specific gravity with compensation for temperatures between 60 and 100°F. Abnormally high amounts of substances such as glucose and protein will elevate refractometer readings. Another indirect method is the **colorimetric method of reagent strips**. This method offers further convenience in that the test area is included on the reagent strip used to measure a number of urinary analytes. The reagent area that measures specific gravity has three primary ingredients: a polyelectrolyte, an indicator, and buffers. The polyelectrolyte is sensitive to the number of ions in the urine specimen. When the concentration of electrolytes in the specimen increases (high specific gravity), the pK_a of the polyelectrolyte in the reagent strip is decreased, thus the pH decreases. The bromthymol blue indicator changes color from blue-green to green to yellow-green, indicating the pH change caused by increasing ionic strength (and increasing specific gravity) and is empirically related to specific gravity. This method also offers the advantage of not being affected by the concentration of glucose and protein in the specimen.

pH

The **pH** of the specimen is an important measurement. Remember that the kidneys and lungs are the two major organs that regulate the acid-base balance of the body. The lungs excrete carbon dioxide while the kidneys regulate the excretion of nonvolatile acids produced by the normal metabolic processes of the tissues. Acidity of urine is primarily due to acid phosphates, with only a minor portion contributed by organic acids such as pyruvic, lactic, and citric acids. These are excreted in urine as salts, primarily sodium, potassium, calcium, and ammonium salts. The kidney regulates the selective excretion of various cations (positively charged ions) to maintain normal acid-base balance. This is chiefly accomplished through reabsorption of a variable amount of sodium ion by the tubules and tubular secretion of hydrogen and ammonium ions in exchange.

EXPECTED VALUES. Normal kidneys are capable of producing urine that can vary from a pH of **4.5 to 8**. A pH < 7 indicates an acid urine and a pH > 7 indicates alkaline urine. A pH of 7 is considered neutral.

CLINICAL SIGNIFICANCE. When evaluating the significance of a particular pH, it is important to remember that normal kidneys can produce widely varying pH levels. Significance must be determined in conjunction with other values and with the clinical picture. An **acid urine** with a pH < 6 may be excreted by patients on high protein diets. Some medications will produce acid urines as well. Patients with acidosis and/or uncontrolled diabetes mellitus excrete urine containing large amounts of acid. Alkaline urine is frequently excreted after meals as a normal response to the secretion of hydrochloric acid in the gastric juice. It also occurs in individuals consuming diets high in vegetable, milk, and other dairy products as well as with some medications. Renal tubular acidosis is a disease of the kidney in which the renal tubules are unable to adequately excrete hydrogen ions, although severe systemic acidosis is present in the body. Urinary pH in these patients usually remains neutral and never falls below 6. A similar defect occurs in Fanconi syndrome. Highly alkaline urines may represent either urinary tract infection or possible bacterial contamination of an old specimen with urea-splitting organisms.

MEASUREMENT. pH is the measure of hydrogen ion concentration. It is usually measured using a reagent strip. The reaction area is impregnated with two separate indicators—methyl red (alkaline indicator) and bromthymol blue (acid indicator). Together these indicators provide a wide spectrum of color changes from orange to green to blue in the pH range of 5 to 8.5 in response to changes in hydrogen ion concentration of the specimen. Since urine can become alkaline on standing as a result of the loss of carbon dioxide and the conversion of urea to ammonia by certain bacterial organisms, pH should be measured on a fresh specimen for accurate results. The specimen should be refrigerated if analysis will be delayed.

Glucose

Glucose is the sugar most commonly found in urine, although other sugars, such as lactose, fructose, galactose, and pentose, may also be found under certain conditions. The presence of detectable amounts of glucose in urine is called **glycosuria**. Glycosuria occurs whenever the blood glucose level exceeds the reabsorption capacity of the renal tubules (called the renal threshold), that is, when the glomerular filtrate contains more glucose than the tubules are able to reabsorb.

EXPECTED VALUES. Glucose is not expected to be at a detectable level in normal urine.

CLINICAL SIGNIFICANCE. Glycosuria may be either benign or pathologic. Renal glycosuria occurs with normal blood glucose levels because tubular reabsorption is below normal and thus permits some glucose to "spill" into the urine. This is a benign condition that may be seen after a heavy meal or in conjunction with emotional stress. Diabetes mellitus is the pathologic state that is the chief cause of glycosuria. It is associated with a marked increase in urine glucose and usually with increased urinary volume as well (because increased amounts of water are required to excrete the high levels of glucose present).

MEASUREMENT. The most frequently used reagent strip tests for the presence of glucose are of two types—enzymatic and reduction tests. Enzymatic tests are based on the action of glucose oxidase on glucose. Glucose oxidase catalyzes the oxidation of glucose to gluconic acid and hydrogen peroxide. In the presence of peroxidase, the peroxide will oxidize an indicator which produces a color change. This method is specific for glucose because other sugars cannot act as a substrate for glucose oxidase. Reduction tests are based on the reduction of certain metal ions, such as copper, by glucose. This method is nonspecific for glucose because the reaction may be brought about by any reducing substance present in the urine— other reducing sugars, ascorbic acid, uric acid, etc. The nonspecificity of this method can be both an advantage and a disadvantage—an advantage in that reducing sugars other than glucose can be detected, such as galactose in infants with galactosemia, and a disadvantage in that reducing substances other than sugars (such as ascorbic acid) are detected. The copper reduction test is also the basis for testing with Clinitest tablets and Clinistix reagent strips. The practice of good laboratory medicine requires the screening of urine specimens from children below established ages with a reduction test to permit the detection of galactosemia, a severe condition that will result in rapid physical and mental deterioration and early death if not detected and properly treated. The combination of the use of an enzymatic glucose oxidase method on the routinely used reagent strip for the specific detection of glucose and the use of copper reduction methods for the screening of infants and very young children is a practical and prudent approach. Reduction tests may also be warranted in other instances in which disorders involving reducing sugars other than glucose are suspected. Lactose may appear in the urine of lactating women, usually a temporary condition corrected when lactation ends. Children and adults who are deficient in intestinal lactase may excrete lactose. Fructose sometimes occurs in the urine of patients with hepatic disorders. Pentose is associated with certain types of drug therapy and with some hereditary conditions, both considered benign. Galactose, as described earlier, is a reducing sugar present in galactosemia that must be detected early in order to prevent rapid deterioration and death.

Ketone Bodies

Ketone bodies are intermediary products of fat metabolism. Normally the body completely metabolizes fats to carbon dioxide and water. Whenever there is inadequate carbohydrate in the diet or a defect in carbohydrate metabolism or absorption, the body metabolizes increasing amounts of fatty acids. When this increase is large, fatty acid utilization is incomplete and intermediary products of fat metabolism appear in the blood and are excreted in the urine. These products are the three ketone bodies: acetoacetic acid, acetone, and betahydroxybutyric acid. Acetone and betahydroxybutyric acid are derived from acetoacetic acid. All three are present in the urine of patients with ketonuria in the relative (although variable) proportions of 20 % acetoacetic acid, 2 % acetone, and 78 % betahydroxybutyric acid.

EXPECTED VALUES. No ketone bodies are expected in normal urine.

CLINICAL SIGNIFICANCE. Diabetes mellitus is the most important disorder in which ketonuria occurs. Glucose metabolism is sufficiently impaired that fatty acids are utilized to meet the body's energy requirements. If untreated or inadequately treated, excessive amounts of fatty acids are metabolized, which results in the accumulation of ketone bodies in the blood (ketosis) that are excreted into the urine (ketonuria). The ketone bodies acetoacetate and betahydroxybutyrate are acids and can cause systemic acidosis. Progressive diabetic ketosis is the cause of diabetic acidosis, which can eventually lead to coma and even death. The term *ketoacidosis* is used to designate the combined ketosis and acidosis of diabetes. Ketonuria also accompanies the restricted carbohydrate intake that occurs in association with fevers, anorexia, gastrointestinal disturbances, fasting, starvation, and cyclic vomiting. Ketonuria can also be seen following anesthesia and as a result of some neurologic disorders.

MEASUREMENT. Because all three ketone bodies are excreted in urine, a general test that indicates the presence of one of the three is usually satisfactory for the diagnosis of ketonuria. Although specific tests exist for the determination of each substance, they are not often used because the methods are more cumbersome and less sensitive. Nitroprusside reacts with acetoacetic acid (but poorly with acetone) in the presence of alkali to produce a purple-colored compound. This is the basis for a number of tests. The reagent strip method is the simplest. The reagent area is impregnated with sodium nitroprusside and alkaline buffers. Color changes indicate the presence or absence and varying concentrations of ketone bodies. This method is sensitive to acetoacetic acid (from which both acetone and betahydroxybutyric acid are derived), but does not react with acetone or betahydroxybutyric acid.

Protein

About one-third of normal urinary **protein** is albumin. The majority of normal proteins in urine are globulins, primarily alpha-1 and -2 globulins with smaller amounts of beta- and gamma-globulins. The albumin in urine appears identical to that in serum; the globulins in urine have a lower MW than the corresponding serum globulin, but are closely related antigenically. Trace quantities of other proteins are also found. A high MW protein, Tamm-Horsfall protein, occurs in small amounts in normal urine and may occur in higher concentrations in nephrosis. It is not found in serum and is thought to originate in the kidney. It forms the basic matrix of urinary casts.

EXPECTED VALUES. An average of about 40 to 80 mg of protein are excreted daily (higher amounts are sometimes considered normal). Normal amounts excreted will not be detected on the urine reagent strip in a random specimen, thus the reference range for protein in a urinalysis is 0.

CLINICAL SIGNIFICANCE. **Proteinuria** refers to an increased amount of protein in the urine. It is one of the most important indicators of renal disease. Detection of protein in the urine along with microscopic examination of the urinary sediment forms the basis of the differential laboratory diagnosis of renal disorders. Proteinuria may at times reflect extrarenal disease as well. The proteins excreted in disease states are typically related to the serum proteins and, in severe cases, they *are* the serum proteins. Smaller proteins, such as albumin and alpha-1 globulin, are more readily excreted than larger proteins. Albumin constitutes between 60% and 90% of protein excreted in most disease states. Proteinuria depends on the nature of the clinical and pathologic disorder and on the severity of the disease. It may be intermittent or continuous. Transient, intermittent proteinuria is usually caused by physiologic or functional conditions rather than by renal disorders. **Minimal proteinuria**, excretion of < 0.5 g of protein per day, is associated with glomerulonephritis, polycystic disease of the kidneys, renal tubular disorders, the healing phase of acute glomerulonephritis, latent or inactive stages of glomerulonephritis, and various disorders of the lower urinary tract. **Moderate proteinuria**, daily excretion of between 0.5 and 3 or 4 g (the upper limit for classification of moderate proteinuria varies among sources/experts), is found in the vast majority of renal diseases as well as in all the disorders listed for marked proteinuria. It is also found in chronic glomerulonephritis, diabetic nephropathy, multiple myeloma, toxic nephropathy, pre-eclampsia, and inflammatory, malignant, degenerative, and irritative conditions of the lower urinary tract, including the presence of calculi. **Marked proteinuria**, excretion of >3 or 4 g per day, is typical of nephrotic syndrome, but also occurs in severe glomerulonephritis, nephrosclerosis, amyloid disease, systemic lupus erythematosus, and severe venous congestion of the kidney produced by renal vein thrombosis, congestive heart failure, or constrictive pericarditis. **Functional proteinuria** refers to protein excretion in association with fever, excessive exercise, or emotional stress and is induced by renal vasoconstriction in these cases.

MEASUREMENT. A number of tests are available for the determination of protein, both qualitative and quantitative measurements. The discussion here will be limited to the simple colorimetric reagent strip test used in routine urinalysis. Testing by electrophoretic methods is a more complicated and accurate procedure useful in further identifying abnormalities detected by simpler methods. This procedure separates the various protein components and quantitates each. The colorimetric reagent strip test is based on the ability of proteins to alter the color of some acid-base indicators without affecting the pH of the solution. When an indicator, such as tetrabromphenol blue, is buffered at pH 3, it is yellow in solutions without protein but, in the presence of protein, the color will change to green and then to blue with increasing protein concentration. Table 2–1 lists the type of protein found in various conditions and Table 2–2 provides examples of conditions resulting in the various levels of proteinuria.

Blood

Although protein is the most important indication of renal dysfunction, the presence of **blood** in the urine (excluding blood as a contaminant) is also an indication of damage to the kidney or urinary tract. Recall that blood cells are not able to pass through the intact glomerular membrane. Blood may be present as intact cells or as free hemoglobin. Usually the presence of free hemoglobin indicates that the cells have ruptured because of traumatic passage through the kidney and urinary tract to the bladder or because of exposure to dilute urine in the bladder causing them to hemolyze. Free hemoglobin is excreted from the blood into the urine only in special cases, such as hemolytic transfusion reaction or other conditions causing *in vivo* lysis of red cells (such as hemolytic anemias). The presence of red cells in the urine is referred to as hematuria; the presence of hemoglobin in the urine is called hemoglobinuria.

EXPECTED VALUES. Normally there is no detectable amount of occult blood in the urine.

CLINICAL SIGNIFICANCE. The presence of blood in the urine most likely indicates bleeding in the urinary tract. This may occur in a variety of renal disorders, infectious disease, neoplasms, or trauma affecting any part of the urinary tract. Free hemoglobin is likely in any of the above disorders as well. Free hemoglobin may indicate hemolytic transfusion reaction, hemolytic anemia, or paroxysmal hemoglobinuria or may appear in various poisonings and following severe burns. Positive chemical tests without the presence of red cells can also indicate myoglobinuria as a result of traumatic muscle injury. A specific test for myoglobin is available. The significance of hemoglobinuria, with or without intact red cells, is summarized in Table 2–3.

TABLE 2–1. Conditions Associated with Various Urinary Proteins

Condition(s)	Urinary Protein
Strenuous physical exercise Emotional stress Pregnancy Infections Glomerulonephritis Newborns (first week)	Albumin
Glomerulonephritis Tubular dysfunction	Globulins
Hematuria/hemoglobinuria	Hemoglobin
White cells in urine Epithelial cells in urine	Nucleoproteins
Severe renal disease	Fibrinogen
Multiple myeloma Leukemia	Bence Jones (determined by electrophoresis)

TABLE 2–2. Conditions Resulting in Proteinuria

Proteinuria	Conditions
Minimal	Exercise Fever Hypertension Renal tubular dysfunction Polycystic kidneys Lower urinary tract infection Hemoglobinuria
Moderate	Congestive heart failure (may be marked) Mild diabetic nephropathy Chronic glomerulonephritis Pyelonephritis Pre-eclampsia Multiple myeloma
Marked	Congestive heart failure (may be moderate) Nephrotic syndrome Acute glomerulonephritis Severe chronic glomerulonephritis Severe diabetic nephropathy

MEASUREMENT. The reagent strip method is the most direct and the simplest method. The reagent area is impregnated with tetramethylbenzidene and buffered organic peroxide. The composition forms a green to dark blue compound when hemoglobin catalyzes the oxidation reaction of tetramethylbenzidene with a peroxide. Many strips distinguish between intact red cells and hemoglobin by the color pattern—solid versus speckled.

TABLE 2–3. Causes of Hemoglobinuria

Hemoglobinuria with	Possible Causes
Intact red cells in sediment No casts present	Menstrual contamination Vigorous exercise Trauma to urinary tract Cystitis Calculi (stones) Kidney tumors Malignant hypertension Sickle cell (disease or trait)
Intact red cells in sediment Red cell or granular casts noted Proteinuria present	Acute glomerulonephritis Chronic glomerulonephritis Lupus nephritis Polyarteritis Goodpasture Syndrome Allergic nephropathy
No intact red cells in sediment	Delayed examination (esp. if dilute urine) Hemolytic transfusion reaction Hemolysis of transfused red cells Hemolytic disorders (immune and nonimmune) Presence of myoglobin (no hemoglobin present; suspect in cases of crushing injury or other severe muscle trauma; also present in alcholic or congenital myopathy. Serum creatine kinase levels high)

Adapted from Sacher RA, McPherson RA. *Widmann's Clinical Interpretation of Laboratory Tests,* 10th ed. Philadelphia, FA Davis, 1991

 TIME FOR REVIEW. After studying the preceding sections, you should be able to respond correctly to the following:

■ List two methods for the determination of specific gravity.

■ A low specific gravity may indicate a loss of effective _____ ability of the kidney.

■ List three possible causes of an elevated specific gravity.

■ pH is the measure of _____ ion concentration.

■ The _____ and _____ are the major organs that regulate acid-base balance of the body.

■ List two possible causes for an acid urine and for an alkaline urine.

■ Define glycosuria. Give an example of benign glycosuria and pathologic glycosuria.

■ What is the rationale for utilization of glucose oxidase reagent strips for routine urinalysis and the addition of a copper reduction test on young children? What does the copper reduction test detect that the glucose oxidase test does not?

■ When and how are ketone bodies formed?

■ List the three ketone bodies and two situations in which ketones are detected in urine.

■ _____ reacts with acetone and acetoacetic acid in the presence of alkali to produce a purple-colored compound.

■ Which protein is predominantly excreted in most disease states?

■ Define and give two examples of minimal proteinuria, moderate proteinuria, marked proteinuria, and functional proteinuria.

■ Describe the basis for the colorimetric reagent strip test for protein.

■ Review the tables in this section.

■ List two causes of intact red cells in the urine and two causes of free hemoglobin in the urine.

■ Distinguish between hematuria and hemoglobinuria.

■ Although hemoglobin may be present in urine as a result of traumatic passage through the urinary system or as a result of exposure to dilute urine, it is only excreted from the blood to the urine in conditions in which there is _____ of red cells.

Check your responses by reviewing the preceding pages.

Bilirubin

The presence of **bilirubin** in urine indicates the presence of hepatocellular disease or of intra- or extrahepatic biliary obstruction. It can be an early sign of these disorders and may appear before other symptoms, such as jaundice or clinical illness, and thus can be a useful diagnostic tool. Bilirubin is **formed by the breakdown of hemoglobin** in the reticuloendothelial cells of the spleen and bone marrow. It is linked to albumin in the bloodstream and then transported to the liver. The albumin-bound form of bilirubin is called **indirect** (or unconjugated) bilirubin; it is **not soluble in water** and therefore is not found in urine. In the liver cells, the indirect bilirubin is conjugated with glucuronic acid. This bilirubin is called **direct** (or conjugated) bilirubin; it **is water soluble**. Because direct bilirubin is water soluble, it can be excreted in the urine. Direct bilirubin is excreted from liver cells into the bile and then into the intestinal tract through the bile duct. It is converted, by bacterial action, in the intestinal tract to urobilinogen.

EXPECTED VALUES. Bilirubin is excreted in such small amounts (about 0.02 mg/dL) that it is normally not detected by reagent strip testing in urine. The reference value is 0.

CLINICAL SIGNIFICANCE. Bilirubin excretion in urine will reach significant levels in any disease process that increases the amount of direct (conjugated) bilirubin in the blood. An increase in the amount of indirect (unconjugated) bilirubin will not change the amount of bilirubin in the urine (is not water soluble and cannot be excreted in urine). Bilirubin may be found in some liver diseases due to infectious or hepatotoxic agents. In such cases, the liver cells are unable to excrete all of the direct bilirubin in the bile and sufficient amounts are returned to the bloodstream to elevate blood levels and cause bilirubinuria. In obstructive biliary tract disease, biliary stasis interferes with the normal excretion of direct bilirubin via the intestinal tract and causes a buildup in the bloodstream with resulting bilirubinuria.

MEASUREMENT. The reagent strip test area is impregnated with stabilized diazotized 2,4-dichloroaniline, which reacts with bilirubin in urine to form a brownish to purplish colored azobilirubin compound. Ictotest tablets, which are highly sensitive to bilirubin, are sometimes used to confirm positive reagent strip test results. It is important to note that bilirubin is an unstable compound and is **very light sensitive.** It will disappear from urine on standing, especially if exposed to light. For most accurate results, the specimen should be tested as soon as possible following collection.

Urobilinogen

Urobilinogen is formed by the conversion of direct bilirubin as describe above. As much as 50 % of the urobilinogen that is formed in the intestines is reabsorbed into the portal circulation and re-excreted by the liver. Small amounts are normally excreted in the urine, but the major excretion is in feces.

EXPECTED VALUES. The normal range in a random sample is less than 2 Ehrlich units/dL.

CLINICAL SIGNIFICANCE. Urinary urobilinogen is *increased* by any condition that causes an increase in the production of bilirubin and by any disease that prevents the liver from normally removing the reabsorbed urobilinogen from the portal circulation. Therefore it is increased when there is excessive destruction of red cells (increased bilirubin), such as with hemolytic anemias and malaria. Urobilinogen is also increased (the liver is unable to normally remove reabsorbed urobilinogen) in infectious hepatitis, toxic hepatitis, cirrhosis, and congestive heart failure. Urobilinogen can be used as a guide in detecting and differentiating liver disease, hemolytic anemia, and biliary obstruction. Urinary urobilinogen is *decreased* or *absent* when normal amounts of bilirubin are not excreted in the intestinal tract, which usually indicates a partial or complete obstruction of the bile ducts. Also, during antibiotic therapy the normal flora of the intestinal tract may be reduced, preventing normal conversion of bilirubin to urobilinogen. Using bilirubin and urobilinogen results together can provide more helpful information for differential diagnosis than either result alone (see Table 2–4).

TABLE 2–4. Bilirubin and Urobilinogen Findings in Selected Conditions

	Hemolytic Disease	Hepatic Disease		Biliary Obstruction
		Early	*Mod.— Severe*	
Urinary urobilinogen	▲	▲	▲	▼ or absent
Urinary bilirubin	0	0	+	+
Serum bilirubin	Direct: N	Direct: N / sl. ▲	Direct: ▲	Direct: ▲
	Indirect: ▲	Indirect: N	Indirect: ▲	Indirect: ▲

▲ = increased; ▼ = decreased; N = normal; 0 = negative; + = positive.

MEASUREMENT. The reagent strip area is impregnated with para-diethylaminobenzaldehyde and an acid buffer solution. They react with urinary urobilinogen, porphobilinogen, and para-aminosalicylic acid to form colored compounds. Excretion is thought to be at the highest rate in early afternoon. As with most analytes, the most accurate results are obtained on a fresh specimen. Drugs containing azo dyes will have a masking effect on the urobilinogen test area of the reagent strip.

Other Measurements

The measurement of **nitrite** in urine is an indirect method for the detection of significant bacteriuria. A *positive* nitrite result always indicates bacteriuria with an organism that contains reductase enzymes that reduce the nitrate in urine to nitrite (nitrates are in the urine as a result of protein metabolism). Common infecting organisms include species of *Escherichia, Enterobacter, Citrobacter, Klebsiella, Proteus,* and *Pseudomonas.* All of these organisms contain the reductase enzyme. The reagent strip is impregnated with a reagent that forms a diazonium compound with nitrite, which in turn couples with another chemical to produce a color change. Thus a positive result is an indication of significant bacteriuria. The converse, however, is not true; a *negative* result does not necessarily rule out significant bacteriuria. A negative result may indicate no bacteriuria, but may also be due to an infecting organism that does not contain the reductase enzyme (and thus cannot reduce nitrate to nitrite). Such organisms are the least common pathogens, however. It is also possible to get a negative result in the presence of bacteriuria if urine has not remained in the bladder long enough for the bacteria to convert nitrate to nitrite. This can usually be avoided by testing a first morning specimen.

Leukocyte esterase detects the esterase released from white cells in the urine. The presence of a significant number of white cells in the urine usually indicates bacteriuria or a urinary tract infection. Granules of neutrophilic leukocytes release esterases into the urine that can be detected chemically. Esterase splits an ester to form a pyrole compound which reacts with a diazo reagent to form a highly colored azo dye. Color intensity is proportional to the amount of enzyme and thus to the number of white cells. It is important to correlate other indications of urinary tract infection such as a high pH or positive nitrite and microscopic examination for bacteria.

 TIME FOR REVIEW. After studying the preceding sections, you should be able to respond correctly to the following:

■ The presence of bilirubin in the urine indicates the presence of conditions falling into two categories. List these.

■ Bilirubin is formed from the breakdown of what substance?

■ Distinguish between direct and indirect bilirubin, including which form is water soluble and thus may be excreted in the urine.

■ Why is it important to test for bilirubin as soon as possible after specimen collection?

■ How is urobilinogen formed?

■ Conditions causing an increase in urinary urobilinogen may be grouped into two general categories. List these and provide an example of each.

■ What condition is usually indicated by an absence of urinary urobilinogen?

■ What is indicated by a positive nitrite result?

■ List three possible causes of a negative nitrite result.

■ What is detected by the leukocyte esterase test?

Check your responses by reviewing the preceding pages.

■ MICROSCOPIC EXAMINATION

Qualitative or semi-quantitative evaluation of urine sediment provides adequate information for the majority of diagnostic and clinical needs. However, further evaluation may be required in evaluating the course and progression of renal disease. Examination of sediment is more reliable when the urine is relatively concentrated (another reason to use first morning specimens). If the specimen is too dilute, the cellular elements may be lysed and the amount of sediment obtained, even after centrifugation, may not be representative. Urine should be fresh and examined without excessive delay to prevent cellular deterioration. The microscopic examination of urinary sediment can provide evidence of renal disease as opposed to lower urinary tract infection and an indication of the type and activity of a renal disease condition.

Sediment preparation variables (volume centrifuged, centrifuge time and speed, volume of sediment examined) should be as standardized as possible in order to achieve reliable and reproducible results. Following physical examination and chemical testing of the specimen, a volume (usually 10 to 15 mL for a representative sampling) of well-mixed urine is centrifuged at a standard time and speed. The supernatant is then poured off and the sediment resuspended in the remaining urine. The resuspended sediment is placed on a slide with a cover and examined microscopically. Initial examination is on **low power** to scan the entire slide, locate any casts (they tend to congregate near coverslip edges), locate elements that are present in only a few fields, and quantitate some elements (those reported per low power field [lpf]). **High power** examination is used to identify cell types, crystals, and other elements, delineate various types of casts, and quantitate some elements (those reported per high power field [hpf]). A minimum of 10 to 15 fields are to be examined to ensure accurate, representative results. To quantitate elements, the elements are counted in at least ten fields and the average number reported. Ranges are often used in this reporting. **Varying intensity of the light source** is required because some elements are more easily recognized in subdued light and others in brighter light. In fact, some elements may be missed entirely if this technique is not used.

A number of elements will be discussed here in terms of their clinical utility. This discussion will not address the microscopic appearance and identification of these elements as this is beyond the scope of this text. Microscopic and reagent strip test results should be correlated.

Blood

Red cells (erythrocytes) in the urine can indicate a variety of renal and systemic diseases. More than 3 red cells per high power field is considered abnormal. Increased numbers of red cells in the urine may be present in:

- *renal disease*—including glomerulonephritis, calculus, tumor, acute infection, tuberculosis, trauma (including biopsy), and a variety of other renal disorders

- *lower urinary tract disease*—including acute and chronic infection, calculus, stricture, and hemorrhagic cystitis
- *extrarenal disease*—acute appendicitis, acute febrile episodes, malaria, subacute bacterial endocarditis, and other disorders
- *toxic reactions*—due to drugs such as sulfonamides, salicylates, and anticoagulants
- *physiologic causes*—very strenuous exercise

When increased numbers of red cells are found in conjunction with red cell casts (discussed later), bleeding may be assumed to be renal in origin. In the absence of casts or proteinuria, increased red cells are suggestive of a bleeding site that is distal to the kidney. Red cells become large and swollen in dilute urine and tend to lyse or dissolve in urine that is alkaline or dilute. In concentrated urines they may be small and crenated. Red cells must be distinguished microscopically from yeast cells, some forms of urate crystals, and oil droplets.

The presence of large numbers of **white cells** (leukocytes; usually segmented neutrophils; "segs") is called pyuria and usually indicates bacterial infection in the urinary tract, but may be seen in almost all renal diseases and diseases of the urinary tract. White cells may be transiently increased during fever and following strenuous exercise. When microscopic findings include white cell casts or mixed white cell-epithelial casts, increased white cells are considered to be renal in origin. Moderate numbers of white cells in conjunction with white cell casts may reflect either bacterial (acute and chronic pyelonephritis) or non-bacterial (acute glomerulonephritis, nephritis) renal disease. Numbers of 30 or more white cells per high power field suggest an acute infection. Calculi at any level may result in increased white cells due either to stasis induced infection or inflammatory response. Acute or chronic localized inflammatory processes such as cystitis, prostatitis, and urethritis also result in increased white cells in the urine. Gross pyuria may indicate the rupture of a renal or urinary tract abscess. Large numbers of lymphocytes in a patient with a kidney transplant may indicate early tissue rejection. A few white cells in a urine specimen is not an abnormal finding; up to 5 cells per high power field is considered a normal finding.

Leukocytes are rapidly lysed in hypotonic (dilute) urine and in alkaline urine. About 50% of the white cells present will be lost after standing more than 2 hours. This provides another example of the inaccuracies that can result from delays in delivery or testing of specimens when the specimen is not refrigerated. Such inaccuracies may, of course, lead to erroneous diagnoses and/or inappropriate treatment.

Epithelial Cells

Epithelial cells found in the urine vary in significance and appearance based on the location of their origin.

Squamous epithelial cells are of the least significance and are frequently found in normal urine, especially in females, in whom the majority are contaminants from the vagina or vulva. The distal third of the urethra is lined with squamous epithelial cells which may appear in the urine.

Renal tubular epithelial cells (RTEs) originate, as the name implies, in the renal tubules. Small numbers of tubular cells may be seen in normal urine as a result of the sloughing of aging cells. RTEs from the proximal or distal tubules usually occur singly and may be seen in increased numbers in cases of acute tubular necrosis and with toxicity of certain drugs and heavy metals. RTEs from the collecting tubules may be found in acute tubular necrosis, renal transplant rejection, and other ischemic injuries to the kidney. They may also be found in malignant nephrosclerosis, and in acute glomerulonephritis accompanied by tubular damage. Ingestion of various drugs and chemicals may also be implicated.

Transitional epithelial cells line the urinary tract from the renal pelvis to the proximal two-thirds of the urethra. A few may be found in normal urine. If large clumps or "sheets" of these cells are present (in the absence of other explanations such as catheterization), the need for a cytologic examination is suggested because of possible transitional cell carcinoma.

Casts

Cast formation usually occurs in the distal convoluted tubule of the nephron and may also occur in the ascending loop of Henle or in the collecting duct. Four requirements for the formation of casts are:

1. acidic conditions
2. high salt concentration
3. reduced urine flow
4. protein

Casts are formed as translucent, colorless gels from protein in the nephrons. Tamm-Horsfall protein forms the matrix of all casts. Very few, if any, casts are found in normal urine and increased numbers usually indicate that kidney disease is widespread and that many nephrons are involved. Casts begin to disintegrate in dilute and alkaline urine or in the presence of bacteria (which may contribute to the alkalinity). The size and shape of casts are dependent upon the site of formation. Casts may be classified according to their matrix, inclusions, pigments, and cells present as shown in Table 2–5.

Hyaline casts are formed of the gel of Tamm-Horsfall protein and are translucent, requiring variations of light intensity in brightfield microscopy for detection. An occasional hyaline cast is not considered a significant finding. Increased numbers may indicate damage to the glomerular capillary membrane permitting leakage of proteins through the glomerular filter in renal disease. They may be transiently increased with fever, exercise, emotional stress, congestive heart failure, and diuretic therapy.

Waxy casts are more easily visualized because of their high refractive index. The presence of waxy casts is significant. They are believed to reflect the final dissolution of the granules in granular casts (discussed on the following page). Because time is required for the granules to lyse, waxy casts imply localized nephron

TABLE 2–5. Classification of Casts

Classification	Type of Casts
Matrix	Hyaline (variable in size)
	Waxy (often broad)
Inclusions	Granules (cell debris; proteins)
	Fat globules (trig., chol.)
	Hemosiderin granules
	Crystals (rare)
	Melanin granules (rare)
Pigments	Hemoglobin
	Bilirubin
	Myoglobin
	Drugs
Cells	Red cells
	White cells
	Renal tubular
	Mixed cells
	Bacteria

obstruction and oliguria. They are commonly associated with tubular inflammation and degeneration and are observed most frequently in patients with chronic renal failure. They may also be found in acute and chronic renal allograft rejection. When waxy casts are unusually broad (termed broad waxy cast), they are known as renal failure casts. These casts imply advanced tubular atrophy and/or dilation, reflecting end stage renal disease.

Granular casts are not uncommon. The granules may be small (fine) or large (coarse) and represent plasma protein aggregates that pass into the tubules from damaged glomeruli or cellular remnants from cellular casts. There does not appear to be any advantage to separating granular casts into the classifications of fine granular and coarse granular, but the casts are often reported in this manner. Granular casts appear with glomerular and tubular diseases and may be seen in renal allograft rejection. They may be seen in pyelonephritis, viral infections, and chronic lead poisoning. Because the origin of the granules in these casts is disintegration of cellular elements in cellular casts, they may theoretically be found in any condition in which cellular casts are found.

Fatty, hemosiderin, and crystal casts are also types of inclusion casts and are not commonly seen. *Fatty casts* have fatty material from lipid-laden renal tubular cells incorporated into the cast matrix and may be seen with heavy proteinuria and in the nephrotic syndrome. *Hemosiderin casts* result from hemosiderin granules in the tubular cells. Hemosiderin is an iron-containing pigment derived from hemoglobin from the disintegration of red cells. *Crystal casts* indicate deposition of crystals in the tubule or collecting duct. Obstruction occurs and hematuria is regularly seen. It is important that these be distinguished from clumps of crystals that may have formed at room or refrigerator temperatures, as there is much difference in significance and not as much difference in appearance.

Hemoglobin, myoglobin, and bilirubin casts are pigmented casts and are also not frequently encountered. *Hemoglobin casts* accompany red cell casts and glomerular disease. They are less commonly seen with tubular bleeding and hemoglobinuria. *Myoglobin casts* occur with myoglobinuria following acute muscle damage and may be associated with acute renal failure. *Bilirubin casts* are seen in the urine with obstructive jaundice.

Finding *red cell casts* in the urine is very significant. They are generally diagnostic of glomerular disease or renal parenchymal bleeding. Glomerular damage (most frequently due to immune injury) allows erythrocytes to escape into the tubule. If, in addition, the conditions are met for cast formation, red cell casts form in the distal nephrons. If many red cells are present, the matrix may not be visible. However, there may also be delicate hyaline casts with only a few cells visible in the matrix assisting in identification. When stasis has occurred in the nephron, a red cell cast may degenerate and appear in the urine as a reddish-brown, coarsely granular cast (hemoglobin cast). Disorders that may be suggested by the presence of red cell casts in the urinary sediment are acute glomerulonephritis, IgA nephropathy, lupus nephritis, subacute bacterial endocarditis, and renal infarction. They are rarely seen in pyelonephritis.

TABLE 2–6. Casts Found in Various Conditions

Type of Cast	Conditions
Hyaline	Strenuous exercise Congestive heart failure Diabetic nephropathy Chronic renal failure (although not predominant type, seen in glomerulonephritis and pyelonephritis)
Red cell	Acute glomerulonephritis Lupus nephritis Goodpasture syndrome Subacute bacterial endocarditis Renal infarct
White cell	Acute pyelonephritis Interstitial nephritis
Epithelial	Tubular necrosis Cytomegalovirus infection Heavy metal or salicylate toxicity Transplant rejection
Granular	Nephrotic syndrome Pyelonephritis Glomerulonephritis Transplant rejection Lead toxicity
Waxy	Severe tubular atrophy Renal failure Transplant rejection

Leukocytes generally enter the tubular lumen from the interstitium through and between the tubular epithelial cells. Therefore, diseases associated with *white cell casts* are those in which white cell exudates and interstitial inflammation are present—the most common being pyelonephritis. They may also be seen in glomerular disease, interstitial nephritis, lupus nephritis, and in the nephrotic syndrome.

Renal tubular epithelial cell casts are seen in urine with acute tubular necrosis, viral disease (eg, cytomegalovirus), or exposure to a variety of drugs. In transplants, these cells and casts constitute one of the more reliable criteria for detecting acute allograft rejection after the third postoperative day. It can be difficult to distinguish between white cell casts and renal tubular epithelial cell casts.

Mixed cell casts contain two distinct cell types. When the cell type cannot be reliably distinguished in a cast, it is generally reported simply as a *cellular cast*. However, some inferences as to the cell type may be drawn from the predominant surrounding cells in the sediment. *Broad casts* are defined as those with a diameter 2 to 6 times that of normal casts and indicate tubular dilation and/or stasis in the distal collecting duct. They represent a poor prognosis and may be of any cast type. Table 2–6 summarizes the various conditions in which different types of casts are found.

 TIME FOR REVIEW. After studying the preceding sections, you should be able to respond correctly to the following:

■ List four variables involved in the preparation of urine sediment.

■ Why is initial examination of the sediment on low power important?

■ High power examination is used to:

■ List three general categories of conditions in which red cells may be found in increased numbers in the urine and give an example of each.

■ What impact does alkaline, dilute urine have on:

  ■ red cells

  ■ concentrated urine

■ What is pyuria and what does it usually indicate?

■ Which of the leukocytes is usually present in pyuria?

■ What effect does dilute, alkaline urine have on white cells?

■ List three types of epithelial cells found in urine. Note the least significant of the three.

■ List three instances in which renal tubular epithelial cells may be found in the urine.

■ List the four conditions necessary for the formation of casts.

■ Identify the cast most likely to be seen in or most commonly associated with each of the instances listed:

following strenuous exercise: _____

in chronic renal failure: _____

in pyelonephritis: _____

in glomerulonephritis or renal bleeding: _____

in end stage renal disease: _____

in acute allograft rejection: _____

■ Which casts result from the disintegration of the cellular elements in cellular casts?

■ Glomerular damage allowing erythrocytes to escape into the tubules is most frequently caused by:

Check your responses by reviewing the preceding pages.

Crystals

A variety of **crystals** may appear in the urine. The type of crystal and the quantity varies with the pH of the urine. Crystals are identified by their appearance, by the pH of the urine, and by the solubility characteristics of the crystal. For the most part, crystals are of limited clinical significance, but some are indicative of pathology. A brief discussion of some of the more commonly seen crystals and crystals found in abnormal urine follows. Table 2–7 provides a summary of some selected crystalline and amorphous materials, including the pH of the urine in which they are found and their solubility characteristics.

TABLE 2–7. Characteristics of Urinary Crystals

Substance	Urine pH			Solubility Characteristics and Comments
	Acid	Neutral	Alkaline	
Ammonium biurate	-	+	+	Soluble at 60°C with acetic acid; soluble strong alkali; change to uric acid in conc .hydrochloric acid (HCl)
Amorphous phosphate	-	+	+	Insoluble with heat; soluble with acetic acid or dilute HCl
Amorphous urate	+	+	-	Soluble in dilute alkali and at 60°C or lower
Ampicillin	+	-	-	
Bilirubin	+	-	-	Soluble in acid, alkali, acetone, chloroform
Calcium carbonate	-	+	+	Soluble in acetic acid with effervescence
Calcium oxalate	+	+	-	Soluble in dilute HCl
Cholesterol	+	+	-	Very soluble in hot alcohol, or ether or chloroform
Cystine	+	-	-	Soluble in alkali (esp. ammonia) and dilute HCl, insoluble in boiling water and acetic acid
Radiographic media	+	-	-	Soluble in 10% NaOH, urine will have very high specific gravity by some methods
Triple phosphate	-	+	+	Soluble in dilute acetic acid
Sulfonamides	+	-	-	
Tyrosine	+	-	-	Soluble in alkali and in dilute mineral oil; relatively heat stable; insoluble in alcohol
Uric acid	+	-	-	Soluble in alkali and with heat; insoluble in acetic acid

Crystals found in *normal acid urine* include *amorphous urates* of calcium, magnesium, sodium, and potassium. The amorphous material precipitates in concentrated urine of a slightly acid pH as small granules that may form clumps and adhere to fibers and mucus threads. *Uric acid* crystals have a variety of shapes and are often colored a yellow or reddish-brown. In rare cases, they are colorless and similar to cystine in appearance. *Calcium oxalates* are relatively common crystals that are typically quite small octahedrons resembling envelopes, although they may be larger or appear as dumbbell or ovoid forms. They sometimes appear in clusters.

In *normal alkaline urine, amorphous phosphates* of calcium and magnesium may be found. These are colorless granules that may be seen in clumps or masses. *Ammonium biurate* crystals are also found in alkaline urine, but are also seen in neutral urine and occasionally in slightly acid urine. These are yellow-brown spheres with irregular projections, often referred to as "thorn apples" because of their characteristic appearance. *Calcium carbonate* crystals are uncommon, small granules or colorless spheres. They form pairs or fours. *Triple phosphate* crystals are fairly common. They are variable is size. They are colorless, three- to six-sided prisms with oblique ends and are often called "coffin lids."

Crystals in *abnormal urine* include *cystine,* colorless refractile plates found in acid urine. These crystals are among the most important found in urine and occur in patients with cystinuria and may be associated with cystine calculi. *Tyrosine* crystals are uncommon, fine silky needles that may be arranged in sheaves or clumps, particularly after refrigeration. They, along with leucine crystals, are occasionally seen in patients with severe liver disease. *Leucine* crystals are rare, yellow, oily appearing spheres with radial and concentric striations. They often appear with tyrosine.

The clinical significance of other crystals is variable. *Phosphates* have little, if any, significance; they are often seen in infected urine of alkaline pH. Large numbers of *uric acid* crystals and *urates* may reflect increased nucleoprotein turnover (especially during chemotherapy) or may provide some evidence for the nature of small stones lodged in the ureters. They may also signal the urate nephropathy of gout. *Oxalate* crystals in large numbers may reflect severe chronic renal disease or may reflect the increased absorption of oxalates from food following small bowel diseases and resection, notably Crohn's disease. *When unusual crystals are noted, it is important to first check the patient's drug therapy and radiographic procedures.* Various forms of *sulfonamide* crystals may be seen in the urine, depending upon the nature of the therapy, although the advent of soluble sulonamides has reduced the frequency of this occurrence. *Ampicillin* may crystallize in the urine under conditions of high dosage. Urinary crystals are also seen following radiographic procedures using diatrizoate dyes.

Bacteria and Parasites

Bacteria in the urine may or may not be significant. Normal urine contains no bacteria, so if proper, careful technique is used to collect the specimen and it is protected from contamination, the presence of bacteria in significant numbers may indicate urinary tract infection. Rod-shaped bacteria, bacilli, are more commonly seen since the enteric organisms are most often found in urinary tract infection. Bacilli are generally easier to recognize in urine than cocci, which can resemble amorphous material. If urinary tract infection is present, many leukocytes will usually be seen in the sediment as well. Thus, the presence or absence of white cells may help to differentiate between infection and contamination. It is important to remember that bacteria will multiply in urine at room temperature giving falsely elevated amounts. Refrigeration slows this process.

The majority of the **parasites** seen in urine are contaminants from fecal or vaginal material. *Trichomonas vaginalis* is the most frequently seen parasite in urine (vaginal contamination). In patients with schistosomiasis due to *Schistosoma haematobium,* typical ova are shed directly into the urine accompanied by erythrocytes from the bladder.

Other Findings

Yeast cells (*Candida albicans*) may be indicative of urinary moniliasis, especially in diabetics. However, they are frequently seen as a contaminant in the urine of females with vaginal yeast infection. Yeast is also a common contaminant from the skin and air. Yeast cells can be difficult to distinguish microscopically from erythrocytes, but are more round and variable in size than red cells. The presence of budding in some of the yeast cells assists in the differentiation. If identification is in doubt, acetic acid may be added to the sediment on the slide: red cells will lyse in the presence of the acetic acid and the yeast cells will remain intact.

Spermatozoa may be seen in the urine following nocturnal emissions or sexual intercourse.

A variety of **contaminants and artifacts**, such as cotton threads, hair, starch granules, and oil droplets, may be seen in the urine and must be distinguished from significant elements in the sediment. Short fibers from disposable diapers are easily confused with casts. Unlike casts, however, these fibers polarize brightly. Oil droplets from catheter lubricants may be confused with cells, especially red cells, but are structureless.

 TIME FOR REVIEW. After studying the preceding sections, you should be able to respond correctly to the following:

■ List three characteristics used to identify crystals.

■ List the two crystals that may be seen together in severe liver disease.

■ Which crystal may be seen in gout?

■ List two crystals that may be found in normal acid urine and two that may be found in normal alkaline urine.

■ What aspects of the patient's history may be important when unusual crystals are noted in the urine? Why?

■ Name the crystal that may be present in large numbers in severe renal disease or in Crohn's disease.

■ Review the tables in this section.

■ List two possible explanations for the presence of bacteria in the urine and one aid in differentiating the two.

■ What type of bacteria are most often seen in the urine?

■ What impact will remaining at room temperature for an extended period have on bacteria present in the urine sample?

■ List two sources of contamination from which most parasites seen in the urine originate.

■ What parasite is most commonly seen in the urine?

■ Which cell are yeast cells easily confused with? How can the two be differentiated?

■ Why must attention be given to contaminants and artifacts in the urinary sediment? Provide an example.

Check your responses by reviewing the preceding pages.

OTHER TESTS OF RENAL FUNCTION

■ GENERAL INFORMATION

Urinalysis is the initial and most cost effective screen for the evaluation of renal function. However, additional testing is needed for most abnormalities. The major functions of the kidney can be used to assess renal status (ie, how well that function is performed):

Waste elimination: As the kidneys fail, acutely or chronically, the end products of nitrogen accumulate (increases of non-protein nitrogen), and is reflected in a rise in blood urea nitrogen (BUN) and serum creatinine. The end result is uremia—a state in which the kidneys fail to eliminate the waste products of metabolism.

Regulation of volume, acid-base balance, and chemical composition of body fluid: This is another function that can be monitored to assess renal status. The internal cellular composition has to be maintained within narrow limits and is influenced by the surrounding extracellular fluid. The extracellular fluid is regulated by the respiratory and renal systems. The lungs establish partial pressures and concentration of blood gases and the kidneys regulate the concentrations of nonvolatile substances. Thus, abnormalities in water balance, electrolyte concentration, and acid-base status may reflect disturbances in renal function.

■ RENAL CLEARANCE STUDIES

Normal kidney function is dependent on the following four aspects of renal physiology:

1. Renal blood flow must be appropriate
2. Glomerular filtration should be adequate
3. Renal tubular function should be normal
4. No significant obstruction to urinary outflow

Overall renal function and some aspects of its physiology can be determined by simultaneously measuring concentrations of substances in both the blood and the urine. An ideal substance for this purpose would:

- have small molecules not bound by protein.
- be freely filtered by the glomeruli.
- be neither reabsorbed nor secreted by the tubules.

Both endogenous and exogenous substances may be used for this purpose. Inulin is an excellent exogenous substance used in clearance studies, but because it is not practical for clinical use it is used primarily in a research environment. The most commonly used endogenous substance for the assessment of glomerular filtration rate (GFR) is creatinine. **Creatinine** is a degradation product of creatine that is formed at a fairly constant rate by muscle (the major storage site of creatine phosphate). Thus production and excretion are directly related to muscle mass. Although creatinine is freely filtered by the glomeruli and is not reabsorbed by the tubules, there is some tubular secretion of creatinine in small amounts. For this reason, the **creatinine clearance** may, in some cases, overestimate the GFR. Another reason creatinine is used in clearance studies is that it is not routinely affected by diet (an exception is large quantities of canned meats).

MEASUREMENT. The creatinine clearance requires collection of a 24-hour urine specimen. Clear and thorough instructions to the patient are essential in order to ensure an appropriately collected specimen. The accuracy and precision of the collection are important and complete, carefully timed collection is essential.

Refrigeration throughout the collection period is required; failure to do so may give falsely low results.

A blood specimen is collected either at the beginning or the end of the 24-hour urine collection period for determination of serum creatinine. The concentration of creatinine in the urine and in the serum is determined using the Jaffe reaction, which uses an alkaline picric acid solution to produce a bright orange-red complex.

The creatinine clearance, expressed in milliliters per minute (mL/min), is determined using the urine creatinine concentration, the serum creatinine concentration, the volume of the specimen, and the time period of the collection. In addition, a correction is necessary to account for differences in body surface area (and thus muscle mass) using a standard body surface area and the patient's body surface area. The patient's body surface area is determined from formulas that relate height and weight to body surface area or, more simply, from a nomogram providing the same relationship.

The formula used to calculate a creatinine clearance is:

$$\text{Creatinine Clearance mL/min} = \frac{\text{U mg/dL}}{\text{S mg/dL}} \times \text{V mL/min} \times \frac{1.73}{\text{A}}$$

where

$\quad$ U $\;=\;$ urine creatinine concentration in milligrams per deciliter

$\quad$ S $\;=\;$ serum creatinine concentration—expressed in the same units as the urine concentration

$\quad$ V $\;=\;$ volume—first determine the volume per minute based on the 24-hour volume (there are 1440 minutes in 24 hours)

$\quad$ 1.73 $\;=\;$ standard body surface area

$\quad$ A $\;=\;$ patient's body surface area determined based on the patient's height and weight

LIMITATIONS. As the GFR increases in renal disease, tubular secretion relative to glomerular load becomes a larger proportion of the clearance, making the estimate of GFR by creatinine clearance more uncertain. GFR is increased in pregnancy and exercise may also cause increased creatinine clearance. Another variable to consider is drug interference. For example, salicylates, cimetidine (Tagamet), procainamide, and trimethoprim interfere with tubular secretion of creatinine, so while the GFR may not change, the creatinine clearance is lowered and may confuse the interpretation of the GFR based on this test result. Ascorbic acid, ketones (acetoacetic acid), and numerous cephalosporins may influence creatinine measurements by some methods. Icteric samples and samples with significant amounts of lipemia and hemolysis may interfere with the determination of creatinine levels. In spite of the many variables influencing creatinine clearance, this estimate of GFR has good clinical utility.

Reference Range: female: 60 to 115 mL/min
                    male: 70 to 135 mL/min

SERUM CREATININE

As noted earlier, creatinine is a waste product of creatine. Recall that creatine is important in muscle metabolism, providing storage of high energy phosphate. The serum concentration of creatinine is relatively constant and is somewhat greater in males than in females. It is measured using the Jaffe reaction as described above.

CLINICAL SIGNIFICANCE.

Elevated: renal diseases and insufficiency with decreased GFR (uremia or azotemia if severe); urinary tract obstruction; reduced renal blood flow including congestive heart failure, shock, and dehydration; diseases that increase creatine concentration including skeletal muscle necrosis or atrophy, trauma, rapidly progressing muscular dystrophy, myasthenia gravis.
Decreased: debilitation; decreased muscle mass; inadequate dietary protein.

LIMITATIONS. With reduced renal blood flow, the serum creatinine rises less quickly than the BUN and decreases more slowly with dialysis (however, also has advantages over BUN because it is not so dependent on diet, hydration, and protein metabolism as the BUN). The creatinine may only become significantly abnormal when about half the nephrons have stopped functioning in chronic, progressive renal disease. Increased results can be seen from non-creatinine substances, including numerous medications. Those substances listed as influencing or interfering with creatinine measurements by some methods on the previous page are, of course, considerations as well.

Reference Range: 0.5 to 1.3 mg/dL

BLOOD UREA NITROGEN (BUN)

The BUN is not measured on whole blood, but rather on serum or plasma. Urea is a major end product of protein and amino acid metabolism and is generated in the liver through the urea cycle. It enters the blood to be distributed to all intra- and extracellular fluids. Most of the urea is ultimately excreted by the kidneys, but minimal amounts are found in sweat and minimal amounts are degraded by bacteria in the intestines. Urea nitrogen reflects the ratio between urea production and clearance, so elevated BUN levels can be due either to increased production or to decreased excretion. The BUN is only a rough guide to renal function as it varies widely in health and is influenced by a variety of factors, including dietary intake of protein and the state of hydration. BUN is usually measured by an indirect method that generates ammonium from urea using the enzyme urease. The ammonium produced can be detected by a subsequent chemical reaction and quantitated.

CLINICAL SIGNIFICANCE.

Elevated: chronic glomerulonephritis; pyelonephritis and other causes of chronic renal disease; acute renal failure; decreased renal perfusion (as in shock); urinary tract obstruction; severe congestive heart failure; dehydration.

Decreased: normal pregnancy; decreased protein intake; IV fluids; some instances of liver disease.

LIMITATIONS. The BUN may not be significantly increased until the GFR is decreased by at least 50%. It is a highly variable substance and is influenced by a number of factors, including diet and hydration status. Citrate or fluoride can inhibit urease, resulting in negative interference with this method.

Reference Range: 8 to 23 mg/dL

■ COMBINED USAGE OF BUN AND CREATININE

Although most clinicians prefer creatinine to BUN as a *single* test to assess renal functioning, a better picture may be gained when the two measurements are used together for several reasons.

1. One assay may confirm the other.
2. The ratio from both measurements (BUN/creatinine ratio) may suggest an etiology:

    In renal parenchymal damage, both usually rise together maintaining the ratio.

    An increased ratio is seen in excess urea production from gastrointestinal bleeding, catabolic drugs, and decreased urine flow.

    Low ratios are commonly seen in patients consuming a low protein diet; they are also seen in chronic hemodialysis; in pregnancy (GFR is increased, which has greater affect on BUN than creatinine).
3. Urea concentrations may correlate better with uremic symptoms than creatinine alone.

A better understanding of the patient's prognosis may be gained from serial determinations of both analytes. A consistent increase, not explicable by other causes, suggests deteriorating renal function. Rapid changes suggest acute illness or exacerbation of a chronic disorder and reduction may indicate improvement.

■ TUBULAR FUNCTION

Tubular functions vary among the different tubule segments. For clinical purposes, tubular function may be evaluated by *comparing the amounts of certain substances found both in the serum and the urine.* Such substances include the standard electrolytes, glucose, phosphates, hydrogen ions, and bicarbonate, among others. With knowledge of the functions of the different tubule segments, the comparison of these measurements can be of diagnostic value. For instance, defects in the function of the proximal tubule may result in the presence of glycosuria with a normal serum glucose level and dysfunction of the distal tubule may result in inappropriate secretion of bicarbonate, sodium, and potassium.

■ CONCENTRATING ABILITY

An evaluation of renal concentrating ability may detect renal damage that has not progressed to a level of severity sufficient to be detected by an elevation in serum levels of BUN and creatinine. The ability to effectively concentrate urine is dependent upon the normal functioning of the collecting tubules, the loop of Henle, and the renal medulla. A significant relationship exists between urinary volume and urinary concentration.

Osmolality, a measure of osmotic concentration, refers to the concentration of dissolved substances in a defined unit of the liquid (or solvent; eg, water) in which the substance is dissolved. It can be measured in both the serum and the urine. Comparing the two can provide an indication of disorders (renal or prerenal) that cause hyperosmolarity states. A common method of measurement is freezing point depression.

A simple approach to the evaluation of renal concentrating ability involves measurement of the **specific gravity** and osmolality on a first morning urine specimen. If random checks of first morning specimens do not provide evidence of adequate concentrating ability (ie, inadequate concentration reflected by decreased specific gravity and osmolality), further testing should be performed under conditions of regulated fluid intake. Conditions affecting urine volume and conditions that impair concentrating ability are summarized in Tables 2–8 and 2–9.

TABLE 2–8. Conditions Impacting Urine Volume

▼ Volume (Ologuria)	▲ Volume (Polyuria), Acute	▲ Volume (Polyuria), Chronic
Dehydration	Overhydration	Diabetes insipidus
Hypovolemic shock	Diabetes mellitus	Chronic renal failure
Hypotension	Diuretic therapy	Diabetes mellitus
Massive edema or ascites	Diuretic phase of recovery from renal failure	Glucocorticoid deficit or excess
Heat stroke		Hyperparathyroidism
Nephrotoxic drugs		Salt-losing nephritis
Malignant hypertension		Compulsive water drinking
Eclampsia		
Obstruction		
Acute glomerulonephritis		

Adapted from Sacher RA, McPherson RA. *Widmann's Clinical Interpretation of Laboratory Tests,* 10th ed. Philadelphia, FA Davis, 1991

TABLE 2–9. Impaired Concentrating Ability

Condition	Examples
Renal diseases	Pyelonephritis Acute or chronc glomerular failure Renal tubular acidosis Nephrogenic diabetes insipidus
Metabolic disturbances	Osmotic diuresis (esp. diabetes mellitus) Hypokalemia Hypercalemia Lithium use Alcohol use Prolonged overhydration Severe hypoproteinemia
Systemic diseases (affecting renal medulla)	Multiple myeloma Amyloidosis Sickle cell disease or trait

Adapted from Sacher RA, McPherson RA. *Widmann's Clinical Interpretation of Laboratory Tests,* 10th ed. Philadelphia, FA Davis, 1991

■ CLINICAL PRESENTATION AND LABORATORY FINDINGS IN SELECTED DISORDERS

Renal disease results from a variety of causes. Often the patient's history and clinical presentation are suggestive of a particular renal disorder and the cause of the disease, with laboratory analyses used to confirm or rule out a suspected diagnosis. A variety of laboratory findings are beneficial, with definitive diagnosis sometimes requiring a renal biopsy. Clinical manifestations and laboratory findings for selected renal diseases are summarized in Table 2–10. As this information is presented in a summary format, it is important to note that the information presented may not include a comprehensive listing of all notable symptoms or laboratory findings and that the patient's physician is best able to determine the appropriate diagnostic approach and treatment regimen.

TABLE 2–10. Findings in Selected Renal Disorders

Condition	Clinical Findings	Laboratory Findings	Comments
Glomerulonephritis Acute (AGN)	Bloody urine Peripheral edema Hypertension Recent/concurrent infection with group A beta-strep Back pain Oliguria	Red cell (most diagnostic) Hematuria Mild-mod, proteinuria White cells (often) If post-strep, ASO titer may be ▲ and complement C3 ▼ ▲ bun (50% of cases) Renal function tests basically normal or show varying degrees of impairment	Higher incidence in childhood and relatively benign with permanent damage uncommon Lower incidence in adults, but higher percentage develop chronic renal disease

Chronic	Similar to AGN, but runs slowly progressive/ intermittent course	Stage dependent:
		  Early: mild hematuria
		    mild proteinuria
		    slow ▼ in urine conc.
		    progressive ▼ in GFR
		  Terminal: mod. proteinuria
		    granular casts
		    waxy casts
		  (terminal stage has same findings as in renal failure)	

Rapidly progressive	Seen as a severe form of AGN	Many hyaline and epith casts Red cell casts Mod. marked proteinuria Anemia Renal function tests show both glomerular and tubular destruction Renal biopsy shows epith cell proliferation, filling of space between Bowman's capsule and glomerular tuft	May/may not be preceded by AGN Sometimes difficult to distinguish from nephrotic syndrome Death often results within weeks/months
Pyelonephritis	Spiking fever Dysuria Back pain	Mild proteinuria White cells (often with clumping) White cell casts (diagnostic if found) Positive URN culture (doesn't distinguish from lower UTI)	
Nephrotic syndrome (includes two clinical disorders)	Edema	Marked proteinuria Hyaline and epith casts Variable hematuria Fat bodies/fatty casts (most characteristic) ▲ serum cholesterol ▼ serum albumin ▲ serum alpha-2-globulin Glomerular lesions	
Acute tubular acidosis	Oliguria or near anuria	Mod. proteinuria Epith casts Mild-mod. hematuria Broad, waxy casts Fixed sp. Grav. (~1.010) ▲ BUN	May result in acute or sudden renal failure, most often secondary to hypotension Also seen in intravascular hemolysis (ex. hemolytic transfusion reactions)

TIME FOR REVIEW. After studying the preceding sections, you should be able to respond correctly to the following:

■ List two functions of the kidneys that can be monitored to assess renal status.

■ The abbreviation GFR is used to indicate _____.

■ List the four aspects of renal physiology on which normal kidney function depends.

■ List three characteristics of an ideal substance for use in clearance studies.

■ What endogenous substance is most commonly used for clearance studies?

■ Why is a correction for body surface area important in the calculation of creatinine clearance?

■ What advantages does serum creatinine have over BUN in the assessment of renal function?

■ Creatinine is a waste product of _____.

■ List two causes of an elevated serum creatinine level and of a decreased serum creatinine level.

■ BUN is a major end product of _____.

■ List two causes of an elevated BUN and two causes of a decreased BUN.

■ Explain why using BUN and creatinine measurements together may provide a better diagnostic picture and more information regarding prognosis.

■ A simple initial approach to the evaluation of renal concentrating ability involves what two measurements?

■ A measure of the concentration of a dissolved substance in a defined unit of the liquid in which the substance is dissolved is _____.

Check your responses by reviewing the preceding pages.

2. SELF TEST

Choose the best response by circling the appropriate letter. The answer key may be found in the appendices.

1. **The basic structural and functional unit of the kidney is**
   - **A.** the glomerulus
   - **B.** the nephron
   - **C.** the loop of Henle
   - **D.** Bowman's capsule

2. **These substances *do not* pass through the undamaged glomerular membrane:**
   - **A.** red cells
   - **B.** glucose
   - **C.** urea
   - **D.** amino acids

3. **Substances are removed from the filtrate and returned to the blood by reabsorption in the**
   - **A.** bladder
   - **B.** glomerulus
   - **C.** tubules of the nephron
   - **D.** capillary network in Bowman's capsule

4. **The best specimen for a urine culture is**
   - **A.** catheterized
   - **B.** voided
   - **C.** placed in preservatives
   - **D.** timed

5. **The necessity to excrete large amounts of dissolved solids results in**
   - **A.** variations in ADH secretion
   - **B.** reabsorption of water
   - **C.** oliguria
   - **D.** polyuria

6. **A common cause of a hazy or cloudy urine appearance is**
   A. a low specific gravity
   B. an acidic pH
   C. the presence of amorphous or cellular elements
   D. a positive bilirubin

7. **A specific gravity of 1.002 could indicate**
   A. dehydration following vomiting and diarrhea
   B. ineffective concentrating ability of the kidneys due to tubular damage
   C. the presence of abnormally high amounts of glucose and protein
   D. insufficient intake of fluids

8. **Which of the following patients would be expected to have a urinary pH of 5?**
   A. a patient with insulin-dependent diabetes
   B. a patient with untreated urinary tract infection
   C. a patient whose renal tubules are unable to adequately excrete hydrogen ions
   D. a patient who is a vegetarian

9. **A negative glucose oxidase reagent strip test and a positive Clinitest copper reduction test most likely indicates**
   A. a false negative glucose oxidase test
   B. a false positive copper reduction test
   C. the presence of glucose
   D. the presence of galactose

10. **Ketone bodies are formed as a result of**
    A. abnormal production of amino acids in urinary proteins
    B. increased metabolism of fatty acids due to insufficient carbohydrates or defective carbohydrate metabolism
    C. the body's inability to utilize high levels of stored fatty acids
    D. increased excretion of proteins due to inflammatory or degenerative conditions of the lower urinary tract

11. **The predominant protein excreted in most disease states is**
    A. albumin
    B. alpha-1 globulin
    C. alpha-2 globulin
    D. beta globulin

12. **Functional proteinuria may result from**
     A. nephrotic syndrome
     B. acute glomerulonephritis
     C. diabetic nephropathy
     D. excessive exercise

13. **A positive dipstick result for blood with no red cells noted on the microscopic examination may be explained by any of the following** *except*
     A. traumatic passage of red cells through the kidney
     B. conditions causing *in vivo* lysis of red cells
     C. elevated specific gravity
     D. exposure of red cells to dilute urine

14. **Bilirubin is formed by the breakdown of**
     A. urobilinogen
     B. protein
     C. hemoglobin
     D. carbohydrates

15. **Bilirubinuria may be present in each instance listed** *except*
     A. obstructive biliary disease
     B. increased serum levels of indirect bilirubin
     C. increased serum levels of direct bilirubin
     D. liver disease resulting from an infectious agent

16. **A positive nitrite test indicates the presence of**
     A. bacteria
     B. white cells
     C. elevated protein levels
     D. red cells

17. **The leukocyte usually found in pyuria is the**
     A. lymphocyte
     B. monocyte
     C. neutrophil
     D. eosinophil

18. **Pyuria may be seen in almost all renal diseases and diseases of the urinary tract, but usually indicates**
     A. chronic pyelonephritis
     B. acute glomerulonephritis
     C. transplant rejection
     D. bacterial infection of the urinary tract

19. **The cast most likely to be seen as a result of strenuous exercise is the**
    A. red cell cast
    B. hyaline cast
    C. white cell cast
    D. broad waxy cast

20. **The cast most commonly associated with glomerular damage is the**
    A. red cell cast
    B. hyaline cast
    C. white cell cast
    D. broad waxy cast

21. **The cast reflecting end stage renal disease is the**
    A. red cell cast
    B. hyaline cast
    C. white cell cast
    D. broad waxy cast

22. **A crystal often appearing with tyrosine crystals in severe liver disease is**
    A. calcium oxalate
    B. uric acid
    C. amorphous phosphates
    D. cystine

23. **Blood urea nitrogen (BUN) is a major end product of**
    A. fatty acid metabolism
    B. carbohydrate metabolism
    C. protein metabolism
    D. bilirubin metabolism

24. **The endogenous substance most commonly used to evaluate glomerular filtration rate (GFR) is**
    A. creatinine
    B. urea nitrogen
    C. inulin
    D. uric acid

25. **An ideal substance for use in clearance studies would be**
    A. large, protein-bound molecules
    B. reabsorbed in the tubules
    C. secreted in high quantities by the tubules
    D. freely filtered by the glomeruli

26. Osmolality is a measure of
  A. glomerular dysfunction
  B. concentration of dissolved substances
  C. degree of proteinuria
  D. epithelial cell proliferation

3. THE COMPLETE BLOOD COUNT

The complete blood count, or CBC, is one of the most frequently requested laboratory tests. This test provides a wealth of information and may be beneficial in the diagnosis and treatment of a number of conditions. Uses include, but are not limited to, detection and evaluation of anemia, evaluation of reactions to inflammations and infections, detection and evaluation of leukemias, evaluation of peripheral blood cell characteristics, and polycythemia evaluation. A CBC report typically includes a white cell count (WBC), red cell count (RBC), hemoglobin, hematocrit, red cell indices and morphology, a WBC differential, platelet count or estimate, and platelet morphology.

THE PARAMETERS

Parameters included on the CBC may differ somewhat among laboratories. A typical list of CBC parameters and units of measure is provided below with each parameter defined briefly. Additional information is provided in the next section, Methods of Measurement.

WBC (10^3/mL): white cell count; measure of the number of white cells in a given volume

RBC (10^6/mL): red cell count; measure of the number of red cells in a given volume

HGB (g/dL): hemoglobin; iron containing substance in red cells that carries oxygen

HCT (%): hematocrit; packed red cell volume

MCV (fL): mean cell volume

MCH (pg): mean cell hemoglobin

MCHC (g/dL): mean cell hemoglobin concentration   } red cell indices

RDW (%): red cell distribution width; a measure of anisocytosis

PLT (10^3/mL): platelet count; measure of the number of platelets in a given volume

MPV (fL): mean platelet volume

Neut (% and/or 10^3/mL): neutrophils
Lymp (% and/or 10^3/mL): lymphocytes
Mono (% and/or 10^3/mL): monocytes   } automated WBC differential
Eos (% and/or 10^3/mL): eosinophils
Baso (% and/or 10^3/mL): basophils

METHODS OF MEASUREMENT

Virtually all laboratories provide a CBC with some sort of automated analyzer. Many laboratories use highly automated, multi-channel instruments, but even the smallest of laboratories usually has at least semi-automated methods. The automated analyzers are generally used for measurement and calculation of the parameters with microscopic examination (leukocyte differential, evaluation of cellular morphology, etc) as follow-up based on results or as requested.

Manual counts of white cells, red cells, and platelets may be performed using the microscopically ruled counting chambers of a hemacytometer and special diluting fluids. The number of cells are then calculated using a formula based on the dilution made, the area and volume of the counting chamber used, and the number of cells counted. Manual cell counting procedures are more frequently used to enumerate cells in fluid specimens (cerebrospinal fluid, synovial fluid, etc) and are not commonly used in peripheral blood counts except in some confirmatory processes.

Details of methodologies employed by the automated analyzers are beyond the scope of this text and only a basic overview of the principles of measurement is provided. The instruments perform measurements by electronic means based on two primary principles. In the first, **electrical impedance**, cells passing through an aperture through which a current is flowing will cause changes in the electrical resistance. The cells are suspended in a diluting fluid that will conduct electrical current. The number of electrical pulses determines the cell count and the size of the pulses is proportional to the volume of the cell. Red and white cells are counted using different instrument "channels" and the diluting fluid used for white cells lyses, or destroys, the red cells.

In the second, **light scattering**, electro-optical analyzers use a light-sensitive detector to measure the amount of light scatter as cells pass through a flow cell on which a laser light is focused. When cells interrupt the beam of light, the light is scattered in all directions and sensed by photodetectors in specific "sensing zones." Analysis of the amount and type of light scatter (including diffraction, refraction, and reflection) provides a determination of cell counts and information about the size of the cells counted. As with light impedance methodology, white cell counts are performed on a different diluted portion of the blood sample in a fluid that lyses the red cells. The highly automated devices include extensive microcomputer processing of the electrical signals after analog/digital conversion.

Hemoglobin is usually measured (whether on an automated analyzer or by manual techniques) using a form of the cyanmethemoglobin method. In this two-step process, a fluid is used to dilute and lyse the red cells and form a cyanmethemoglobin compound that is then read spectrophotometrically at 540 nm. The mean cell volume (MCV) of red cells is determined on the basis of voltage pulses formed during counting of the red cells.

Parameters not measured directly are calculated based on directly measured parameters.

Hematocrit: Using the direct measurements obtained for the hemoglobin and MCV, the hematocrit is calculated using the formula

$$RBC \times MCV = HCT$$

MCH: The mean corpuscular hemoglobin (MCH) is derived from the hemoglobin and red cell count:

$$\frac{HGB \ (g/dL)}{RBC \ (millions/\mu L)} \times 10$$

MCHC: Mean cell hemoglobin concentration (MCHC), the average concentration of hemoglobin in a given volume of cells calculated by

$$\frac{HGB \ (g/dL)}{HCT \ \%} \times 100$$

Automated analyzers flag results that are questionable or that require verification or microscopic analysis of the blood sample. Various notations are used to alert the technologist to possible abnormalities and indicate the suspected nature of the abnormality. Each laboratory should establish a set of review criteria as the basis for confirmation of automated results, for performance of a manual differential, and for review by a supervisor or pathologist. Examples of such criteria are provided in Figs. 3–1 and 3–2 and in Table 3–1.

When a manual WBC differential is indicated, a specially stained blood smear is examined microscopically. A total of 100 white cells are counted, each cell categorized based upon morphologic characteristics, and cells of each type reported as a percentage of the total white cell count. The manual differential also includes a review of the morphologic characteristics of white cells, red cells, and platelets for the presence of abnormalities or significant variations as discussed in later sections of this chapter.

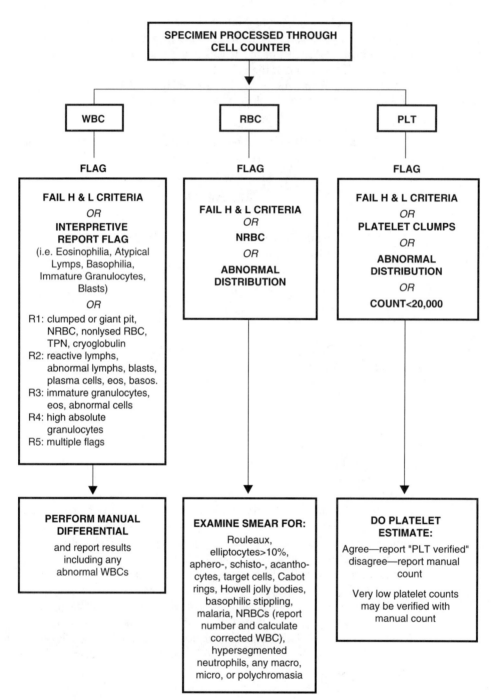

FIGURE 3–1. Flow chart for follow-up of automated CBC results. *(Courtesy Ephraim McDowell Regional Medical Center.)*

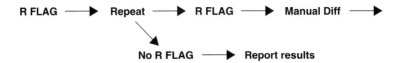

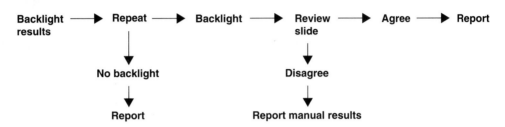

FIGURE 3–2. CBC review criteria. Flags may vary among instruments. *(Courtesy Ephraim McDowell Regional Medical Center.)*

TABLE 3–1. Review of CBC Results

For Supervisor Review	For Pathologist Review
RBC <2.5 Million or >5 Million	WBC <2500 or >25,000
Hemoglobin >16 or <8	Hemoglobin <6 or >16
Hematocrit >50	Any granulocyte younger than a metamyelocyte
MCV <75 or >100	Before atypical cells are signed out
WBC <4000 or >25,000	Lymphocytosis >50% [PT >5 yrs] or >75% [PT <5 yrs]
Significant increase or decrease in platelets	Absolute lymphocyte count >10,000
	Monocytosis >15%
Atypical cells of any line	Basophils >3%
Nucleated red cell precursors	Nucleated red cell Precursors
	Moderate or marked anisocytosis or poikilocytosis
	Howell-Jolly Bodies
	Diffuse or punctate basophilia >10%
	Any cell suspicious for malignancy

Criteria for review may vary among laboratories and with different instruments. Review may be requested for any reason and should be sought any time questions/uncertainties exist. When immediate review is not possible and results must be reported, report should note "pending supervisor/pathologist review." (*Courtesy of Ephraim McDowell Regional Medical Center.*)

ERYTHROCYTES

Several of the parameters on a CBC report are related to the erythrocytes: red cell count, hemoglobin, hematocrit, MCV, MCH, MCHC, and RDW. This section focuses on erythrocytes (red cells; RBCs) in regard to their maturation cycles, appearance, abnormal forms, and alterations in disease states. Hemoglobin and the red cell indices will be discussed as well.

■ FUNCTION

Erythrocytes, commonly referred to as red cells or RBCs, provide the means for the transport of hemoglobin, which carries oxygen. Oxygen is bound to hemoglobin in the erythrocyte and carried from the lungs throughout the body, where it is used by the cells for aerobic metabolism. (Hemoglobin is produced in the precursor cells of the erythrocytes.) The erythrocyte also functions to aid in the removal of the waste product carbon dioxide.

■ PRODUCTION AND DEVELOPMENT

In order to better understand the role of red cells and how this role relates to disease states, a basic understanding of red cell development is important. A detailed explanation of this complex process is beyond the scope of this text. However, a brief discussion is provided.

Red cells are formed in the bone marrow from **pluripotential stem cells** (early cells with the potential to develop into any of the cellular components of blood). The pluripotential stem cell may become either a lymphoid stem cell (from which lymphocytes are formed in the bone marrow and thymus) or a **hematopoietic stem cell** (hematopoiesis is the production and development of blood cells) from which the other cellular components of blood are formed. Following stimulation by certain influences, the hematopoietic stem cell becomes a committed **erythroid progenitor cell**, or a cell "committed" to the production, through a number of maturation phases, of mature erythrocytes. A number of nuclear and cytoplasmic characteristics are used to identify and distinguish the red cell precursors, which are not normally seen in the peripheral blood. These characteristics are not dealt with in this text, but the last two developmental stages are briefly described.

The earliest recognizable precursor to the mature red cell is called the *pronormoblast.* It is followed in the developmental cycle by the *basophilic normoblast,* the *polychromatophilic normoblast,* the *orthochromatic normoblast,* and the *reticulocyte,* which is followed by the mature *erythrocyte.* The orthochromic normoblast stage is reached after the last mitosis. The nucleus becomes small and dense and mitosis is no longer possible. The cytoplasm contains more abundant hemoglobin than the previous stage and remains slightly *polychromatophilic* (literally, stainable with more than one type of stain—on the stained peripheral smear, the cell appears less red-pink than the mature cell and retains more of a bluish tinge). This **nucleated red cell** may sometimes be seen in the peripheral blood under some of the conditions described later.

Following this stage of development, the nucleus and a small rim of the cytoplasm are ejected and the next cell in the developmental cycle, the **reticulocyte**, is seen. The reticulocyte is also polychromatophilic and retains RNA in the cytoplasm. This cell may also be seen in the peripheral blood in some situations, particularly those conditions resulting in increased red cell production.

Reference Ranges

The number of red cells considered to be "normal" varies with a number of factors, including not only (as with all laboratory measurements) the methodology used, but also gender and age (for example, newborns have significantly larger numbers of red cells, particularly during the first week, than older children and adults) and altitude (Table 3–2).

TABLE 3–2. Selected Reference Ranges for RBC Count

Age	RBC Range ($10^6/\mu L$)
1 Day	5.25–5.35
2 Months	3.70–3.80
1 Year	4.40–4.48
10 Years	4.75–4.85
Adult male	4.73–5.49
Adult female	4.15–4.87

Ranges from Jacobs DS, et al. *Laboratory Test Handbook*, 2nd ed. Cleveland, LexiComp Inc., 1990.

■ MORPHOLOGY

In a normal, healthy individual mature erythrocytes range, on average, from 6 to 8 microns (µ) in diameter. If not crowded together on a blood smear, they appear as circular, homogeneous discs with a center that is somewhat paler than the periphery of the cell. Although there is some variation even in normal subjects, the cells are generally of nearly uniform size and shape. In a variety of disorders that are discussed later, red cells will vary in their hemoglobin content, size, shape, structure, and staining properties (Table 3–3).

Hemoglobin Content

The hemoglobin content of red cells can be roughly judged by the depth of staining on the peripheral blood smear when the red cells are examined as a part of the differential or in follow-up to abnormal or questionable findings from the automated analysis of the sample. If the amount of hemoglobin is diminished, the central pale area becomes larger and paler, a state known as *hypochromia;* cells exhibiting this characteristic are referred to as *hypochromic.* The **mean corpuscular hemoglobin** (MCH—the hemoglobin content of the average red cell) and the **mean corpuscular hemoglobin concentration** (MCHC—the average concentration of hemoglobin in a given volume of packed cells) are usually decreased when hypochromia is noted.

TABLE 3–3. Red Cell Abnormalities on Peripheral Smear

Type of Abnormality	Specific Abnormality	Microscopic Observations (related measurements)	Selected Conditions[1] Producing Abnormality
Abnormalities related to size	Microcytosis (MCV <80)	Significantly smaller red cells	Iron deficiency anemia; thalassemia
	Macrocytosis	Significantly larger red cells (MCV >100)	B_{12} or folate deficiency; severe liver disease
	Anisocytosis	Significant variation in red cell size (elevated RDW)	Variety of conditions, esp. anemia with reticulocytosis
Abnormalities related to hemoglobin	Hypochromia	Larger central pallor zone (▼ MCH; more severe ▼ MCHC also)	Iron deficiency anemia; thalassemia
	Polychromasia	Red cells stained diffusely blue and slightly larger than normal (increased reticulocyte count)	Conditions resulting in increased red cell production (characteristic staining indicates cell still has some RNA)
	Hyperchromia	Decreased or absent central pallor zone (increased MCHC)	Spherocytosis; hemolytic anemia
Abnormalities related to cell shape	Poikilocytosis	Significant variation in shape Abnormally shaped cells	Sickle cell disease; red cell membrane disorders
	Spherocytosis[2]	Spherical cells w/o biconcavity, lacking central pallor (increased MCHC)	Hereditary membrane defect; immune hemolysis; microangiopathic hemolysis
	Leptocytosis[3]	Red cells with peripheral HGB area and hypochromic ring surrounding central area of NGB-target cell	Iron deficiency; thalassemia; hemoglobinopathies
	Schistocytosis[3]	Fragmented cells; helmet shaped cells	Conditions causing membrane damage—micro-angiopathic hemolysis, DIC, severe burns, etc
	Elliptocytosis[2]	Elliptical, oval, or sausage shaped cells	Hereditary membrane defect or acquired in some anemias—iron deficiency, megaloblastic, thalassemia
	Stomatocytosis[2]	Elongated, slit-like central pallor zone—mouth shaped	Hereditary anomaly affecting membrane transport of sodium; severe liver disease
	Dacrocytosis[3]	Teardrop or pear shaped cells that may have bluntly pointed projection	Myelofibrosis; PA; thalassemia; and in cells with inclusions such as Heinz bodies
	Acanthocytosis[2]	Small, densely stained cells with irregularly spaced thorn-like projections	Hereditary anomaly; alcoholic cirrhosis; post-splenectomy

[1]Conditions provided as examples; listing is not all-inclusive.
[2]Abnormality results from an inherited or acquired defect of the red cell membrane.
[3]Abnormality results from excessive physical trauma in the cardiovascular system.

Hyperchromic cells stain more deeply with less central pallor. Hyperchromia in megaloblastic anemia is seen because the cells are larger and thicker, thus they have an increased hemoglobin content (elevated MCH), but the hemoglobin concentration (MCHC) is normal. The hyperchromia seen in sideroblastic anemia results from a reduced surface to volume ratio—the hemoglobin content (MCH) is normal, but the hemoglobin concentration (MCHC) is usually increased as a result of the reduced surface/volume ratio.

Cells exhibiting normal staining intensity are called **normochromic**. Red cells that contain residual RNA will stain with a blue-gray tint called **polychromasia** or **polychromatophilia**. The residual RNA indicates that the cell is immature and has only been in the blood 1 to 2 days. When these cells are stained with a special stain (supravital stains) such as methylene blue, precipitated RNA can be observed. Cells in which the precipitated RNA is visible when stained in this manner are reticulocytes. Increased polychromasia implies reticulocytosis, which may be seen in a variety of conditions, but is most marked in hemolysis and in acute blood loss. The increased number of immature red cells in the peripheral blood is indicative of increased red cell production.

Size

Cells that are abnormally small are called **microcytes** (microcytic cells) and those that are abnormally large are **macrocytes** (macrocytic cells). Some variation in the size of cells is normal, but an abnormal amount of variation is referred to as **anisocytosis**. Anisocytosis is seen in most of the anemias and when marked anisocytosis is noted, both microcytes and macrocytes are usually present. The **RDW** (red cell distribution width), provided by a number of automated analyzers, is an indicator of the presence and relative amount of anisocytosis present—the higher the RDW, the greater the level of anisocytosis detected. The terms *microcytic* and *macrocytic* are more meaningful in terms of volume rather than cell diameter. The **mean cell volume** (MCV) is either measured directly on automated analyzers or calculated using the hematocrit and the red cell count. In some instances the MCV may be normal even though many of the cells have a decreased diameter. In spherocytosis, for example, the cells may have a decreased diameter but a normal volume because the cells are thicker than normal red cells.

Shape

Some variation in the shape of red cells is normal. Increased variation in shape is noted in terms of **poikilocytosis**. A variety of abnormal shapes may be seen, a number of which are defined below, but any abnormally shaped cell is referred to as a *poikilocyte*.

As implied by the name, *elliptocytes* are elliptical. Up to 10 % of red cells in normal individuals may be elliptical; amounts above this are considered abnormal. In a dominant hereditary condition called *elliptocytosis*, the majority of red cells are elliptocytes. Increased numbers of elliptocytes may also be seen in iron deficiency anemia, megaloblastic anemias, sickle cell anemia, and in myelofibrosis with myeloid metaplasia.

Spherocytes are nearly spherical as opposed to the normal biconcave discs and they have a smaller than normal diameter. The central pale area is smaller, or absent. They are found in hereditary spherocytosis, some cases of acquired hemolytic anemia, and in some conditions where there has been direct physical or chemical injury to the cells (such as heat).

Target cells (leptocytes) are thinner than normal. When they are stained, a peripheral rim of hemoglobin is seen with a dark, central hemoglobin-containing area, resembling a "target." Target cells are found in obstructive jaundice, after splenectomy, in hypochromic anemias, and in hemoglobin C disease.

Schistocytes are cell fragments and can indicate the presence of hemolysis such as in megaloblastic anemia and severe burns. These cell fragments are often called by names derived from their microscopic appearance: helmet cells and burr cells, for example.

Acanthocytes have irregular spicules with bulbous, rounded ends and are seen in hereditary or acquired abetalipoproteinemia and some cases of liver disease.

Echinocytes (Crenated Cells) have regular contractions and can commonly occur as an artifact from smear preparation as well as in some physiologic conditions.

As indicated by the name, *teardrop cells (Dacrocytes)* are generally tear shaped but may also be pear shaped with a blunt pointed projection. When a red cell contains a rigid element, such as a Heinz body, the part of the cell with the inclusion cannot pass through small splenic sinus openings and is left behind. The cell is stretched beyond its ability to regain its shape as it squeezes through the small opening and the tear or pear shaped cell results. These cells are typically seen in myeloid metaplasia because of the enlarged spleen, but are also seen in some forms of anemia as well as in other conditions.

Inclusions

Red cells may exhibit **basophilic stippling**, which is characterized by the presence of irregular basophilic (stains with basic dyes; appearance is dark blue) granules that may be fine or coarse. The cell containing these granules may stain normally in color or exhibit polychromasia. Fine basophilic stippling is commonly seen with increased production of red cells. Coarse basophilic stippling can be seen in lead poisoning or other diseases with impaired hemoglobin synthesis, in megaloblastic anemia, and in other severe forms of anemia.

Howell-Jolly bodies are remnants of nuclear chromatin and appear as smooth, round bluish dots within the red cell. Howell-Jolly bodies are seen singly in megaloblastic and hemolytic anemias and after splenectomy. Multiple bodies in a single cell are usually indicative of megaloblastic anemia or another form of abnormal erythropoiesis. It is not unusual to find these bodies in the later stages of maturing blast cells in erythrocyte development.

Cabot rings also indicate abnormal erythropoiesis. These are bluish, thread-like rings or convolutions (figure-of-eight, loop shaped) and are occasionally formed by double or several concentric lines.

Heinz bodies are round refractile inclusions not visible on a standard Wright's stained smear. They result from abnormal hemoglobin precipitation and may be a single large body or several small ones. They are best seen with a supravital stain and care must be exercised to avoid confusing red cells containing Heinz bodies with reticulocytes. They are not seen in normal individuals (except in cases of acute poisoning with certain agents) because they are removed from the red cell by the spleen. If the spleen has been removed or is atrophied, the inclusions are seen frequently. Heinz bodies may also occur in hereditary deficiency of some enzymes.

Nucleated red cells, as mentioned previously, are precursors to the mature erythrocyte. The erythrocyte is unlike most other mammalian cells in that it does not contain a nucleus in its mature form. The presence of these cells in the peripheral blood of very young infants is normal, but in the healthy adult, they are found only in the bone marrow. They may appear in the peripheral blood circulation in certain disease states where their presence generally indicates a significantly increased demand has been placed on the bone marrow. Especially large numbers are found in hemolytic disease of the newborn (erythroblastosis fetalis) and in an anemia called Thalassemia major (discussed in erythrocytic disorders).

RED CELL MASS DISORDERS

Normally, red cell production and the circulating red cell mass remain at a relatively constant level regulated by the erythropoietic mechanism. When the red cell mass is significantly decreased or increased, clinical problems occur. Anemia is associated with decreased red cells. Most disorders of the erythrocyte can be classified into one of the many anemias.

■ ANEMIAS

Anemias, conditions of decreased red cell mass, can be divided into *absolute abnormalities* and *relative abnormalities*. In absolute conditions there is a true decrease or increase in the red cell mass. Relative anemia results from a fluid shift from the extravascular to the intravascular compartment, which expands the plasma volume and dilutes the red cell mass (an increase in volume rather than an actual decrease in red cells). Relative anemia is often seen in pregnancy and in individuals with diseases involving high protein levels. A decrease in plasma volume results in relative erythrocytosis even though the red cell mass is normal. This can be seen in conditions associated with dehydration. The presence of anemia or erythrocytosis points to an underlying pathophysiologic process.

The term *anemia*, as generally used in clinical medicine, refers to a reduction below normal of the hemoglobin, hematocrit, and the number of red cells. When anemia is detected, the presence of an underlying disease process is suggested. Determining a definitive diagnosis can be quite complicated as there are a number of possible mechanisms that result in anemia.

The anemias can be divided into four major groups:

1. *hypoproliferative anemia*—decreased bone marrow production
2. *maturation disorders*—ineffective marrow production
3. *hemolytic disorders*—increased red cell destruction
4. *blood loss anemia*

In each case, the condition is in excess of the marrow's ability to replace the loss.

Classifications

Once detected, classifying the anemia is usually beneficial in helping to establish a definitive diagnosis. The three basic formats used are

1. *etiologic:* underlying pathophysiologic mechanisms
2. *morphologic:* using red cell indices and microscopic examination of red cell morphology
3. *physiologic:* based on the bone marrow ability to respond with increased erythropoiesis

ETIOLOGIC CLASSIFICATION. Classification according to etiology is often difficult as there may be multiple causative factors. Further, anemia is often complicated by another disease process making definitive etiologic classification even more difficult. Table 3–4 shows a few of the etiologic classifications, types of anemias in each, and the primary causative mechanisms.

TABLE 3–4. Etiologic Classification of Anemia

Anemia Category	Examples	Primary Causes
Relative anemia	Pregnancy; Hyperproteinemia; Intravenous fluids	Increased plasma volume
Defective hemoglobin synthesis	Iron deficiency	Excess loss; increased requirements; deficient intake; defective absorption
	Sideroblastic anemia	Enzymatic defect in heme synthesis
	Anemia of chronic disease	Defective iron utilization: infection; inflammation; neoplasm
	Thalassemia syndromes	Imbalanced globin synthesis
Vitamin B_{12} or folate deficiency	Vitamin B_{12} deficiency	Inadequate dietary intake; defective absorption; increased requirements; defective production of intrinsic factor
	Folate deficiency	Inadequate dietary intake; defective absorption; increased requirements; impaired utilization—folate antagonists

Impaired marrow/ stem cell function	Bone marrow injury
	  Primary aplastic anemia
	  Secondary aplastic
		Reduced hematopoietic tissue
		  Idiopathic defect
		  Injury by drugs, infectious agents, etc

	Bone marrow replacement Myeloplastic anemia	Infiltration with abnormal tissue: leukemia, lymphoma, storage disease, etc
	Ineffective hematopoiesis Myelodysplastic anemias	Disorder of stem cell: abnormal proliferation and maturation
	Decreased marrow stimulation	Reduced secretion of hematopoietin

Adapted from Lotspeich-Steiniger C, Stiene-Martin A, Koepke J. *Clinical Hematology: Principles, Procedures, Correlations.* Philadelphia, Lippincott, 1992

MORPHOLOGIC CLASSIFICATION. This system uses red cell size and hemoglobin content as determined by the red cell indices (MCH, MCV, MCHC—RDW also used sometimes in conjunction with MCV) and microscopic examination of red cell morphology to classify anemias into four categories:

1. normocytic, normochromic
2. microcytic, hypochromic
3. microcytic, normochromic
4. macrocytic, normochromic

Although widely used and accepted, this method has been criticized as lacking sensitivity and standardization; however, review of red cell morphology continues to be important in the classification of anemias. Table 3–5 shows classifications based on MCV and gives examples of each. It is beneficial to understand both classification systems since some anemias have more than one mechanism and go through more than one morphologic stage.

TABLE 3–5. Morphologic Classification of Anemia

Classification	Examples

Microcytic (MCV < 80)	Commonly microcytic
	   iron deficiency
	   thalassemias
	   hereditary sideroblastic anemia
	Occasionally microcytic
	   anemia of chronic disease
	   hemoglobinopathies

Macrocytic (MCV >100)	Commonly macrocytic
	   folic acid deficiency
	   B_{12} deficiency
	Occasionally macrocytic
	   liver disease
	   hemolytic anemia
	   blood loss anemia

Normocytic	Commonly normocytic
	   hypoproliferative anemia
	   hemolytic anemia
	   hemoglobinopathies
	   blood loss anemia
	   anemia of chronic disease
	   acquired sideroblastic anemia
	Occasionally normocytic
	   early iron deficiency
	   refractory anemia

PHYSIOLOGIC CLASSIFICATION. As previously mentioned, physiologic classification is based on the marrow's ability to respond with increased erythropoiesis. Erythrocyte production is assessed using the reticulocyte count, sometimes with additional mathematical calculation to correct for reticulocytes being shifted out of the marrow early and remaining in the circulation longer.

Megaloblastic Anemias

The megaloblastic anemias are a major subgroup of the anemias caused by abnormal nuclear development. These anemias are characterized by large, oval red cells, which are usually detected by seeing an increased MCV on the CBC. Megaloblastic anemias are generally classified as macrocytic, normochromic.

The most common cause of megaloblastic anemia is vitamin x and folate deficiency. Vitamin B_{12} and folate are important components in DNA synthesis. A deficiency in B_{12} causes defective DNA synthesis by preventing the appropriate conversion of a number of substances, including folate, and by preventing the catabolism of another substance. The defect in DNA synthesis results in megaloblastic erythropoiesis and anemia. A deficiency of folate, whether as a result of being "trapped" in the conversion process because of B_{12} deficiency, insufficient dietary intake, or other causes, also results in defective DNA synthesis and megaloblastic anemia. B_{12} deficiency may result from a variety of causes, including dietary deficiency, with small bowel bacterial overgrowth, malabsorption of B_{12}, and deficiencies or defects in intrinsic factor. Possible causes of folate deficiency include dietary deficiency, alcoholic cirrhosis, folate antagonists (some anti-malarial and chemotherapy agents), pregnancy, and infant malnutrition. Conditions that lead to intestinal atrophy can cause a deficiency of both B_{12} and folate.

Pernicious anemia (PA) is also a megaloblastic anemia and is perhaps the most representative form. PA is associated with B_{12} deficiency as a result of an atrophy of the stomach lining. This atrophy results in a reduction or elimination of the secretion of intrinsic factor (IF), which protects B_{12} from destruction in the gastrointestinal tract before it can be absorbed in the ileum. PA is almost always an acquired disorder although there are rare cases of congenital PA inherited as an autosomal recessive trait. In congenital cases, the stomach lining is normal and the defect in B_{12} absorption is due either to an inherited lack of IF production or to an abnormality in the structure of IF.

LABORATORY FINDINGS IN MEGALOBLASTIC ANEMIA. Findings on the CBC are very similar in all cases of megaloblastic anemia regardless of the underlying cause. Additional testing may be necessary to definitively establish the cause of the anemia. The red cell count is, of course, decreased with the degree depending upon when the diagnosis is made—anemia may range from mild to severe. The MCV is increased. With mild to moderate anemia the MCV may increase to 110 and with severe anemia ranges from 110 to 130 with some even higher values seen. An increased MCH is also usually seen, as the hemoglobin content is increased in proportion to the cell size. The MCHC, however, usually remains normal. Microscopically the red cells are large (increased MCV) and oval with little or no central pallor (increased MCH). Anisocytosis is commonly seen which results in an increased red cell distribution width (RDW).

Poikilocytosis is also present, with the most common poikilocyte being the large, oval cells (macro-ovalocytes). Other poikilocytes may include teardrop cells and cell fragments. In more advanced anemia, red cell inclusions, particularly Howell-Jolly bodies and basophilic stippling, may be seen. Large, abnormal nucleated red cells may be noted on the peripheral smear as well. The white cell count is normal in the early stages, but will gradually decline as the condition progresses. Microscopically, giant neutrophils and bands are common. Hypersegmentation of the nucleus of the neutrophil is a characteristic finding and a classic indicator of megaloblastic anemia (neutrophils may have five to ten lobes; normal neutrophils have fewer than five nuclear lobes). Platelet counts usually fall with the red cell count and the platelets may be granule deficient, making them stain poorly. Reticulocytes are larger than normal and counts may show an inadequate marrow response to the anemia. Table 3–6 shows the biochemical differentiation of B_{12} and folate deficiencies.

Pernicious anemia has other distinguishing laboratory features, including a moderate decrease in red cell survival. The serum B_{12} level is decreased. Erythrocyte folate is decreased, but serum folate levels are normal or elevated. Serum iron is moderately increased in progressive stages and total iron binding capacity may be slightly reduced. PA patients may demonstrate neurologic disturbances, the severity of which is not directly related to the degree of anemia. Abnormal neurologic findings are less common today (about 30% of patients) because of earlier diagnosis and treatment.

TABLE 3–6. Differentiation of B_{12} and Folate Deficiency

Condition	Serum B_{12}	Serum Folate	Red Cell Folate
B_{12} deficiency	⇓⇓⇓	N or ⇓	⇓ or ⇓⇓
Folate deficiency	N or ⇓	⇓⇓⇓	⇓⇓⇓
B_{12} and folate deficiency	⇓	⇓	⇓⇓⇓

N = Normal; ⇓⇓⇓ = markedly decreased; ⇓⇓ = moderately decreased; ⇓ = decreased.

TIME FOR REVIEW. After studying the preceding sections, you should be able to respond correctly to the following:

■ The term used to describe an increased amount of variation in red cell size is

_____ .

■ Increased variation in the shape of red cells is described in terms of

_____ .

■ The presence of nucleated red cells in the peripheral circulation of an adult generally indicates _____ .

■ Megaloblastic anemia is characterized by large, oval red cells often detected by an increased _____ on the CBC.

■ The most common cause of megaloblastic anemia is _____ .

■ Describe typical laboratory findings in megaloblastic anemia.

■ Review Table 3–6 (Differentiation of B_{12} and Folate Deficiency).

Check your responses by reviewing the preceding pages.

Abnormal Iron Metabolism Anemias

Iron is necessary for the synthesis of normally functioning hemoglobin. When the supply of iron available for hemoglobin synthesis is decreased, anemia will occur. The anemia may be due to a deficiency of iron (iron deficiency anemia), to a defect in the release of stored iron (anemia of chronic disorders), or to a defect in the utilization of the iron in the early red cell, the erythroblast (sideroblastic anemia).

Iron deficiency anemia develops gradually because the body maintains iron in a stored condition as *ferritin.* As the demand for iron increases or as iron is lost, the stored iron is used. If the increased demand or loss of iron continues beyond the ability of the stored iron to serve as adequate replacement, iron deficiency occurs. The deficiency may be caused by varying factors such as:

- *increased physiologic demands:* periods of rapid growth in infants and children (red cell mass increases 30-fold from infancy to adulthood) and during pregnancy and lactation.
- *inadequate intake:* from an iron-deficient diet or from inadequate absorption.

- *chronic blood loss:* menstrual flow, gastrointestinal bleeding, regular blood donation, chronic hemolysis (disorders such as the rare condition paroxysmal nocturnal hemoglobinuria).

The clinical presentation of iron deficiency anemia is similar to that of any other form of anemia (see Clinical Signs and Symptoms of Anemia later in this text) with the usual range of symptoms, including fatigue, breathlessness, and dizziness. These symptoms are all due to the reduction in oxygen delivery to the tissues and thus could represent any form of anemia. Because of the gradual onset of iron deficiency anemia, which allows the body's compensatory mechanisms to minimize the symptoms, the anemia may be moderate or even severe before the patient seeks treatment. Particularly with iron deficiency of chronic blood loss, patients may present with symptoms related to their primary condition instead of the anemia (eg, a man complaining of epigastric pain associated with ulcers or a woman noting menorrhagia, with the anemia detected as a part of the investigation of these conditions).

LABORATORY FINDINGS. Table 3–7 summarizes laboratory tests that assist in the diagnosis of iron deficiency. Table 3–8 shows the sequential changes in selected laboratory values as iron deficiency develops. In this table the normal individual is depicted, followed by stage I, in which iron stores have been depleted in response to either increased demands of excessive loss of iron. In stage II, iron deficient ery-

TABLE 3–7. Laboratory Tests Aiding in Diagnosis of Iron Deficiency

Most frequently required tests	CBC (including red cell morphology)
	Serum ferritin
	Reticulocyte count 7 to 10 days after initiation of iron therapy
Occasionally required tests	Serum iron
	TIBC
	Percent transferrin saturation

TABLE 3–8. Sequential Changes in Iron Deficiency Development

Test	Normal (Adequate Iron Stores)	Stage I (Iron Depleted)	Stage II (Iron Deficient Erythropoiesis)	Stage III (Iron Deficient Anemia)
Serum ferritin	>12	<12	>12	<12
Serum iron	65–165	~115	<60	<40
TIBC	300–360	~360	~390	~410
Hemoglobin	Normal	Normal	Normal	⇓⇓⇓
Red cell morphology	Normal	Normal	Normal	Microcytic Hypochromic
MCV	Normal	Normal	Normal	⇓⇓⇓

thropoiesis (red cell production) occurs and is followed by stage III, in which anemia results from the iron deficiency.

When iron deficiency anemia has developed (stage III), the CBC reflects a decreased hemoglobin and hematocrit. These may be significantly decreased (hgb < 8 g/dL; hct < 24%) before the patient complains of anemia-related symptoms. The MCV, MCH, and MCHC are all reduced in severe iron deficiency anemia and the red cells appear microcytic and hypochromic microscopically. In severe cases, only the outer rim of the red cell may be visible. Moderate anisocytosis may be seen, with some cells in the normal size range, with an elevated RDW. Poikilocytosis is also present, with a variety of abnormal cell shapes observed microscopically. Platelet counts are often increased to close to twice the reference range, but may be normal or even decreased in some cases.

Analysis of iron status is useful in identifying the stages of iron deficiency and in diagnosis, as well as in measuring the response to therapy. Serum ferritin levels can be particularly useful as this measurement reflects iron storage levels and is decreased before hematologic changes and symptoms occur. It is important to note, however, that ferritin levels are increased in inflammation and can mask iron deficiency. If inflammation is present and iron deficiency is suspected, other measures of iron status should be employed. As a rule of thumb, when ferritin concentrations are > 80 to 100 ng/mL in the presence of inflammation, iron deficiency can usually be ruled out. Serum iron, total iron binding capacity (TIBC), and transferrin saturation are useful values. Serum iron and transferrin saturation decrease as iron loss progresses and the TIBC increases as a result of the lack of iron available for transport.

Reticulocyte counts are not particularly useful in the diagnosis of iron deficiency, but are used to monitor the response to iron therapy. Iron therapy should result in an increase in the reticulocyte count within a few days, with a peak reached between 7 and 10 days after the initiation of therapy.

Anemia of chronic disorders is fairly common, being second only to iron deficiency anemia, and may be the most common form found in hospital populations. This type of anemia is found in association with chronic disorders of more than 1 or 2 months duration. Causes include infectious diseases such as tuberculosis, pneumonia, osteomyelitis, pelvic inflammatory disease, and subacute bacterial endocarditis; noninfectious, inflammatory diseases, including rheumatoid arthritis, systemic lupus erythematosus, and thermal injury; and malignant diseases such as leukemia, Hodgkin's disease, and carcinomas. The mechanism resulting in anemia is uncertain, but may be a decrease in release of stored iron, shortened red cell survival, or impaired marrow response in red cell replacement.

The clinical presentation of these patients generally involves symptoms and physical findings related to the primary disorder (the infectious, inflammatory, or malignant process). Laboratory findings include a slightly reduced hemoglobin (often 1 or 2 g below the patient's usual level, which in some cases, will still be within the normal reference range). The red cells are generally normocytic and normochromic, but hypochromic cells may be seen. Microcytosis (small red cells; decreased MCV) is not common, but if present is not usually as pronounced as that seen in iron deficiency anemia. Mild to moderate anisocytosis may occur, but poikilocytosis is generally minimal. Serum iron levels are low, usually similar to those found in iron deficiency anemia. However, the TIBC is decreased in chronic disorders, but increased in iron deficiency. Serum ferritin levels are elevated in this type of anemia as opposed to the decrease seen in iron deficiency. Ferritin levels can be useful in differentiating the two anemias. However, no specific tests are recommended for the diagnosis of anemia of chronic disorders because it is secondary to a disease process that is the primary focus of diagnosis and treatment protocols.

Sideroblastic anemias include a diverse group of anemias with abnormal iron kinetics resulting in an excess accumulation of iron. These anemias may be hereditary or acquired (secondary to drugs or toxins, including lead intoxication). Despite differing etiologies, the sideroblastic anemias all share the common feature of ringed sideroblasts (iron deposits in the normoblast red cell precursor) in the bone marrow, which are identified with a special staining process. The variety of sideroblastic anemias and their associated clinical and laboratory findings will not be discussed in this text. However, the laboratory tests most frequently required to diagnose these anemias are the CBC with red cell morphology, serum ferritin, and bone marrow studies with the Prussian blue stain procedure.

Anemia of abnormal iron metabolism may also result from lead intoxication in both children and adults. The elevated lead levels cause a variety of injuries resulting in a reduction of the red cell mass. Among these injuries are inhibited activity of enzymes necessary for heme synthesis and injury to the red cell membrane. Common symptoms include abdominal pain, constipation, vomiting, and muscle pain. Neurologic and psychological symptoms are less frequent. The anemia associated with lead intoxication is usually mild to moderate with the red cells appearing slightly to moderately hypochromic and microcytic (decreased MCH and MCV, respectively). Basophilic stippling is present in many cases and the reticulocyte count is slightly increased. The chemistry measurements reflecting iron storage, such as ferritin, are normal in lead intoxication as opposed to the other anemias in the abnormal iron metabolism group. Lead levels are, of course, vital in the diagnosis of lead intoxication. Other serum and urine chemistries may also be useful. Treatment of the lead intoxication is of primary importance in the patient demonstrating anemia as a result of lead intoxication.

Hemoglobinopathies

Hemoglobin, the iron containing pigment of the red cells that functions to carry oxygen from the lungs to the tissues, has many variants. In fact, there are hundreds of abnormal hemoglobins. When hemoglobin variants (or abnormal hemoglobins) are produced, the patient is said to have a *hemoglobinopathy*. Hemoglobinopathies are caused by structural abnormalities in the polypeptide chains (abnormalities may be in the alpha, beta, gamma, or delta chains, but beta is most common) resulting from altered DNA. These disorders may or may not result in clinical and laboratory abnormalities, and a number of laboratory tests are needed to identify and distinguish hemoglobin variants. It is beyond the scope of this study to discuss the classifications and diagnosis of the large number of hemoglobinopathies. The most common hemoglobin variant, hemoglobin S, will be discussed as an example of the hemoglobinopathies.

Sickle cell anemia is an inherited disorder resulting from homozygous (SS) inheritance of a codominant gene. Heterozygous inheritance (AS) is termed *sickle cell trait.* Hemoglobin S results from a mutation in an amino acid in the beta chain. With the exception of this one amino acid, hemoglobin S is the same structurally as the normal hemoglobin A. The anemia associated with hemoglobin S derives its name from the characteristic "sickle" shape of the red cells at decreased oxygen levels. When oxygenated, hemoglobin S is fully soluble and the erythrocytes are not "sickled." When oxygen decreases at the tissue level, sickling occurs as a result of a change in the hemoglobin molecule that causes it to become rigid. The sickled cells impede the blood flow to organs and tissues, which causes tissue death, organ infarction, and pain. Hemolysis is common as the abnormally shaped cells are destroyed prematurely both by the phagocytic system (especially the spleen) and by their inability to pass through the microcirculation (cells are too rigid). This increased destruction brings about a response by the bone marrow to increase erythropoiesis.

Symptoms of sickle cell anemia can be very severe and every organ in the body is affected. For example, the sequestration of sickled cells in the liver may cause hepatomegaly and liver malfunction; iron deposition in the heart as a result of frequent transfusions can lead to heart failure, and cardiomegaly may appear early in childhood; infarcts may occur in the kidneys; and infarcts in lung tissue may occur as a result of infections and sickle cell occlusion.

Abnormal splenic function and splenomegaly may begin even in infancy. As a consequence of sickle occlusion, later in childhood, splenic infarction and fibrosis occur. The spleen eventually shrivels and becomes nonfunctional. As a result of the multiple organs affected, symptoms include pain of many types. Fatigue, weakness, pallor, and other general symptoms of anemia result from chronic hemolysis of red cells. Between the ages of 10 and 20, growth and sexual maturation lag behind in sickle cell anemia patients.

Many symptoms are related to *sickle cell crises,* which are caused by any situation that causes excessive deoxygenation (infection, obstetric delivery, dehydration, violent exercise, high altitudes, etc). Sickle cell crises occur as a result of vaso-occlusive disorders caused by the rigid sickle cells: development of microthrombi, vascular occlusions, infarctions in joints and extremities and in major organs which can lead to organ failure.

Infectious crises are one of the major causes of death in sickle cell anemia, with *Streptococcus pneumoniae* being the major infectious agent in children. Sickle cells may also accumulate in the joints and in the shafts of bones, causing severe joint pain. As noted, every organ in the body is affected by this disorder. The following list briefly describes the impact of this disease on some of the major organs.

Spleen: When sickle cells become trapped in the microcirculation of the spleen, splenic sequestration crises occur. The spleen becomes larger as more cells are trapped, and hypovolemia (decreased blood volume) can result. In some cases, shock and even death result from this crisis, usually in children under age 6. Splenic enlargement and abnormal splenic function can begin in infancy. Later in childhood, as a result of sickle occlusion, splenic infarction and fibrosis occur. The spleen eventually shrivels, becoming nonfunctional.

Liver: Liver malfunction and hepatomegaly may occur as a result of sickle cell sequestration in the sinusoids of the liver. This condition may be seen in both children and adults, and can also result in jaundice and hyperbilirubinemia.

Heart: Particularly in patients requiring frequent transfusions, iron deposits may occur in the heart and can lead to heart failure. Enlargement of the heart may be seen in early childhood.

Lungs: Tissue may become necrotic in the lungs as a result of blocked blood supply by sickle cell occlusion or from infections.

Kidneys: Necrosis following loss of blood supply to tissue in the kidneys may also occur and result in hematuria and a loss of concentrating ability of the kidneys.

LABORATORY FINDINGS. The anemia in sickle cell disease is generally severe with hemoglobin levels between 5 and 9g. The red cell indices are usually typical of normochromic, normocytic cells. Anemia and other symptoms are generally not evident until about 6 to 9 months of age. Anisocytosis and an increased RDW are common findings. The most important poikilocyte is the sickle cell, which may be present in abundance or only noted in an occasional microscopic field depending upon the current status of the patient. Target cells are generally seen in large numbers and ovalocytes and cell fragments may also be noted. When red cells have gone back and forth several times between the normal and the sickle state, they usually become irreversibly sickled and appear as dense elliptocytes with areas where the hemoglobin has shrunk away from the cell membrane. Other findings on the peripheral blood smear include polychromasia, nucleated red cells (rare to many), basophilic stippling, and, in cases where the spleen is nonfunctional, Howell-Jolly bodies and Pappenheimer bodies. The reticulocyte count is increased in the range of about 8% to 16%. It is common to see an increased white count with an increase in the percentage of neutrophils. It is also common to see an increase in platelets because a fibrotic spleen cannot pool platelets in the manner of a normal spleen. However, during a vasoocclusive crisis, the platelet count will be decreased.

Hemoglobin electrophoresis is necessary to confirm the presence of hemoglobin S with quantitation used to distinguish sickle cell disease from other hemoglobinopathies. Abnormalities in some chemistry parameters may be noted as a result of the hemolytic component of sickle cell disease: an increase in LD, and indirect bilirubin.

Individuals with sickle cell trait (heterozygous AS inheritance) generally have no anemia and have normal red cell morphology (few target cells and occasional sickle cells sometimes seen), and rarely, if ever, require treatment. The presence of sickle cell trait can be determined by quantitative hemoglobin electrophoresis.

Hemolytic Anemias (Increased Red Cell Destruction)

A number of anemias result from the increased destruction of red cells. These anemias of increased erythrocyte destruction may be hereditary or acquired disorders. These anemias will not be discussed in this text beyond the information provided in Tables 3–9 and 3–10, which present the classification of these hemolytic anemias and summarize laboratory findings. Note that in Table 3–10 only one or two examples are provided for each type of anemia, although, in some cases, many others may also be representative of that classification.

TABLE 3–9. Hemolytic Anemia Classification

Intrinsic[1] Hemolytic Anemias	Extrinsic[1] Hemolytic Anemias
Hereditary	**Hereditary**
Due to membrane defects—hereditary spherocytosis	Abetalipoproteinemia
Due to enzyme defects—g6pd deficiency	
Due to hemoglobinopathies—thalassemia	
Acquired	**Acquired**
Paroxysmal nocturnal hemoglobinuria	Immune mediated
	Mechanical, thermal, or chemical damage

[1]Intrinsic hemolytic anemias involve some sort of defect in the red cell itself; extrinsic refers to factors outside the red cell that damage normal red cells.

TABLE 3–10. Laboratory Findings in Hemolytic Anemias

Test/Observation	Result
Appearance of serum/plasma	Color may indicate presence of free hemoglobin
CBC[1]	⇓ RBC; ⇓ HGB; ⇓ HCT (MCV sometimes increased)
Peripheral smear[1]	Polychromasia with morphology specific to underlying disease
Reticulocyte count[1]	⇑
Urinalysis	⇑ Urobilinogen; + hemoglobin
Bilirubin, unconjugated[1]	⇑
Prussian blue stain of urine sediment	+ Hemosiderin; + ferritin
Occult blood, feces	– (Result should be negative in hemolytic anemia; a positive result is indicative of gastrointestinal bleeding)

[1]Recommended for initial screening. The test results in this table are for hemolytic anemias in general. For differential diagnosis, additional testing may be performed as indicated by the initial screening test results.

Key: + = positive; – = negative; ⇑ = increased; ⇓ = decreased.

Blood Loss Anemia

Blood loss anemia may be acute or chronic. If a quantity of blood sufficient to result in anemia is lost over a short period of time, acute post-hemorrhagic anemia occurs. The blood loss may be from the circulation externally, into the gastrointestinal tract, or into a tissue space or body cavity. The most prominent symptoms following a sudden blood loss are those associated with depletion of blood volume (hypovolemia). These symptoms are relieved by absorption of fluid from the tissues or by artificial fluid replacement returning the volume to previous levels. When the volume is returned to normal, the anemia becomes apparent, with the earliest hematologic change being a transient fall in the platelet count, which may become elevated within an hour. A moderate increase in the neutrophilic leukocytes with a left shift may occur in 2 to 5 hours. A decrease in the hemoglobin and hematocrit are not seen immediately, but fall slowly as the tissue fluids move into the circulation to compensate for the lost blood volume. The full extent of red cell loss may not be evident from the fall in hemoglobin and hematocrit until 2 or 3 days after the hemorrhage.

Initially the resulting anemia is normocytic and normochromic. The MCV and MCHC are also normal and only minimal anisocytosis and poikilocytosis are present. In 3 to 5 days, as increases in erythropoietin stimulate increased erythrocyte production in the marrow, reticulocytes can be found in the peripheral circulation, peaking at about 10 days. During this time transient macrocytosis (increased MCV) and increased polychromasia may be noted. Nucleated red cells may also be seen. About 2 to 4 days after the blood loss, the white count returns to normal and in about 2 weeks the morphologic changes in the red cells disappear.

In chronic post-hemorrhagic anemia, the blood loss is in small amounts over an extended period of time. The clinical features present in acute blood loss are not present and significant anemia does not usually develop until stored iron is depleted. The red cells are regenerated at a slower rate as well. Laboratory findings may include a normal or slightly increased reticulocyte count and an anemia that is at first normochromic and normocytic. Gradually the newly formed red cells become microcytic and then hypochromic. (Since chronic blood loss leads to iron deficiency anemia, the laboratory findings will be the same when iron deficiency develops.) The leukocyte count is normal or slightly decreased and the platelets are commonly increased (later in severe iron deficiency, the platelets are likely to be decreased). It is important, of course, to identify and treat the cause of the blood loss.

■ SYSTEMATIC EVALUATION OF ANEMIA

A systematic approach integrating both clinical and laboratory findings can be very beneficial in the diagnosis of anemia and in the identification of underlying causes. A number of anemias were presented in the previous section. In this section the roles of both the clinician and the laboratorian in the evaluation of anemia will be discussed to aid in the understanding of how to evaluate red cell abnormalities from a laboratory standpoint when a disorder is discovered, but not yet diagnosed.

One of the best examples of the importance of laboratory studies in the diagnosis of disease can be seen in the close relationship between clinical anemia and hematologic studies. As detailed in the preceding section, anemia may result from decreased synthesis of red cells and hemoglobin, from increased destruction of red cells, or from acute or chronic blood loss. From the laboratorian's point of view, the most useful classification of anemias is based on the red cell indices, especially the MCV and MCHC, with these studies being further reinforced by examination of red cell morphology on a stained peripheral blood smear. In some cases, the laboratory characterization of red cell abnormalities has been used to name the condition (eg, sickle cell anemia; macrocytic anemia, microcytic anemia). The clinician plays a vital role in obtaining and evaluating the patient's medical history and physical examinations and requesting and evaluating appropriate laboratory studies.

Identifying the cause of anemia is accomplished by integrating clinical information with the results from laboratory studies. The exact diagnosis is not always obvious to the physician from the patient's symptoms and medical history. Clues provided in the patient's history may suggest some specific causes of anemia and indicate laboratory studies that would be useful in the diagnostic process. The physical examination may also provide important information as to the cause of the anemia. These clues and the anemia that may be associated with each are summarized in Tables 3–11 and 3–12.

TABLE 3–11. Patient History and Common Associations in Anemia

History	Associated Anemia
Chronic hepatic, renal, or other diseases (eg, cancer)	Anemia of chronic disease
Alcoholism	Folate deficiency
Vegetarian diet	Iron deficiency
Bleeding (gastrointestinal, menorrhagia, etc)	Iron deficiency
Exposure to toxic chemicals	Hypoplastic[1] or aplastic[1] anemia
Chronic drug ingestion	Megaloblastic, hypoplastic,[1] aplastic[1] anemia

[1]These anemias were not discussed in the previous section on abnormalities.

Adapted from Lotspeich-Steininger C, Stiene-Martin A, Koepke J. *Clinical Hematology: Principles, Procedures, Correlations.* Philadelphia, Lippincott, 1992

The clinical signs and symptoms of anemia are a result of the reduced oxygen delivery to the tissues. The development of symptoms is primarily dependent upon three factors: the causative disorder, the degree of change in blood volume, and the reduction in the oxygen-carrying capacity of blood with the consequent disturbances in cell nutrition and function. These symptoms are related to the lowered concentration of hemoglobin and to the blood volume and thus are dependent on the rate of change in these levels.

TABLE 3–12. Physical Signs and Common Associations in Anemia

Physical Signs	Associated Anemia
Spleen enlargement	Hemolytic anemia, chronic liver disease, leukemia, lymphoma
Liver enlargement	Hemolytic anemia, metastatic carcinoma
Jaundice	Hemolytic anemia, anemia associated with chronic liver disease
Leg ulcers (black patient)	Sickle cell anemia
"Spooned" nails	Iron deficiency anemia
Neurologic defect	Megaloblastic (vitamin B_{12}) anemia
Lymph node enlargement	Anemia secondary to leukemia, lymphoma, or infection
Bone tenderness	Anemia secondary to myeloma or metastatic carcinoma

Adapted from Lotspeich-Steininger C, Stiene-Martin A, Koepke J. *Clinical Hematology: Principles, Procedures, Correlations.* Philadelphia, Lippincott, 1992

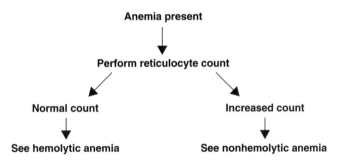

FIGURE 3–3. Hemolytic versus nonhemolytic anemia.

Common physical findings are pallor, rapid pulse, and low blood pressure. A slight fever, some dependent edema, and systolic murmurs may be noted. Patients generally complain of becoming easily fatigued and of dyspnea on exertion. Patients may also report faintness, vertigo, palpitation, and headache. Additional clinical findings can be characteristic of the particular type of anemia present. In the patient who is otherwise in reasonably good health, and in whom the anemia develops slowly, hemoglobin concentration may be as low as 6 g/dL without producing any discomfort or physical signs as long as the patient is at rest. The body is able to compensate for anemia to some degree by adjustments in cardiac output, respiratory rate, and the oxygen affinity for hemoglobin.

A logical systematic approach in the evaluation of anemia allows for the most efficient usage of laboratory resources and avoidance of unnecessary cost to the patient as a result of tests that may not be useful or delays in diagnosis and initiation of effective treatment. Such an approach is depicted in Fig. 3–3 and Tables 3–13 and 3–14. The flow charts provide a tool for arriving at a possible diagnosis in a step-by-step fashion with each question being contingent upon the answer to the preceding question.

TABLE 3–13. Nonhemolytic Anemia Evaluation

Are Red Cells:		
Macrocytic?	**Normocytic?**	**Microcytic/Hypochromic?**
Consider: Folate deficiency; B$_{12}$ deficiency; pernicious anemia (PA); liver disease (see Table 3–3 and tests in preceding section)	Consider: Acute blood loss; chronic infection; renal disease; bone marrow failure (supporting history, symptoms, lab studies)	Consider: Iron deficiency (see Tables 3–5 and 3–6; note that iron deficiency anemia may also result from chronic blood loss)

Adapted from Lotspeich-Steininger C, Stiene-Martin A, Koepke J. *Clinical Hematology: Principles, Procedures, Correlations.* Philadelphia, Lippincott, 1992

TABLE 3–14. Hemolytic Anemia Evaluation

Which Poikilocytes Are Observed on Peripheral Smear?			
Sickle Cells	**Target Cells**	**Spherocytes**	**None/Insignificant**

Consider:
Sickle cell disease
(perform sickle cell
screen; HGB
electrophoresis to
confirm and to
distinguish between
disease and trait)
	Consider:
	Hemoglobinopathies,
	including sickle cell
	disease, thalassemia,
	hemoglobin C and others
	(HGB electrophoresis;
	sickle cell screen may be
	performed initially if desired)
		Consider:
		Hereditary
		spherocytosis,* burns
		or toxins, or antibody
		coated⁺ cells
		Perform tests:
		  *osmotic fragility
		  ⁺direct antiglobulin
			Consider:
			Autoimmune hemolytic
			anemia,* paroxysmal
			nocturnal hemoglobinuria,⁺
			RBC enzyme deficiency,
			sickle cell disease
			Perform tests:
			*for detection/ID of
			autoantibody
			⁺to show abnormal sensitivity
			to complement
			≠RBC enzyme assays
			sickle screen and HGB
			electrophoresis

NOTE: Correlation of history and clinical findings with the results of laboratory findings is essential in the differential diagnosis of anemia, as in other disease states. In some instances, particularly when history and clinical findings strongly suggest a probable cause of anemia, a group of laboratory studies may be requested together rather than in a step-wise fashion based on results of previous testing. Additional laboratory studies may be desired. Clinical judgment must always be used in developing diagnoses.

Adapted from Lotspeich-Steininger C, Stiene-Martin A, Koepke J. *Clinical Hematology: Principles, Procedures, Correlations.* Philadelphia, Lippincott, 1992

This process begins with establishing the presence or absence of anemia using parameters from the CBC: the hemoglobin, the hematocrit, and the red cell count. Obviously, if anemia is not detected at this initial stage, alternative causes for the patient's history and symptoms should be investigated because the charts provide for the investigation and evaluation of anemia only. When anemia is detected, a determination is made as to whether the anemia is a hemolytic anemia or a non-hemolytic anemia. The reticulocyte count serves as a simple, but useful test for this determination as the red cells most recently released from the bone marrow are counted. With increased peripheral hemolysis, increased numbers of reticulocytes will be found.

At this point in the decision-making process, the blood film examination is an important tool. These results may already be available if a CBC was utilized for the initial determination of the presence of anemia (as opposed to the hemoglobin and hematocrit only). Additional laboratory tests may be necessary to arrive at a definitive diagnosis following this step. In some instances, bone marrow studies may be beneficial in the evaluation of anemia. This examination is not, however, frequently employed because little additional information of significance is provided by bone marrow studies in most cases of anemia.

 TIME FOR REVIEW. After studying the preceding sections, you should be able to respond correctly to the following:

■ Explain why anemia may be severe before patients with iron deficiency anemia seek treatment.

■ List the three laboratory tests most frequently needed to aid in the diagnosis of iron deficiency anemia.

■ Review Table 3–8 (Sequential Changes in Iron Deficiency Development).

■ Sideroblastic anemias result in excess accumulation of _____ .

■ The most common hemoglobin variant is _____ .

■ Homozygous inheritance of the hemoglobin variant above results in _____ and heterozygous inheritance results in _____ .

■ Describe the impact of sickle cell disease on three organs in the body.

■ Name the test used to confirm the presence of hemoglobin S.

■ Describe laboratory findings in sickle cell disease.

■ Hemolytic anemias result from _____ .

■ Review Tables 3–6 (Differentiation of B_{12} and Folate Deficiency) and 3–7 (Laboratory Tests Aiding in Diagnosis of Iron Deficiency).

■ Blood loss anemia may be _____ or _____ .

■ The clinical signs and symptoms of anemia are the result of:

■ A patient's history may suggest a possible cause for the presence of anemia. What cause of anemia is suggested by the following?

   vegetarian diet

   alcoholism

   menorrhagia

■ The presence of anemia with neurologic defects noted on physical examination is suggestive of _____ .

■ The _____ serves as a simple, useful test to assist in distinguishing between hemolytic and non-hemolytic anemias.

■ Review the systematic approach to the evaluation of anemia and all tables in this section.

Check your responses by reviewing the preceding pages.

■ INCREASED RED CELL MASS

The term **erythrocytosis** denotes conditions in which there are too many red cells in the circulation. Conditions of increased red cell mass can be divided into absolute or relative abnormalities in the same manner as the anemias or conditions of decreased cell mass. In **absolute** conditions there is a true increase in the red cell mass associated with a variety of causes, including **primary** conditions such as polycythemia vera and **secondary** conditions in response to a variety of triggers. Absolute secondary increases may be termed *appropriate,* as seen in response to the presence of hypoxia resulting from high altitude or from disease processes such as pulmonary or cardiovascular conditions, or *inappropriate* as seen in response to renal disorders that interfere with renal blood flow or extrarenal tumors that trigger inappropriate erythropoiesis. The term inappropriate is applied because the increased red cell production is not in response to a generalized hypoxia, as is the case in appropriate responses.

Relative erythrocytosis, though not a true hematologic disorder, must be distinguished from absolute erythrocytosis, which is a hematologic disorder. Relative erythrocytosis refers to conditions in which the red cell mass *appears* to be increased as a result of another condition, but in which the actual red cell mass is within an acceptable range. This apparent increase in red cell mass can result from the decreased plasma volume seen in dehydration and has also been described as a spurious condition in certain individuals experiencing stress.

Polycythemia vera, an absolute erythrocytosis resulting from a stem cell defect, is characterized by an increase in all the cellular elements and thus may be classified as a myeloproliferative disorder rather than an erythrocytic disorder. It is discussed here in terms of an erythrocyte disorder because the increase in red cell mass is generally the most problematic manifestation of the disorder and is most often the basis for treatment of the condition. Patients often present complaining of dizziness and headaches and may be noted to have a ruddy and somewhat cyanotic appearance. Hypertension is common and affected individuals may also complain of a ringing in the ears, pruritis, (severe itching) and gastrointestinal pain. Physical examination often reveals an enlarged spleen and enlargement of the liver is not uncommon. Gout may be present as a result of high uric acid levels produced by a rapid turnover of red cells. Because other conditions may produce erythrocytosis, its presence alone is not diagnostic of polycythemia vera and other conditions of increased red cell mass must be ruled out before the diagnosis is made. Table 3–15 provides some of the laboratory findings in polycythemia vera.

TABLE 3–15. Selected Laboratory Findings in Polycythemia Vera

Test	Findings
RBC	↑↑
HGB	↑ or ↑↑
HCT	↑ or ↑↑
WBC	↑ or ↑↑
PLT	↑ or ↑↑ (abnormal platelets and abnormal aggregation may be seen)
MCV	N to sl. ↓
MCHC	N to sl. ↓
Reticulocytes	N to sl. ↑
B_{12}	N to ↑
B_{12} binding	↑
Iron	↓
Ferritin	↓
LAP score	usually ↑
Erythropoietin	↓ to N
Peripheral smear	occ. NRBC; thick smear/"crowded" cells—dilution may be required for better film
Bone marrow	Hypercellular; ↑ normoblasts/megakaryocytes (some large, abnormal), ↓ or absent iron

Key: ↑ = increased; ↓ = decreased; N = normal; sl. = slightly.

TABLE 3–16. Polycythemia Vera Diagnostic Criteria

Category A	Category B
1. ↑ RCM: male >36 ml/kg female >32 ml/kg	1. Platelet count >400 × 10⁹/L
2. Arterial O_2 Saturation > 92%	2. WBC >12 × 10⁹/L (fever and infection absent)
3. Splenomegaly	3. ↑ LAP >100 (fever and infection absent)
	4. ↑ B_{12} >900 ng/ml or ↑ unbound B_{12} binding capacity >2200ng/ml

RCM = red cell mass; tested for by method using radioactive labeling of red cells.
N = normal; ↑ = increased; ↑↑ = very increased; ↓ = decreased
Diagnosis may be made if the patient has not been diagnosed with the disease longer than 4 years and has had no prior treatment other than phlebotomy and:
    1. All category A characteristics present *OR*
    2. Characteristics 1 and 2 from category A and any two characteristics from category B are present.

Lotspeich-Steininger C, Stiene-Martin A, Koepke J. *Clinical Hematology: Principles, Procedures, Correlations.* Philadelphia, Lippincott, 1992

A set of criteria for the diagnosis of polycythemia vera was developed by the 1967 Polycythemia Study Group and is summarized in Table 3–16.

Treatment often consists of therapeutic phlebotomy to reduce the red cell mass, and myelosuppressive drugs may also be indicated. Radiation is used in some instances to reduce the proliferation of red cells and platelets. Continued phlebotomy may cause further iron deficiency, but iron deficiency is a desired outcome to limit increases in the red cell mass. Existing thrombocytosis (increased platelets) may be aggravated by repeated phlebotomy.

Progression of the disease is variable, with the disease transforming into acute myelogenous leukemia in a notable number of patients and to acute lymphocytic leukemia in some others. In some cases, normal cellular elements are virtually eliminated and increasing anemia results from ineffective erythropoiesis. A megaloblastic crisis with platelet counts at critically low levels may also develop. The most common development is a reactive response, secondary to the polycythemia, that results in myelofibrosis (a replacement of the bone marrow with fibrous tissue) and myeloid metaplasia (conversion of myeloid tissues/cellular elements to abnormal forms) that are increasing and irreversible. These conditions may be called the "spent phase" of polycythemia vera or post-polycythemic myeloid metaplasia (PPMM). Death may result from thrombosis, hemorrhage, acute leukemia, or infection.

LEUKOCYTES

Leukocytes (white cells; WBCs) are colorless, nucleated cells in the peripheral blood functioning as the body's main line of defense against foreign substances. The number of leukocytes found in the peripheral blood is much smaller than the number of erythrocytes. The peripheral blood serves as a means of transport of leukocytes to the tissues.

In this section the formation, classification, and identification of leukocytes will be discussed briefly. The section's focus will be on the function of the different cell types and on nonmalignant leukocyte abnormalities. Malignant abnormalities are discussed briefly in Chapter 4.

Function

Leukocytes function to defend the body against substances recognized as foreign such as bacteria and viruses. Although leukocytes work together as a group, each cell type has its own specific function. Some white cells act as **phagocytes** and engulf and destroy foreign substances, while others are involved in the **production of antibodies**. Both functions are important and each depends upon the other to provide an efficient and effective immune response. As each cell type is introduced, the function(s) of that particular cell type will be discussed.

Formation

The details of leukocyte formation and the precursors in each cell line are beyond the scope of this text. However, leukocytes are believed to be formed from a "totipotent" stem cell that gives rise to a partially committed lymphoid stem cell (from which immunocytes arise) and a partially committed myeloid stem cell (from which phagocytic leukocytes—as well as red cells and platelets—are formed). The bone marrow is the principal site of granulocyte production, but lymphocytes are normally formed in lymphoid tissues throughout the body as well as in the bone marrow.

Classification

The five types of leukocytes normally found in the peripheral blood are **neutrophils** (band forms and segmented forms—"segs"), **eosinophils**, **basophils**, **lymphocytes**, and **monocytes**. A variety of criteria may be used to classify these cells (Table 3–17). For example, cells may be classified based on granularity (granulocytes and nongranulocytes), nuclear segmentation (polymorphonuclear and mononuclear), or function (phagocytes and immunocytes).

TABLE 3–17. Leukocyte Classification

Granularity		Nuclear Segmentation		Function	
Granulocytes	Nongranulocytes	Polymorphonuclear	Mononuclear	Phagocytes	Immunocytes
Neutrophils	Lymphocytes	Neutrophils	Lymphocytes	Neutrophils	Lymphocytes
Eosinophils	Monocytes	Eosinophils	Monocytes	Eosinophils	
Basophils		Basophils		Basophils	
				Monocytes	

Identification

Leukocytes are identified based upon their microscopic appearance on a stained blood smear. Cells may be identified based on their reactions to the different dyes in the stain. Criteria used to identify the various cells include cell size, the ratio of the nucleus to the cytoplasm, characteristics of the cytoplasm (ie, color, presence or absence of granules, color and size of granules), and nuclear characteristics (ie, shape, color, chromatin pattern, and presence or absence of nucleoli).

Granulocytes are named according to their staining properties. For instance, the granules in eosinophils stain a bright orange-red because of their affinity for an acidic dye, eosin, in the stain. The granules in basophils, on the other hand, have an affinity for the basic dye, methylene blue, and stain a dark purple-blue. Granules in neutrophils show minimal affinity for either of the dyes (neutral), staining a light pink-purple or pink-tan. Because of these staining properties, the pH of the staining solution is critical to a properly stained smear, and a properly stained smear is essential for proper cell identification.

One of the most reliable criteria, particularly in determining cellular maturity, is the chromatin pattern of the nucleus. In immature cells, chromatin is finely granular and distributed evenly, with few, if any, aggregates. As the cell matures, the chromatin is more coarsely granular, with medium to large aggregates distributed irregularly.

Criteria for identification must be applied carefully and must be evaluated together because the stages of cell maturation evolve one to another without sharp, distinctive dividing lines between stages. It is possible for a cell to demonstrate some of the characteristics of two maturation cycles and lack one or more criteria for a particular stage. As many features as possible must be used in order to make the best decision possible.

Methods of Measurement/Usage

Leukocytes may be enumerated by either manually (hemacytometer counting chamber) or by a variety of semi- and fully automated methods, as described previously. White cell counts are beneficial for a variety of conditions, including bacterial and viral infections, diagnosis and evaluation of leukemic states, and evaluation of myelopoiesis. By automated methods, white cells must be distinguished from nucleated red cells and platelet aggregates.

An elevated white cell count does not necessarily signify the presence of a pathologic process. For example, counts from actively crying babies can show **leukocytosis** (increased number of leukocytes) with a *left shift* (greater than normal number of less mature cells), as can any stressful situation that leads to an increase in endogenous epinephrine production in newborns, children, or adults. Leukocyte counts from different vascular sources (capillary, venous, arterial) in newborns are not necessarily equivalent.

The types of leukocytes are differentiated and reported in terms of percentages on a *differential* leukocyte count. Many automated methods are capable of reporting partial or complete differentials with special "flags" to alert technologists to the possible presence of abnormal cells requiring microscopic examination. Manual differentials are performed by microscopic examination of a specially stained blood film.

Reference Ranges

White cell counts are age dependent and significant variation may occur within and between subjects. The counts of individual healthy subjects may vary based upon a number of factors, including stress and exercise. As with all reference ranges, each laboratory should ensure that the reference range used is appropriate based on the methodology used and on its population (see Table 3–18 for sample white cell reference ranges).

TABLE 3–18. White Cell Reference Ranges

Age	Range (10^9/L)
12 Hours	13.0–38.0
1 Year	6.0–17.5
6 Years	5.0–14.5
Adult	4.5–11.0

Adapted from Lotspeich-Steininger C, Stiene-Martin A, Koepke J. *Clinical Hematology: Principles, Procedures, Correlations.* Philadelphia, Lippincott, 1992

Variation in differential counts, often not clinically significant, may relate to differences in sex, race, physiologic state, and method of analysis. Reference ranges provided with reports should be specific to the methodology employed. Further variation can occur with manual differentials performed by different technologists (especially when from different laboratories), particularly in regard to the classification of bands ("stabs"), because differing criteria for identifying the less mature cell may be used; technologists within the same institution follow the same criteria, however. When only 100 cells are examined (out of several thousand), as is commonly the case with a manual differential, large statistical variation can occur. More significant variation occurs with age (see Table 3–19 for examples of reference ranges for selected ages). Note that most variation is seen between the neutrophil population (segs and bands) and the lymphocyte population, while the monocyte, eosinophil, and basophil populations remain relatively constant.

TABLE 3–19. Age Variation in the Differential Leukocyte Count

Age	Segs	Bands	Lymphs	Monos	Eos	Basos
12 Hours	53	15.2	24	5.3	2.0	0.4
6 Years	43	8	42	4.7	2.7	0.6
14 Years	48	8	37	4.7	2.5	0.5
Adult	51 ± 15	8 ± 3	34 ± 10	4	2.7	0.5

Number of cells in percentage.

Adapted from Jacobs DS, et al. *Laboratory Test Handbook,* 2nd ed. Cleveland, LexiComp Inc, 1990

■ PHAGOCYTES

The phagocytic leukocytes include **neutrophils**, **monocytes**, **eosinophils**, and **basophils**, each of which is discussed in this section. Phagocytic cells have the ability to ingest and *destroy* particulate substances such as bacteria, viruses, cellular debris and other foreign materials. These cells are the body's first line of defense and their concentration and appearance can provide insight into a variety of conditions. However, they must be evaluated in light of the interrelationship of all the cells and their functions, particularly since the phagocytic cells spend only a short time in the vascular space. The presence of immature cells provides indicators of disease and marrow stress.

Neutrophils

The neutrophil has a segmented nucleus and cytoplasm containing pinkish purple or pink-tan granules. It is the most common leukocyte found in the peripheral blood. The maturation cycle of the neutrophil is made up of six stages:

1. myeloblast
2. promyelocyte

3. myelocyte
4. metamyelocyte
5. band (stab)
6. mature segmented neutrophil (poly; PMN)

These stages are also referred to as the *granulocytic series* or granulocytes. The morphologic characteristics used to identify the immature forms of the series will not be discussed in this text. However, it is essential that laboratorians recognize the early forms of the series as they are present in a number of conditions. The life span of the neutrophil is about 9 to 10 days from myeloblast to cell death. During this time the cell is in three main parts of the body passing from the bone marrow to the peripheral blood and from the peripheral blood to the tissues. This movement is not a reversible process (ie, the neutrophils do not re-enter the peripheral circulation after entering the tissues).

The function of the neutrophil is to *protect the body from infection* in conjunction with other leukocytes. This is accomplished by *phagocytosis,* which involves locating, ingesting, and killing foreign invaders. The process of phagocytosis includes five steps: motility, recognition, ingestion, degranulation, and killing.

1. **Motility:** The neutrophil's motility is a result of *pseudopods* that are filled with filament networks that are polymers of a muscle protein. Adenosine triphosphate (ATP) provides the energy for contraction of these fibers. During locomotion the neutrophil acquires a distinctive asymmetric shape resembling a hand mirror. The neutrophil is guided (or drawn) to the invading organism by a process called *chemotaxis.* Chemotaxis involves the release of chemical stimuli as a result of interactions between tissues and invading organisms. The released substances result in the migration of the neutrophil toward the source of the stimulus. More simply stated, tissues that have been invaded by a foreign substance signal the neutrophils (likened to the "soldiers" of the body) to rid them of the "invaders." Without such a signal, the neutrophils' migration is random.

2. **Recognition:** Once the neutrophils reach the invasion site, they must be able to recognize the "enemy" in order to attack the offending substance. Some bacteria can be recognized by neutrophils without special assistance, but others are more difficult to recognize because they have a capsule. In such cases, the neutrophil is assisted by antibodies (especially immunoglobulin G, or IgG) and complement substances that coat the organism to make it recognizable. Substances that act in this manner to "point out" the "enemy" to the neutrophils are called *opsonins.* Some have been shown to further assist the neutrophil by not only coating the invader, but also binding it to the phagocytic cell for ingestion.

3. **Ingestion:** Once the neutrophil travels to the site of the invasion and recognizes the foreign substance, its pseudopods flow around the particle and fuse together to completely surround it. The membrane of the neu-

trophil becomes sticky, allowing it to adhere firmly to the foreign particle. This process of ingesting the invader takes place whenever the neutrophil comes into contact with a substance it recognizes as foreign
whether the contact was a result of random migration or of guided
migration in response to chemotactic stimuli.

4. **Degranulation:** The granules of neutrophils contain enzymes that, for
the most part, aid in killing ingested substances. When a particle has
been ingested, the neutrophilic granules migrate to the area and release
their contents.

5. **Killing:** In addition to the granular enzymes that help destroy the foreign particle, the neutrophil produces toxic substances, by metabolizing
oxygen, to kill the invader. These substances are also toxic to the host
cell. Several detoxification mechanisms keep these substances in check.
The toxic substances are sealed off from the rest of the cell in the area
where the particle was ingested. Other enzymes convert, detoxify, and
destroy any toxic substances that do escape into the cell.

A disease process can result when anything interferes with any of the steps
described in phagocytosis. A patient with such a disorder may suffer from recurrent infections. The rare congenital disorder, Chediak-Higashi syndrome, is a
defect in locomotion and ingestion that renders patients very susceptible to infections. Corticosteroids taken in high dosages for long periods can inhibit the ability of the neutrophil to migrate, its adhesiveness, and the ability to ingest. Alcohol
also has been shown to inhibit locomotion and ingestion. Some systemic illnesses
(rheumatoid arthritis, multiple myeloma, systemic lupus erythematosus, diabetes
mellitus) can impair neutrophilic function by decreasing the chemotactic response
or ingestion.

Monocytes

Monocytes are often classified with lymphocytes based on their similar morphologic characteristics. In terms of function, however, the monocyte is more closely
related to the granulocytic series because its primary function is *phagocytosis.* The
monocyte also plays other roles in the immune response, including participation
in *humoral immunity* (antibody production). The *macrophage,* a phagocytic cell
found in the tissues and in body fluids, is the tissue cell counterpart of the blood
monocyte. The monocyte appears to be the precursor cell of most macrophages.

The early, immature cell forms in the monocytic series are the monoblast and
the promonocyte, both of which are quite difficult to identify morphologically. In
fact, monoblasts may be impossible to distinguish from myeloblasts. Monocytes
are formed in the bone marrow from the same progenitor cell that forms neutrophils. They stay in the peripheral blood for only about 70 hours before moving
into the tissues.

Mature monocytes, although similar in diameter to neutrophils, often appear
larger than the other leukocytes on a stained blood film because it has a strong tendency to adhere and spread on a glass slide. Monocytes may be confused with large

lymphocytes, especially reactive or variant cells. The nuclear chromatin pattern is best used to distinguish monocytes and lymphocytes. In monocytes the chromatin is loosely woven and linear and the nucleus stains somewhat lighter. The lymphocytic chromatin is compact and lumpy. Additional distinguishing characteristics include a lighter staining cytoplasm than the lymphocyte; a nucleus that is often lobulated or kidney-bean shaped while that of the lymphocyte is usually round or oval; more abundant cytoplasm and lower nuclear/cytoplasmic ratio than the lymphocyte.

Phagocytosis is the primary function of the monocyte and is accomplished in a manner similar to that described for the neutrophil. The neutrophil is generally a more efficient phagocyte than the monocyte and monocytic motility is slower than that of the neutrophil. However, when the particle to be ingested is large in relation to the cell, the monocyte is more efficient than the neutrophil. The two cells may work together, with the neutrophil arriving at the invasion site in the tissue first and the monocyte arriving later to ingest cellular debris at the site of tissue damage.

Mononuclear phagocytes also play a role in **cellular and humoral immunity** in close association with T-lymphocytes. They phagocytize and degrade antigens then "present" them to the T-cells, which then secrete a substance to activate resting macrophages. The activated macrophages kill the microorganism and liberate substances to "turn off" the T-lymphocyte reactions (or signal that the "mission" is accomplished). Macrophages also release a substance to stimulate T-cells to replicate in response to an antigen. They also secrete substances to regulate the inflammatory response and numerous components of the complement system. In animal and culture studies, activated macrophages have been shown to kill several types of tumor cells. Whether this also occurs *in vivo* is not yet known.

Eosinophils

Although the eosinophil is a phagocyte, its role is less pronounced than that of the neutrophil and is primarily involved in the *control of parasitic infections and hypersensitivity reactions*. The eosinophil is formed in the bone marrow and follows the same maturation stages as the neutrophil. It can first be distinguished from the neutrophil at the promyelocyte stage.

The mature eosinophil is easily identified by the characteristic appearance of its bright reddish orange cytoplasmic granules. More immature forms of the eosinophil are difficult to distinguish from each other because the size and number of these granules can mask other morphologic features. However, it is rarely clinically important to distinguish the various maturation stages because of the relatively low percentage of eosinophils. Classification as mature or immature forms is generally sufficient.

Eosinophils function as phagocytes in a manner similar to that of neutrophils, but move more slowly and have less intracellular killing ability. They remain in the tissues longer than the neutrophil and are found mostly in the skin or mucosal surfaces of the respiratory and gastrointestinal tracts. They respond to a number of chemotactic factors, but seem most responsive to histamines and antigen-antibody complexes. Another important eosinophilic function is the ability to damage larval stages of parasitic helminths. The eosinophil attaches to antibody coated parasites, extends projections over its surface, and releases the contents of its granules to break down the parasite which is then phagocytized by other eosinophils.

Basophils

The basophil is the least common leukocyte and is formed in the bone marrow, with a maturation cycle paralleling that of the neutrophil except that the nucleus does not always segment. Because so few basophils are present in either marrow or peripheral blood, staging is usually not done, with distinction only being made between mature and immature forms. The large, dark staining granules of the basophil make the mature form easily recognizable.

Although basophils are phagocytes, their phagocytic ability is substantially less than that of either the neutrophil or the eosinophil. They ingest sensitized red cells and antigen-antibody complexes. The granules of the basophil synthesize and store histamine, the release of which serves as a chemotactic factor for the eosinophil. The most important function of the basophil is their role in *immediate hypersensitivity reactions.* Basophils have specific receptor sites for IgE, the immunoglobulin important in allergic or hypersensitivity reactions, which trigger degranulation in the presence of the appropriate antigen. Clinical manifestations of this immediate hypersensitivity reaction include allergic rhinitis, some forms of bronchial asthma, urticaria, and anaphylaxis to drugs, insect stings, and other antigens. Basophils also play a role in delayed hypersensitivity reactions mediated by lymphocytes. T-lymphocytes stimulated by an antigen generate substances that cause the basophil to release histamine. Basophils account for from 5 % to 15 % of the infiltrating cells in allergic contact dermatitis and skin allograft rejection and a smaller percentage in tuberculin and other delayed hypersensitivity reactions (Lotspeich-Steininger, et al, 1992).

■ IMMUNOCYTES

The lymphocytes are important in the response to disease, to recovery, and to health maintenance. They are formed in lymphoid tissues, including the bone marrow, thymus, lymph nodes, spleen, tonsils, and numerous foci of subendothelial and subepithelial lymphocytes, monocytes, and macrophages. These sites of formation are classified functionally into primary lymphoid organs (PLO) and secondary lymphoid tissue (SLT). The PLO supplies partially differentiated lymphocytes to the SLT where lymphocytes are produced in response to antigens. Lymphopoiesis in the PLO is continuous and not antigen dependent. A detailed explanation of primary and secondary lymphopoiesis is beyond the scope of this text, where the focus will be on the function of the lymphocyte.

Lymphocytes differ from other normal blood cells in three distinguishing physiologic characteristics.

1. They are **not obligate end cells** (a mature cell committed to perform a function and die). For example, granulopoiesis produces end cells—neutrophils—which die in the completion of their function. Lymphopoiesis, on the other hand, produces a continuous supply of incompletely differentiated cells (PLO) to peripheral tissue where, in response to antigenic stimulation, they either transform into cells that die in fulfilling their function (called *effector* or *end cells*) or they may undergo blastic transformation to produce new lymphocytes that will react with the appropriate antigen.

2. They are a **heterogeneous** (having unlike natures, as opposed to homogeneous) group of cells. Some lymphocytes become **T cells**, immunocompetent cells in cellular immunity. Others develop into **B cells**, which function in humoral immunity (antibody production). Another group of lymphocytes, known as natural killer (NK) cells, are capable of lysing a variety of cells. The fraction of cells that do not develop along either the T or B cell line are called *non-T, non-B cells*. These groups of lymphocytes appear identical on routine stains with light microscopy, but can be differentiated with special procedures based on differences in maturation, surface and biochemical markers, and responses to stimulation.

3. They **migrate in more than one direction**. The lymphocytes generally spend several hours to days in tissue and then migrate to the peripheral blood and back to the lymphatic tissue. Other blood cells that migrate tend to go in one direction only and do not return to the blood. The migration of mature lymphocytes from blood to lymphoid tissue and back to the blood (called *recirculation* and taking place over a period of hours) is, in addition to the migration of immature, dividing cells from the marrow to the thymus and to peripheral tissue, which requires a long period of time.

Functional characteristics of the lymphocytes are specific to the various types of cells found in the lymphocyte population. The primary function of the immune system as a whole is to *recognize a foreign antigen and generate an appropriate immune response.* The interaction between T and B cells with each other and with other cell systems plays an important role in the immune response. The manner in which each lymphocyte group carries out its role in this response is quite complex. However, the basic function of the various cell types in the lymphocyte population can be summarized to provide a general understanding of how they work to provide protection to the body against foreign invaders. Table 3–20 summarizes the functions of B cells, T cells (note that T lymphocytes are divided into additional cell subsets), and non-B, non-T cells (also consisting of subgroups of cells). An effective and competent immune response is dependent on the heterogeneity, quantitative balance, and interaction of the subpopulations of lymphocytes with each other and with other cells.

TABLE 3–20. Summary of Lymphocyte Functional Characteristics

Cell Type	Summary of Function
B Cells	Differentiate into plasma cells, which produce antibodies (immunoglobulins) in response to stimulation by foreign antigens. The antibody binds to the antigen, beginning a succession of events including adherence of immune complex to leukocytes, complement activation, and neutralization of toxins and viruses.
T Cell, helper	Helper T cells proliferate in response to soluble antigens and produce a substance to induce other T cells. They also help B cells in the production of antibody by increasing antigen expression.
T Cell, suppressor	Suppressor T cells are important to keeping the immune response in check. By recognition of specific substances, these cells function to repress the responses of both T and B cells when further response is not needed.
T Cell, delayed hypersensitivity (DHTL)	The DHTLs respond to particulate and soluble antigens and produce substances (chemotactic lymphokines) that confine and activate macrophages. They are involved in reactions such as that to the TB skin test and to poison ivy.
T Cell, cytotoxic	Cytotoxic T cells destroy antigen-specific target cells on contact and have the ability to recycle to fulfill their function.
Natural killer (NK) cells[1]	NK cells react spontaneously against a variety of cells. Their functions include recognition and lysis of certain tumor cells and virus infected cells; resistance to some bacterial, fungal, and parasitic agents; immune regulation; regulation of hematopoiesis; natural resistance to allogenic grafts. Their activity is enhanced by interferon. They may fulfill an important early function before antibody-dependent mechanisms are mobilized.
Killer (K) cells[1]	K cells do not react specifically with cell membrane antigens (as NK cells do), but effect binding and cytotoxicity by way of antibodies already bound to the target cell (antibody-dependent cell-mediated cytolysis).
Lymphokine activated killer cells[1]	Require activation by lymphokines before acting on targeted cells.

[1]Non-T, non-B lymphocytes.

TIME FOR REVIEW. After studying the preceding sections, you should be able to respond correctly to the following:

■ Classify the five types of leukocytes according to:

   nuclear segmentation:

   function:

■ Which two leukocyte populations vary most with age?

■ List the phagocytic leukocytes.

■ Define phagocytosis.

■ List and briefly describe the five steps included in phagocytosis.

■ Define chemotaxis and explain its role in the motility of neutrophils.

■ The granules of the neutrophil contain _____ .

■ List two mechanisms by which toxic substances, metabolized to destroy foreign particles, are prevented from harming the host cell.

■ The   tissue   cell   counterpart   of   the   blood   monocyte   is   the
_____ .

■ _____ is the primary function of the monocyte, but it also plays a role in cellular and _____ immunity.

■ Eosinophils are primarily involved in the control of _____ and _____ .

■ The least common leukocyte is the _____ .

■ List the most important function of the basophil.

■ List at least three organs and/or tissues involved in lymphopoiesis.

■ List three distinguishing physiologic characteristics of the lymphocyte as compared to other normal blood cells.

■ Match the lymphocyte with the appropriate functional description.

___ Repress T and B cell responses.

___ Become plasma cells and produce antibodies.

___ Destroy target cells on contact.

___ Induce other T cells and help B cells.

___ Lysis of tumor and virus-infected cells. Enhanced by interferon.

___ Antibody-dependent cell-mediated cytolysis.

___ Produce substances to activate and confine macrophages. Involved in TB skin test reactions.

___ Require activation by lymphokines.

a. B cells   e. T cytotoxic
b. T helper   f. Natural killer
c. T suppressor   g. Killer
d. DHTL   h. Lymphokine activated

Check your responses by reviewing the preceding pages.

LEUKOCYTE ABNORMALITIES

A variety of abnormalities may be seen in the leukocytes, including both malignant and nonmalignant conditions. The nonmalignant abnormalities will be the focus of this section. Nonmalignant leukocytic abnormalities may be either *reactive* or *inherited* disorders and may be abnormalities of quantity or number (**quantitative abnormalities**) or morphologic abnormalities (**qualitative abnormalities**). Nonmalignant qualitative abnormalities must be distinguished from those seen in malignant conditions.

■ REACTIVE DISORDERS

When leukocytes fulfill their function of protecting the body against foreign invaders, they undergo changes, both quantitative and qualitative, that are visible on microscopic examination in the laboratory. These changes are referred to as *reactive* or *toxic changes* and are the most common leukocyte abnormality seen in the laboratory. Again, the disorders covered in this section are nonmalignant abnormalities.

Quantitative Disorders of Neutrophils

Prior to beginning a discussion of quantitative abnormalities, a review of terms may be beneficial. **Leukocytosis** refers to an increase in the total number of leukocytes, or white cells, and may be caused by an increase of one or more of the cell types normally found in peripheral blood or by the presence of abnormal cells. A decrease in the total number of leukocytes is referred to as **leukopenia**. Leukopenia may result from a decrease in neutrophils (*neutropenia*) or lymphocytes (*lymphopenia*) or from a decrease in all cell types (*pancytopenia*). Because the number of monocytes, eosinophils, and basophils normally found in the peripheral circulation is so low, individual decreases in these cell types do not produce leukopenia.

Neutrophilia refers to an increase in the *absolute neutrophil count.* The absolute neutrophil count is the product of the total leukocyte count and the percentage of neutrophils, including all stages of maturity. The primary causes of neutrophilia are **infection**, **inflammation**, and **malignancy**. Reactive neutrophilia may be either acute and transient or chronic and often includes an increased number of immature neutrophils such as bands and metamyelocytes. This increase in immature forms is referred to as a **left shift**.

The degree of neutrophilia seen in infection depends on a variety of factors: the virulence of the organism, the patient's age, and the patient's overall health/resistance. Children usually develop more significant neutrophilia than adults, while elderly patients, those with nutritional deficits, and those who have had marrow replacement may produce only moderate responses or none at all with the same infection. Bacterial infections, especially when caused by cocci, can result in striking neutrophilia. However, not all bacteria cause neutrophilia and some actually suppress neutrophil production and cause neutropenia (discussed later). Neutrophilia may also be seen with inflammatory responses to tissue injury or destruction such as is seen in rheumatoid arthritis, colitis, myocardial infarction, burns, drugs, surgical or traumatic wounds, and a variety of other conditions. In these instances, the dead or dying cells release substances that act as chemotactic agents or stimulate the marrow to release and/or form new cells. Inflammatory responses may also occur in the presence of neoplasms and in metabolic disorders such as diabetes, renal dysfunction, or liver disease. In metabolic disorders, toxic circulating substances may be produced that will stimulate the neutrophils to respond. The mechanism by which some drugs cause neutrophilia is unclear, but in some cases may result from direct stimulation of hematopoiesis.

Not all neutrophilia is pathologic. Physiologic neutrophilia, sometimes referred to as *pseudoneutrophilia,* may be seen in response to certain physical stimuli such as exercise, pregnancy and labor or to emotional stimuli such as panic, rage, or stress. This neutrophilia is transient, usually lasting only a few hours, and generally does not include a significant number of immature forms. Table 3–21 summarizes the causes of reactive neutrophilia.

Neutropenia, a decreased number of neutrophils, is the most common cause of leukopenia. Neutropenia may result from a decrease in the production of neutrophils, an increase in the destruction of neutrophils, or sequestration.

Table 3–21. Conditions Causing Reactive Neutrophilia

Cause	Examples
Infections	Pyogenic bacteria; some viruses, fungi, spirochetal and rickettsial organisms
Inflammatory response: tissue destruction	Serosal; visceral; blood cell destruction; posttraumatic (surgical or accidental); thermal or chemical injury; drugs or venoms causing tissue injury; parasitic invasions
Other inflammatory responses	Neoplastic growth; metabolic disorders; acute hemorrhage
Drugs	Corticosteroids; lithium
Pseudoneutrophilia (physiologic)	Physical or emotional stimuli

Decreased production may be inherited or acquired, but inherited forms are rare and include a variety of poorly understood syndromes. Acquired forms are common. It results from injury or destruction to stem cells suppressing the bone marrow and causing a decrease in all cell types. Moderate to severe marrow suppression can be caused by ionizing radiation, chemicals like benzene, and a number of cytotoxic drugs used in the treatment of malignancies. Vitamin B_{12} or folate deficiency causes ineffective hematopoiesis that can lead to a decrease in all cell types. Marrow replacement by tumor, fibrous tissue, or hematopoietic malignancy also result in neutropenia. Neutropenia is sometimes seen as a pre-leukemic manifestation.

Neutropenia can also be caused by an **increase in the destruction of neutrophils** resulting from infections, immune mechanisms, or hypersensitivity states. An infection that overwhelms the capacity of the bone marrow to produce neutrophils results in them being consumed or recruited to the tissues faster than they can be replaced. This is most frequently seen in patients with little or no marrow reserves—debilitated patients, elderly persons, and infants. Typhoid, paratyphoid, and brucellosis are bacterial infections that are commonly associated with neutropenia. Neutropenia may also be seen in viral infections (measles, infectious hepatitis, infectious mononucleosis) and is often noted in the early stages of the disease. Destruction of neutrophils may also be increased as a result of antibodies directed against the neutrophils in acquired autoimmune neutropenia and in some collagen vascular diseases such as lupus erythematosus. Drug hypersensitivity is another cause of increased destruction and may lead to severe neutropenia. Removal of the causative drug generally results in prompt recovery.

Sequestration is a third mechanism of neutropenia. When the spleen is enlarged, regardless of the cause of the enlargement, neutropenia (usually mild) can result. Neutrophils may also be sequestered in the pulmonary vasculature.

Qualitative Disorders of Neutrophils

Qualitative disorders refer to the alterations in morphology of the neutrophil in response to infection, inflammation, or stress and are often called *toxic changes.*

Qualitative, or toxic, changes include a left shift (increased numbers of circulating immature forms—nonsegmented or immature neutrophils) and morphologic changes that indicate maturation abnormalities, altered functional activity, or degenerative changes.

A *left shift* may be mild, moderate, or severe depending upon the demand placed on the bone marrow. Release of the cells stored in the marrow results in larger numbers of bands and perhaps metamyelocytes. If marrow stimulation continues, neutrophil production is accelerated and myelocytes may be seen along with an occasional promyelocyte. In individuals with overwhelming infections promyelocytes and some blast forms may also be seen.

Morphologic changes indicating activation or degenerative changes are divided further into alterations of the cytoplasm of the cell and alterations of the nucleus. Cytoplasmic abnormalities are more commonly seen, or at least more prominently reported and discussed, than nuclear abnormalities in toxic neutrophils.

Toxic granulation is one of the more frequently reported cytoplasmic abnormalities in neutrophils. It is believed that these are primary granules, normally present in the cell, but altered as a result of neutrophilic stimulation by foreign antigens, with a resulting change in staining properties making them more visible. These granules are larger and darkly staining and tend to cluster together in the cell. Not all neutrophils will be affected or affected equally. Other abnormalities must not be confused with toxic granules (artifactual granules resulting from staining technique, metachromatic granules seen in some genetic disorders of mucopolysaccharide metabolism, or Alder-Reilly bodies seen in an inherited anomaly by the same name).

Dohle bodies are found in segmented and band form neutrophils, where they appear as pale blue or grayish, round or elongated bodies usually seen close to the cell membranes. These cytoplasmic inclusions are nonspecific and may be found in a variety of conditions, including pregnancy. They are usually seen 1 to 3 days after an infection, burn, surgery, or other trauma, and then disappear. It is important to differentiate between the transient Dohle body appearing after infection or tissue damage and the larger spindle-shaped inclusion seen in the May-Hegglin anomaly (a rare inherited disorder).

Vacuolation of the cytoplasm can be caused by autophagocytosis (self) or by phagocytosis of extracellular material. Autophagocytosis can be caused by drugs (sulfonamides and chloroquine), by prolonged storage of cells, or by degranulation on exposure to high doses of radiation or other toxins. The phagocytic vacuoles seen following ingestion of extracellular material are usually larger and less evenly distributed than those resulting from autophagocytosis. They are commonly seen in septic processes.

Other cytoplasmic abnormalities include *degranulation,* a normal function of activated or injured neutrophils; *cytoplasmic pseudopods,* rare granule free protrusions of cytoplasm giving the neutrophil an amoeboid look and seen most commonly in association with cytotoxic agents—either therapeutic or released by other cells; and *cytoplasmic swelling,* caused either by actual osmotic swelling or the increased adhesiveness to glass of stimulated neutrophils.

Reactive **nuclear abnormalities** include hypersegmentation of the nucleus, nuclear pyknosis, and ringed nuclei. A *hypersegmented neutrophil* is one in which the nucleus is segmented into a larger than usual number of lobes. The generally accepted criterion for classification of a neutrophil as hypersegmented is more than five nuclear lobes. A hypersegmented nucleus is not necessarily of increased size, but may be larger than usual in some instances. Hypersegmented neutrophils may be seen in long term, chronic infections and are associated with folate deficiencies.

Pyknosis is the term applied to a dense and shrunken nucleus most often seen in conditions of sepsis. The cells containing such a nucleus are likely cells that are near the end of their life span. *Ringed nuclei* may be seen in toxic states, in malignant myeloproliferative disorders, and sometimes in extreme leukocytosis with a significant left shift. Cytoplasmic and nuclear abnormalities are summarized in Table 3–22.

Table 3–22. Cytoplasmic and Nuclear Abnormalities in Toxic Neutrophils

Cytoplasmic Abnormalities		Nuclear Abnormalities	
Toxic granules	Large darkly staining granules resulting from neutrophilic stimulation by foreign antigens. Must be distinguished from artifactual granules (staining technique) and granules seen in a genetic disorder.	Pyknosis	Shrunken, dense nuclei seen most frequently in septic conditions. Probably in cells that are about to die.
Dohle bodies	Cytoplasmic inclusions of ribosomal RNA. Nonspecific finding (ie, occur in variety of conditions, including pregnancy). Transient. Usually seen 1 to 3 days after incident such as infection, burn, or surgery and then disappear. Cause unknown—may reflect sudden storage pool release.	Hypersegmentation	Nuclei having more than the usual number of lobes (>5). May be large or normal size. Common in long-term, chronic infections. Can reflect folate deficiency or a degenerative process.
Vacuolation	Caused by phagocytosis. Seen in infections; especially common in septic processes caused by bacteria or fungi.	Projections	Hair-like projections more commonly found in band forms. May be seen in metastatic carcinoma or after irradiation.
Degranulation	Normal function of activated or injured neutrophils. Often accompanied by disruption of cellular membrane.	Ringed nuclei	Seen in toxic states and in malignant myeloproliferative disorders. Small numbers of ring-like nuclei may be seen in infections when leukocytosis is significant and bands are increased to 30% or more.

Table developed based on information from Henry JB. *Clinical Diagnosis and Management by Laboratory Methods,* 19th ed. Philadelphia, Saunders, 1996; Lotspeich-Steininger C, Stiene-Martin A, Koepke J. *Clinical Hematology: Principles, Procedures, Correlations.* Philadelphia, Lippincott, 1992; and Sacher RA, McPherson RA. *Widmann's Clinical Interpretation of Laboratory Tests,* 10th ed. Philadelphia, FA Davis, 1991

Quantitative Disorders of Eosinophils

An increase in the number of eosinophils—**eosinophilia**—may result from malignancy, or from a rare inherited disorder with a benign eosinophilia, or may be a reactive disorder. Reactive eosinophilia is most commonly associated with **parasitic invasion of tissue or hypersensitivity disorders**. An eosinophilic response may also be seen in collagen-vascular disorders, neoplastic disorders, and in some immune deficiency states. Eosinophils have capabilities for suppressing most helminth organisms (trematodes, nematodes, and cestodes) that invade and cause tissue destruction. There is a significant correlation between the eosinophil count and parasite death. The attraction of the eosinophil to the parasite is directed by T lymphocytes and is antibody dependent. Parasites are killed through eosinophilic degranulation. Comparable eosinophil activity is not characteristic of protozoal infections. In allergic reactions, the eosinophil acts to modulate the inflammatory response caused by degranulation of basophils or mast cells.

Eosinopenia is quite difficult to detect using routine methods, but may result from **production abnormalities** and from the **depression of eosinophil levels** seen with glucocorticoids, prostaglandins, and epinephrine. It is a **characteristic finding in most acute bacterial infections** (cause unknown) and the reappearance of eosinophils in the peripheral blood is usually a sign of recovery from the infection. Eosinopenia is also known to result from the administration of ACTH if adrenal function is normal.

Qualitative Disorders of Eosinophils

It is extremely rare to see immature eosinophils in the peripheral blood as a result of a reactive disorder, even when the number of eosinophils is greatly increased. However, some evidence of stimulation and activity may be seen morphologically. These **morphologic changes** include **degranulation** (the most prominent alteration), **vacuolation** (seen occasionally and of unknown significance), and **hypersegmentation of the nucleus** (may be seen in long-term chronic infections and defined as having three or more lobes, as eosinophils, unlike neutrophils, normally have only two nuclear lobes).

Reactive Disorders of Basophils

Basopenia has been described in acute infections, stress, hyperthyroidism, and increased levels of glucocorticoids. However, with normal circulating levels so low, the detection of basopenia is beyond the capability of most laboratories. **Basophilia** is seen in many of the disorders that cause eosinophilia (basophils and eosinophils have a common stem cell) and is most frequently cited in immediate hypersensitivity reaction, long-term foreign antigen stimulation, hypothyroidism, ulcerative colitis, and estrogen therapy. Both basophilia and basopenia are, of course, quantitative disorders. In terms of qualitative abnormalities, **degranulation** is the only morphologic alteration that may be detected in basophils, but can be difficult to evaluate because the granules are water soluble and may be lost during the staining process. Degranulation is associated with antigen-related stimulation and can also be seen after ingestion of a fatty meal. No immature forms of the cell are seen in reactive disorders.

Quantitative Disorders of Monocytes

Monocytosis (increased absolute number of monocytes) often accompanies neutrophilia in many of the conditions previously discussed as causes of neutrophilia (monocytes and neutrophils have a common stem cell). However, the monocytosis is often not noticed in the presence of the more conspicuous neutrophilic response.

Monocytosis may be seen in a variety of acute bacterial infections, but is more frequently associated with tuberculosis, subacute bacterial endocarditis (SBE), and syphilis. In tuberculosis, the increase in monocytes is probably due to their role in granuloma formation in the cellular response to the infecting bacillus. In some cases of SBE, monocytes may remain in the peripheral blood to mature into circulating histiocytes or macrophages, which is a significant finding discussed further in the qualitative disorder section. Inflammatory reaction to tissue destruction in conditions varying from surgical trauma and tumors to gastrointestinal diseases and tetrachlorethane poisoning may also result in absolute monocytosis. Relative monocytosis is frequently seen as a signal of recovery from agranulocytosis or marrow hypoplasia, because monocytes are released into circulation before neutrophils because of the minimal marrow storage of monocytes. Table 3–23 summarizes the causes of reactive monocytosis. **Monocytopenia** may be seen in overwhelming infections that also cause neutropenia and following the administration of glucocorticoids.

TABLE 3–23. Causes of Reactive Monocytosis

Cause	Examples
Bacterial infections	Tuberculosis Subacute bacterial endocarditis Syphilis
Inflammatory responses	Surgical trauma Tumors Collagen vascular disease Gastrointestinal disease Tetrachlorethane poisoning
Recovery from relative neutropenia	

Qualitative Disorders of Monocytes

Reactive morphologic changes in monocytes result from the basic monocyte responses to stimuli, including the appearance of immature monocytes and the transformation of monocytes into histiocytes or macrophages. These morphologic changes providing evidence of phagocytic activity include:

- an increase in the volume of the cytoplasm and in the ability of the cell to spread

- increased numbers of granules
- increased cytoplasmic vacuolation
- intracellular debris
- irregular cytoplasmic borders

The shape of the monocytes nucleus may also change, with transformation from a rounded nucleus to an oval shape, or it may become a long, thin band-like shape.

◼ REACTIVE DISORDERS OF LYMPHOCYTES

Lymphocytic proliferation and the finding of reactive lymphocyte morphology is the result of a normal lymphocyte response to antigen stimulation and reflects a benign lymphoproliferative process. The morphology of such lymphocytes is well known, yet distinguishing benign from malignant disorders can be quite difficult, with additional testing sometimes needed and often only clinical findings establishing the difference.

A variety of terms have been used to describe the nonmalignant, "reactive" changes in lymphocytes, including *variant lymphs, atypical lymphs, reactive lymphs, virocytes, Downey cells,* and several others. The term **reactive lymphs** is used in this discussion. It is important to note that a few reactive lymphs is a normal finding on a peripheral blood smear.

Morphology
There is morphologic variation even among lymphocytes classified as reactive. This variation is sufficient to divide the reactive lymphs into three types, but it is not common to do so in routine hematologic studies. Reactive lymphs are generally increased in size, with the amount of the increase highly variable. The cytoplasm may be quite abundant. Cytoplasmic alterations may consist of vacuoles and an indented appearance around the periphery of the cell. The cytoplasm may be pale or a bright blue, may have a "foamy" appearance, or may contain azurophilic granules.

Because both reactive and malignant lymphocytosis can exhibit immature looking cells, distinguishing the two requires skill and experience. A major difference can be seen in the heterogeneity of reactive lymph morphology versus a more homogeneous morphology in malignancies. In reactive lymphocytosis, both large and small cells, basophilic and pale cells, and cells with varying nuclear characteristics are seen in the same specimen. Malignancies are usually more homogeneous, with all abnormal cells being quite similar. This distinction is significant, but may not be sufficient to distinguish malignant and benign conditions.

Table 3–24 summarizes causes of lymphocytosis with and without the appearance of reactive lymph morphology (Lotspeich-Steininger et al, 1992). The discussion of reactive lymphs that follows is presented based upon the clinical condition resulting in the observed changes.

TABLE 3–24. Causes of Lymphocytosis

Type of Lymphocytosis	Causes
Absolute lymphocytosis with reactive lymphs	Infectious mononucleosis Acute viral hepatitis Cytomegalovirus (CMV) infections

Relative lymphocytosis with reactive lymphs	Toxoplasmosis
	Viral-related disorders
	  measles
	  mumps
	  chicken pox
	  rubella
	  viral pneumonia
	Immune disorders
	  drug reactions
	  idiopathic thrombocytopenia
	  autoimmune hemolytic anemia
	Nonviral infections
	  tuberculosis
	  syphilis
	  malaria
	  typhus
	  brucellosis
	  rickettsia
	  diphtheria

Absolute lymphocytosis with normal lymphs	Acute infectious lymphocytosis Bordetella pertussis infection
Relative lymphocytosis with normal lymphs	Neutropenia

From Lotspeich-Steininger C, Stiene-Martin A, Koepke J. *Clinical Hematology: Principles, Procedures, Correlations.* Philadelpia, Lippincott, 1992.

Infectious Mononucleosis

Infectious mononucleosis (IM) is an acute, contagious viral disease caused by the Epstein-Barr virus (EBV) that primarily affects teenagers and young adults. It is a self-limited benign condition, but serious complications can occur. When occurring in adults over 40, the illness is generally more severe.

The major diagnostic laboratory findings for IM are found in the hematology and serology areas, although other findings may also be indicative of the disease. Serologically, the classic finding is the **presence of the heterophile antibody as indicated by a positive monotest**. In hematology, the classic findings are an **absolute lymphocytosis with more than 20% reactive lymphs**. Tests specific for the EB virus are also available. The reactive lymphs usually appear about 4 to 5 days after the onset of the illness and remain for 30 days or more. IM can be particularly difficult to diagnose in the first few days of the illness before lymphocytosis and reactive lymphs are present. In fact, during the first few days lymphopenia may be present.

The lymphocytes found in IM include a mixture of normal and reactive lymphs; monocytes and eosinophils may also be increased, but these findings are not as significant as the morphologic changes in the lymphocytes. Reactive lymphs found in IM vary in size and shape; nuclear content; and cytoplasmic features and may include all three types of reactive lymphs. The most predominant type of reactive lymphs are those classified as type II (type II is also sometimes called the IM cell), which appear as large, irregularly shaped cells with coarse chromatin and abundant cytoplasm. The cytoplasm is often indented by surrounding cellular structures. Few vacuoles are present and the cytoplasm is pale with basophilia radiating from the nucleus and around the periphery of the cytoplasm.

Of course, reactive lymphs are also present in a number of other conditions, so the percentage of reactive lymphs can be helpful in distinguishing IM from other illnesses. A percentage of 40 % or more is strongly suggestive of IM. (See the virology section of the Microbiology chapter for additional detail.) If serologic findings do not confirm a suspected case of IM, (cytomegalovirus) infection or toxoplasmosis should be suspected (although the lymphocytosis in toxoplasmosis is usually relative rather than absolute).

Cytomegalovirus Infection

Cytomegalovirus (CMV) infections closely resemble IM in terms of both clinical presentation and laboratory hematology findings. Clinically, however, CMV patients generally do not have tonsillitis or enlarged lymph nodes as do IM patients. In terms of laboratory findings, although an absolute lymphocytosis with reactive lymphs is present in both IM and CMV, CMV patients do not exhibit the heterophile antibody. Tests for IgM and IgG antibodies specific for CMV are also available. The reactive lymphocytes seen in both cases are very similar; therefore distinction between the two must be made using serologic differences and clinical findings.

Acute Infectious Lymphocytosis

This condition is contagious, benign, self-limited, and most frequently seen in children between 1 and 10 years of age. Patients are generally asymptomatic, but may exhibit fever, upper respiratory infection, diarrhea, and abdominal pain. The causative agent has not been definitively established. A classic and striking feature of this condition is an extreme lymphocytosis, with leukocyte counts usually between 40 and 50 x 10^9/L, but sometimes exceeding 100 × 10^9/L. The leukocytosis is due to a marked proliferation of T lymphocytes. The lymphocytes are small "resting" lymphocytes with an absence of reactive lymph morphology.

Bordetella pertussis Infection

In this condition the leukocytosis and lymphocytosis are more pronounced than in any other febrile illness except IM. Normal looking lymphocytes make up 70 % to 90 % of the leukocytes on the peripheral blood smear. Like acute infectious lymphocytosis, the lymphocytosis is absolute without the presence of reactive lymphocytes.

Lymphocytic Leukemoid Reaction

When a condition produces a lymphocytic leukocytosis so marked that it gives the impression of a possible leukemia, it is called a *lymphocytic leukemoid reaction*. This may be true in some cases of IM especially with white cell counts of 50×10^9/L (giving the impression of acute lymphocytic leukemia), in infectious lymphocytosis (similar to chronic lymphatic leukemia), and in children who are critically ill with *Bordetella pertussis*.

Toxoplasmosis

Infection with *Toxoplasma gondii* is similar in clinical presentation to IM. Laboratory findings differ in that the lymphocytosis is relative instead of absolute (even though both conditions result in reactive lymphs) and the heterophile antibody is not present. Clinical symptoms can also help to distinguish the two as the lymphadenopathy in toxoplasmosis is more generalized than in IM and sore throats and splenomegaly are less common.

■ HEREDITARY DISORDERS

There are a number of nonmalignant, inherited disorders of leukocytes. These disorders include abnormalities of granulocyte morphology, abnormalities of granulocyte function, defects in the killing of microorganisms, disorders of the monocyte-macrophage system, and disorders of immune leukocytes. A few such disorders are briefly defined here.

Pelger-Huet Anomaly

This anomaly of the granulocyte nucleus is characterized by hyposegmentation of the nucleus—generally appearing with two symmetric, rounded lobes attached by a fine filament or failing to segment at all and appearing as a peanut or dumbbell shape. The cells appear to function normally. An acquired (pseudo) form of this anomaly has been associated with malignant myeloproliferative disorders and infections or malignancies that have metastasized to the bone.

May-Hegglin Anomaly

This is a rare syndrome characterized by leukopenia, variable thrombocytopenia, giant platelets, and gray-blue spindle-shaped cytoplasmic inclusions in granulocytes and monocytes that resemble Dohle bodies (Dohle bodies are smaller and found only in neutrophils). Patients are generally in good health, with about 30 % developing some sort of hemorrhagic problem.

Alder-Reilly Anomaly

The presence of abnormally large azurophilic granules, resembling severe toxic granulation, characterize this condition. These granules, however, occur not only in granulocytes, but may also be found in lymphocytes and monocytes. Cellular function does not appear to be affected. This condition may be seen in association with storage diseases in which mucopolysaccharides accumulate in the cytoplasm of tissue and blood cells.

Job's Syndrome

In this uncommon condition the directional motility of phagocytes is impaired, so the cells respond very slowly to chemotactic agents. Patients suffer from persistent boils and staphylococcal abscesses (hence the name of the condition likening patients to the biblical Job). The mechanism for the poor phagocytic response is unknown, but may be related to elevated IgE levels.

Chediak-Higashi Syndrome

This syndrome affects not only humans, but at least five other species: mink, cattle, mice, cats, and killer whales. It is manifested in all affected species in essentially the same manner. First recognized because of giant cytoplasmic granules in phagocytes and lymphocytes, the disease has been extensively studied because of the availability of animal models. Affected individuals show partial albinism and greater susceptibility to a number of common infectious agents (primarily due to abnormal phagocytosis), and have hemorrhagic tendencies. In later stages, an enlarged spleen, liver failure, lymphadenopathy with lymphoma type morphology, and neuropathy can develop. The cause of death is usually an overwhelming infection.

Chronic Granulomatous Disease

Phagocytes are able to ingest, but not kill, certain organisms in this condition, which can be inherited either as a sex-linked trait or as an autosomal recessive trait. The clinical picture is variable, but may include recurrent chronic pyogenic infections with healing that is often accompanied by granuloma (an accumulation of masses of cells [macrophages, lymphoid cells]) formation. Recurrent pneumonia is common and is often the cause of death.

Mucopolysaccharidoses

This term is used to describe a group of related genetic deficiencies of enzymes that break down mucopolysaccharides. Syndromes include Hunter, Hurler, Scheie, and others. Because of the characteristic facial and skeletal features, Hurler and Hunter syndromes were given the name *gargoylism*. The severity and expression of the syndromes depends upon the extent of the deficiency and in which tissues the abnormal product accumulates. Cells in affected tissues have a swollen appearance and clearing of their cytoplasm. In the peripheral blood and the bone marrow, metachromatic granules like those described for Alder-Reilly are seen in the leukocytes.

B Cell Deficiencies

The function of B cells can be assessed by the level of serum immunoglobulins and by the ability of the patient to produce immunoglobulins against antigens not normally encountered. (Recall that B lymphocytes are responsible for humoral immunity, or antibody production.) Two types of B cell deficiencies can be inherited: infantile sex-linked agammaglobulinemia and common variable hypogammaglobulinemia. The infantile agammaglobulinemia is transmitted by the mother to male children and becomes obvious at about 6 months of age, when protection by maternal IgG is lost. All classes of immunoglobulins are either absent or very low and the child contracts a series of bacterial infections, failing to develop immunity to any. Peripheral lymphocytes are usually normal, but consist almost exclusively of T cells that are normal in function. Patients are treated with antibiotics and passive immunization with pooled human gamma globulin. Variable hypogammaglobulinemia is a more common defect in which one or a combination of immunoglobulins are either absent or decreased. A decreased resistance to infectious agents is seen only in patients with absent or decreased IgG. A decrease in production of IgA (both serum and secretory) is characterized by a malabsorption syndrome with noninfectious diarrhea and is closely associated with autoimmune disorders such as collagen diseases and thyroiditis.

T Cell Deficiencies

T cell status can be evaluated by a number of methods, including assessment of hypersensitivity responses, history of normal recovery from viral agents, and measurement of the number of circulating T cells. Inherited deficiencies arise either from failure of development of the thymus (where T lymphocytes form) or from a blockage of the stem cell that would become a T lymphocyte in the thymus. An example of a T cell deficiency is Nezelof syndrome, which results from a block in or near the stem cell and thus an inability to produce lymphocytes to populate the thymus. Affected children are susceptible to repeated yeast, fungal, and viral infections.

Severe Combined Immunodeficiency Disease

In this condition there is a failure of both humoral and cellular immunity and, until recently, affected individuals rarely survived beyond infancy. There are many variants of this condition including sex-linked agammaglobulinemia (seen only in males; a defect in the helper cellular immune mechanism leading to agammaglobulinemia); Swiss-type agammaglobulinemia (the loss of both B and T cell functions); and Wiskott-Aldrich syndrome (sex linked; inadequate T-cell response and deficiency of IgM).

The leukocyte disorders discussed in this text have included only those disorders that are nonmalignant in nature. Certainly malignant disorders of leukocytes are significant and of considerable interest, but are beyond the scope of this study. (Malignant disorders are discussed briefly in the following chapter.) Table 3–25 lists some of the nonmalignant conditions affecting the various leukocyte populations.

TABLE 3–25. Conditions Affecting Leukocyte Populations

	Neutrophilia	Neutropenia	Lymphocytosis	Lymphocytopenia	Monocytosis	Eosinophilia
Physiologic responses	Exercise Acute stress Childbirth Extreme heat/cold					
Infectious diseases	Bacterial (systemic or severe local infection) Some viruses (especially herpes viruses) Some rickettsial diseases (especially Rocky Mountain spotted fever) Some fungi	Some bacterial (ex. typhoid, tularemia, brucellosis) Viruses (mumps, IM, hepatitis, influenza) Malaria Overwhelming infection of any kind	Some bacterial (whooping cough, brucellosis, occ TB, secondary syphilis) Viral (IM, CMV, mumps, hepatitis) Toxoplasmosis	Advanced TB	TB Syphilis Hepatitis Subacute bacterial Endocarditis	Parasitic infection
Inflammatory processes	Rheumatoid arthritis Rheumatic fever Acute gout Vasculitis Hypersensitivity rxns.	Some collagen disorders (eg, LE)	Ulcerative colitis Immune diseases		Ulcerative colitis Rheumatoid arthritis Lupus	Some collagen disorders
Metabolic disorders	Uremia Diabetic ketoacidosis Eclampsia Thyroid "storm"		Hypoadrenalism Occ hyperthyroidism	Hyperactive adrenal Pituitary gland tumor		
Tissue necrosis	Ischemic damage Burns Many carcinomas/sarcomas				Some cancers	Necrosis of solid tumors
Drugs and/or chemicals	Epinephrine Lithium Histamine Heparin Digitalis Heavy metals Toxins and venoms	Radiation Cytotoxic drugs Benezene		Therapeutic steroids Immunosuppressives		
Other		Hyperspenism Liver disease Severe B_{12}/folate deficiency		Immunodeficiency Renal failure Disorders of intestinal mucosa Any severe debilitating illness	Some lymphomas Regional enteritis	Allergies Some skin disorders (such as psoriasis, eczema)

TIME FOR REVIEW. After studying the preceding sections, you should be able to respond correctly to the following:

■ Briefly define the following terms:

leukocytosis:

leukopenia:

left shift:

reactive neutophilia:

■ List two causes of transient, physiologic neutrophilia.

■ List three mechanisms that may result in neutropenia.

■ _____ is one of the more frequently reported cytoplasmic abnormalities in neutrophils and results from stimulation by a foreign antigen.

■ A _____ neutrophil has more than five nuclear lobes and may be seen in folate deficiencies and in chronic infections.

- Reactive eosinophilia is associated most commonly with _____ invasion or _____ disorders.

- List three morphologic changes seen in qualitative disorders of the monocyte.

- Distinguish between absolute and relative increases in a cell population.

- Absolute lymphocytosis with more than _____% reactive lymphs is a classic finding in IM.

- A _____ _____ reaction is the term used to describe conditions that produce a marked lymphocytosis giving an initial impression of leukemia.

- _____ is a hereditary granulocytic anamoly characterized by nuclear hyposegmentation (usually two lobes).

- B lymphocytes function in _____ immunity, while T lymphocytes are important in _____ immunity.

- _____ describes a group of genetic conditions in which the enzymes that break down mucopolysaccharides are deficient (Hunter and Hurler syndromes, for example).

- Review the tables presented in this section.

Check your responses by reviewing the preceding pages.

PLATELETS

Platelet counts are typically included on the routine CBC along with the mean platelet volume (MPV). Though often considered a third type of blood cell found in the peripheral circulation (red cells and white cells being the other two), platelets are not true intact cells. Instead, platelets are very small fragments (1 to $4\mu m$) of the giant megakaryocyte. They function as a part of the coagulation process, with direct or indirect influence on a variety of aspects of hemostasis and thrombosis.

Maturation Cycle

Platelets, also called **thrombocytes**, are derived from the cells of the megakary-ocytic system. Cells of this series, at all levels of maturity, are generally seen only in the bone marrow and not expected in the peripheral blood. The least mature cell in the maturation cycle is the **megakaryoblast** derived from a hematopoietic progenitor cell. Megakaryoblasts are about 15 to $50\mu m$ in diameter, with an irregular shape and blunt protrusions of its diffuse blue cytoplasm.

Megakaryoblasts mature to become **promegakaryocytes**, with an even larger volume (20 to $80\mu m$) and an increasing number of nuclear lobes. Bluish granules, not present in the blast stage, become apparent around the nucleus in this stage. Following the promegakaryocyte is the **megakaryocyte**, an even larger cell that has abundant cytoplasm containing small, reddish blue granules and multiple nuclei.

The **metamegakaryocyte** is the fourth stage of this maturation cycle and is a giant cell several times the size of a mature granulocyte. This is the stage from which platelets are produced (some megakaryocytes with four or more nuclei may also produce platelets) and platelets may be seen adhering to the cell membrane. Cytoplasmic platelet fragments are "shed" into the bone marrow sinus, where individual platelets result from further dissolution. Each cell may shed 1,000 to 4,000 platelets to be released into the circulation. Platelets have a relatively short life span, remaining in the circulation about 5 to 10 days, with old or damaged platelets removed by the spleen.

Structure

Although relatively small and without a nucleus (anucleate), the platelet has a complex structure. A detailed discussion of platelet structure is beyond the scope of this text; briefly a description of the four major areas of the platelet is as follows:

1. **Peripheral zone:** surface coat, plasma membrane, and submembrane area
2. **Submembrane area:** separates the internal side of the cell wall from the organelles in the inner cell body
3. **Sol-gel zone:** underlies the submembrane filaments and regulates arrangement of internal organelles like musculoskeletal system
4. **Organelle zone:** major portion of platelet; influences its function in response to stimuli; contains granules, mitochondria, lysosomes

Function

Platelets play an important role in the coagulation process (a separate chapter is devoted to coagulation testing). They respond following stimulation that results from interaction with injured vascular surfaces, plasma proteins, and other cells in the circulation. Platelets respond to such stimulation by

- *adhesion:* adhering or sticking to the wall of an injured vessel to form a barrier against blood loss.

- *release:* contents of alpha-granules released following weak stimulus and with greater stimulus, contents of dense granules also released; released substances assist platelet aggregation and serve to activate the coagulation system; release stimulated by variety of substances including collagen, thrombin, epinephrine, and thromboxane A_2 (a vasoconstrictor).
- *aggregation:* clumping together; induced by ADP (from dense granules), thrombin, and thromboxane A_2.

In addition to their role in the initiation of the coagulation process, platelets participate in thrombin generation and provide a surface on which clotting factors can bind to activate coagulation factors II and X. Factors II, VII, IX, and X, the vitamin K dependent factors, all interact with platelets (more detail on coagulation factors is provided in Chapter 15).

The full clinical significance of platelet size (reflected by the measurement of MPV) is not fully known. In general, large platelets represent younger platelets with better hemostatic function than older platelets. Evidence also suggests that the MPV correlates with bleeding tendency in patients with thrombocytopenia in that the bleeding tendency is significantly less with higher MPV values. This finding would be consistent with the larger, younger platelets having better hemostatic function and thus thrombocytopenic patients with less bleeding than might be anticipated based solely upon the number of platelets present. With this in mind, the MPV may be of some benefit in evaluating the need for platelet transfusion. The MPV may be useful when immune thrombocytopenia purpura is suspected in acute presentations of thrombocytopenia. However, platelets with increased MPV are seen in a variety of thrombocytopenic conditions, including Bernard-Soulier syndrome and myeloproliferative disorders. Large platelets may also indicate altered platelet production, as in the May-Hegglin anomaly. Small platelets (lower MPV) are seen in autoimmune thrombocytopenia, leukemia, and the Wiskott-Aldrich syndrome.

Methods of Measurement

Platelet counts and the MPV are determined by electronic means as described under Methods of Measurement in Chapter 2. Counts may also be determined manually using a special diluting fluid and a hemacytometer counting chamber. Platelet estimation from a stained peripheral smear is typically included in the performance of a manual differential or may be performed as follow-up to flagged or suspicious automated results. The estimation is beneficial in verifying an unexpected automated count and in detecting invalid counts resulting from clumped platelets.

A *platelet estimation* may be performed by examining ten consecutive oil immersion fields in an area of the slide where red cells are slightly overlapping and counting the number of platelets observed in relation to the number of red cells present in the same field. The average number of platelets observed per oil immersion field is calculated and multiplied by a standard ratio or automated platelet count to platelets per oil immersion field previously established by the laboratory for each type of microscope and instrument in use. For example, if this ratio has been established as 17 and an average of eight platelets per oil immersion field was observed, the platelet estimate would be 136,000. In general terms, however, with a normal platelet count (150,000 to 400,000), a field containing 200 red cells should contain approximately 6 to 18 platelets. It is important that each laboratory establish standardized methods for the estimation of platelet counts from the peripheral smear. The information regarding platelet estimation given here is provided solely for the purpose of understanding the platelet estimation.

Reference Ranges

Platelet count: 150 to 400 × 10^3/μL [10^9/L], or 150,000 to 400,000
Mean platelet volume (MPV): 7.4 to 10.4 fL

Platelet counts under 50,000 may be considered a **critical value** in some situations and counts below 20,000 are considered critical. Values above one million may also be considered critical.

PLATELET ABNORMALITIES

Platelet disorders may be *quantitative* (abnormal number of platelets) or *qualitative* (defect in function of platelets) and may be *inherited* or *acquired.* Some disorders are *primary* in nature, while others are *secondary,* or occur as a result of another condition or disease process.

■ QUANTITATIVE DISORDERS

Thrombocytopenia refers to a *decreased number of platelets* and is a relatively common disorder. The number of circulating platelets may be reduced for a variety of reasons or a combination of causes including:

- decreased production
- increased destruction (immune or nonimmune)
- sequestration in the spleen

Decreased production of platelets may result from production defects that impact more than one cellular element (such as that seen in aplastic anemia) and from any condition, hereditary or acquired, that results in **bone marrow hypoplasia** (radiation; chemotherapy drugs; Fanconi syndrome—a genetic aplastic anemia; some viral infections, particularly with infection to stem cells). The production defect may also effect only the megakaryocytic series, as is seen in response to certain drugs and in an inherited syndrome that involves absent, decreased, or abnormal megakaryocytes in the bone marrow. A deficiency in *thrombopoietin* (a substance that is to platelets what erythropoietin is to red cells) also causes thrombocytopenia as a result of insufficient or absent megakaryocyte maturation and platelet production. Other causes of thrombocytopenia from decreased production include space-occupying lesions in the bone marrow in which the abnormal cells replace normal bone marrow elements; ineffective thrombopoiesis resulting from alcohol abuse, megaloblastic conditions, severe iron deficiency anemias, and paroxysmal nocturnal hemoglobinuria (discussed in more detail later); and conditions such as May-Hegglin, Wiskott-Aldrich, and Bernard-Soulier syndromes (discussed in the Selected Platelet Disorders section).

Platelets may be destroyed or lost at an accelerated rate. **Increased destruction** may result from both immune and nonimmune processes. Nonimmune causes of platelet destruction include some cases of sepsis, drugs that may cause platelet clumping within the body, extensive burns, and disseminated intravascular coagulation (DIC; discussed in Chapter 15). Immune processes leading to increased destruction of platelets are generally related to increased immune antibodies (immunoglobulins) or complement. A decreased platelet count that results from these immune processes is termed an **immune thrombocytopenia**. Immune thrombocytopenias may result from alloantibodies (as may be seen as a result of multiple transfusion or in neonates as a result of placental crossing of maternal antibodies directed against antigens on fetal platelets) or from autoantibodies in an autoimmune process as in immune thrombocytopenia purpura (ITP; formerly called idiopathic thrombocytopenia purpura).

Normal splenic functions include removal of old and/or damaged platelets from the circulation and sequestering (or segregating and setting aside) a portion of the normal, undamaged circulating platelets for mobilization when needed. Thrombocytopenia results when the spleen sequesters increased numbers of normal, undamaged platelets. Conditions in which the spleen is enlarged can result in the majority of the circulating platelets being sequestered in the spleen and a resultant decrease in the number of circulating platelets. This **increased sequestration** may be the cause of thrombocytopenia in Gaucher's disease and in sarcoidosis.

Thrombocytosis refers to an abnormally increased platelet count. Such increases may be benign (transient increases seen in response to vigorous exercise or other physiologic stress) or pathologic and may be classified as a primary condition or as secondary to another condition such as iron deficiency, hemolytic anemia, acute blood loss, major surgical procedures or other tissue injuries, and post-splenectomy. *Secondary thrombocytosis* is generally without significant complications (hemorrhage or thrombosis) because the increase is usually temporary and platelet counts return to normal within a relatively short time. *Primary thrombocytosis* is seen in a number of myeloproliferative disorders, including polycythemia vera (discussed in the section on erythrocyte abnormalities). In such disorders, the bone marrow contains an increased number of megakaryocytes (which will mature and produce more platelets) even with the high number of circulating platelets.

■ PLATELET FUNCTION (QUALITATIVE) DISORDERS

Defects in the normal functioning of platelets may be hereditary or acquired and may occur as a primary process or secondary to another condition. Upon initial presentation, disorders of platelet function clinically resemble a thrombocytopenia; however, platelets are normal in number. Therefore, a qualitative defect should be suspected in a patient presenting with symptoms such as easy bruising, nose bleed, menorrhagia, or other bleeding tendencies, but yielding a platelet count that is within or very near the normal reference range.

The platelet response to stimuli, as previously described, includes an **adhesion** to injured vessel walls, **aggregation** or platelet clumping, and the **release** of substances required for the coagulation process. Functional abnormalities may be classified in terms of these responses as well. Normal platelet adhesion is dependent upon membrane receptors on the platelet itself as well as the availability of certain plasma proteins in adequate concentration. Defects of platelet adhesion occur when either is lacking, as demonstrated by the following two examples.

- *Bernard-Soulier Syndrome:* platelets lack the membrane receptor required for binding with von Willebrand factor (vWF) resulting in an inability to adhere to substances, like collagen, exposed in vessel injury.
- *von Willebrand's Disease:* deficiency of plasma protein factors VIII:vWF or VIII:Ag renders platelets unable to effectively adhere to vessel wall; these factors "link" the platelet to the wall.

The ability of platelets to change shape and aggregate in response to ADP requires an adequate concentration of fibrinogen and glycoprotein complexes on the platelet membrane. **Defective aggregation** is seen in conditions where fibrinogen is absent (afibrinogenemia) or reduced and where the glycoprotein complexes are absent or insufficient in number. An inherited disorder called *Glanzmann's thrombasthenia* is an example of such a defect: in type I (most severe), platelets lack the glycoprotein complexes as well as intraplatelet fibrinogen, and in type II, fibrinogen concentration is decreased and the percentage of the normal number of glycoprotein complexes is reduced.

Release defects may result from a defect in or an absence of platelet granules, or a deficiency in the substances stored in and released from the granules (called storage pool defects), or be due to a defective secretion of granule contents. **Acquired defects** of platelet function may be secondary to a variety of substances, including aspirin and other nonsteroidal anti-inflammatory agents, penicillin, alcohol, and some dietary components. Functional platelet defects may also be seen in vitamin B_{12} or folate deficiencies, myeloproliferative disorders, uremia, and disseminated intravascular coagulation (DIC). Table 3–26 summarizes some of the quantitative and qualitative platelet abnormalities.

TABLE 3–26. Platelet Abnormalities

Quantitative	Qualitative	
Thrombocytopenia	**Adhesion Defects**	
Decreased Production	Bernard-Soulier Syndrome	
Aplastic anemia	Uremia	
Leukemia	DIC	
Megaloblastic anemia	von Willebrand's Disease	
Metastatic carcinoma		
	Aggregation Defects	
Increased Destruction/Loss	Glanzmann's thrombasthenia	
(nonimmune)	Afibrinogenemia	
Severe hemorrhage		
DIC	**Release Defects**	
Sepsis	Storage pool disease	
(immune)	Wiskott-Aldrich Syndrome	
Neonatal purpura	Uremia	
ITP	Aspirin	
Post-transfusion purpura	Alcohol	
Increased Splenic Sequestration		
Thrombocytosis	**Inherited**	**Acquired**
Primary	Bernard-Soulier	Uremia
Polycythemia vera	Glanzmann's	Aspirin
Essential thrombocythemia	von Willebrand	Alcohol
Chronic granulocytic leukemia	Afibrinogenemia	DIC
	Wiskott-Aldrich	
Reactive		
Iron deficiency anemia		
Acute blood loss		
Hemolytic anemia		
Rheumatoid arthritis		
Hodgkin's disease		

■ TESTS OF PLATELET FUNCTION

The ability of platelets to effectively fulfill their intended role in the coagulation process is dependent not only upon the number of platelets present, but also on the *quality* of the platelets or their ability to function as intended. A number of tests of varying complexity are available for the evaluation of platelet function. Some of these tests are briefly described below.

BLEEDING TIME. The bleeding time is the time required for a wound of standardized length and depth to stop bleeding; it is a simple test sensitive to abnormalities of both number and function, but primarily used in evaluation of platelet adhesion; prolonged in thrombocytopenia, von Willebrand's disease, severely decreased or absent fibrinogen, and in other platelet disorders. Its general reference range is 2 to 9 minutes (method and age dependent).

PLATELET FACTOR ASSAYS. These are assays available for platelet factor III (PF3) activity (the ability of platelets to provide a surface for factor binding); and platelet factor IV (PF4) and beta-thromboglobulin (proteins in alpha-granules that can bind heparin). They are not widely used; PF4 and beta-thromboglobulin assays are considered research procedures.

PLATELET AGGREGATION TEST. In this test a standardized concentration of an aggregating substance (eg, ADP, epinephrine, thrombin, ristocetin reagent) is added to a suspension of platelet-rich plasma and changes in light transmission are measured; it is a useful aid in the diagnosis of hereditary and acquired disorders.

VON WILLEBRAND FACTOR ASSAY. von Willebrand factor (vWF) functions to assist in platelet aggregation; the amount of factor present is determined by comparing platelet agglutination results for a patient sample to a standard curve.

CLOT RETRACTION. This test is rarely performed because more sophisticated tests are available. It measures platelet ability in achieving a firm clot that retracts (shrinks and pulls away from the sides of the test tube) a given amount in a defined time period at 37°C. Soft, watery clot that does not retract may indicate lack of or defective platelets. It is also dependent on the presence of calcium and ATP, normal fibrinogen concentration, and absence of fibrinolysins.

■ PRESENTATION AND CLINICAL FINDINGS

Common manifestations of thrombocytopenia and disorders of platelet function include petechiae, easy bruising, and bleeding. Petechiae and purpura result from even the smallest of injuries because capillaries or other damaged vessels cannot be immediately sealed off. The point at which a given patient will bleed in terms of platelet count or function varies, however, significant bleeding does not usually occur with functional platelets at a count > 50,000 or 60,000 and as platelet counts approach or fall *below 20,000,* spontaneous bleeding is likely. More common sites of bleeding include mucous membranes (nose, mouth) and the gastrointestinal, urinary, and respiratory tracts. Bleeding may also occur at the site of surgical or other wounds, and menorrhagia is not an uncommon finding. Bleeding in the central nervous system can be fatal.

■ LABORATORY FINDINGS AND TREATMENT APPROACHES

By definition, thrombocytopenic disorders include a laboratory finding of a decreased platelet count and thrombocytosis an increased platelet count. The treatment of platelet disorders is dependent upon the cause of the abnormality in number and/or function and may involve treatment of an underlying condition from which the platelet abnormality results or removal of a substance (such as a drug) causing an abnormality. General laboratory findings and treatment approaches are discussed briefly.

In addition to the obvious decreased platelet count, laboratory findings in thrombocytopenia include an increased bleeding time as a result of the low number of platelets, and if performed, the clot retraction test will be abnormal.

In ITP (formerly referred to as idiopathic—of unknown etiology—and now considered to be an immune disorder), which may be either acute or chronic, platelet counts are typically < 50,000 with an increased number of large platelets. Antibodies bound to the surface of the platelet can be demonstrated in most cases. The anti-platelet antibody in this condition is usually an IgG antibody, but may also be seen with IgA or IgM antibodies.

Thrombocytopenia resulting from nonimmune destruction of platelets, such as that occurring in DIC, hemolytic uremia syndrome (HUS), or thrombotic thrombocytopenia purpura (TTP), produces additional laboratory findings specific to the condition. The CBC findings in all three conditions are similar and may include anemia, increased anisocytosis, and many red cell fragments. LD and bilirubin levels are likely to be increased as a result of the intravascular hemolysis. In HUS and TTP the fibrinogen, PT, and PTT are usually normal as opposed to DIC, which includes a decreased fibrinogen and increased PT and PTT levels. (DIC is discussed in greater detail in Chapter 15.)

The goal of treatment in thrombocytopenia, of course, is to raise the platelet count. Therapy is indicated until the count reaches a level sufficient to maintain hemostasis—not necessarily a level that falls within an established reference range. Depending on the type and cause of thrombocytopenia, as well as other factors, treatment may involve administration of immunosuppressant drugs such as corticosteroids; splenectomy; platelet transfusion; plasmapheresis; and withdrawal of drugs causing thrombocytopenia.

Using splenectomy as a treatment of thrombocytopenia removes a major source of platelet storage and destruction as well as a site of antibody synthesis. Corticosteroids may be effective in immune thrombocytopenias because of their immunosuppressant effect. They also can have a beneficial effect on vascular integrity.

Platelet transfusions may be given in instances in which a malignancy or treatment with chemotherapeutic drugs results in thrombocytopenia. The decision to administer platelets is made with consideration of the potential risks, including allergic reactions, transfusion-transmitted infectious disease, and sensitization. Transfusions are generally reserved for those patients who are at significant risk. Platelet transfusion is not an effective therapy in patients in whom the underlying immune process will result in destruction of the infused platelets.

Patients who have received long-term support with platelet transfusion, such as those with aplastic anemia or acute leukemia, may develop *alloimmunization.* This means that these patients have developed an antibody (in this case an *allo*antibody, an antibody against an antigen different from their own antigens—as opposed to an *auto*antibody, developed against a "self" antigen) that will "attack" and destroy infused platelets bearing the offending antigen. Such patients are said to be "refractory" to platelet transfusion. It can be quite difficult to find platelets suitable for transfusion in these cases, with family members often being the more suitable donors (unless bone marrow transplantation from a family member is anticipated). Alloimmunization is suspected when administration of platelets does not result in the expected increment of platelet increase following transfusion. Infusing a large quantity of platelets can temporarily reduce the antibody level and allow the excess platelets to halt bleeding. The level of the antibody can be reduced prior to platelet transfusion by *plasmpheresis.*

Treatment may not be required in acute ITP because spontaneous remission occurs within about 6 months in 90% of cases (Stein, 1993). ITP in pregnancy raises special considerations requiring close monitoring and management as the antibody responsible for platelet destruction in the mother is most likely an IgG antibody. IgG antibodies are able to cross the placenta, meaning neonatal thrombocytopenia is possible. Although this thrombocytopenia generally disappears within 2 months of birth, it can present significant birth complications (including intracranial hemorrhage in the infant) as a result of the trauma of vaginal delivery. Cesarean section may be considered. A platelet count can be performed early in labor from blood obtained from a scalp vein to aid in making this decision.

Thrombotic thrombocytopenia purpura and HUS present different treatment concerns in that platelet thrombus formation is characteristic of these conditions. Drugs that have an inhibitory effect on the ability of platelets to aggregate may be given. Exchange transfusion, exchange plasmapheresis, or plasma infusion can remove or reduce immune complexes and replace plasma factors. Platelet transfusion is not effective for these conditions and in fact may be contraindicated because of the likelihood of life-threatening hemorrhage.

Many cases of thrombocytosis are reactive and thus transient in nature and unlikely to require treatment. Platelet thrombus formation may occur in some types of thrombocytosis. When thrombus formation is considered a possibility, aspirin may be given to reduce the adherance of platelets and reduce the likelihood of thrombus formation.

 TIME FOR REVIEW. After studying the preceding sections, you should be able to respond correctly to the following:

■ List and describe the three ways platelets respond to the stimulus of vascular injury.

■ Substances released from platelet granules assist _____ and activate the _____ .

■ Define the following terms

thrombocytosis

thrombocytopenia

MPV

■ List the three mechanisms that result in thrombocytopenia.

■ Disorders of platelet function are (quantitative/qualitative) disorders.

■ List two tests of platelet function and briefly describe what the test measures.

■ Discuss reasons why platelet transfusion might not be used to treat thrombocytopenia.

■ Describe how the following therapies may be effective in the treatment of thrombocytopenia:

corticosteroid administration

splenectomy

plasmapheresis

■ Alcohol and aspirin may result in abnormalities of platelet _____.

■ Review the tables provided in this section.

Check your responses by reviewing the preceding pages.

3. SELF TEST

Choose the best response by circling the appropriate letter. The answer key may be found in the appendices.

1. **Which of the following cell types is *not* classified as a phagocyte?**
   A. neutrophils
   B. eosinophils
   C. monocytes
   D. lymphocytes

2. **Monocytes and lymphocytes are classified together when the grouping is based on**
   A. nuclear segmentation and/or granularity
   B. function and/or granularity
   C. function and/or nuclear segmentation
   D. phagocytosis and/or antibody production

3. **The two leukocyte populations that vary most with age are the**
   A. eosinophils and monocytes
   B. neutrophils and lymphocytes
   C. neutrophils and monocytes
   D. lymphocytes and basophils

4. **The ingestion of foreign substances such as bacteria, viruses, and cellular debris and the subsequent destruction of the foreign material is called**
   A. motility
   B. chemotaxis
   C. phagocytosis
   D. humoral immunity

5. **The release of chemical stimuli that results in a phagocytic cell being "drawn" to a foreign substance is called**
   A. degranulation
   B. chemotaxis
   C. stimulation
   D. recognition

6. **Neutrophilic granules contain**
    A. pseudopods for locomotion
    B. oxygenated hemoglobin
    C. substances that stimulate antibody production
    D. enzymes that aid in killing ingested substances

7. **The tissue cell counterpart of the blood monocyte is the**
    A. eosinophil
    B. macrophage
    C. immunocyte
    D. stem cell

8. **Eosinophils are primarily involved in**
    A. control of protozoal and bacterial infections
    B. control of viral and parasitic infections
    C. control of parasitic infections and hypersensitivity reactions
    D. control of bacterial infections and hypersensitivity reactions

9. **The least common peripheral blood cell with a role in immediate hypersensitivity reactions is the**
    A. basophil
    B. eosinophil
    C. lymphocyte
    D. monocyte

10. **The lymphocytes that become plasma cells and produce antibodies are**
    A. T helpers
    B. B cells
    C. T suppressors
    D. lymphokine activated

11. **The lymphocytes that repress T and B cell responses are**
    A. T helpers
    B. B cells
    C. T suppressors
    D. lymphokine activated

12. **The lymphocytes that induce other T cells and assist B cell functions are**
    A. T helpers
    B. B cells
    C. T suppressors
    D. lymphokine activated

13. **A neutrophilic left shift refers to the presence (in peripheral blood) of**
    A. nucleated red cells
    B. an increased number of segmented neutrophils
    C. neutrophils with liberal social policies
    D. an increased number of immature neutrophils

14. **Decreased production, increased destruction, or sequestration of neutrophils may all lead to**
    A. an inflammatory response
    B. neutropenia
    C. neutrophilia
    D. leukocytosis

15. **A cytoplasmic abnormality found in toxic neutrophils as a result of phagocytosis and especially common in septic processes is**
    A. degranulation
    B. hypersegmentation
    C. vacuolation
    D. Dohle bodies

16. **A nuclear abnormality found in neutrophils that can be seen in chronic infections or may reflect a folate deficiency is**
    A. degranulation
    B. hypersegmentation
    C. vacuolation
    D. Dohle bodies

17. **Reactive eosinophilia is most commonly associated with**
    A. overwhelming bacterial infections
    B. decreased production of eosinophils
    C. administration of ACTH
    D. parasitic invasion and hypersensitivity

18. **A finding commonly seen in conjunction with an increased number of eosinophils is**
    A. monocytosis
    B. monocytopenia
    C. basophilia
    D. basopenia

19. **A finding commonly seen in conjunction with an increased number of neutrophils, although not as conspicuous as the neutrophilic response, is**
    A. monocytosis
    B. monocytopenia
    C. basophilia
    D. basopenia

20. **The presence of a few reactive lymphs on a peripheral blood smear is**
    A. indicative of a preleukemic condition
    B. highly suggestive of infectious mononucleosis
    C. a normal finding
    D. an early indication of an immune disorder

21. **Absolute lymphocytosis with reactive lymphocytes in excess of 40% is**
    A. indicative of a preleukemic condition
    B. highly suggestive of infectious mononucleosis
    C. a normal finding
    D. an early indication of an immune disorder

22. **Absolute lymphocytosis with a very high white count and with normal lymphocytes is most indicative of**
    A. infectious mononucleosis
    B. acute infectious lymphocytosis
    C. viral-related disorders
    D. cytomegalovirus infections

23. **Relative lymphocytosis in the presence of reactive lymphs may be seen in a number of disorders, including**
    A. infectious mononucleosis
    B. acute infectious lymphocytosis
    C. viral related disorders
    D. cytomegalovirus infections

24. **A hereditary leukocyte disorder that is assessed by the level of serum immunoglobulins or the patient's ability to produce antibodies is**
    A. B cell deficiency
    B. T cell deficiency
    C. mucopolysaccharidoses
    D. Chediak-Higashi syndrome

25. **A condition in which there is a failure, to some extent, of both the humoral and cellular immune responses is called**
    A. Job's syndrome
    B. Pelger-Huet anomaly
    C. chronic granulomatous disease
    D. severe combined immunodeficiency

26. **The term used to describe an increased amount of variation in erythrocyte size is**
    A. poikilocytosis
    B. anisocytosis
    C. hypochromia
    D. polychromasia

27. **Increased variation in the shape of erythrocytes is described in terms of**
    A. poikilocytosis
    B. anisocytosis
    C. hypochromia
    D. polychromasia

28. **The presence of nucleated red cells in the peripheral circulation of an adult generally indicates**
    A. a normal peripheral blood finding
    B. a decreased production of red cells
    C. a significant increased demand on the bone marrow
    D. the presence of schistocytes

29. **The most common cause of megaloblastic anemia is**
    A. iron deficiency
    B. B_{12} and folate deficiency
    C. chronic bleeding
    D. abnormal iron metabolism

30. **Choose the laboratory findings most consistent with a megaloblastic anemia.**
    A. decreased red cell count; decreased MCV and MCH; normal MCHC; presence of anisocytosis and poikilocytosis; normal platelet count; elevated reticulocyte count
    B. decreased red cell count; decreased MCV and MCH; normal MCHC; no anisocytosis and poikilocytosis; elevated platelet count; decreased reticulocyte count; basophilic stippling
    C. increased red cell count; increased MCV and MCH; normal MCHC; presence of anisocytosis and poikilocytosis; normal platelet count; elevated reticulocyte count; hypersegmentation of nucleus of neutrophils
    D. decreased red cell count; increased MCV and MCH; normal MCHC; presence of anisocytosis and poikilocytosis; decreased platelet count; large reticulocytes; hypersegmentation of nucleus of neutrophils

31. **Choose the condition best described by these laboratory findings: marked decrease in serum B_{12} level; increased serum folate; marked decrease in erythrocyte folate level.**
    A. vitamin B_{12} deficiency
    B. folate deficiency
    C. vitamin B_{12} and folate deficiency
    D. iron deficiency anemia

32. **Three lab tests most commonly required to aid in diagnosis of iron deficiency anemia are**
    A. serum iron; TIBC; CBC
    B. MCV; serum iron; percent transferrin saturation
    C. serum ferritin; CBC; reticulocyte count
    D. serum iron; cholesterol; hemoglobin electrophoresis

33. **Findings most descriptive of the last stage in development of iron deficiency anemia are**
    A. significantly decreased hemoglobin and MCV with microcytic, hypochromic cells; decreased serum ferritin and iron levels; increased iron binding capacity
    B. significantly decreased hemoglobin and MCV with macrocytic, normochromic cells; increased serum ferritin and iron levels; increased iron-binding capacity
    C. significantly decreased hemoglobin; increased MCV with microcytic, hypochromic cells; decreased serum ferritin and iron levels; normal iron-binding capacity
    D. significantly decreased hemoglobin and MCV with macrocytic, hypochromic cells; increased serum ferritin; decreased iron levels; increased iron-binding capacity

34. Sideroblastic anemia results in the excess tissue accumulation of
    A. folate products
    B. iron
    C. hemoglobin
    D. bilirubin

35. The most common hemoglobin variant is
    A. C
    B. F
    C. S
    D. Y

36. The test used to confirm the presence of sickle cell disease is
    A. CBC
    B. finding of sickled cells on microscopic examination
    C. reticulocyte count
    D. hemoglobin electrophoresis

37. Hemolytic anemias result from
    A. increased red cell production
    B. increased red cell destruction
    C. abnormal iron metabolism
    D. folate deficiency

38. Along with a decreased red cell count, hemoglobin and hematocrit, which laboratory findings are most consistent with a hemolytic anemia?
    A. increased reticulocyte count; decreased serum bilirubin; elevated urinary urobilinogen; presence of hemoglobin in urine
    B. increased reticulocyte count; increased serum bilirubin; elevated urinary urobilinogen; presence of hemoglobin in urine
    C. decreased reticulocyte count; increased serum bilirubin; decreased urinary urobilinogen; presence of hemoglobin in urine
    D. decreased reticulocyte count; decreased serum bilirubin; elevated urinary urobilinogen; presence of hemoglobin in urine

39. A patient's history reveals a strict vegetarian diet and physical examination shows a "spooned" appearance to the nails. A CBC reveals the presence of a microcytic, hypochromic anemia. The anemia, pending confirmation by additional testing, is most likely a result of
    A. iron deficiency
    B. B_{12} deficiency
    C. hemolytic anemia
    D. folate deficiency

40. The presence of anemia with neurologic defects noted on physical examination is most likely
    A. iron deficiency anemia
    B. hemolytic anemia
    C. sideroblastic anemia
    D. megaloblastic B$_{12}$ deficiency anemia

41. A simple, useful test aiding in the distinction between hemolytic and nonhemolytic anemias is the
    A. CBC
    B. reticulocyte count
    C. hemoglobin electrophoresis
    D. sickle cell screen

42. An anemic patient with a normal reticulocyte count and microcytic, hypochromic cells has findings consistent with
    A. megaloblastic anemia
    B. pernicious anemia
    C. iron deficiency anemia
    D. acute blood loss

43. Thrombocytopenia may result from all of the following *except*
    A. increased destruction
    B. increased thrombopoietin
    C. increased splenic sequestration
    D. decreased production

44. Bleeding time elevation would be expected in
    A. polycythemia vera
    B. essential thrombocythemia
    C. immune thrombocytopenia purpura
    D. thrombocytosis

45. The thrombocytopenia seen in DIC results from
    A. increased destruction
    B. decreased production
    C. increased splenic sequestration
    D. decreased platelet antibodies

46. A condition in which primary thrombocytosis is seen in conjunction with an increase in other cellular elements is
    A. immune thrombocytopenia purpura
    B. aplastic anemia
    C. Hodgkin's disease
    D. polycythemia vera

47. Normal platelet function due to a deficiency in a component of the factor VIII plasma protein required to link platelets to vessel walls results in
    A. von Willebrand's disease
    B. ITP
    C. Bernard-Soulier syndrome
    D. polycythemia vera

4. MYELOPROLIFERATIVE AND LYMPHOPROLIFERATIVE DISORDERS

This chapter includes a basic discussion of hematopoietic malignancies, or "clonal" leukocyte disorders. The term *malignancy* is used to refer to the growth and proliferation of clones of abnormal cells. These abnormal, malignant blood cells are not responsive to the usual control and feedback mechanisms and thus, in the absence of effective intervention, continue unchecked growth that significantly impairs the ability of normal cells to survive. Normal blood cell survival may be impeded by the malignant cells as they fill all available space, crowding out the normal cells, or by substances produced by malignant cells that inhibit the growth of normal cell populations. As a result, anemia (from inhibited red cell growth and proliferation) and thrombocytopenia (from inhibited growth and proliferation of platelets) are common laboratory findings in malignant leukocyte disorders. Much investigatory effort has been directed toward determining the cause of the initial cellular transformation that results in malignancy. Although it is difficult to specifically identify a causative agent in most cases, malignant transformations have been linked to various environmental, chemical, and viral agents, and to genetic susceptibility. In some cases a combination of agents is implicated.

Knowledge of several terms used to describe blood cell malignancies is important to an understanding of a discussion of these disorders. Blood cell malignancies in which the abnormal cells are found in both the bone marrow and in the peripheral circulation are referred to as **leukemias**. If the abnormal cells are found only in the bone marrow, the condition may be referred to as an *aleukemic leukemia*. The leukemias are identified based on the stem cell line from which the abnormal cells arise. Malignant transformations in the **myeloid stem cell line** result in **myeloproliferative disorders**, or **myelogenous leukemias**. This group of disorders includes proliferation of abnormal granulocytes, monocytes, megakaryocytes, or erythrocytes. Malignant transformation in the **lymphoid stem cell line** results in **lymphoproliferative disorders** involving B or T lymphocytes. Lymphoproliferative disorders may be leukemias or, if the neoplastic cells are confined to a solid tumor in the lymphatic tissues (eg, lymph nodes), **lymphomas**.

Leukemias are further classified as acute or chronic. Although these terms were originally applied in terms of the life expectancy of individuals diagnosed with the

149

conditions (ie, weeks or months for acute and a few years for chronic), they have been retained despite the significant changes in life expectancy achieved with advances in treatment. Today, the terms *acute* and *chronic* are an indication of the percentage of blast cells found in the peripheral circulation and/or bone marrow. Conditions are generally considered **chronic** when the number of blasts in the peripheral blood is < 10% and as acute when > 25 to 30% blasts are found in the peripheral blood. Blast forms between 10% and 30% in the peripheral blood are not as clearly delineated and may be classified as subacute, chronic, or as a chronic condition that is transforming to an acute one (Lotspeich-Steininger, 1992). Findings from other hematologic tests and the clinical history may be helpful in such cases. Acute leukemias are subdivided into **FAB** (France, America, Britain) **classifications** that include morphologic and other criteria. Such a detailed classification has not been developed for the chronic leukemias.

MYELOPROLIFERATIVE DISORDERS

Myeloproliferative disorders include a group of related diseases that are characterized by the uncontrolled growth and proliferation of one or more types of cells from the myeloid stem cell line. The conditions in this group of disorders generally share some common features:

1. occurrence with higher incidence in adults
2. clinical presentation
   symptoms related to anemia
   recurrent infections
   bleeding or thrombotic tendencies
   splenomegaly; sometimes massive
3. laboratory findings
   mild to moderate normocytic, normochromic anemia (except polycythemia vera)
   diffuse red cell polychromasia
   poikilocytosis; dacrocytes are predominate poikilocyte (esp. prominent in anogenic myeloiod metaplasia)
   elevated serum uric acid levels
   elevated serum vitamin B_{12} levels
   elevated serum LDH
   elevated leukocyte alkaline phosphatase (LAP) (except in chronic myelogenous leukemia)

Although the term *leukemia* is generally associated with white cell malignancies, a broader definition includes any type of blood cell malignancy. Myeloid leukemias may involve one or more cell types of the granulocyte, monocyte, megakaryocyte, or erythroid cell lines.

Acute Non-lymphocytic Leukemia

Acute non-lymphocytic leukemia (ANLL), also called *acute myelogenous* (or myeloid) leukemia (AML), is a progressive malignancy that is rapidly fatal if undetected or untreated. Immature cells that are undifferentiated or partially differentiated are predominate and the numbers of normal myeloid elements are reduced, eventually replaced by the unchecked growth of the leukemic cells. Death usually results as a consequence of the decreased number or absence of normal cells, producing anemia, bleeding, and impaired resistance to infection. ANLL varies significantly in incidence among different age groups. Although relatively rare in childhood and adolescence, it is the most common form of acute leukemia in adulthood.

Because ANLL is a general term used to describe all acute leukemias that do not involve lymphocytes, the ANLLs may be quite heterogeneous in terms of specific cell types and morphology. This heterogeneity allows the ANLLs to be further subdivided based on FAB criteria (Table 4–1). Appropriate classification of leukemia into as specific a category as possible is important in terms of treatment decisions and prognosis. The **classification** criteria refer to pretreatment characteristics, as cytotoxic therapy can alter morphology. A variety of techniques are employed to classify leukemias, including morphologic characteristics, various staining properties, cytochemical tests, and immunochemical antigen analysis. The FAB classification criteria include a determination of the number of blast cells present as a percentage of the total of all nucleated cells or of the total of all nonerythroid cells. Two types of blasts are defined based on morphologic characteristics:

1. *Type I:* no cytoplasmic differentiation or cytoplasmic granules; prominent nucleoli.
2. *Type II:* more differentiated than type I with few cytoplasmic granules and lower nuclear:cytoplasmic (N:C) ratio.

Clinical signs of ANLL are related to the varying degrees of bone marrow failure seen in this group of disorders. Patients may present with anemia, leukopenia, or thrombocytopenia. Symptoms include those associated with anemia (eg, fatigue, weakness, pallor, dyspnea); with leukopenia (eg, fever, infection); and with thrombocytopenia (ie, bruising, purpura, bleeding). Other symptoms may be indicative of organ infiltration and include splenomegaly, hepatomegaly, lymphadenopathy, and bone tenderness. The FAB subtype M3 is associated with a high incidence of coagulation disorders, especially an unusually high incidence of disseminated intravascular coagulation (DIC). Tissue infiltrates (particularly of the gums) and central nervous system involvement are characteristic of FAB subtypes M4 and M5.

Laboratory diagnosis of ANLL usually begins with a demonstration of immature cells in the peripheral blood, often (but not always) with an elevated white cell count above 50,000. ANLL patients may also present with white cell counts < 5,000 or with normal white cell counts, but the cells are abnormal and show

TABLE 4–1. Summary and Classification of Acute Non-lymphocytic Leukemias

FAB	Descriptive Diagnostic Term	Origin	Predominate Morphology/Criteria	~% of ANLL	Unique Clinical Features	Cytochemical Reactions				
						SBB/ Perox.	PAS	α-NA	α-NB	Napthol-ASD Chloroacetate
M1	Acute myeloblastic leukemia (AML) without maturation	Myelocytic	Predominately myeloblasts; ≥ 30% of all nucleated cells are type I and II blasts; ≥90 of all nonerythroid cells are blasts	20%		+	+	Neg	Neg	+
M2	Acute myeloblastic leukemia (AML) with maturation	Myelocytic	Myeloblasts with other immature granulocytes; ≥30% of all nucleated cells are blasts; <90% of all nonerythroid cells are blasts and ≥10% are promyelocytes or more mature forms	30–35%		++	+	Neg/+	Neg/+	++
M3	Acute promyelocytic leukemia (APL), hypergranular	Myelocytic	Promyelocytes with conspicuous granules; Auer rods often present; ≥30% blasts and abnormal hypergranular promyelocytes	16%	DIC	+++	±/++	Neg/+	Neg	+++
M3V	Acute promyelocytic leukemia (APL), hypogranular		Promyelocytes without prominent granules; Auer rods rare; ≥30% blasts and abnormal microgranular promyelocytes							
M4	Acute myelomonocytic leukemia (AMML)	Myelocytic and Monocytic	Characteristic cells have monocytic type nucleus and myelocytic type cytoplasm; ≥30% of all nucleated cells are type I and II blasts; >80% nonerythroid cells are monoblasts, promonocytes, or monocytes	15–20%	Tissue infiltration (esp. gum tissue); CNS involvement	++	Neg/++	++/+++	++	++
M4E	Acute myelomonocytic leukemia with eosinophilia		Same as M4, but with increased and abnormal eosinophilia							
M5A	Acute monocytic leukemia (AMoL) without maturation (monoblastic)	Monocytic	Predominantly monoblasts without granulocytic type cytoplasm; ≥ 30% of all nucleated cells are blasts; ≥ 80% of nonerythroid cells are monoblasts, promonocytes, or monocytes; ≥80% of monocytic cells are blasts	10–12%	Tissue infiltration (esp. gum tissue); CNS involvement		++	+++	+++	Neg/+
M5B	Acute monocytic leukemia (AMoL) with maturation		Predominantly nonblast form monocytes without granulocytic type cytoplasm; ≥30% of all nucleated cells are blasts; ≥80% of nonerythroid cells are monocytes, promonocytes, or monocytes; <80% of monocytic cells are blasts							
M6	Erythroleukemia (EL)	Erythocytic and Myelocytic	Megaloblastic pronormoblasts and myeloblasts present with other cells; ≥50% of all nucleated cells are erythroblasts; ≥30% of nonerythroid cells are blasts	3–4%		++	++	++	Neg/+	Neg
M7	Megakaryocytic leukemia (ML)	Megakaryocytic	Immature megakaryocytes; ≥30% of all nucleated cells are megakaryoblasts or leukemic cells	3%[1]	Myelosclerosis	++	++	+	Neg/+	Neg

[1] Sources vary from < 1% up to 10%; Neg = negative; ± = weak reaction/few cells positive; + = moderate positive reaction; ++ = moderately strong positive reaction; +++ = strong/most cells positive; SBB = Sudan Black B; α-NA = alpha napthyl acetate; α-NB = alpha napthyl butyrate; PAS = Periodic Acid Schiff; data for table compiled from various sources.

morphologic immaturity. Examination of bone marrow cells is performed as confirmation and to aid in categorizing the immature cells as lymphocytic or non-lymphocytic. Differentiation of blast cells requires considerable knowledge and expertise and may be particularly difficult based solely on morphologic criteria (Table 4–2). Further characterization of the cell types based on morphology and other characteristics allows the leukemia to be placed in the appropriate FAB subgroup. Table 4–1 summarizes the characteristics of the ANLLs including the FAB classification.

TABLE 4–2. Morphologic Differences in Myeloblasts and Lymphoblasts

	Cell Size	Amount Cytoplasm	Nucleoli	Chromatin	Auer Rods
Myeloblast	Larger	Moderate	Prominent; usually ≥2	Fine, lacy pattern	Present in up to 50% of cases
Lymphoblast	Smaller	Scant	Indistinct; usually <2	More dense	Not present

Modified from Sacher RA, McPherson RA. *Widmann's Clinical Interpretation of Laboratory Tests,* 10th ed. Philadelphia, FA Davis, 1991

Chronic Myeloproliferative Disorders

The chronic myeloproliferative disorders are a group of four related clonal disorders of the hematopoietic stem cell. These syndromes are characterized by the uncontrolled growth and proliferation of multipotent (pleuripotent) cells that are capable of differentiation along a particular cell line to maturity. The four chronic myeloproliferative disorders are

1. **Chronic myelogenous leukemia** (CML): pleuripotent cells differentiate along granulocytic cell line
2. **Polycythemia vera** (PV): differentiation along erythroid cell line (this disorder is discussed in Chapter 3)
3. **Agnogenic myeloid metaplasia** (AMM): also called *myelofibrosis* or *myelofibrosis with myeloid metaplasia* (MMM)
4. **Essential thrombocythemia** (ET): differentiation along megakaryocytic cell line

Chronic myelogenous leukemia occurs more frequently in the adult population with increased incidence after age 50. Because CML often begins insidiously, it is not uncommon for the condition to first be detected on the basis of a routine CBC. Common early **symptoms** include fatigue, malaise, abdominal fullness, and shortness of breath with mild exertion. Splenomegaly is almost always present, with progressive enlargement. Hepatomegaly is also common. The sensation of abdominal fullness resulting from hepatosplenomegaly often results in loss of appetite (patient feels full after ingesting small quantities) and a consequent weight loss.

Patients generally have an increased metabolic rate and may experience night sweats and low-grade fever. Bone tenderness, especially of the sternum, is a common finding. Lymphadenopathy may also be present, but is more commonly seen in juvenile CML than in adult cases.

White cell counts generally reveal a marked leukocytosis with counts ranging from 50,000 to 600,000 and higher prior to initiation of therapy. Anemia is usually mild and normocytic/normochromic. More than half (Ravel 1990) of CML patients have somewhat elevated platelet counts (usually 450,000 to 600,000) upon initial diagnosis. Few patients exhibit thrombocytopenia, but bleeding disorders may result from qualitative platelet defects. The characteristic differential in CML reveals the full spectrum of granulocytic cells from myeloblasts (usually only 1% to 5%), promyelocytes (usually < 10%), myelocytes, metamyelocytes, bands, and mature neutrophils. The majority of the cells seen on the peripheral smear have matured to at least the myelocyte stage. Myelocytes and neutrophils both outnumber other cell types (bimodal distribution; Henry, 1996). Eosinophilia and basophilia are usually noted and monocytosis is present in many patients. The bone marrow is markedly hypercellular, with most cells being of the granulocytic series. The proportions of cells in the various stages of maturity are similar to those seen in the peripheral blood, although the average stage of maturity is earlier. The **Philadelphia chromosome**, an abnormal chromosome resulting from translocation of a portion of chromosome 22 onto chromosome 9, is found in a majority of CML cases.

Many cases of CML undergo an **acute blastic transformation** or acute blast crisis during which the chronic, stable condition accelerates to an acute condition in which increasing numbers of immature cell forms and blasts are seen. As this transformation progresses, the laboratory picture may be virtually the same as that seen in ANLL (AML). In acute blastic transformation, thrombocytopenia may be severe and produce significant bleeding tendencies. The trigger or initiating event(s) for blastic transformation is (are) unknown.

Although **differential diagnosis** of CML is generally not complicated, it is important that it be distinguished from leukemoid reactions. **Leukemoid reaction** is a term applied to a benign leukocytosis with a left shift (increased numbers of immature cells), and sometimes thrombocytosis, that may be seen in response to infection or tissue necrosis and can mimic leukemia. Table 4–3 summarizes the distinguishing features of these two conditions.

The majority of CML patients respond to chemotherapeutic agents. Bone marrow transplantation is an option for some patients. However, the higher rate of serious, often fatal, complications (eg, severe graft versus host disease, septic complications) in older patients usually precludes transplantation for patients > 40 to 50 years of age (Lotspeich-Steininger, 1992)—the age group in which the disease is most likely to be found. The median survival rate for patients with CML is 40 months (Lotspeich-Steininger, 1992; Sacher, 1991). Median survival for patients in acute blastic transformation is 3 months with treatment and 6 weeks or less without treatment (Sacher, 1991). CML patients without the Philadelphia chromosome (Ph[1]–) have a worse prognosis than those who are Ph[1]+ (Lotspeich-Steininger, 1992).

TABLE 4–3. Differentiation of CML and Leukemoid Reactions

	CML	**Leukemoid Reaction**
Blasts	Usually 1% to 5%	Uncommon
White cell count	Markedly elevated	Moderately elevated
Anemia	Mild; normocytic and normochromic	Absent
Platelet count	Usually increased (450,000 to 600,000)	Usually normal to slightly increased
LAP/NAP[1]	Decreased[1]	Normal or increased
Splenomegaly	Present in almost all cases	Usually absent
Philadelphia chromosome	Present in most cases	Absent

[1]Leukocyte (or neutrophil) alkaline phosphatase; underlying infection in CML will alter results.

Agnogenic (idiopathic) **myeloid metaplasia** (AMM), alternately referred to as *myelofibrosis with myeloid metaplasia* (MMM) and *idiopathic myelofibrosis,* is an uncommon condition that may sometimes be confused with CML. (Table 4–4 lists some aids in distinguishing the two conditions.) This condition is characterized by replacement of the bone marrow with fibrous tissue, unregulated proliferation of granulocytic precursors, and enlargement of the spleen and liver due to a proliferation of granulocytes in these organs. Like CML, AMM is a condition for which the onset is usually insidious, that occurs most often after age 50, and in which patients may first present with symptoms including fatigue, weight loss, and abdominal fullness. Splenomegaly, often marked, is generally present. Hepatomegaly is common and lymphadenopathy may be present in occasional cases. Mild to moderate anemia is often present and is usually normocytic and normochromic, although some red cells may be hypochromic and show basophilic stippling (Henry, 1996).

Peripheral blood smears reveal prominent dacrocytes along with a notable degree of anisocytosis and poikilocytosis. Other common findings on the peripheral smear, especially as the disease progresses, include nucleated red cells, often

TABLE 4–4. Differentiation of CML and AMM

	CML	**AMM**
Nucleated red cells	Occ/few	Often numerous
Dacrocytes	Few	Numerous; prominent feature
Abnormal platelets	Occ	Numerous
Megakaryocyte fragments	Occ	Numerous
LAP	Decreased	Normal to increased
Ph[1]	Often present	Absent

LAP = leukocyte alkaline phosphatase; Ph[1] = Philadelphia chromosome; occ = occasional data compiled from various sources.

in numbers above that expected for the degree of anemia present; giant platelets and other platelet abnormalities, including agranularity; megakaryocyte fragments, and immature neutrophils with an occasional myeloblast. White blood cell counts may be normal, but are usually moderately increased, with the typical count for AMM falling in the 12,000 to 50,000/mm^3 range (Ravel, 1995). Platelet counts are usually normal or decreased, but increased counts are occasionally seen. Patients may develop a significant thrombocytopenia as a consequence of splenic sequestration and resultant purpura and bleeding tendencies. Platelet function may also be abnormal and produce bleeding disorders even in the presence of a normal or increased platelet count.

Bone marrow aspiration is often difficult to impossible (dry tap) in AMM, especially later in the disease, and a surgical biopsy may be necessary to obtain a marrow sample. In early stages, the bone marrow may show normal cellularity, but often shows hypercellularity, with panmyelosis and increased megakaryocytes with numerous atypical, dysplastic forms. Later in the course of the disease the marrow shows extensive replacement with fibrous tissue. Osteosclerosis (hardening of the bone) may develop in the end stages of AMM and is demonstrated by increasing bone density.

Patients who are asymptomatic at diagnosis generally have a survival period of about 5 years. However, a significant number of patients present in the later stages of the disease and often survive < 1 year (Sacher, 1991). Most patients die from complications of marrow failure, including hemorrhage, infections, and cardiac complications. Some patients, especially those with a longer period of survival, terminate in acute leukemia.

Essential thrombocytosis is characterized by a proliferation of the cells of the megakaryocytic line resulting in significantly elevated platelet counts, often > 1 million/μL. This is one of the least common myeloproliferative disorders and has a better prognosis than the other conditions in this group. The prognosis is particularly good in younger patients. Patients may present with either bleeding tendencies (as a result of abnormal platelet function), especially bleeding of the gastrointestinal tract or mucous membranes, or with thrombotic symptoms related to the marked elevation in the number of platelets. About half of patients have a mild splenomegaly.

The most prominent laboratory finding is the markedly increased platelet count, with the peripheral smear showing large aggregates of platelets, giant platelets, and a number of abnormal, bizarre platelet shapes. Poikilocytosis may be present, particularly if splenic function is impaired. Bone marrow examination typically reveals a marked increase in the number of megakaryocytes with significant platelet debris and large masses of aggregated platelets.

The term **myelodysplastic syndrome** is used to refer to a group of disorders characterized by ineffective hematopoiesis, abnormal cellular maturation, and a hypercellular bone marrow. Unstable growth may be seen in the development of the erythroid cell line (*dyserythropoiesis*), the granulocytic cell line (*dysgranulopoiesis*), or the megakaryocytic cell line (*dysmegakaryocytopoiesis*). Abnormalities may occur in any one or in a combination of these cell lines. In contrast to the hypercellularity of the bone marrow, varying degrees of cytopenia are present in the peripheral blood, reflecting the ineffective cellular growth and maturation. These conditions are sometimes referred to as preleukemic because of the number of cases that eventually progress to an acute leukemic condition. However, less than half of these cases actually evolve into an acute leukemia. The five myelodysplastic syndromes defined by FAB nomenclature are summarized in Table 4–5.

LYMPHOPROLIFERATIVE DISORDERS

The lymphoproliferative disorders include conditions in which there is unregulated growth and proliferation of cell in the lymphoid cell line. These conditions may be acute or chronic and include both leukemias and lymphomas (see the distinction earlier in this chapter). Lymphoproliferative disorders can be subdivided based on several criteria:

- functional characteristics: into T cell disorders or B cell disorders
- morphology: FAB classifications
- immunologic characteristics
- cytochemical reactions

Acute Lymphoproliferative Disorders

In acute lymphoproliferative disorders, there is little cellular differentiation to maturity with blast forms predominating. **Acute lymphoblastic leukemia** (ALL) is primarily a disease of childhood with the greatest frequency between the ages of 2 and 10 years (Lotspeich-Steininger, 1992). Although the onset of ALL is clinically similar to that of other acute leukemias, the onset is typically much more sudden. The **signs and symptoms** of ALL (eg, anemia, granulocytopenia, thrombocytopenia) are often related to the replacement of normal bone marrow cells with the abnormal lymphoid cells characteristic of these conditions. Patients commonly present with fatigue, malaise, and pallor as a result of anemia. Easy bruising, petechiae, or bleeding may be present depending upon the degree of thrombocytopenia. Chills and fever may be present, as granulocytopenia increases the patient's susceptibility to infections. **Physical examination** commonly reveals a generalized lymphadenopathy. Splenomegaly and hepatomegaly are common findings. A number of other symptoms may be present as a consequence of tissue infiltration by the abnormal cells. Such infiltrates may occur in a variety of tissues throughout the body with resultant symptoms (eg, bone and large joint pain from infiltrates in bone or joint tissues; neurologic symptoms like headache, nausea, vomiting, cranial nerve paralysis, and increased intracranial pressure resulting from meningeal infiltrates).

In terms of **laboratory findings**, many ALL patients have an increased white cell count, some markedly so, but counts may also be normal or leukopenic. Immature lymphocytes and lymphoblasts predominate on the peripheral smear

TABLE 4-5. Myelodysplastic Syndromes

FAB Term	Other Terms	Laboratory Findings	Comments
Refractory anemia (RA)	Chronic erythemic myelosis	Anemia; normocytic/normochromic or macrocytic Decreased reticulocytes Hypercellular bone marrow (may be normocellular) Erythroid hyperplasia/dyserythropoiesis in marrow < 5% blasts	Least likely of syndromes to transform into acute leukemia More common in elderly
Refractory anemia with ringed sideroblasts (RARS)	Acquired idiopathic sideroblastic anemia	Findings as in RA above with: Ring sideroblasts in ≥ 15% of erythroid cells Anemia usually hypochromic, microcytic Serum iron and % saturation usually increased	About 10% of cases transform to acute leukemia
Refractory anemia with excess blasts (RAEB)	Acute myeloproliferative syndrome	Anemia Cytopenia of two or three cell lines < 5% peripheral blasts and 5% to 10% of marrow blasts Hypercellular marrow; variable erythroid or granulocytic hyperplasia Pseudo Pelger-Huet seen in some cases	About 30% transform to ANLL, thus RAEB sometimes called subacute leukemia
RAEB in transformation	Primary acquired panmyelopathy with myeloblastosis (PAMP)	Similar to RAEB, but with > 5% circulating blasts and 20% to 30% marrow blasts More severe anemia Auer rods	Advanced stage of RAEB More refractory to chemo than ANLL Intermediate between RAEB and ANLL
Chronic myelomonocytic leukemia	Subacute myelomonocytic leukemia	Absolute moncytosis with many atypical or immature monocytes < 5% blasts Frequent neutrophilia with abnormal morphology Marrow picture similar to RAEB but often with increased promonocytes/other monocyte precursors	

Data for table compiled from various sources.

and very few neutrophils are observed. A normochromic anemia, often pronounced, is typically present with reticulocytopenia and moderate to marked thrombocytopenia. Lymphoblasts are the predominant cell in the bone marrow and erythroid and granulocytic cells are significantly decreased. **Definitive laboratory diagnosis** of ALL requires **cytochemical testing** with Sudan Black B or peroxidase. Blasts are negative in both of these tests as well as with naphthol ASD chloroacetate esterase.

Acute lymphoblastic leukemia is divided into three **FAB classifications** (L1, L2, L3) based on morphologic characteristics, including cell size, characteristics of the nucleus (chromatin, nuclear shape, presence and appearance of nucleoli), and cytoplasmic characteristics (amount, appearance, vacuolization). Of the three types, **L1**, which has small homogeneous cells with scanty cytoplasm and either inconspicuous or indistinct nucleoli, has the best prognosis. **L3**, or Burkitt's type, has larger, fairly uniform cells with prominent vacuolization of a deeply basophilic cytoplasm and one or more prominent nucleoli, and has the worst prognosis. **L2** has a prognosis intermediate between L1 and L3 and has large heterogeneous cells with an irregularly shaped nucleus, variable amounts of cytoplasm, and one or more nucleoli that are often large.

Acute lymphoblastic leukemia can also be classified using monoclonal antibodies to detect various **immunological cell markers**. This system divides ALL into four immunophenotypes. A combination of cytochemical techniques and immunologic markers can be used to divide ALL into six subgroups as summarized in Table 4–6.

An increased knowledge of the acute lymphoblastic leukemias and a variety of improved treatment options have greatly improved the prognosis for ALL. Prior to 1950, 80% of children with ALL died within 8 months of diagnosis (Sacher, 1991). Today children survive for significantly longer intervals, often with disease-free intervals of a year or more, and about half eventually achieve a long-term disease-free state requiring no further therapy. Whether treatment is chemotherapy or bone marrow transplantation, the objective is to eradicate every malignant cell to prevent a recurrence of the disease. Bone marrow transplantation, if it is to be used as a treatment approach, is usually performed during the first remission. Achieving the goal of complete eradication of malignant cells is not without risk and is often accompanied by severe pancytopenia, leaving the patient with significant anemia and vulnerable to infection (granulocytopenia) and bleeding tendencies (thrombocytopenia). Thus patients require close monitoring during therapy and may require transfusion support and aggressive antibiotic therapy.

Chronic Leukemic Lymphoproliferative Disorders

In chronic leukemias involving the lymphoid cell line, greater differentiation and maturity of cells are observed. Three separate disorders make up this group, but the vast majority involves the unregulated growth and proliferation of B lymphocytes. Only a small percentage of disorders in this group involve proliferation of T lymphocytes, but those that do generally have a poorer prognosis and response to therapy (Lotspeich-Steininger, 1992). The malignant B cells have a much longer survival rate than do normal B cells, which contributes (along with an increased rate of production) to their massive accumulation.

TABLE 4–6. ALL Subgroups Based on Immunologic Cell Markers and Cytochemical Testing

Subgroup	Immunologic Cell Markers	Cytochemical Testing	FAB	Comments
Unclassified ALL (uALL)	Cells lack T cell antigens, common ALL antigen, sheep RBC receptors, and surface immunoglobulins	Negative reaction with acid phosphatase and α-napthyl acetate esterase	L1/L2	10% of childhood cases 40% of adult cases
Common ALL (cALL)	Cells lack T cell antigens, sheep RBC receptors, and surface immunoglobulins	Negative reaction with acid phosphatase and α-napthyl acetate esterase	L1/L2	75% of childhood cases; 40% of adult; highest remission rate; longest remission after chemo
Pre-T ALL	Cells lack sheep RBC receptors and surface immunoglobulins; has T cell antigens	Positive acid phosphatase; negative α-napthyl acetate esterase	L1/L2	
T ALL	Has T cell antigens and sheep RBC receptors; lacks common ALL antigens and surface immunoglobulins	Positive acid phosphatase and weakly positive with α-napthyl acetate esterase	L1/L2	Many patients have mediastinal mass; very high white cell count common; higher rate of CNS involvement; poorer prognosis
Pre-B ALL	Cells lack T cell antigens, sheep RBC receptors and surface immunoglobulins; has cytoplasmic immunoglobulin (only pre-B and B have this marker) and common ALL antigen	Negative reaction with acid phosphatase and α-napthyl acetate esterase	L1/L2	
B ALL	Cells lack T call antigens, sheep RBC receptors, and common ALL antigens; has cytoplasmic and surface immunoglobulins	Negative reaction with acid phosphatase and α-napthyl acetate esterase	L3	< 5% of cases; poor prognosis

Percent of cases from Lotspeich-Steininger C, Stiene-Martin A, Koepke J. *Clinical Hematology: Principles, Procedures, Correlations.* Philadelphia, Lippincott, 1992.

Chronic lymphocytic leukemia (CLL) occurs nearly exclusively in adults over the age of 40 (usually in those > 50 or 60) and comprises about 30 % of all leukemia cases (Ravel, 1995). Occurring twice as frequently in men as in women, the disease begins insidiously and progresses slowly over several years. It is commonly diagnosed as a result of findings in a routine examination or unexpected findings during the course of examination or treatment for other conditions. In other instances, **symptoms** including enlarged lymph nodes, fatigue, weakness, and, in more advanced stages, bruising, fever, persistent infections, anorexia, and weight loss may prompt the patient to seek medical attention. Hepatosplenomegaly may also be present. In most cases of CLL, the proliferating B cells have no detectable immunologic activity and thus are functionally inert. As these non-functional cells crowd out the normal B cells, immune function is impaired, leaving the individual at heightened risk of infection. Impaired function involves both humoral immunity (recall the role of B cells in immunoglobulin production) and cellular immunity (accumulation of inert B-cells impedes movement of granulocytes and monocytes in an immune response).

Laboratory findings include a white cell count that is typically between 30 and 200 × 10^9/L (Henry, 1996), but may occasionally be significantly lower or markedly higher. The majority of lymphocytes observed on the peripheral smear are small and relatively normal in appearance, although there may be some variation in nuclear chromatin. Anemia and thrombocytopenia are not evident until later stages of the disease and although the percentage of neutrophils on a differential count from a peripheral smear is likely to be decreased, absolute numbers are typically normal until later in the disease. **Marrow findings** may be equivocal early in CLL because marrow infiltration occurs slowly. When a sustained peripheral lymphocytosis is present, 30 % or more of lymphocytes in the bone marrow is considered diagnostic for CLL (Lotspeich-Steininger, 1992).

Symptoms, laboratory findings, and the expected length of survival are dependent upon the clinical stage of the disease at the time of diagnosis. The clinical stages of CLL are summarized below (Sacher, 1991).

10 to 20 year survival	Stage 0:	peripheral and marrow lymphocytosis only
	Stage I:	lymphadenopathy present (along with lymphocytosis)
	Stage II:	additional finding of splenomegaly, hepatomegaly, or both
< 5 year median survival	Stage III:	additional finding of anemia (hemoglobin < 11 g/dL)
	Stage IV:	additional finding of thrombocytopenia (plt. count < 100,000/mm^3)

Chronic lymphocytic leukemia is treated with agents aimed at controlling proliferation of the lymphocytes and preventing marrow replacement, as the eradication of all malignant cells is not possible because of the widespread proliferation before the disease becomes apparent. Therapy involves chemotherapeutic agents to reduce the number of abnormal cells in the blood and the tissues. The concurrent destruction of normal red cells, granulocytes, and platelets may produce anemia, granulocytopenia, and thrombocytopenia with related symptoms and complications. Radiation may be used for enlarged lymph nodes or splenomegaly not sufficiently responsive to chemotherapy. Leukapheresis may be employed to reduce the number of circulating lymphocytes in some cases (Lotspeich-Steininger, et al, 1992).

Prolymphocytic leukemia (PLL) is an uncommon, but aggressive chronic leukemic lymphoproliferative disorder. It is rapidly progressive, with survival rates typically < 1 year. Like the other chronic disorders with which it is grouped, PLL typically occurs in older adults. It is somewhat more frequent in males. Unlike CLL, the onset of PLL is rather acute. Patients characteristically present with a marked elevation of the white cell count in conjunction with anemia and thrombocytopenia. The proliferating cells are most often prolymphocytes and have potential for rapid growth. PLL patients commonly have striking enlargement of the spleen. Hepatomegaly may also be present, but lymphadenopathy is not a common finding. Nearly complete bone marrow replacement by prolymphocyte infiltration is a typical finding. PLL has a poor prognosis and is less responsive to treatment than CLL (Lotspeich-Steininger et al, 1992).

Hairy cell leukemia (HCL), also called *leukemic reticuloendotheliosis,* is a third chronic leukemic lymphoproliferative disorder. Its name is indicative of the distinctive morphology of the proliferating cell, which has a number of fine, hair-like cytoplasmic projections. These cells, usually B cell subgroups, have a uniform, loose and lacy chromatin pattern, similar to that of monocytes, and one or two small, sometimes inconspicuous nucleoli. This disorder can mimic CLL, but differentiation is essential due to distinct differences in treatment. Hairy cells contain a specific acid phosphatase isoenzyme that is resistant to tartrate inhibition (ie, positive tartrate resistant acid phosphatase [TRAP] test), unlike the cells in CLL. Patients characteristically have splenomegaly that may be marked. Symptoms include those characteristic of related disorders such as weakness, fatigue, anemia, bleeding tendencies, and infection. A feeling of abdominal fullness may result from splenomegaly and hepatomegaly. Lymphadenopathy may be present. Pancytopenia or cytopenia in two cell lines is a consistent laboratory finding. Bone marrow aspiration is difficult in most cases of HCL as a result of fibrous tissue in the marrow. Examination reveals variable cellularity and an increase in reticulin fibers. Large numbers of hairy cells are typically present. Splenectomy is a beneficial treatment in most cases, especially for patients in whom cytopenia is severe, as cells may be sequestered in this organ. Interferon may induce remission (Henry, 1996), but aggressive use of the alkylating chemotherapeutic agents typically used in lymphoid disorders may be inadequate in reduction of the tumor burden, with benefits outweighed by their toxicity worsening cytopenia (Lotspeich-Steininger, 1992). Median survival is 5 to 6 years (Henry, 1996).

Lymphomas

The term *lymphoma* is used to refer to a group of malignant neoplasms involving unregulated growth of lymphoid cells and primarily involving lymphoid tissues, particularly the lymph nodes and the spleen. Lymphomas usually begin in the lymph nodes, but may originate in the spleen or gastrointestinal tract (Henry, 1996). Other lymphoid tissues are involved as the disease progresses. The lymphomas are divided into two groups: Hodgkin's disease and non-Hodgkin's lymphomas.

Hodgkin's disease involves a cellular infiltrate with greater morphologic variability than that seen with other lymphomas. The cells found in the lymph nodes in Hodgkin's disease are predominately normal in appearance or normal cells reacting to the presence of the neoplasm, rather than the neoplastic cells themselves (Henry, 1996; Lotspeich-Steininger, 1992). The neoplastic cell is a large, multinucleated cell with large eosinophilic nucleoli and is called the **Reed-Sternberg cell** for the two men who initially characterized this distinctive cell. Definitive diagnosis of Hodgkin's disease is made only by lymph node biopsy, although some laboratory data may be suggestive of the disease.

Hodgkin's disease may occur at virtually any age, but is seen with greater frequency in the 15 to 35 year age group, with increased incidence also occurring after age 50. Patients commonly present with enlarged but painless lymph nodes, most frequently in the neck. Patients who present with symptoms of fever, weight loss, and night sweats (B symptoms) are likely to have a poorer prognosis than those who are asymptomatic. The disease is sometimes detected based on the presence of a mediastinal mass revealed on a chest x-ray.

Based on cellular morphology, Hodgkin's disease is divided into four subgroups (see Table 4–7) in what is called the Rye classification system. All of these subtypes have the diagnostic Reed-Sternberg cell, but differ in terms of the number of these cells present and the degree of lymphocyte infiltration, as well as in terms of prognosis.

Overall, about 85% of Hodgkin's disease cases result in long-term remission with treatment (Sacher, 1991). Patients are typically monitored at regular intervals for evidence of relapse.

Hodgkin's disease typically starts in one group of lymph nodes and spreads to adjacent lymph nodes in a regular, predictable manner, and in advanced cases, to non-lymphatic tissues. This orderly, predictable progression is beneficial to the clinical staging of the disease at the time of diagnosis. The stage at which Hodgkin's disease is detected has prognostic and therapeutic implications. There are four major **clinical stages** (stage 3 is further divided). Each stage may be further clarified by the addition of a suffix (A to indicate a lack of symptoms; B to denote the presence of symptoms, including fever, night sweats, and weight loss) and/or of a subscript (E indicating extralymphatic disease involvement; or S denoting splenic involvement). Table 4–8 summarizes the clinical stages of Hodgkin's disease, with corresponding treatments and cure rates.

As noted previously, Hodgkin's disease must be diagnosed on the basis of a lymph node biopsy. Laboratory testing cannot be used to establish or rule out this diagnosis. However, certain findings are often associated with this condition. A mild normochromic, normocytic anemia may be present in early stages of the disease and become more severe in later stages. Moderate leukocytosis, often accompanied by eosinophilia, is typical of early stages with leukopenia more common in later stages. Platelet counts are generally normal or increased early in the disease

TABLE 4–7. Hodgkin's Disease Subgroups

Subgroup	Characteristics	Reed-Sternberg Cells	Prognosis	% of Cases
Lymphocyte predominant	Abundant lymphocytes; diffuse infiltrate of mature cells; no fibrosis; scanty granulocytes and plasma cells	Few	Best; 95% at 5-year survival	7
Nodular sclerosis	Birefringent bands of collagen enclosing nodules of lymphoid tissue; moderate lymphocytes, granulocytes, and plasma cells; RS cells in clear zone—called *lacunar cells*, an RS variant	Ocasionally; lacunar variant present	Second best; 85% at 5-year survival	68
Mixed cellularity	Diffuse lymphocyte infiltrate; moderate lymphocytes, granulocytes, and plasma cells	Numerous	Third best; 65% at 5-year survival	23
Lymphocyte depletion	Few lymphocytes; diffuse fibrosis and decreased cellularity	Occasionally numerous; bizarre shaped	Worst; 20% at 5-year survival	2

Five-year survival rates from Lotspeich-Steininger C, Stiene-Martin A, Koepke J. *Clinical Hematology: Principles, Procedures, Correlations.* Philadelphia, Lippincott, 1992

TABLE 4-8. Clinical Stages of Hodgkin's Disease

Stage	Description	Treatment	Approximate Cure Rate
I	One group of lymph nodes involved	IA and IB usually responsive to radiation alone	~90%
II	Two or more groups of lymph nodes involved; either both above diaphragm or both below diaphragm	IIA usually responsive to radiation alone; IIB may be responsive to radiation alone or may require chemotherapy	IIA: ~90% IIB: ~70%; relapse rate higher with radiation alone
III	Lymph node regions both above and below diaphragm involved III$_1$: abdominal involvement only in upper abdomen above renal artery III$_2$: abdominal involvement below renal artery	IIIA (subgroup 1 or 2): radiation with chemotherapy; may respond to radiation alone, but relapse is higher IIIB: combination chemotherapy	IIIA: 70% IIB: 80%
IV	Diffuse extranodal involvement (including bone marrow and liver) in sites not contiguous with lymph nodes	Combination chemotherapy	55–70% free of disease after 5 years

Treatment and cure rates from Lotspeich-Steininger C, Stiene-Martin A, Koepke J. *Clinical Hematology: Principles, Procedures, Correlations.* *Philadelphia, Lippincott, 1992* with thrombocytopenia more likely with disease progression. Hodgkin's disease, as well as non-Hodgkin's lymphomas, may produce a false positive result in rapid screening tests for infectious mononucleosis.

Non-Hodgkin's lymphomas are more common in the United States than Hodgkin's disease (Lotspeich-Steininger, 1992) and occur most frequently in older adults. The lymphomas in this group vary in terms of the size of the proliferating cell, the presence or absence of nodularity, and the degree of cellular differentiation. These variations, along with the complexity of lymphocyte differentiation and the lymphocyte subtypes, has resulted in a number of classification systems, ranging from those that are relatively simple and practical to those that are quite complex. The Rappaport classification system introduced over 30 years ago (Henry, 1996) provided a simple, but practical system of classification with prognostic and therapeutic relevance. This system classifies the lymphomas based on two criteria (the type of cell in the infiltrates and the histiopathologic morphology—diffuse or nodular) into three types, designated as lymphocytic lymphoma, histiocytic lymphoma, and undifferentiated lymphoma.

Increased knowledge led to more classification systems and attempts to better describe the diverse histology seen in these disorders, to allow greater accuracy in terms of functional characteristics, and to classify the different immunologic subtypes. In an effort to reduce the confusion arising from the array of classification systems, a group of experts brought together by the National Cancer Institute (NCI) developed an **International Working Formulation** aimed at translating between the different classifications and at integrating the advantages of various systems. This system resulted in improved agreement in the classification of lymphomas and is widely, though not universally, accepted. Other classification systems continue to be developed based, in many cases, on new knowledge of the lymphomas but are not yet widely accepted. For instance, the Working Formulation was published in 1982 before universal recognition of the importance of T lymphocytes and B lymphocytes to a system of classification (Henry, 1996). In addition, new entities have been described during this time period. The non-Hodgkin's lymphomas (NHLs) are discussed here in terms of the classification in the Working Formulation. In this system, the lymphomas are classified based on clinical outcome (which is highly dependent on histologic patterns) and ranked in terms of the aggressiveness of the disease. This system results in three grades: low, intermediate, and high, with each grade composed of distinct types of lymphomas. Table 4–9 summarizes the NHLs using Working Formulation grades.

Diagnosis of non-Hodgkin's lymphomas must be made by lymph node biopsy. Blood counts are usually normal in these conditions. Thrombocytopenia may be present in come cases. Some patients with follicular or small cell lymphomas may develop an autoimmune hemolytic anemia (Lotspeich-Steininger, 1992).

TABLE 4–9. Non-Hodgkin's Lymphomas with Working Formulation Classification

Grade	Lymphoma with Cell Type and Morphology	Infiltrate Pattern	Initial Marrow Involvement	Median Survival	Comments
Low	Small lymphocytic (SL); small lymphocytes with clumped chromatin-like normal mature lymphs	Diffuse	Frequent; early	5–7 yrs	Slow growing; lymph nodes may be enlarged long before diagnosis, at which time disease is often in stage 3 or 4
	Follicular, predominately small cleaved cell (FSC); lymphocyte with less condensed nuclear chromatin, scant cytoplasm, and clefted or indented nucleus	Nodular			
	Follicular, mixed small cleaved and large cell (FM); mixture of large and small cleaved lymphs; large non-cleaved lymphs with multiple nucleoli also present	Nodular			
Intermediate	Follicular, predominantly large cell (FL); large, cleaved lymphocytes predominate with large, non-cleaved lymphocytes also present	Diffuse	Less frequent, especially with DM and DL	1.5–3 yrs; DL may be longer	More rapid lymph node enlargement; extranodal involvement (except marrow) more common
	Diffuse, small cleaved cell (DSC); small lymphocytes with scanty cytoplasm and irregular, often cleaved, nuclear membrane	Diffuse			
	Diffuse mixed (DM); mixture of small and large lymphocytes	Diffuse			
	Diffuse, large cell (DL); large cleaved and non-cleaved lymphocytes with moderately abundant cytoplasm and (usually) multiple nucleoli	Diffuse			
High	Large cell immunoblastic (IBL); large lymphocytes with oval nuclei; ≥ 1 prominent nucleoli; three subtypes: plasmacytoid—eccentric nucleus, clear cell-central nucleus and clear cytoplasm, polymorphous—small lymphs with twisted nucleus and larger lymphs with clear cytoplasm	Diffuse	Occasional	1.3 yrs.	May involve B or T cells; fast developing; rapidly fatal if not treated; responds poorly to chemo; survival is often < 1 year
	Lymphoblastic (LBL); lymphocytes with scanty cytoplasm and fine chromatin; nucleus may be convoluted (about half of cases) or round	Diffuse	~ 50% of cases	2 yrs.	Usually involves T cells; may evolve into T cell ALL; may respond to chemo, but relapse is common
	Small, non-cleaved cell (SNC); lymphs intermediate in size between small, cleave lymphs and large lymphs; multiple, small nucleoli; divided into Burkitt's type (cells uniform in size and shape) and non-Burkitt's (cells more heterogenous in size and shape and usually larger than cells in Burkitt's)	Diffuse	Occasional	0.7 yrs.	Aggressive malignancy; involves B cells; sensitive to chemo, but poor prognosis with relapse; high rate of CNS involvement; organ involvement common

Data for table compiled from Henry JB. *Clinical Diagnosis and Management by Laboratory Methods*, 19th ed. Philadelphia, Suanders, 1996; Lotspeich-Steininger C, Stiene-Martin A, Koepke J. *Clinical Hematology: Principles, Procedures, Correlations*. Philadelphia, Lippincott, 1992; Ravel R. *Clinical Laboratory Medicine: Clinical Application of Laboratory Data*, 6th ed. St Louis, Mosby, 1995; and Sacher RA, McPherson RA. *Widmann's Clinical Interpretation of Laboratory Tests*, 10th ed. Philadelphia, FA Davis, 1991

4. SELF TEST

Choose the best response for each item. The answer key may be found in the appendices.

1. **Myeloproliferative and lymphoproliferative disorders are so named based on**
    A. the stem cell line from which the abnormal cells arise
    B. results of serum chemistry tests
    C. the organs within the body in which infiltrates are commonly found

2. **A lymphoproliferative disorder in which the neoplastic cells are confined to a tumor in the lymph nodes would be classified as a/an**
    A. acute leukemia
    B. chronic leukemia
    C. lymphoma
    D. aleukemic leukemia

3. **Myeloproliferative disorders generally occur with higher incidence in**
    A. childhood
    B. adulthood
    C. incidence is similar in all age groups

4. **Current designations of acute leukemia and chronic leukemia are based on**
    A. period of survival following diagnosis
    B. response to treatment with chemotherapeutic agents
    C. number of blast cells in the peripheral blood and/or bone marrow
    D. the clinical stage of the condition at the time of diagnosis

5. **This condition describes a group of related acute leukemias involving cells of the myelocytic, monocytic, erythroid, or megakaryocyte cell lines. Immature cells that are undifferentiated or partially differentiated are predominate.**
    A. ALL
    B. ANLL
    C. CML
    D. AMM

6. This acute nonlymphocytic leukemia is the most frequently occurring of the leukemias in this group. In this condition, ≥ 30% of all nucleated cells are blasts, < 90% of all nonerythroid cells are blasts, and ≥ 10% are promyelocytes or more mature forms.
   A. acute myeloblastic leukemia with maturation (M2)
   B. acute promyelocytic leukemia (M3)
   C. acute myelomonocytic leukemia (M4)
   D. acute myeloblastic leukemia without maturation (M1)

7. This chronic condition begins so insidiously that it is not uncommon for it to be detected based on results of a CBC performed for other reasons. White cell counts are typically markedly elevated and a normochromic, normocytic anemia is common. The majority of patients with this condition have the Philadelphia chromosome and many undergo an acute blastic transformation.
   A. ANLL
   B. CLL
   C. CML
   D. AMML

8. A benign leukocytosis with an increased number of immature cell forms (left shift) that is seen in response to infection is called
   A. acute blastic transformation
   B. leukamoid reaction
   C. aleukemic leukemia
   D. preleukemia

9. This condition is characterized by a proliferation of the cells of the megakaryocytic line resulting in significantly elevated platelet counts, often > 1 million/µL. This is one of the least common myeloproliferative disorders and has a better prognosis than the other conditions in this group.
   A. anogenic myeloid metaplasia
   B. idiopathic thrombocytopenia
   C. acute megakaryocytosis
   D. essential thrombocytosis

10. In this acute lymphoproliferative disorder, blast forms predominate and there is little cellular differentiation. It is primarily a disease of childhood and typically has a quite sudden onset. Leukocytosis, anemia with reticulocytopenia, and moderate to marked thrombocytopenia are common findings.
   A. ANLL
   B. AMM
   C. ALL
   D. CLL

11. Of the three FAB classifications of the condition described in question 10, which has the best prognosis?
   A. L1
   B. L2
   C. L3
   D. prognosis does not differ significantly among the three

12. A combination of cytochemical testing and detection of immunologic markers can be used to divide acute lymphocytic leukemia into six subgroups. Which of these subgroups is seen in the greatest percentage of childhood cases and has the highest remission rate?
   A. unclassified ALL
   B. common ALL
   C. T cell ALL
   D. B cell ALL

13. This ALL subgroup has a higher rate of CNS involvement, and lacks the common ALL antigen and surface immunoglobulins. Many patients have a mediastinal mass and very high white cell counts.
   A. unclassified ALL
   B. common ALL
   C. T cell ALL
   D. B cell ALL

14. The majority of chronic leukemic lymphoproliferative disorders involve the unregulated growth and proliferation of
   A. B cells
   B. T cells
   C. an equally mixed population of B and T lymphocytes
   D. distinction between B and T lymphocytes cannot be made in these cases

15. This chronic leukemic lymphoproliferative disorder can mimic CLL, but must be distinguished because of differences in treatment. The cells in this condition contain an acid phosphatase isoenzyme that is resistant to tartrate inhibition (have a positive TRAP test). Marked splenomegaly is common and bone marrow aspiration is usually difficult. Splenectomy is beneficial in many cases. The characteristic cells of this condition have fine cytoplasmic projections, for which the disease is named.
    A. prolymphocytic leukemia
    B. acute lymphocytic leukemia
    C. hairy cell leukemia

16. Hodgkin's disease is classified as a/an
    A. acute leukemia
    B. chronic leukemia
    C. lymphoma
    D. myelodysplastic syndrome

17. The most common subgroup of Hodgkin's disease is
    A. nodular sclerosis
    B. mixed cellularity
    C. lymphocyte predominant
    D. lymphocyte depletion

18. The Hodgkin's disease subgroup with the *best* prognosis is
    A. nodular sclerosis
    B. mixed cellularity
    C. lymphocyte predominant
    D. lymphocyte depletion

19. The Hodgkin's disease subgroup with the *worst* prognosis is
    A. nodular sclerosis
    B. mixed cellularity
    C. lymphocyte predominant
    D. lymphocyte depletion

20. A definitive diagnosis of a lymphoma is made based on
    A. bone marrow biopsy
    B. laboratory test results
    C. clinical findings and laboratory test results
    D. lymph node biopsy

21. When Hodgkin's disease is diagnosed with involvement in two lymph node regions above the diaphragm and the patient exhibits no symptoms in addition to the lymph node enlargement, the clinical stage of the disease is
    A. IE
    B. IA
    C. IIA
    D. IIB

22. This non-Hodgkin's lymphoma is an aggressive malignancy involving B lymphocytes that has a high rate of CNS involvement. The lymphocytes observed in this lymphoma are intermediate in size between the small, cleaved cells and the large lymphocytes and are divided into Burkitt's and non-Burkitt's types. Which Working Formulation grade includes this lymphoma?
    A. low
    B. moderate
    C. high

23. This high grade lymphoma usually involves T cells and may evolve into a T cell acute lymphocytic leukemia.
    A. lymphoblastic lymphoma (LBL)
    B. immunoblastic lymphoma (IBL)
    C. mixed T cell lymphoma (MTL)
    D. follicular, large cell lymphoma (FL)

5. LIVER FUNCTION TESTS

Before undertaking a study of the tests of hepatic function and the clinical significance of test results, it is important to have a basic understanding of the anatomy and physiology of the hepatic system. Although some of the information provided may be a review for you, this knowledge forms an important basis for understanding, evaluating, and using the results from tests of liver function.

■ MAJOR FUNCTIONS

The hepatic system is one of the major systems involved in the regulation of body functions. It is structured to receive large supplies of blood to carry out multiple functions. The major functions of the liver are as follows:

- major role in metabolism of fat, carbohydrates, and protein
- bilirubin metabolism and bile production
- detoxification of both endogenous and exogenous substances

Hepatocytes make many proteins—both enzymes and transport proteins—required to carry out the functions of the liver as well as some of the constituents necessary for an appropriately functioning clotting system (prothrombin and fibrinogen). The liver also serves as a storage area for a variety of vitamins and other substances.

■ BASIC ANATOMY AND PHYSIOLOGIC FUNCTIONING

The liver is one of the largest organs in the body. It is located in the upper right quadrant of the abdomen under the diaphragm and extends up under the ribs. The liver consists of two lobes and is made up of small lobules composed of hepatic cellular plates. The lobules are the functional units of the liver. A tough fibrous sheath, called Glisson's capsule, completely covers the liver. Strands of connective

173

tissue originating from the capsule enter the liver parenchyma and form the supporting network of the organ and separate the functional units (lobules).

Bile canaliculi run between the cells in the cellular plates. These bile passages converge and open in to each other, finally leading into the hepatic duct, the excretory channel of the liver. The hepatic duct receives the cystic duct and the union of these two ducts forms the common bile duct (ductus choledochus), which enters the duodenum. The gallbladder (vesica fellae) lies under the inferior surface of the liver on the end of the cystic duct. The bile leaving the liver enters the gallbladder, where it undergoes concentration, primarily through the absorption of fluids by the gallbladder mucosa. When bile is needed in the intestine for digestive purposes, the gallbladder contracts and the sphincter (a ring of smooth muscle at the terminal end of the common bile duct) relaxes, permitting escape of the bile. The sphincter is usually contracted, which closes the duodenal entrance and forces bile into the gallbladder after leaving the liver.

Hepatic sinusoids, which receive blood from the portal vein and hepatic artery, lie on opposite sides of the hepatic cells. They are lined with highly phagocytic cells, called Kupffer cells, that remove cellular debris, bacteria, and other foreign particulate matter from the blood stream. The blood supply to the liver is from the hepatic artery, a branch of the celiac artery, and the hepatic portal vein that drains the intestine. After flowing through the hepatic sinusoids, the blood is emptied into the central vein and from there flows into the hepatic vein (Figs. 5–1 to 5–3).

Because it receives blood from the portal vein, the liver is the first organ to receive blood from the intestines, where the blood has absorbed the final products of digestion and decomposition products. Through a variety of enzymatic activities, the liver is able to:

- oxidize fats, carbohydrates, and proteins for energy
- produce compounds for storage and later use from fat, carbohydrates, and protein
- use fat, carbohydrate, and protein to make other needed compounds

In *carbohydrate metabolism,* the liver removes glucose from the blood, from which it synthesizes glycogen, which is then stored. Glucose not stored as glycogen or used to form amino acids is converted to fatty acids, carbon dioxide, and water. The liver is also primarily responsible for the metabolism of galactose. The liver deaminates amino acids, forming ammonia, which is converted to urea in *protein metabolism.* It also incorporates amino acids into proteins and synthesizes essential proteins, including albumin, some globulins, and clotting factors such as prothrombin and fibrinogen. In *fat metabolism* the liver is responsible for the production of phospholipids, lipoproteins, and cholesterol.

A major role of the liver lies in the *detoxification* (biotransformation) of various substances absorbed into the blood from the intestines. It has an important role in the detoxification of many drugs, including most barbiturates and sedatives, which are inactivated by the liver. The effectiveness and toxicity of these and

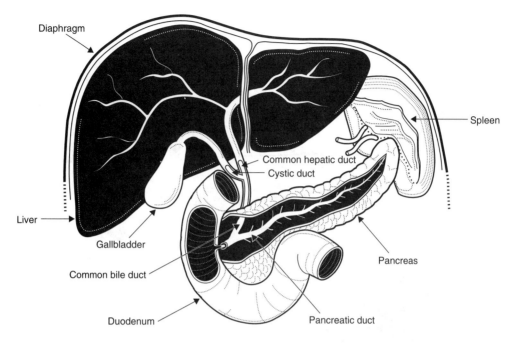

Diaphragm

Spleen

Liver

Gallbladder

Common bile duct

Duodenum

Common hepatic duct

Cystic duct

Pancreas

Pancreatic duct

FIGURE 5–1. Location and basic features of the liver.

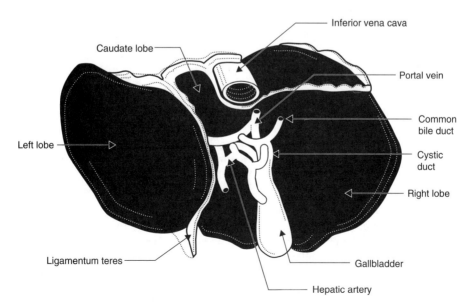

Inferior vena cava

Caudate lobe

Portal vein

Common bile duct

Cystic duct

Left lobe

Right lobe

Ligamentum teres

Gallbladder

Hepatic artery

FIGURE 5–2. Features of the liver.

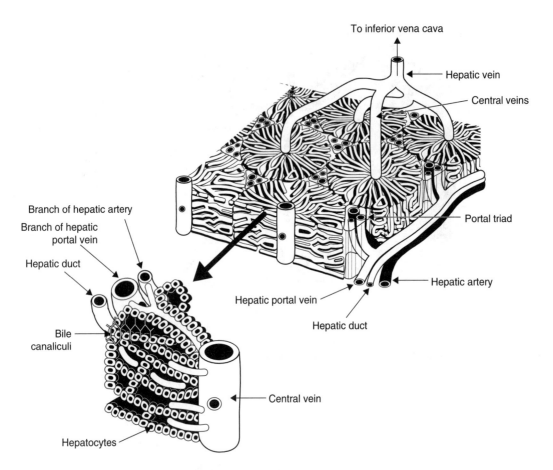

FIGURE 5–3. Liver lobules.

other drugs are highly dependent upon the status of the liver. In addition, the liver inactivates hormones, including corticosteriods, aldosterone, and estrogen. Pathophysiologic levels of these hormones may be due to the liver's inability to inactivate them.

As explained in Chapter 2, bilirubin is a by-product of the heme portion of red cells released when these cells are destroyed. To review the liver's role in *bilirubin metabolism,* recall that indirect (unconjugated) bilirubin, which is not soluble in water, is bound with albumin and transported to the liver. In the liver, indirect bilirubin is combined with glucuronic acid to form a water-soluble compound, direct (conjugated) bilirubin, which is secreted into the bile. The bilirubin in bile is secreted into the duodenum and broken down by bacterial action in the intestines to form urobilinogen. Small amounts of urobilinogen are excreted into the urine, but the major excretion is in feces and as much as 50 % is reabsorbed into the portal circulation.

The liver is also the source of the anticoagulant heparin, the source of red cells in the fetus, and the main site for the production of plasma proteins. In addition, it is responsible for storage of vitamin B_{12} and the fat-soluble vitamins A, D, E, and K. The liver is one of the main sources of body heat and plays a role in the regulation of blood volume.

TESTS OF HEPATIC STATUS

The role of laboratory determinations in assessing the status of the liver has been continuously evolving and has changed dramatically over the past 50 years. The most widely used tests in the 1950s are no longer available, having been replaced by more specific indicators of cellular integrity and function. Most testing is now performed by automated instruments, often in panels, so details of test performance and the chemical reactions involved will not be dealt with in this text. Rather, the focus will be on what the determinations measure, what the results signify, and how to interpret the results in different settings.

As with tests of renal function in Chapter 2, knowledge of the organ's normal functions leads to methods for monitoring its status in health and disease. In the case of the liver, the activity of several enzymes, the concentrations of several proteins, and substances synthesized or stored by the liver can be used to estimate the status of the liver, including the integrity of hepatocellular organelles and membranes, the ability to synthesize or convert various compounds, and the ability to excrete bile.

■ ENZYMES

Measurement of most substances is based on the determination of their concentration in serum or the amount excreted in urine or bile in a given time. Enzymes, however, are measured by their activity or how rapidly or extensively they perform their catalytic functions. Activity depends on a number of factors, including inhibitors, promoters, cofactors, energy supply, and substrate concentrations. For this reason, results of enzyme determinations are not concentrations, but rather are expressed in terms of substrate consumed or end product made. This is referred to as *enzyme activity.*

Aminotransferases

The aminotransferases are enzymes that catalyze the transfer of an amino group of one amino acid to a ketoacid to form a different amino acid. These enzymes include aspartate aminotransferase, or AST (SGOT), and alanine aminotransferase, or ALT (SGPT). The activity of these enzymes has been used as an indicator of hepatocellular damage for many years.

AST reversibly transfers the amino group of aspartic acid to alpha-ketoglutaric acid to form oxalacetic acid and glutamic acid. It has a blood half life of 17 hours and is present in many organs other than the liver, including the heart and muscle. In the liver, 80% of the AST is found in the mitochondria of the cells (Henry, 1996).

ALT reversibly transfers the amino group of alanine to alpha-ketoglutamic acid to form pyruvic acid and glutamic acid. It has a blood half life of 47 hours and is found primarily in the liver. ALT is not found in the same intracellular location as AST, but is located elsewhere in the cytoplasm. The different locations of these enzymes has led to observations about their role in the diagnosis and prognosis of liver disease—ie, with mild hepatocellular injury more cytoplasmic ALT and AST are released; with severe injury, mitochondrial damage would result in release of mitochondrial AST, increasing the AST:ALT ratio.

CLINICAL SIGNIFICANCE. Elevations in both ALT and AST may be seen in any condition involving hepatocellular injury.

ALT:
- more specific for liver injury than AST because AST is also found in heart and muscle
- more sensitive for detection of injury to hepatocytes than for biliary obstruction
- useful for hepatic cirrhosis
- screening test for hepatitis
- increased in Reye syndrome
- usually increased to greater degree than AST in acute or chronic viral hepatitis
- less sensitive than AST to alcoholic liver disease
- in children with acute lymphoblastic leukemia, high ALT on diagnosis is associated with a rapidly progressive disease

AST:
- low in uremia
- increased in cirrhosis
- elevated in chronic alcohol ingestion, hepatitis, and Reye syndrome
- increased in other liver diseases such as hemachromatosis and chemical toxicity
- increased in some instances of cholecystitis
- peaks about 24 hours after myocardial infarction; returns to normal in 3 to 4 days

AST/ALT Ratio:
- normally 1 or slightly more
- often < 1 in acute hepatocellular injury
- value of 3 or 4:1 can be found with near normal ALT in alcoholic liver disease

AST:ALT ratios are highest in alcoholic liver disease, but are often somewhat elevated in cirrhosis. The ratio is commonly reduced with viral hepatitis.

Acetaminophen hepatotoxicity can also produce an AST that is greater than the ALT by a considerable margin. Mild to severe coagulopathy is characteristicly present as well. (In alcoholics, even apparently moderate doses of acetaminophen have caused severe hepatoxicity.)

LIMITATIONS. A number of drugs, including heparin therapy, cause ALT increases and may warrant evaluation for hepatotoxicity. Grossly hemolyzed specimens may generate spurious results for ALT and falsely elevated AST. Increases in AST are not specific for liver damage and must be evaluated in conjunction with other test results and the patient's clinical picture.

Reference Range: AST = 8 to 38 IU/L; ALT = 8 to 48 IU/L.

 TIME FOR REVIEW. After studying the preceding sections, you should be able to respond correctly to the following:

■ List three major functions of the liver, briefly describing its role in each.

■ List the two aminotransaminases.

■ Why is ALT more specific for liver injury than AST?

■ Which of the aminotransaminases is:

  most sensitive to alcoholic liver disease?

usually higher in viral hepatitis?

at peak 24 hours after myocardial infarction?

■ The AST:ALT ratio is:

normally _____ .

highest in _____ .

commonly reduced with _____ .

Check your responses by reviewing the preceding pages.

Gamma Glutamyl Transferase

Gamma glutamyl transferase, or GGT, is an enzyme that regulates the transport of amino acids across cell membranes by catalyzing the transfer of a glutamyl group from glutathione to a free amino acid. This biliary enzyme is most useful in the diagnosis of obstructive jaundice, intrahepatic cholestasis, and pancreatitis. It is more responsive to biliary obstruction than are the transaminases. It is a sensitive test for detecting hepatocellular injury, but it does not differentiate well among the various liver diseases. GGT activity generally parallels that of alkaline phosphatase (discussed below) in many liver diseases. However, GGT has no origin in bone or placenta, unlike alkaline phosphatase, so age beyond infancy does not influence GGT levels. Unlike AST, it is not elevated in skeletal diseases. The GGT is most often used in conjunction with other test results when evaluating hepatic status.

CLINICAL SIGNIFICANCE. The highest GGT values are obtained in obstructive liver disease or in chronic cholestasis due to primary biliary cirrhosis or sclerosing inflammation of the bile ducts. These values may be ten times or more the upper limit of the normal reference range. In addition, GGT levels are:

- useful in screening for alcoholism (with mean cell volume [MCV] of red cells)—generally increased in alcoholics even without liver disease
- commonly elevated in cirrhosis and hepatitis, but may not be elevated in acute hepatitis; transaminases rise higher in acute viral hepatitis
- increased in hepatoma and carcinoma of pancreas
- useful in diagnosis of metastatic carcinoma in liver—increasing levels relate to tumor progression and decreasing levels to response to treatment
- increased in systemic lupus erythematosus
- increased with hyperthyroidism/decreased with hypothyroidism
- increased in some obese persons without apparent liver disease
- may be increased with large doses of some medications, particularly acetaminophen, with no apparent liver disease
- commonly elevated in infectious mononucleosis
- treatment of hypertriglyceridemia may lead to decreased GGT

LIMITATIONS. GGT does not discriminate well among the various liver diseases and may not be elevated in acute hepatitis. Although it may be considered useful in the diagnosis of metastatic carcinoma in the liver, it should be noted that one study resulted in 19 % of patients with progressive disease having normal values and 4 % of patients with no evidence of tumor with elevated values. It is best used in conjunction with additional laboratory tests. Serial determinations may be useful in some cases.

Alkaline Phosphatase

The alkaline phosphatase enzyme is located in several tissues. In addition to the liver, it is also present in the bone, kidney, intestine, and placenta. The isoenzymes of alkaline phosphatase (AP), separated based on heat stability, may be useful in determining the source of an increase in total AP. Heating the serum to 56°C causes significant inactivation of the AP of bone origin. Hepatic, bone, and renal AP are similar molecules, but the forms found in the intestine and placenta are distinctive. Serum AP activity of intestinal origin is found only in persons of blood groups O and A who are secretors of ABH red cell antigens and carry the Lewis red cell antigen.

Most of the AP present in the serum of normal individuals is from the liver and bone. In the serum, AP is present as either unbound isoenzymes or as complexes with lipoproteins (rarely with immunoglobulins). AP is excreted into the bile. The role of this enzyme differs depending upon its site; its role in the liver has not been clearly determined.

CLINICAL SIGNIFICANCE. When bile flow is impaired or when space-occupying lesions develop, AP rises rapidly and values may exceed ten times the upper limit of the normal reference range.

If bile flow is stopped completely because of intrahepatic or obstructive cholestasis, AP rises to twice or more the upper normal limit, generally in parallel to the increases seen in serum bilirubin levels. With partial obstruction the AP rises as much as with complete obstruction, but the bilirubin level will not rise as much.

A moderate elevation of AP is seen in most instances of jaundice resulting from hepatic injury, which might reflect a minor component of cholestasis. When cholestasis is relieved, AP levels return to normal more slowly than the bilirubin. There is debate as to the reasons for increased AP in cholestasis, but evidence seems to support an increase in enzyme synthesis by the hepatocytes over reduced biliary secretion. However, both mechanisms likely contribute.

Moderate increases may be seen in viral hepatitis, but greater increases would be seen in the transaminases. Increases may be seen in a variety of other conditions, including diabetes mellitus and diabetic hepatic lipidosis; pancreatitis; carcinoma of the pancreas; infectious mononucleosis; and congestive heart failure. Many drugs elevate AP—large doses of estrogen, birth control agents, methyltestosterone, phenothiazines, oral hypoglycemic agents, erythromycin, or any drug producing hypersensitivity or toxic cholestasis.

Other causes of elevated AP include bone growth, healing fractures, acromegaly (a chronic disease characterized by elongation and enlargement of the bones of the extremities and certain bones in the head), osteogenic sarcoma, Paget's disease (skeletal disease of the elderly with chronic bone inflammation causing thickening and softening of bones), and bone metastases. The increase in these instances would be of the bone fraction and are unrelated to liver function.

Intestinal AP is increased in cirrhosis and in a variety of intestinal disorders. Levels are increased during pregnancy (placental); a marked decline in an elevated AP of pregnancy is seen with placental insufficiency and imminent fetal demise.

Alkaline phosphatase may be decreased in some cases of hypothyroidism and in a few patients with pernicious anemia. Some drugs lower AP activity—clofibrate, azathioprine, estrogen and estrogen in combination with androgens.

LIMITATIONS. Results are most accurate on a fasting specimen, as AP elevation may occur 2 to 4 hours after a fatty meal (especially in Lewis positive secretors). Increases are also found in stored specimens. Reference ranges are dependent not only on method, but also on sex and age (bone fraction increased with bone growth). Used alone, AP levels can be misleading. To be useful in the evaluation of hepatic status, the AP must be used in conjunction with other laboratory measures and with the patient's clinical picture.

■ BILIRUBIN

The liver plays an important role in bilirubin metabolism and the excretion of file. As explained in the discussion of the functions of the liver, indirect (unconjugated) bilirubin, which is not soluble in water, is bound with albumin and transported to the liver. In the liver the indirect bilirubin is combined with glucuronic acid to form a water soluble compound, direct (conjugated) bilirubin, which is secreted into the bile. The bilirubin in bile is secreted into the duodenum and broken down by bacterial action in the intestines to form urobilinogen. Small amounts of urobilinogen are excreted into the urine, but the major excretion is to the feces. As much as 50% of the urobilinogen is reabsorbed into the portal circulation.

The *diazo reaction,* which distinguishes between direct and indirect bilirubin, is the most widely used bilirubin method. The names *direct* and *indirect* are derived from the way the two fractions react with a diazo reagent. Conjugated bilirubin reacts immediately with the reagent and thus was called "direct reacting," whereas unconjugated bilirubin reacts with the reagent only after the addition of alcohol and was called "indirect reacting." The majority of current methods measure total bilirubin and direct bilirubin with the difference between the two being calculated and reported as indirect method. However, newer techniques, not in common use, have identified another bilirubin fraction called *delta bilirubin.*

CLINICAL SIGNIFICANCE. (Note that this discussion does not pertain to bilirubin levels seen in newborns [normally higher than those for adults] or to details of increases seen in hemolytic disease of the newborn.) Total bilirubin levels are elevated in liver diseases such as hepatitis, inflammation of the bile ducts, cirrhosis, and primary or secondary neoplasia. Elevations are also seen in alcoholism (usually with high AST, GGT, and MCV), biliary obstruction, and infectious mononucleosis. A moderate increase may be seen in anorexia or with 36 hours or more of fasting. Levels may be elevated in pernicious anemia, hemolytic anemias, hemolytic disease of the newborn (erythroblastosis fetalis), and other neonatal jaundice, after the transfusion of several units of blood in a short period of time, and in hemolytic transfusion reactions as a result of increased red cell destruction.

Hyperbilirubinemia of unconjugated (indirect) bilirubin is seen with pigment overproduction in hemolytic disorders as well as with defects in liver uptake or conjugation. With hemolytic anemia, a rise in indirect bilirubin results from abnormally high hemoglobin levels and a subsequent rate of bilirubin formation exceeding the ability of the liver to conjugate it. A familial hyperbilirubinemia, *Gilbert's disease,* results in an elevation of indirect bilirubin with a normal direct bilirubin. These patients are unable to compensate for the increased bilirubin load above the normal conjugated bilirubin level. In this syndrome, indirect bilirubin accounts for 90% to 99% of the total bilirubin level, whereas, in normal individuals, the percentage is 72% to 90% (Henry, 1996).

In hepatic disease, hyperbilirubinemia is caused by impaired excretion of conjugated bilirubin with enhanced reflux into the serum. The conjugated bilirubin makes up 75% to 80% of the elevation. Bilirubin is elevated in biliary obstruction and the increase is greater than and out of proportion to the transaminases (also true of AP).

A large number of drugs may also be implicated, including diphenylhydantoin, azathioprine, phenothiazines, erythromycin, penicillin, sulfonamides, oral contraceptives, anabolic-androgenic steroids, and several others.

LIMITATIONS. As with other tests of hepatic status, the bilirubin is most useful when evaluated as one component of liver assessment. Differential diagnosis of liver diseases requires total and direct bilirubin levels along with other tests of hepatic function. If serum is very hemolyzed or lipemic, results may be affected.

Reference Range: 0.2 to 1.0 mg/dL (total; adult).

■ SERUM PROTEINS

The evaluation of the levels of several serum proteins may also be of benefit in assessing hepatic status. Two major serum proteins, albumin and globulin, are more frequently used than a number of "special" proteins.

Albumin

Albumin is synthesized by the liver and serves as the transport protein for many substances, both endogenous and exogenous. It is the main osmotic colloid in the plasma. The liver's synthetic rate of albumin can be almost doubled when the level of serum albumin falls. Liver diseases can lead to low albumin values either by altering synthesis, by increasing degradation, or by promoting extra-vascular loss. Alcohol ingestion may also contribute to decreased albumin production in patients with cirrhosis.

When the serum albumin is decreased and the globulins (particularly gamma) are increased, chronic liver disease is generally suspected. Albumin may be low in patients with ascites even with a normal rate of synthesis. Other disease process-es may be additional causes of hypoalbuminemia in patients with liver disease. These diseases include chronic inflammatory diseases, renal disease with albu-minuria, protein losing conditions, and malnutrition. Most measurements of albu-min are based on its ability to bind with dyes (such as bromphenol blue) after it has been separated from globulins.

Reference Range: 3.2 to 4.5 g/dL.

Globulins

Globulins are a group of proteins made up of the fractions alpha-1, alpha-2, beta, and gamma. These distinctions are made based upon electrophoretic patterns. In terms of liver disease, alpha-1 and gamma are the important fractions. Alpha-1-globulin is mostly antitrypsin, which will be discussed later. Gamma-globulin is immune globulin (Ig) or antibody protein and is divided further into G, A, and M fractions. Gamma globulins are produced by plasma cells which are derived from the B lymphocytes. Most come from lymphoid tissue, although some may be formed by these cells in the liver.

Total gamma globulins are increased in most chronic liver diseases, but the level of each fraction is dependent on the particular type of liver disease. The highest total values (almost always > 2.5 and sometimes exceeding 6 g/dL) are seen in autoimmune chronic hepatitis. Most of this increase is gamma fraction G (IgG). Very high levels are also seen in myeloma. Chronic hepatitis B is also associated with a globulin increase, mostly IgG, but at levels less than twice the normal. Chronic hepatitis C often has normal levels of gamma globulins, but may show slight increases. Chronic alcoholic liver disease results in elevations of the level seen with hepatitis B, however, the increase is due both to IgA and IgG fractions.

A slight elevation in IgA may also be seen in biliary obstruction. Primary biliary cirrhosis is associated with elevations in IgM that may be as much as five times the upper normal limit.

The level of gamma globulin or its subfractions will roughly reflect the activity of the liver disease with values returning to normal (or close to normal) when effective therapy is instituted. Total globulin levels are generally provided from a calculation using total protein and albumin measurements (total protein – albumin = globulin), while the fractions are determined by protein electrophoresis and immunoelectrophoresis.

Alpha-1-Antitrypsin

Alpha-1-antitrypsin comprises about 90 % of the alpha-1-globulin fraction and is a circulating inhibitor of proteolysis. It is a glycoprotein synthesized in the liver. A deficiency of this protein is associated with both liver and lung disease. The genotypic expression of various allotypes is used to determine a deficiency of the antiprotease activity of this protein.

A test report includes phenotypes and interpretation, the details of which are beyond the scope of this text. Briefly, however, the phenotype is determined using a special immunoelectrophoresis method. Over 75 alleles have been described and expression is codominant. The majority of the U.S. population is phenotype PiMM (normal phenotype)—homozygous for the protease inhibitor M protein. The ability to inhibit proteases is directly related to the level of this protein in all allotypes. Two other proteins, Z and S, are present in other phenotypes. The heterozygous genotype PiMZ indicates an intermediate deficiency and the homozygous PiZZ indicates severe deficiency (homozygous ZZ is the most pathologic of the genotypes). Other genotypes include PiSS, PiSZ, and a rare null genotype Pi—. Z and S are considered mutant proteins. Because of codominant inheritance, measurable activity of antiprotease is present in all genotypes except for the null genotype. If the normal homozygous MM genotype activity is called 100 % activity, MZ is about 58 %, SS about 60 %, MS 80 %, and ZZ about 15 % (Henry, 1996). Hereditary deficiencies are associated with chronic obstructive pulmonary disease, hepatic cirrhosis, and hepatoma. This deficiency, one of the most frequent inborn metabolic errors, usually produces cholestasis early in childhood and may lead to cirrhosis in adolescence or adult life. Cholestasis with neonatal hepatitis is found in some neonates with alpha-1-antitrypsin deficiency.

Other Special Proteins

Other special proteins that may be useful in the evaluation of hepatic status are **ceruloplasmin** (a copper-containing glycoprotein synthesized in the liver; serves as an oxidase; deficient in Wilson's disease, resulting in copper accumulation in the hepatocytes, cornea, and brain); **alpha-fetoprotein** (useful in detecting primary hepatocellular carcinoma); collagen (used to monitor the degree of hepatic fibrosis, which may determine the extent of liver disease; may be useful in distinguishing some subgroups of liver disease); and **fibronectin** (helps determine the rate of removal of particulate debris from circulation; decreased in parenchymal liver disease/advanced cirrhosis). Table 5-1 shows the changes in serum proteins for selected liver diseases.

TABLE 5–1. Affect of Selected Liver Diseases on Serum Proteins

	Albumin	Alpha-Globulin	Beta-Globulin	Gamma-Globulin
Acute hepatitis	N or Sl. ↓	N or Sl. ↑	Sl. ↑	↑ (IgG and IgM)
Chronic active hepatitis	↓↓	N	↑	↑↑ (IgG)
Biliary cirrhosis	↓	↑	↑↑	↑ (IgM)
Extrahepatic biliary obstruction	N	N or Sl. ↑	↑	N

N = normal; SL. = slightly; ↑ = increased; ↓ = decreased; ↑↑ = markedly increased; ↓↓ = markedly decreased

From Sacher RA, McPherson RA. *Widmann's Clinical Interpretation of Laboratory Tests,* 10th ed. Philadelphia, FA Davis, 1991

CLOTTING FACTORS AND TESTS

Assessment of hemostasis can be useful in the evaluation of the liver. (See Chapter 13 for a more detailed discussion of coagulation tests.) Because it makes most of the coagulation factors, the liver plays an important role in hemostasis. With the exception of the von Willebrand factor, all of the coagulation proteins are synthesized in the liver. In light of this, it is not surprising that as many as 75% of patients with liver disease have coagulation defects, the manifestation of which ranges from ecchymoses to severe bleeding.

The factors synthesized in the liver include fibrinogen; prothrombin; factors V, XI, XII, and XIII; and the vitamin K dependent factors II, VII, IX, and X. The antihemophilic factor (VIII) is synthesized both in the liver and the spleen. Important inhibitors are also synthesized in the liver, the most important of which is antithrombin III, which is responsible for neutralizing thrombin.

The overall hemostatic defect(s) in liver disease is quite complex and will vary depending upon several factors:

- type of liver disease
- degree of impairment in synthesis of factors and inhibitors
- degree of increased consumption of factors in circulation (intravascular clotting or fibrinolysis)
- degree of hepatic clearance of factors and inhibitors

Disseminated intravascular coagulation (DIC), causing increased consumption of clotting factors and platelets, is often seen with liver disease (as well as in a number of other conditions; see Chapter 13). DIC in liver disease is caused by decreased synthesis of inhibitors, decreased clearance of activated factors, or release of tissue thromboplastin from the hepatocytes. Fibrin degradation products (FDP), which are found in DIC, have been found in up to 80% of patients with liver disease who have no evidence of fibrinolysis (dissolution of fibrin by the action of a proteolytic enzyme system).

The possibility of DIC must be considered in any patient with a condition known to be associated with this disorder and who begins to bleed. The diagnosis must be made as soon as possible, particularly in the acutely ill patient. DIC may present acutely and catastrophically or in a more chronic form. The most common clinical feature is bleeding from several sites such as venipuncture sites, surgical wounds, the nose, and the gastrointestinal tract. Widespread bruising is common and intramuscular hemorrhages may occur. Tests that may be most useful in making this diagnosis quickly (because of their relative simplicity and time required for analysis) are listed in Table 5–2. Other more complex and time consuming tests are also available. Diagnosis of chronic DIC may be more difficult than acute and may require repeated measurements. See Chapter 13 for additional information regarding DIC.

Platelet deficiency or dysfunction may also be seen in patients with liver disease. Thrombocytopenia (reduced platelets) may result from splenic sequestration or from the presence of platelet antibodies, which may be tested for directly. Alcoholism or acute viral hepatitis can also cause thrombocytopenia. However, spontaneous bleeding as a result of platelet deficiency is not common in liver disease if the platelets are functioning properly (unless count falls to < 20,000).

TABLE 5–2. Selected Laboratory Findings in DIC

Test	Result	Comments
Prothrombin time (PT)	↑	Sensitive to reductions in fibrinogen, factors II (prothrombin), V, VII, X and to FDP
Activated partial thromboplastin time (aPTT)	↑	Main value is as confirmatory test; sensitive to depletion of factors II, V, VIII, IX, X, and XII, and to fibrinogen
Thrombin time	↑ and Poor quality clot	In severe cases, clot may not form at all; affected by fibrinogen concentration and by presence of FDP
Fibrinogen	↓	Slightly more time consuming than above tests
Platelet count	↓	Reduced in acute DIC; may be normal/near normal in chronic cases
Fibrin degradation products (FDP)	Present	Fragments produced from the digestion of fibrin or fibrinogen by plasmin

Vitamin K is required to make precursor proteins functional coagulation factors. The absorption of vitamin K in the gut may be impaired as a result of a deficiency of bile salts in the intestinal lumen. In this case the pro-thrombin time (PT) is prolonged and factors II, VII, IX, and X (vitamin K dependent factors) are reduced. Factor V is not vitamin K dependent, but may be low in severe hepatocellular injury of advanced chronic liver disease because of decreased synthesis. Correction of the PT by administration of vitamin K is usually possible if factor V is normal in patients with cholestatic liver disease. In hepatocellular diseases such as acute hepatitis or cirrhosis, synthesis of vitamin K dependent factors may be impaired even in the presence of adequate vitamin K. In this instance, administration of vitamin K is usually of little value unless there is also a degree of biliary obstruction. In fact, the response of the coagulation factors to vitamin K administration has been used as a tool to differentiate between hepatocellular jaundice and obstructive jaundice.

Plasminogen levels are often found to be reduced in uncomplicated cases of cirrhosis. This may reflect either decreased synthesis, increased consumption, or both. (Plasminogen is a protein from which plasmin is derived. Plasmin acts as a fibrinolytic enzyme—the two are important in the prevention of fibrin clots.) Reduced levels of inhibitors of fibrinolysis may occur in cirrhosis. In forms of liver disease other than compensated cirrhosis, rapid fibrinolysis is the exception rather than the rule. In combination with coagulation abnormalities, anatomic lesions in patients with liver disease, especially cirrhosis, can be associated with bleeding. The most common sites of bleeding in these patients are esophageal and gastric varices.

Cholesterol and Other Lipids

Because the liver plays an important role in fat metabolism, liver disorders can be associated with abnormalities in lipoproteins. Total cholesterol levels may be very high in patients with chronic cholestatic liver diseases. Modestly elevated triglycerides may occur in hepatocellular injury. More severe elevations may be seen in patients with alcoholic fatty liver. Lipoprotein electophoretic patterns are abnormal in liver disease, but there is no characteristic pattern for different diseases of the liver. Many patients with cholestatic liver disease show the same results as in hepatocellular injury. The cholesterol and phospholipids rise greatly and other lipoproteins appear. Patients with primary biliary cirrhosis have very high levels of high density lipoprotein.

Antibodies

A number of antibodies may be helpful in the diagnosis of liver diseases. These will not be discussed in detail here, but include smooth muscle antibody (SMA) and nuclear antibodies (ANA) seen in autoimmune hepatitis, and mitochondrial antibodies (AMA) seen in primary biliary cirrhosis. Other antibodies directed at liver antigens have also been described.

TIME FOR REVIEW. After studying the preceding sections, you should be able to respond correctly to the following:

■ Which biliary enzyme is more responsive to biliary obstruction than the transaminases and is useful as one of the screening tests for alcoholism?

■ The highest GGT values are found in _____ .

■ List at least four tissues/organs in which AP is found.

■ In what condition does AP rise rapidly to as much as ten times or more the upper limit of the normal range?

■ Briefly explain how differentiating the isoenzymes of AP may be beneficial.

■ Briefly describe the role of the liver in bilirubin metabolism, distinguishing between conjugated and unconjugated bilirubin.

■ Why are bilirubin levels elevated in hemolytic anemia, in hemolytic disease of the newborn, after transfusion of many units of blood in a short period, and in hemolytic transfusion reactions?

■ List three additional conditions in which total bilirubin may be elevated.

■ Which serum protein serves as a transport protein for a variety of substances?

■ List the three mechanisms by which liver disease can result in low albumin levels.

■ List the three globulin fractions, denoting the two that are important in liver disease.

■ List the three fractions of gamma globulins.

■ Total gamma globulins are _____ (increased/decreased/normal) in most chronic liver diseases.

■ The highest total gamma globulin levels are seen in what condition?

■ Most of the increase in the above condition is in _____ (IgG/IgA/IgM).

■ What globulin fraction is a glycoprotein synthesized in the liver and acts as an inhibitor to proteolysis? It is _____ (decreased/increased/normal) in liver disease.

■ All of the coagulation proteins are synthesized in the liver *except:*

■ List the vitamin K dependent coagulation factors.

■ What coagulopathy, causing increased consumption of clotting factors and platelets, is often seen with liver disease?

■ Denote the outcome of the tests listed below in DIC.

Pro-thrombin time (PT)

Activated partial thromboplastin time (aPTT)

Fibrinogen

Thrombin time

Platelet count

Fibrin degradation products (FDP)

Check your responses by reviewing the preceding pages.

DIAGNOSIS OF SELECTED LIVER DISEASES

Diagnostic approaches for selected liver diseases are discussed briefly in this section. The information provided is not intended to serve as the sole basis for disease detection and diagnosis, but rather to more effectively bring together the information discussed in the previous section.

■ EVALUATION OF JAUNDICE

Jaundice (icterus) is a condition characterized by yellowness of the skin, conjunctiva, mucus membranes, and body fluids. It is caused by deposition of bile pigment as a result of an elevated serum bilirubin. Jaundice may appear as the only clinical finding or in conjunction with a range of other findings. Its presence does not necessarily indicate abnormal hepatic function. Causes of jaundice vary widely, from a benign, curable disease, such as a gallstone blocking the common bile duct to a much more serious condition, such as carcinoma of the pancreas involving the opening of the bile duct into the duodenum. Therefore, it is important to attempt to locate the cause of jaundice. Causes for jaundice include obstruction of bile passageways, increased destruction of red cells, and disturbances in the function of liver cells.

Cholestasis

In patients with liver disease, jaundice is most often the result of cholestasis. Patients will often provide a history of dark urine (caused by bilirubinuria) and itching. The history and physical examination alone are useful in differentiating intrahepatic and extrahepatic cholestasis. Pain associated with fever and chills usually points to extrahepatic cholestasis. More definitive diagnosis may be obtained with imaging techniques or more invasive procedures. Table 5–3 summarizes laboratory indicators of cholestasis.

Hepatocellular Jaundice

In analyzing laboratory data, it is important to determine whether the degree of cholestasis is compatible with the degree of hepatocellular injury. Although hepatocellular injury can cause cholestasis, if cholestasis is a primary disorder only mild hepatocellular injury is expected (with some exceptions). If bilirubin and AP levels are increased proportionally more than the ALT and AST, the pattern is predominantly cholestatic. It is generally not necessary to confirm the AST as hepatic in origin if the bilirubin is elevated. The degrees of cholestasis and hepatocellular injury vary during the course of liver or biliary tract disease. Table 5–4 summarizes laboratory indicators of hepatocellular injury.

TABLE 5–3. Laboratory Indicators of Cholestasis

Test	Result	Comments
Bilirubin	⇑	With bilirubinuria as well
Alkaline phosphatase	⇑	
GGT	⇑	
Cholesterol	⇑	

TABLE 5–4. Laboratory Indicators of Hepatocellular Injury

Test	Result
ALT	⇑
AST	⇑
Albumin	⇓
Cholesterol	⇓
Pro-thrombin time	⇑
Iron and ferritin may be elevated in acute phase	

■ ASSESSING HEPATOCELLULAR INJURY

Symptoms usually seen in patients with hepatocellular injury include malaise, anorexia, and fatigability. This condition is recognized acutely with rises in aminotransaminase activity—AST more in alcoholic and toxic injuries and ALT more in viral injuries. Cholestasis may be absent to very severe. Minimal rises in AP are generally seen in acute hepatocellular injuries. The broad range of hepatocellular injury in liver disease is divided into acute and chronic based on how long the elevations in enzyme activity persist.

Alcoholic Injury

An increased GGT is usually seen when large amounts of alcohol have been ingested over a long period of time. This is generally accompanied by an elevation in the MCV of red cells. Hepatocellular injury is best detected with AST. Alcoholic hepatitis with fever, upper right quadrant pain, and leukocytosis is frequently associated with an AST up to ten times the upper normal limit. (It is important to note that a similar discrepancy between AST and ALT is seen in some non-hepatic diseases such as acute myocardial infarction, skeletal muscle necrosis, hemolysis, and renal necrosis.) Hyperbilirubinemia, partly from hemolysis and partly from cholestasis, can occur in alcoholic hepatitis. Hypoalbuminemia may be seen and is usually nutritional, but may signal a rapid transition to cirrhosis.

Viral Hepatitis

Bilirubin levels, ALT, and viral markers are the best laboratory guides in following the course of the primary viral hepatitis infections of the liver. Bilirubin rises rapidly and falls slowly, especially if cholestasis is present. ALT rises abruptly and usually falls without a plateau to 100 to 400 IU/L and then fluctuates within this range for varying lengths of time. The longer the ALT remains elevated, especially in hepatitis A and B, the more likely chronicity will develop.

In *hepatitis A* (incubation period 15 to 45 days; average 28 days), elevation of ALT and AST begins before symptoms appear. IgM antibody to hepatitis A (anti-HAV) is usually present by the time the patient is examined and remains for 3 to 12 months. Anti-HAV, non-IgM indicates previous hepatitis A infection. Bilirubin is elevated and usually returns to normal in a few weeks.

Hepatitis B (incubation period 1-6 months; average 2 to 2.5 months) may be detected by viral markers before symptoms occur or ALT and AST begin to rise. The earliest detectable markers are HB_sAG (hepatitis B surface antigen), HBeAG (hepatitis Be antigen), anti-HBc-IgM (hepatitis B core antibody), DNA and DNA polymerase. HB_sAG is detectable for 1 to 15 weeks after the onset of symptoms and will remain if seroconversion does not occur. Anti-HBc-IgM is usually present when the patient is examined. ALT rises shortly before the onset of symptoms. Antibody to the surface antigen (anti-HB_sAG or HB_sAB) reaches a measurable level late in convalescence.

Hepatitis C is extremely variable in clinical and laboratory findings. ALT rises and falls during the illness, but usually is only modestly elevated. Elevations of gamma globulins either do not occur or are mild even when chronic disease develops. The time course for hepatitis C is more prolonged than for the other forms of hepatitis and it is more likely to progress to cirrhosis. A serologic marker for the hepatitis C virus (HCV) has been available for about 6 years. Persisting elevated ALT levels in patients who have apparently recovered from hepatitis B acquired from blood transfusion or needle use may indicate that the patient also acquired hepatitis C at the same time.

When ALT or AST levels remain elevated for longer than 6 months in hepatitis, the disease is classified as *chronic hepatitis.* Table 5–5 summarizes the clinical and laboratory differences among the major forms of chronic hepatitis. The patterns of clinical and laboratory features during the course of the disease may indicate etiology. ALT elevations are from two to ten times the upper normal limit, but, as with acute hepatitis, the degree of elevation is not indicative of the severity or identity of the disease. Laboratory evaluation begins with general screening. The recognition of cholestasis and hepatocellular injury have been discussed previously. The synthetic functions of the liver can be assessed by the levels of albumin and cholesterol and by the pro-thrombin time. Hypergammaglobulinemia indicates inflammation with the highest levels seen in autoimmune chronic hepatitis. Gamma globulin levels are only slightly elevated in chronic hepatitis C, but in chronic hepatitis B and alcoholic liver disease are usually 2.0 to 3.0 g/dL. The extent of hepatic fibrosis cannot be judged by laboratory determinations, but when fibrosis is active, the amount of procollagen II peptide in serum is increased.

TABLE 5–5. Differences Among Major Forms of Chronic Hepatitis

Feature	Chronic Active Hepatitis B	Chronic Hepatitis C	Chronic Active Hepatitis "Autoimmune"
Age	>30 yrs	All ages	<30 yrs (50%)/>50 yrs
Sex	80–90% male	Both equal	80% female
Onset	Abrupt/insidious	Usually insidious	Usually insidious
Asymptomatic cases	Frequent	Frequent	Rare
Bilirubin >5 mg/dL	5–10%	<5%	30–60%
Increased ALT	15–25%	Fluctuates	70–90%
Decreased albumin	20–30%	Late	85–100%
Increased gamma globulin	50%; pronounced in 10%	Uncommon	80%; pronounced in 40%
Prognosis	Slow progression; low mortality; persistence of HB$_s$AG/HBeAG may indicate more severe disease	Very slow progression, but complications of cirrhosis common late	Progression to cirrhosis with portal hypertension and liver failure
Hepatocellular carcinoma	Common	Increasing	Rare

Table complied with data from Henry, 1996; Ravel, 1990; Sacher, 1991.

■ STORAGE DISORDERS

The liver is an important organ for the storage of substances present in the body in large excess. Storage disorders can lead to enlargement of the liver, malfunction, and usually cirrhosis. Two of the more common disorders are discussed here.

Hemochromatosis is a disease of increased iron deposits in various organs. This condition may be due to a primary defect in iron absorption or secondary to erythrocyte formation, liver disease, or dietary iron overload. Hemochromatosis may result in dysfunction of the liver, pancreas, and heart as well as a change in skin color. Laboratory determinations are utilized to assess the iron excess (iron, % saturation, ferritin) as well as hepatic function. Liver biopsy is often an important tool in diagnosing this condition and, when the diagnosis is made early enough, may determine whether the condition is primary or secondary. The disease may lead to fibrosis progressing to advanced cirrhosis.

Wilson's disease is a disorder of copper metabolism in which copper accumulates in the liver, brain, cornea, and kidneys because it cannot be excreted in the bile. Patients may present with cirrhosis, chronic hepatitis, or, rarely, liver failure. In this condition the serum ceruloplasmin (a copper-carrying oxidase protein) is reduced, serum copper levels decreased, and urinary excretion of copper increased. Liver biopsy is often needed to confirm the diagnosis.

 TIME FOR REVIEW. After studying the preceding sections, you should be able to respond correctly to the following:

■ In patients with liver disease, jaundice is most often the result of _____ .

■ Review the tables in this section.

■ Acute hepatocellular injury results in elevations of the aminotransaminases. AST rises more in _____ and ALT more in _____.

■ An increase in what enzyme is usually seen when large amounts of alcohol have been ingested in a short period of time?

■ List two causes of hyperbilirubinemia in alcoholic hepatitis.

■ List the three laboratory tests best used in following the course of primary viral hepatitis infections of the liver.

■ List two liver storage disorders and the substance deposited in the liver in each.

■ List the type of chronic hepatitis (B, C, autoimmune) best identified by each description below.

_____   Frequently asymptomatic and has slow progression. Few individuals have bilirubin levels > 5 mg/dL; one-fourth or fewer have increased ALT levels; and half have increased gamma globulins levels. Significantly more males are affected than females.

_____   Increased gamma globulins are uncommon and both sexes are equally affected. ALT levels fluctuate and albumin is not decreased until late in the illness. Few patients have bilirubin levels > 5 mg/dL.

_____   Most patients have increased gamma globulin, decreased albumin, and increased ALT levels. The illness is rarely asymptomatic and affects more females than males. Bilirubin levels will be > 5 mg/dL in as many as 60 % of individuals with the illness.

Check your responses by reviewing the preceding pages.

■ SYSTEMIC DISEASES

Liver abnormalities may be detected in a number of systemic illnesses and may represent a significant component of the illness, but in some cases is inconsequential. ALT and AST levels can be slightly increased in systemic infection without the liver being directly involved. The liver can be directly infected by some agents including Epstein-Barr virus, cytomegalovirus (CMV), and herpes virus.

Fungal infections may also affect the liver. Liver function can be mildly to severely abnormal in patients with heart disease. Patients with severely impaired cardiac output may develop hepatic ischemia. Inflammatory bowel disorders is associated with a number of hepatobiliary disorders, including gallstones, sclerosing cholangitis, chronic hepatitis, and others. AIDS is frequently accompanied by hepatic abnormalities often attributable to various infections.

DRUGS

There are a variety of medications that can cause abnormalities in the blood related to the liver. Many have been mentioned throughout this text in the discussions of the various laboratory assays. A rise in AST during the first week or two of administration is seen with some commonly used drugs, including aspirin, anticonvulsants, antiarrhythmics, and psychotherapeutic agents. In these cases the increase is more likely an adaptive response as opposed to an adverse effect. Adverse effects on hepatic function as a result of various drugs vary from moderate increases in AST or ALT to chronic hepatitis and cirrhosis. There may be mild increases in AP and GGT or severe and protracted cholestatic jaundice. Although the reactions in some cases are predictable, they may also occur unpredictably. Laboratory determinations cannot be accurately evaluated without a knowledge of the patient's medications and an awareness of the effects of the medication. Drugs known or suspected to affect hepatic function should be administered only with appropriate monitoring of its effects. For most monitoring purposes, AST with total and direct bilirubin measurements are sufficient. Testing should be more frequent during initial treatment and for the first few months.

NUTRITION

The activity of various hepatic enzymes can be affected by nutritional status. Fatty liver with increased ALT and GGT is not uncommon in obese patients. Low albumin and cholesterol levels are seen in severe malnutrition and parenteral alimentation can cause mild AST abnormalities or varying degrees of cholestasis, occasionally progressing to cirrhosis.

5. SELF TEST

Choose the best response by circling the appropriate letter. The answer key may be found in the appendices.

1. **The condition in which the highest AST:ALT ratio is found, sometimes with near normal ALT activity, is**
   A. uremia
   B. Reye syndrome
   C. alcoholic liver disease
   D. chronic viral hepatitis

2. **ALT enzyme activity is more specific for liver injury because**
   A. AST is decreased in cirrhosis
   B. AST is also found in heart and muscle tissues
   C. ALT is less sensitive than AST to alcoholic liver disease
   D. ALT is decreased in biliary obstruction

3. **This biliary enzyme is more responsive to biliary obstruction than the transaminases and although sensitive for the detection of hepatocellular injury, does not differentiate well among liver diseases.**
   A. GGT
   B. ALT
   C. AST
   D. AP

4. **In which condition does alkaline phosphatase rise rapidly to as much as ten times or more the upper limit of the normal reference range?**
   A. chronic viral hepatitis
   B. alcoholic liver disease
   C. uremia
   D. impaired bile flow

5. The increase in total serum bilirubin levels seen in conditions such as hemolytic anemia and hemolytic disease of the newborn, and in hemolytic transfusion reactions, results from
   A. a decrease in the transport of albumin bound bilirubin
   B. an increase in the destruction of red cells
   C. a decrease in the amount of indirect bilirubin
   D. impaired excretion of conjugated bilirubin

6. The serum protein that serves as a transport protein for a variety of substances is
   A. alpha globulin
   B. beta globulin
   C. gamma globulin
   D. albumin

7. Liver disease may result in low albumin levels by all of these mechanisms *except*
   A. accelerated production
   B. increased degradation
   C. altered synthesis
   D. extravascular loss

8. In most liver diseases, the gamma globulins are
   A. decreased
   B. absent
   C. increased
   D. normal

9. This glycoprotein is synthesized by the liver, inhibits proteolysis, and is deficient both in liver and lung disease.
   A. alpha-1 antitrypsin
   B. albumin
   C. gamma globulin
   D. vitamin K

10. Which of the following coagulation factors are *not* synthesized by the liver?
    A. anti-hemolytic factor (Factor VIII)
    B. von Willebrand factor
    C. fibrinogen
    D. prothrombin

11. **The vitamin K dependent factors are**
    A. I, II, VII, VIII
    B. II, III, IV, VII
    C. II, VII, IX, X
    D. VII, VIII, IX, X

12. **The pattern of coagulation test results most representative of disseminated intravascular coagulation (DIC) is**
    A. decreased PT, APTT, thrombin time, fibrinogen, platelet count; negative FDP
    B. increased PT, APTT, thrombin time; decreased fibrinogen, platelet count; positive FDP
    C. increased PT, APTT, thrombin time, fibrinogen, platelet count; positive FDP
    D. decreased PT, APTT, thrombin time; increased platelet count; negative FDP

13. **In patients with liver disease, jaundice is most often the result of**
    A. cholestasis
    B. increased red cell destruction
    C. pancreatic carcinoma
    D. hepatitis

14. **An increase in this enzyme is usually seen when large amounts of alcohol are ingested in a short period of time.**
    A. ALT
    B. AST
    C. AP
    D. GGT

15. **Which set of test results is most indicative of hepatocellular injury?**
    A. increased ALT, AST, PT; decreased albumin and cholesterol
    B. decreased ALT, AST, PT; increased albumin and cholesterol
    C. increased ALT, AST; decreased PT, albumin, and cholesterol
    D. decreased ALT; increased AST, albumin, cholesterol, and PT

16. **The condition that results in increased iron deposits in various organs is**
    A. cirrhosis
    B. alcoholic liver disease
    C. hemochromatosis
    D. viral hepatitis

17. In this form of hepatitis, most patients have increased gamma globulin, decreased albumin, and increased ALT levels. The illness is rarely asymptomatic and it affects more females than males. Bilirubin levels will be > 5 mg/dL in as many as 60% of cases.
    A. chronic active hepatitis "autoimmune"
    B. chronic active hepatitis B
    C. chronic hepatitis C
    D. chronic hepatitis Z

18. This form of hepatitis is frequently asymptomatic and has slow progression. Few individuals have bilirubin levels > 5 mg/dL; one-fourth or fewer have increased ALT levels, and half have increased gamma globulin levels. Significantly more males are affected than females.
    A. chronic active hepatitis "autoimmune"
    B. chronic active hepatitis B
    C. chronic hepatitis C
    D. chronic hepatitis Z

19. Increased gamma globulin levels are uncommon in this type of hepatitis and both sexes are affected equally. ALT levels fluctuate and albumin is not decreased until late in the illness. Few patients have bilirubin levels > 5 mg/dL.
    A. chronic active hepatitis "autoimmune"
    B. chronic active hepatitis B
    C. chronic hepatitis C
    D. chronic hepatitis Z

6. TESTING FOR GLUCOSE ABNORMALITIES

One of the most frequently requested tests in the chemistry department of the laboratory is a glucose or "blood sugar" level. Most often utilized in the diagnosis and monitoring of diabetes mellitus, blood glucose levels are also useful in evaluating disorders of carbohydrate metabolism; acidosis and ketoacidosis; and coma, dehydration, and hypoglycemia. Measurements may also be useful in the work-up of patients appearing to be alcoholic.

CARBOHYDRATE METABOLISM

Carbohydrates are a class of compounds that consist of carbon, hydrogen, and oxygen, with hydrogen and oxygen present in a 2:1 ratio (as in water). They are often represented by the generic formula $C_x(H_2O)_y$, where x represents the number of carbon atoms and y the number of H_2O groups. Carbohydrates are a major supplier of calories in the typical diet. Medically important carbohydrates include the simple six carbon sugars, or hexoses, glucose, galactose, and fructose, and the disaccharides lactose and sucrose.

Dietary glucose is primarily in the form of **disaccharides** (two sugar molecules that are chemically bonded) such as sucrose (glucose + fructose) and lactose (glucose + galactose). Specific enzymes in the small intestine split these bonds to break down the disaccharide into the individual monosaccharides. For example, the intestinal enzyme sucrase breaks down sucrose into its constituent monosaccharides—glucose and fructose. The oxidative **metabolism of glucose yields** a number of intermediate compounds, including lactic acid, with complete oxidation resulting in **carbon dioxide**, **water**, **and energy stored as ATP** (adenosine triphosphate). Any glucose not immediately metabolized to produce energy, is stored in the liver (primarily) or in muscle in the form of glycogen. **Glycogen** is a polysaccharide of numerous glucose residues. In this form it is available to be converted into glucose, which can then be metabolized to produce energy when needed by the tissues. By other metabolic pathways the liver can also convert glucose into fatty acids stored as triglycerides or into amino acids for protein synthesis. When the glucose available is not sufficient to meet energy demands and the level of stored glycogen is depleted, the liver can synthesize glucose from the stored fatty acids or from amino acids. When glucose intake is excessive, glucose not used for immediate energy demands or stored as glycogen is stored as adipose or fat tissue.

REGULATION OF BLOOD GLUCOSE

Almost all cellular and tissue functions are dependent upon the energy produced from glucose metabolism. Although energy can be produced from fatty acid metabolism, the process is less efficient than that of glucose metabolism and has the undesirable effect of producing acid metabolites that can be harmful upon accumulation. Thus maintaining an appropriate blood glucose level is quite important. A number of mechanisms are employed by the body in the regulation of blood glucose levels to maintain the level within relatively narrow limits. A brief explanation of these mechanisms, though quite complex and in some instances not completely understood, follows.

■ LIVER

The liver plays a crucial role in the regulation of blood glucose levels, as can be seen from the preceding summary of carbohydrate metabolism. The liver's impact on blood glucose levels results from the reversible process of converting glucose to glycogen (and, conversely, converting glycogen to glucose) as well as its role in the distribution of glucose to meet the body's energy needs. An additional role of the liver in glucose regulation is to synthesize glucose, a process known as *gluconeogenesis.*

■ HORMONES

A variety of hormones are involved in the regulation of blood glucose levels, particularly the pancreatic hormones. Adrenal, pituitary, and thyroid hormones also play a role in this regulatory process.

Individual hormone producing cell types in the pancreas secrete three major hormones involved in the maintenance of appropriate blood glucose. These **pancreatic hormones** are *insulin, glucagon,* and *somatostatin.* **Insulin** works to lower the blood glucose by increasing the transport of glucose into tissue cells and by stimulating the oxidation of glucose. It also activates the synthesis of fat, glycogen, and protein and exerts a direct effect on the liver by suppressing the conversion of glycogen to glucose. **Glucagon** levels increase by two- or threefold in response to hypoglycemia (low blood glucose level) and decrease in the presence of hyperglycemia (elevated blood glucose level). As suggested by these responses to significant deviation of the glucose from normal values, glucagon acts to raise the blood glucose level. This is believed to be accomplished by glucagon's enhancement of the glycogen to glucose conversion and of gluconeogenesis. The local action of pancreatic **somatostatin** has a regulatory effect on the release of the other pancreatic hormones, insulin and glucagon. In order to better understand the relationship among these pancreatic hormones in the regulation of glucose levels, we can think of insulin and glucagon as acting in opposition to each other or as being in conflict and of somatostatin as the mediator of the conflict. Food intake is intermittent, not constant, and energy needs rise and fall. In this arena, insulin works to lower the blood glucose through the storage of carbohydrates and inhibiting release of stored energy from the liver, fat, and muscle. In a reciprocal fashion, glucagon is working to increase the glucose level during fasting periods by enhancing the conversion of hepatic glycogen to glucose (glycogenolysis) and enhancing gluconeogenesis. Somatostatin mediates these conflicting roles by regulating the amount of each hormone released from the pancreas, thus ensuring that neither acts too aggressively by reaching inappropriate concentrations.

Other hormones act to raise blood glucose levels by varying mechanisms, including the **adrenal** hormones *epinephrine* and *cortisol,* from the adrenal medulla and cortex, respectively, the **pituitary** hormones *ACTH* and *growth hormone,* and the **thyroid** hormone, *thyroxine.* The regulatory influence of hormones on blood glucose level is summarized in Table 6–1.

TABLE 6–1. Hormonal Regulation of Blood Glucose

	Hormone	Action	Effect
Pancreatic	Insulin	Enhances entry of glucose into cells Enhances storage of glucose as glycogen, or conversion to fatty acids Enhances synthesis of proteins and fatty acids Suppresses breakdown of protein into amino acids, of adipose tissue into free fatty acids	Lowers
	Glucagon	Enhances release of glucose from glycogen Enhances synthesis of glucose from amino acids or fatty acids	Raises
	Somatostatin	Suppresses glucagon release Suppresses release on insulin, pituitary tropic hormones, gastrin, and secretin	
Adrenal	Epinephrine	Enhances release of glucose from glycogen Enhances release of fatty acids from adipose tissue	Raises
	Cortisol	Enhances synthesis of glucose from amino acids or fatty acids Serves as insulin antagonist	Raises
Pituitary	ACTH	Enhances release of cortisol Enhances release of fatty acids from adipose tissue	Raises
	Growth hormone	Insulin antagonist	Raises
Thyroid	Thyroxine	Enhances release of glucose from glycogen Enhances absorption of sugars from intestine	Raises

Adapted from Sacher RA, McPherson RA. *Widmann's Clinical Interpretation of Laboratory Tests,* 10th ed. Philadelphia, FA Davis, 1991

ABNORMAL GLUCOSE LEVELS: HYPERGLYCEMIA AND HYPOGLYCEMIA

Abnormalities in any of the many mechanisms involved in the regulation of blood glucose levels will result in abnormal glucose levels that may be persistent or transient. **Hyperglycemia** refers to abnormally elevated blood glucose levels; **hypoglycemia** is the term used to describe a decreased blood glucose.

■ DIABETES MELLITUS

Diabetes mellitus is perhaps the best known cause of hyperglycemia and is the most common cause of *persistent* hyperglycemia. It results from an abnormality in either insulin production or the utilization of insulin and is classified into three distinct entities. Classification of diabetes mellitus involves clinical manifestation, therapy requirements and response, and pathogenesis of the abnormality, as summarized in Table 6–2.

■ DIAGNOSING DIABETES MELLITUS

It is important to note that not all elevated glucose levels are the result of diabetes mellitus. The hyperglycemia seen in diabetes mellitus results from insulin deficiency whether absolute or relative in nature. Levels may be transiently increased as a result of a variety of drugs. Reversible hyperglycemia (resulting from defects in both the utilization of glucose and impaired insulin secretion) is seen in conditions in which there is an increased production of the adrenal cortical hormones involved in carbohydrate and protein metabolism. Certainly diabetes mellitus is generally a primary diagnostic consideration in patients demonstrating an impairment of glucose metabolism, particularly when presenting with the classic symptom triad of polyuria, polydipsia, and polyphagia. However, an awareness of other possible causes can be beneficial when hyperglycemia is present but clinical observations and/or diagnostic data do not support a diagnosis of diabetes mellitus (Table 6–3).

Various criteria for the diagnosis of diabetes mellitus have been proposed in an effort to promote an improved level of standardization in the diagnosis of this condition. Emphasis will be placed on the American Diabetes Association's (ADA) 1998 Clinical Practice Recommendations in this text although clinicians may utilize older methods including the Wilkerson point system or the Siperstein criteria (Table 6–4). In terms of "real world" practice, insulin dependent diabetes mellitus (IDDM) does not frequently present a diagnostic dilemma to be resolved on the basis of rigidly established criteria. The clinical presentation of such patients often includes abnormalities that are so pronounced, perhaps even critical, that the immediate concern is the institution of timely and effective treatment rather than diagnostic deliberations. Diagnostic criteria are more beneficial in non-insulin dependent diabetes mellitus (NIDDM), because of the more gradual development and sometimes more subtle symptoms of this classification of diabetes, and in other situations such as impaired glucose tolerance.

TABLE 6–2. Classification of Diabetes Mellitus (DM)

	Pathogenesis	Clinical Manifestation	Treatment[1]
Insulin dependent (IDDM, or type I)	Inadequate insulin secretion resulting from autoimmune destruction of pancreatic beta cells (site of insulin secretion); genetic susceptibility; antibodies to islet cells and patient's own insulin present in 95% of cases	Poluria[2] Excessive thirst (polydipsia)[2] Polyphagia (excessive eating)[2] Weight loss (common) Often present with markedly increased blood glucose and/or in diabetic ketoacidosis	Insulin therapy Diet plan for consistent food intake and to maintain ideal body weight Patient education Regular physical activity Monitoring treatment effectiveness/compliance: • home blood glucose test ~ 3 times per day • fasting glucose by lab at established frequency • glycosylated hGB every 4-6 months Treatment to prevent or treat complications
Non-insulin dependent (NIDDM, or type II)	Insulin resistance causing excess glucose output in liver & decreased muscle uptake of glucose; an accompanying beta cell defect (impaired insulin secretion) required for overt diabetes to develop	Often asymptomatic with gradual onset of symptoms such as fatigue, blurred vision, and recurrent skin or vaginal infections; may also have polyuria and polydipsia; women may have history of large babies or gestational diabetes	Oral hypoglycemic agents or insulin as indicated Diet plan for weight loss & appropriate meal spacing Patient education Regular physical activity Monitoring treatment effectiveness/compliance: • home blood glucose test with frequency dependent on stability and level of control • fasting glucose by lab at established frequency • glycosylated hGB every 4-6 months Treatment to prevent or treat complications
Other	Secondary to other causes: pancreatic diseases or pancreatectomy; endocrine disorders (acromegaly, Cushing, etc.); some genetic syndromes; variety of drugs	Initial presentation may correspond to underlying condition; common symptoms of hyperglycemia may be noted depending upon the degree of hyperglycemia present	Treatment appropriate for underlying condition and control of hyperglycemia with monitoring as indicated

[1]Treatments for IDDM and NIDDM based on guidelines from Stein VH. *Internal Medicine: Diagnosis and Therapy*, 3rd ed. Norwalk, CT, Appleton and Lange, 1993. All treatment and monitoring regimens should be established by the attending physician in accordance with accepted clinical practices and the patient's condition. Additional data compiled from various sources.
[2]Classic symptoms.

TABLE 6–3. Causes of Hyperglycemia and Hypoglycemia

	Hyperglycemia	Hypoglycemia
Transient	Acute emotional stress Acute physical stress (trauma, burns, etc) Shock Myocardial infarction Convulsions Severe liver disease Pheochromocytoma (adrenal tumor)	Drugs (salicylates, beta blockers) Acute alcohol ingestion Severe liver disease Sepsis Heart failure Glycogen storage disorders
Persistent	Diabetes mellitus Cushing syndrome (adrenal hyperactivity) Acromegaly (pituitary abnormality) Hyperthyroidism Obesity	Insulinoma (excessive insulin production) Addison's disease (adrenal insufficiency) Antibodies to insulin or insulin receptors Exogenous insulin (from tumor production) Galactosemia Hypopituitarism

TABLE 6–4. Summary of Criteria for Diagnosing Diabetes Mellitus in Nonpregnant Adults

System	Criteria
ADA[1]	(three ways to diagnose) 1. symptoms of diabetes plus casual plasma glucose concentration ≥200 mg/dL OR 2. fasting plasma glucose ≥126 mg/dL OR 3. 2-hour oral glucose tolerance test value ≥200 mg/dL (following 75 g glucose dose)
WILKERSON	Two points required for diagnosis, with points derived from GTT results of: fasting >125 = 1 point 1 hr >195 = $\frac{1}{2}$ point 2 hr >145 = $\frac{1}{2}$ point 3 hr >125 = 1 point
SIPERSTEIN	Fasting >140 on two occasions GTT with 1 hr >260 and 2 hr >220

[1]ADA recommendations include a confirmation of either method on a subsequent day in the absence of unequivocal hyperglycemia with acute metabolic decompensation.

Data from American Diabetes Association, *Clinical Practice Recommendations,* volume 21, supplement 1, 1998; Henry JB. *Clinical Diagnosis and Management by Laboratory Methods,* 19th ed. Philadelphia, Saunders, 1996; Ravel R. *Clinical Laboratory Medicine: Clinical Application of Laboratory Data,* 6th ed. St Louis, Mosby, 1995; and Stein JH. *Internal Medicine: Diagnosis and Therapy,* 3rd ed. Norwalk, CT, Appleton and Lange, 1993

A diagnosis of diabetes mellitus is made when abnormal elevations in the blood glucose level are demonstrated under specified and controlled conditions. Although the presence of symptoms consistent with the condition and elevation of fasting blood glucose levels may be sufficient for diagnosis in some cases, abnormalities will be noted in other instances only following the administration of a large carbo-hydrate load (as in the glucose tolerance test [GTT] discussed later in this chapter). Based upon the criteria for the diagnosis of diabetes mellitus established by the National Diabetes Data Group (NDDG), a fasting serum/plasma glucose level at or above 140 mg/dL on more than one occasion is diagnostic for diabetes mellitus. NDDG criteria also allow diagnosis in the presence of unequivocal symptoms of diabetes along with significant elevation of the fasting glucose or a nonfasting glu-cose level above 200 mg/dL. Alternatively, diagnosis may be made based upon a 75 g dose (nonpregnant adult) glucose tolerance test in which the 2-hour sample has a glucose concentration above 200 mg/dL. Thus the ADA criteria establishes three ways to diagnose diabetes, each of which must be confirmed on a subsequent day. Intermediate groups whose glucose levels do not meet the criteria for a diagnosis of diabetes, but who have glucose levels too high to be considered normal are also rec-ognized. Using the fasting plasma glucose level, individuals who have values above 110 mg/dL but below 126 mg/dL are classified as having an impaired fasting glu-cose. Using the oral glucose tolerance test, a corresponding group having a 2-hour glucose that is above 140 mg/dL but below 200 mg/dL is identified as having impaired glucose tolerance. It is important to note that the new 1998 ADA criteria are for diagnosis and do not present changes to the ADA treatment recommenda-tions of fasting glucose < 120 mg/dL and hemoglobin $A_{1C} < 7\%$ as goals. Diabetes in pregnancy presents a threat to both the mother and the unborn child. A later sec-tion discusses gestational diabetes and special considerations during pregnancy.

■ LABORATORY MEASUREMENT OF GLUCOSE

Glucose can be detected and quantitated in a variety of different specimen types using a number of techniques. **Methods of measurement** can be classified in two categories:

1. chemical reactions dependent on the reducing properties of glucose
2. enzymatic methods

Reducing substance methods are not specific for glucose and can yield values that are considerably higher than the actual glucose level. For this reason, glu-cose measurements by this method are no longer used extensively, particularly with automated analyzers. Enzymatic determinations are more specific because they use enzymes specific for glucose such as glucose oxidase or glucokinase. In the **glucose oxidase method**, the reaction of glucose with the oxidase enzyme, which is highly specific, results in gluconic acid and hydrogen peroxide. In the second step in this method, the peroxide formed in the initial reaction reacts with a special reagent that is an oxygen receptor (hydrogen peroxide = H_2O_2; reaction with oxygen receptor yields H_2O) and allows color formation. The sec-ond step of the glucose oxidase method is catalyzed by peroxidase and is less spe-cific than the first step because other reducing substances can interfere. Overall, however, the glucose oxidase method is considered highly specific for the measurement of glucose.

Most automated analyzers currently in use measure the glucose in serum or plasma, whereas home and bedside monitors use whole blood measurements. Glucose is more stable in serum or plasma than in whole blood because the red cells, and to some extent white cells, metabolize glucose. This causes the glucose level in samples to decrease on standing, particularly in the absence of a preservative or refrigeration. Reduction of the glucose level resulting from glycolysis is not of significance when measurements are made immediately upon collection, as is the case with home and bedside glucose meters. The hematocrit level also influences whole blood measurements in that a higher hematocrit will increase the amount of the decrease in glucose (more red cells = greater glycolysis). Significant differences exist between whole blood glucose values and serum or plasma values and this difference must be taken into account when evaluating glycemic control and comparing results the patient obtained by home monitoring and results obtained from the laboratory. In general, serum/plasma levels are considered to be about 10 % higher than whole blood levels, but studies have shown much greater variation, approaching a 50 % difference in values. With very high levels of variation, the technique, quality control, and instrument performance of the home meter should be investigated. Some variation in whole blood measurements may also be seen from different sources (eg, capillary and arterial samples may produce results slightly higher than those seen in venous samples). This difference is magnified and somewhat more significant following carbohydrate loading.

Serum or plasma glucose levels may be measured under different conditions such as those described below.

- *Fasting glucose:* often referred to as fasting blood sugar, or FBS; glucose is measured on a serum or plasma specimen following a 12-hour fast; this type of specimen yields less variable results than specimens collected at other times; reference range: 70 to 110 mg/dL.
- *Random glucose:* not often used diagnostically; more variable than fasting levels; may be markedly elevated in uncontrolled IDDM; upper normal limit for reference range usually 130 to 140 mg/dL, with somewhat higher normal levels possible in patients over 65.
- *2-hour post-prandial:* glucose is measured in serum or plasma specimen collected 2 hours after a meal; sometimes used to monitor control or to screen for abnormalities; diagnostic value debatable especially because conditions—particularly the carbohydrate content of meal—may not be well controlled. Glucose levels at 2 hours after meal have usually returned to approximately normal following a peak elevation at about 60 to 90 minutes.
- *Glucose tolerance test* (GTT): discussed in detail below; involves collection of a fasting specimen, administration of a defined carbohydrate load, and collection of specimens at hourly intervals thereafter for a defined period; careful standardization is important as test interpretation is affected by a variety of factors.

Glucose may also be measured in urine (see Chapter 2) and in other body fluids such as cerebrospinal fluid. Prior to the development of easy-to-use and readily accessible monitors for home monitoring of blood glucose levels, many diabetics used urine glucose testing to assess their level of control. Although this is a simple and inexpensive method of home monitoring, there are a number of disadvantages to relying on urine glucose measurements to evaluate glycemic control. First, urine glucose measurements are more qualitative in nature than quantitative and provide only an indirect indication of the blood glucose level. This measure is indicative of the blood glucose level hours earlier. Further, the renal threshold for glucose "spillage" into the urine is highly variable among individuals and is increased in renal disease—a common complication of diabetes. Home monitoring of blood glucose levels is preferred and should be used, if at all possible, instead of monitoring by urine testing. Urinary glucose levels are not without usefulness, however, and glycosuria may be the first indication of abnormal glucose metabolism in the absence of reported symptoms. (Urine testing for the presence of ketones is also a useful and practical means for the detection of ketonemia.)

■ GLUCOSE TOLERANCE TEST

As the name implies, the glucose tolerance test (GTT) evaluates the ability to "tolerate" or adequately respond to the challenge of a relatively high glucose dose. The dose may be administered orally or intravenously. The oral glucose tolerance test, most commonly employed, is discussed here.

PATIENT PREPARATION. In order for valid, meaningful data to be obtained, strict control of test conditions and precise standardization of test procedures are essential. In the absence of controlled conditions and test standardization, abnormal responses cannot be interpreted correctly with any degree of confidence. Patients scheduled for a GTT should be carefully instructed regarding appropriate preparation and should be informed that failure to adhere to the specified conditions is likely to produce invalid results, making it difficult for their physician to correctly diagnose and treat any abnormality that may be present. Important conditions to be controlled in preparation for GTT testing include the following:

- *Diet:* should include at least 150 g of carbohydrates per day for the 3 days preceding testing (2 additional days if previous diet has been low in carbohydrates); *inadequate food intake invalidates test results.*
- *Medications:* withhold nonessential medications for 3 days prior to testing; insulin secretion is decreased by salicylates, diuretics, and anticonvulsants; oral contraceptives cause resistance to insulin.
- *Alcohol:* no alcohol intake for 3 days prior to testing.
- *Illness:* testing should not be performed on patients with fever (can produce diabetic-like responses in GTT) and should be delayed for 2 weeks following any illness and for 6 weeks following acute myocardial infarc-

tion, burns, trauma, or other conditions causing transient hyperglycemia, known endocrine disorders should be corrected prior to testing.

- *Physical activity:* data may not be meaningful in nonambulatory patients as bed rest may significantly impair glucose tolerance.
- *12 hours prior to testing:* patient must fast (water only) and refrain from smoking and exercising; the same conditions should be observed throughout the test procedure.

TEST PROCEDURE. The test is scheduled to begin in the morning (usually 7 or 8 AM) because glucose tolerance demonstrates *diurnal variation,* with a significant decrease in tolerance in the afternoon. A fasting glucose specimen is collected and analyzed. In the event that the fasting glucose level is significantly elevated, continuation of the procedure is contraindicated because of the risk of dangerous elevations following a high-dose glucose challenge. Further, continuation of the procedure, used to confirm or rule out abnormalities in glucose metabolism, is not warranted diagnostically when a fasting glucose reflects a notable abnormality. When the fasting glucose level is within an acceptable range, a glucose challenge dose is administered by having the patient drink a flavored glucose solution of standardized concentration. Although the amount of glucose given may vary among laboratories, the generally accepted dosage consistent with NDDG recommendations is 75 g for nonpregnant adults and 100 g for pregnant women. Dosages may be calculated, with 1.75 g of glucose administered for every kilogram of body weight. This method is useful for determining the appropriate dosage for children.

When the patient has ingested the glucose laden beverage (beverage should be finished within 5-minutes), blood samples are collected at established intervals—often each hour for a total of 3 hours. Others may follow test protocols that include collection of a specimen at 30 minutes and at 1.5 hours. In some cases, a 5-hour tolerance may be requested, particularly in the investigation of hypoglycemia. Patients should remain within close proximity of collection personnel throughout the test procedure to better facilitate observation for symptoms such as nausea or vomiting, dizziness or weakness, sweating, or fainting. If such symptoms are noted, a blood sample should be collected immediately and tested on a stat basis. Vomiting or fainting should preclude test completion and the test should also be ended in the presence of other significant symptoms. Upon test completion, it is prudent practice to analyze the last specimen prior to releasing the patient to ensure that the blood glucose level is not significantly decreased.

INTERPRETATION OF RESULTS. Shortly after ingestion of the glucose challenge dose, the blood glucose will begin to rise rapidly, reaching a peak level at about 30 minutes (peak may be reached sooner in some individuals or at 1 hour in others). The level then begins to fall steadily, with the rate of decrease less rapid than the rate of increase leading to the peak level. With normal glucose metabolism, the blood glucose level should return to, or approximate, the normal fasting level at 2 hours following ingestion of the glucose. On the basis of the oral glucose tolerance test and following ADA criteria, diabetes mellitus is diagnosed if the 2-hour level is 200 mg/dL or higher. It is interesting to apply the varying diagnostic criteria presented in Table 6.4 (although ADA criteria are recommended) to GTT results such as those provided in Table 6–5.

Diagnoses for patients A, B, C, and D represented by the results in Table 6–5 are provided based on the ADA, Wilkerson, and Siperstein criteria for diagnosis, as indicated in Table 6–6.

Note that only patient A's GTT results are interpreted consistently across the three sets of criteria. The Wilkerson point system results in three of the four patients being diagnosed with diabetes mellitus (only patient A is not) and the Siperstein method results in only one of the four (patient D) being diagnosed. ADA criteria, increasingly becoming the standard for diagnosis, results in a diagnosis of diabetes mellitus in two of the four patients (patients C and D). ADA criteria make a further distinction in which the GTT curve shows evidence of impaired glucose tolerance but lacks a sufficient level of abnormality to warrant a diagnosis of diabetes mellitus. Such results would include a fasting level < 140 mg/dL and one value ≥200 mg/dL. Patient B fits this criterion and would be said to have **impaired glucose tolerance** based on ADA criteria. The use of the GTT in the evaluation of hypoglycemia is explained in a later section devoted to a discussion of hypoglycemia. Gestational diabetes mellitus is diagnosed using different procedures and criteria, also discussed later in this chapter.

TABLE 6–5. Sample GTT Results

	Glucose Concentration (mg/dL)			
Sample	A	B	C	D
Fasting	105	123	135	127
1/2 hour	200	235	275	285
1 hour	150	198	240	263
2 hour	110	147	205	225
3 hour	105	128	170	190

TABLE 6–6. Application of Diagnostic Criteria for Diabetes Mellitus

Patient	NDDG	Wilkerson	Siperstein
A	No	No	No
B	No	Yes	No
C	Yes	Yes	No
D	Yes	Yes	Yes

TIME FOR REVIEW. After studying the preceding sections, you should be able to respond correctly to the following:

■ Glucose in the diet is primarily in the form of two sugar molecules bound together chemically and called _____ .

■ Stored glucose in the liver is in the form of a polysaccharide called

_____ .

■ The pancreatic hormone that works to lower blood glucose levels by increasing transport to tissues and stimulating glucose oxidation is _____ .

■ What is the impact of glucagon on blood glucose level?

■ Pancreatic, thyroid, _____, and _____ hormones are involved in the regulation of glucose levels.

■ Describe the role of the liver in glucose regulation.

■ A temporary elevation in blood glucose is called _____ _____ and may result from acute stress.

■ The most likely cause of persistent hyperglycemia is

_____ _____.

■ List three classic symptoms of IDDM:

■ In the absence of pronounced classic symptoms of diabetes, a diagnosis of diabetes mellitus may be made based on ADA criteria if

fasting glucose level is ≥ _____ mg/dL on two occasions, or GTT yields 2-hour level that is ≥ _____ mg/dL.

■ Which method of glucose measurement is more specific: reducing substance or enzymatic?

■ Explain why home monitoring of blood glucose levels is preferred over urinary glucose measurements.

■ If a bedside glucose test performed on whole blood yielded a value of 410 mg/dL, which of the following values could be reasonably expected based solely on the inherent differences between serum and whole blood levels— serum level: 450 or 370?

■ Review the tables in these sections and practice the application of various criteria for the diagnosis of diabetes mellitus.

Check your results by reviewing the preceding sections.

■ DIABETIC CONTROL AND MONITORING

The **goal of treatment** for diabetes mellitus is not only the *control of blood glucose level,* but also the *prevention of complications* associated with diabetes. Complications include retinopathy, renal disease, neuropathy, peripheral vascular disorders, and myocardial infarction. Treatment is not addressed in this text beyond the summary information provided in Table 6–2. It is widely believed that maintaining strict glycemic control is beneficial in preventing, delaying, or limiting these significant complications. This is of particular importance when diabetes presents in childhood, adolescence, or early adulthood because these patients are exposed to the adverse impact of the illness for such a long period of time. Complications of diabetes may be seen both in IDDM and in NIDDM.

Achieving and maintaining an acceptable level of control is dependent upon a combination of pharmacologic therapy (insulin, oral hypoglycemics), suitable diet, and consistent physical activity. It is essential that patients and, when possible, family members be given information about the illness and are educated regarding

1. their treatment plan:
   types of treatment (insulin or hypoglycemics, diet, exercise)
   importance of strict adherence to prescribed treatment
2. home glucose monitoring:
   test performance and frequency of testing
   quality control and instrument maintenance
   factors influencing results
   what to do when results are above/below certain limits
3. complications of diabetes mellitus, both acute and chronic
4. how to recognize and respond to emergency situations
5. the need to wear a medical alert

Although home monitoring of blood glucose levels is an essential component of the overall monitoring of diabetes, it cannot be relied upon as the sole measure of the level of control achieved for a variety of reasons:

- patient technique may lead to inconsistent or inaccurate measures
- only acute changes are reflected
- improper maintenance and standardization of the home meter may cause invalid results
- results may be fabricated to satisfy the clinician's criteria for adequate control

If periodic laboratory measurement of serum or plasma glucose levels reveals notable discrepancies, patient technique should be observed and any deficiencies corrected and the home meter should be evaluated for appropriate functioning.

Any measure of blood glucose levels, regardless of method, reveals only the current status of control and is best used for assessing acute changes. Evaluation of long-term control is best accomplished using a measure of **hemoglobin A_{1C} (glycosylated or glycated hemoglobin; GHB)**. In a process called *glycosylation,* the beta-chain of hemoglobin forms a bond with glucose. Once a stable bond is formed, this process is irreversible and the hemoglobin/glucose bond is present for the life span of the red cell. Hemoglobin bound in this manner to glucose is referred to as glycosylated hemoglobin. (Most of the hemoglobin in adults is hemoglobin A. A small percentage of the total hemoglobin A is glycosylated and is composed of subcomponents—hemoglobin A_{1A}, A_{1B}, A_{1C}—the majority of which is A_{1C}.) The glycosylated hemoglobin assay measures the percentage of hemoglobin to which glucose has bound and is dependent upon the amount of glucose to which red cells have been exposed and the length of time over which the exposure occurred. It is a reflection of the average glucose concentration over the 6 to 8 week period prior to testing. Thus, measurement of the glycosylated hemoglobin level provides a more accurate measure of long-term control and is useful for monitoring the effectiveness of therapy and the patient's compliance with the prescribed therapeutic regimen. Measurements should be obtained 2 to 3 times per year—every 4 to 6 months. It is not useful to perform the test at intervals of less than 6 weeks, as the test reflects a period of 6 to 8 weeks. (Although hemoglobin A_{1C} has also been used by some practitioners in the diagnosis of diabetes mellitus or to distinguish between transient hyperglycemia and diabetes, these are not generally accepted indications for use of this test.)

When a patient has consistently reported good glycemic control based upon the results of home glucose monitoring, yet has a significant elevation in hemoglobin A_{1C} levels, an effort should be made to determine whether the discrepancy is related to improper patient technique, home meter malfunction, or falsified home monitoring results. If the discrepancy is not attributable to one or more of these factors, causes for false elevations in the hemoglobin A_{1C} level should be considered. Misleading elevations may be seen in the presence of elevated hemoglobin F—fetal hemoglobin—levels (which occur in children under 2 years and in some hemoglobinopathies), with other hemoglobinopathies, and in uremia. A variation of the glycosylated hemoglobin method using boronic affinity chromatography overcomes many of these problems. Reference ranges vary depending upon methodology (electrophoresis, affinity chromatography, elution from resin columns, etc), but generally have an upper limit of 6% or 7%.

A newer test of glucose control is a **fructosamine assay** measuring glycosylated proteins—usually total protein, including albumin and globulins. Although the name appears to imply testing for the sugar fructose, this is not the case. Rather the name results from the fructoseamine that follows the linkage of glucose to protein. The resulting glycosylated product is a stable ketoamine that can be measured by chromatography or colorimetry. Glycosylation of albumin and globulins is similar to that of hemoglobin, but they are present in the serum for a shorter period of time (shorter half-life than hemoglobin). As a result of this shorter half-life, the fructosamine assay (the test may also be referred to as *glycated protein*) evaluates control over a shorter time period of about 2 to 3 weeks as opposed to the 6 to 8 week period of A_{1C} levels. There is some evidence that fructosamine levels are reduced in response to decreased serum protein levels, which may be a limitation of the assay, but is probably only significant in situations where the decreased protein level is caused by a shortened albumin half-life or an increased loss of albumin. Some methods of measurement may be impacted by reducing substances in the serum.

Routine measurement of both fructosamine and hemoglobin A_{1C} is not necessary and either is likely sufficient to assess long-term control. It is important to recognize that fructosamine evaluates control over a shorter time period than hemoglobin A_{1C}, thus, test selection may be made based upon the time period the clinician wishes to assess as well as on test availability and cost. In patients with hemoglobin abnormalities that can result in elevations in the hemoglobin A_{1C} level, measurement of fructosamine is clearly the preferred choice.

■ OTHER LABORATORY MEASUREMENTS RELATED TO DIABETES MELLITUS

A number of additional laboratory assays are employed in diabetes mellitus, particularly in regard to the evaluation of abnormalities of diabetic control, of complications of insulin therapy, and complications of the disease process.

Hypoglycemia is a common and serious complication of insulin therapy characterized acutely by sweating, weakness, and shaking with eventual changes in consciousness. Such symptoms are a result of heightened secretion of epinephrine in response to a rapid decrease in blood glucose. It generally results from insulin overdose, particularly in unstable IDDM. When hypoglycemia develops more gradually, patients may complain of headache, sluggishness, and irritability. Because this is a common complication, it is imperative that patients recognize early symptoms of hypoglycemia. Laboratory analysis of glucose level on a stat basis or bedside testing with a glucose meter may be employed to confirm hypoglycemic status.

Hyperglycemia resulting from nonconformity to an appropriate diet plan or from inappropriate insulin dosage may also be seen in diabetes. Such elevations may be detected in routine home blood glucose monitoring or by laboratory analysis of glucose levels. In some cases, the development of insulin antibodies can result in hyperglycemia and require adjustment of the insulin dosage. Although virtually all patients on insulin therapy eventually develop such antibodies, they usually are not of sufficient titer to result in significant glucose elevations requiring insulin adjustment. Infrequently the insulin antibody titer is very high and the patient becomes resistant to the action of insulin. A suspected diagnosis of **insulin resistance** can be confirmed by laboratory determination of the **insulin antibody titer**.

Marked hyperglycemia and insulin deficiency may result in the most dangerous, sometimes life threatening complication of IDDM, **diabetic ketoacidosis (DKA)**. DKA results from either an absolute or relative insulin deficiency. Absolute insulin deficiency as a cause of DKA may be seen in previously undiagnosed diabetes mellitus or in patients who have missed an insulin dose. Relative insulin deficiency may result from stress hormones. In the presence of insulin deficiency the liver production of glucose increases (by increased gluconeogenesis and glycogenolysis) and the uptake of glucose by the tissues is decreased, resulting in hyperglycemia and subsequent increases in serum osmolality. As a result of this enhanced osmolality, an excessive amount of water, sodium, potassium, calcium, and phosphate are removed from the body through the urine. The metabolism of fat (in gluconeogenesis) results in ketone bodies, which are highly acidic. These ketone bodies are also excreted in the urine. The blood becomes more acidic, resulting in respiratory stimulation that lowers pCO_2. However, with the continuing production of hydrogen ions (H^+), the level of acidity continues to rise. Intracellular dehydration results from a loss of water in red cells in an attempt to equilibrate with the hyperosmolar serum. A depletion of intracellular potassium (K^+) is also related to intracellular dehydration and occurs because K^+ cannot enter the red cells without insulin. Serum levels may be elevated in some cases as a result, although urinary excretion of K^+ is increased.

Clinical signs of DKA include polyuria, polydipsia, hyperventilation, nausea, vomiting, abdominal pain, and tachycardia. A characteristic fruity breath odor may be detected and coma may result. The metabolic acidosis, dehydration, and potassium deficiencies produced in DKA are life threatening and require immediate intervention to correct the hyperglycemia and acidosis and to replenish electrolyte and water loss. DKA is more likely to be seen in IDDM than in NIDDM. It is important to note that other causes of ketoacidosis include starvation and alcohol ingestion and that DKA coma may require differentiation from hypoglycemic coma, nonketotic hyperosmolar coma, and drug-induced comas. Table 6–7 summarizes laboratory findings in various coma producing conditions. This summary of findings does not imply that laboratory assay of all listed parameters is necessary to diagnose such conditions, but rather is provided for the benefit of comparison.

Although not a frequent occurrence, **nonketotic hyperosmolar coma** is seen in NIDDM patients (particularly older patients) and may be precipitated by decreased glucose utilization resulting from infections, surgery, severe burns, cerebrovascular accidents, or the effects of certain drugs (diuretics, high dose corticosteroids, phenytoin). The metabolism of fat that results in the highly acidic ketones seen in DKA is not a part of the clinical picture in nonketotic hyperosmolar coma because these patients have sufficient insulin levels to prevent excessive gluconeogenesis (but not sufficient to prevent marked hyperglycemia). The development of this syndrome is usually more gradual than that of DKA and, as a result, fluid and electrolyte insufficiency may be more pronounced in this syndrome than in DKA. Laboratory findings are summarized in Table 6–7.

TABLE 6–7. Laboratory Findings in Diabetic Ketoacidosis and Other Coma-Producing Conditions

Laboratory Test	Diabetic Ketoacidosis	Hypoglycemia/ Insulin Overdose	Lactic Acidosis	Nonketotic Hyperosmolar Coma	Salicylate or Other Poisoning
Blood/Serum					
Glucose	↓↓	↓↓	N	↑↑↑	N
Ketones[1]	↑↑	O	O	O	O to ↑↑
PH	↓↓	N	↓↓	N	↓
HCO_3	↓↓	N	↓↓	N	↓
NA+	↓	N	N	N or ↑	↓
K+	variable	N	N	N	N
Anion gap	↑↑	N	↑↑↑	N	↑ or ↑↑
Osmolality	↑↑	N	N	↑↑↑	N
BUN	↑	N	N or ↑	↑	N or ↑
Urine:					
Glucose	↑↑	O	O	↑↑↑	O
Other reducing substances	O	O	O	O	↑↑
Ketones	↑↑	O	O or ↑	O	↑

[1]May be requested as serum acetone, although acetone is not the only ketone body detected.

↑ = increased; ↓ = decreased; O = absent; N = normal

Adapted from Sacher RA, McPherson RA. *Widmann's Clinical Interpretation of Laboratory Test,* 10th ed. Philadelphia, FA Davis, 1991

Lactic acidosis results from tissue hypoxia as a consequence of shock, severe anemia, or carbon monoxide poisoning. It may also be seen in diabetes and alcoholism, and in response to some toxins, including methanol and ethylene glycol. Serum lactate measurement is made to confirm diagnosis. Other laboratory findings are listed in Table 6–7.

Of the chronic complications seen in diabetes (retinopathy, neuropathy, nephropathy), only nephropathy lends itself to evaluation by clinical laboratory methods. **Nephropathy** (specifically glomerular damage) is a significant long-term complication of both IDDM and NIDDM, but has a greater incidence in IDDM. Nephropathy is usually not seen (at least at a level detectable by routine laboratory measurements) in IDDM during the first 5 years following diagnosis. However, the same is not true of NIDDM, in which patients may be diabetic for a notable time period before the diagnosis is made. The earliest indication of renal involvement is the presence of protein in the urine (*proteinuria*). The glomerular damage seen in diabetic nephropathy increases the permeability of the glomerulus, resulting in increased excretion of protein (albumin appears before other serum proteins) and a decrease in the glomerular filtration rate (GFR). Proteinuria may be detected on random or timed urine specimens by dipstick protein tests or by testing 24-hour urine specimens for protein (see Chapter 2). However, before overt proteinuria is detectable by standard dipstick protein tests, a stage called microalbuminuria occurs. *Microalbuminuria* refers to a urinary excretion rate of albumin that is higher than normal, but not sufficiently elevated to be detected by routine measurements of albumin. This subclinical stage can now be detected by special immunoassay tests that measure microalbumin either qualitatively (present or not present) or quantitatively (amount present). Early detection is imperative because a significant number of diabetic patients who develop nephropathy progress to end stage renal disease within a relatively few years. Detection of microalbuminuria allows the clinician to institute treatment that may slow the progression of renal damage or prevent further damage. Patients in whom microalbuminuria is detected have an increased likelihood of developing clinical diabetic nephropathy. Thus many consider the measurement of urinary microalbumin to be a standard component of the management of diabetes mellitus and the ADA has recommended the use of this analysis for several years.

■ HYPOGLYCEMIA

Diagnosis of hypoglycemia has been somewhat controversial or confusing depending upon how it is defined. *Chemical hypoglycemia* refers to a blood glucose level < 50 mg/dL regardless of the presence/absence of symptoms. Clinical hypoglycemia generally refers to the presence of symptoms associated with rapidly falling glucose levels or acute hypoglycemia. These symptoms result from the release of epinephrine and include sweating, shaking, weakness, irritability or anxiety, and palpitation. Persisting hypoglycemia can produce symptoms that include lethargy, confusion or bizarre behaviors, fainting, convulsions, or coma. However, symptoms are not consistently present at established glucose levels and conversely, may be present in some individuals at blood glucose levels well above 50 mg/dL. The presence of symptoms of hypoglycemia depends not only on the blood glucose level, but also on how fast the level is dropping, the level of glucose before the level began to drop, and on the level of glucose regulation. In healthy persons blood glucose levels are maintained within relatively narrow limits, but the degree of regulation varies among those with disorders of glucose metabolism. A well-controlled IDDM patient might not experience symptoms of hypoglycemia even with a blood glucose of 40 mg/dL whereas a poorly regulated patient might be symptomatic with glucose levels within the normal reference range. A diagnosis of hypoglycemia can be made with greater objectivity and less confusion if the following criteria are used for diagnosis:

- symptoms of hypoglycemia are present
- serum or plasma glucose is < 50 mg/dL at the time of symptoms
- raising the glucose level to normal range eliminates symptoms

Hypoglycemia may be divided into two categories based upon when it occurs: fasting or postprandial. **Fasting hypoglycemia** may result from a variety of causes, but is almost always of pathologic significance. The most common causes include excessive insulin production or abnormalities in other hormones involved in the regulation of glucose levels. One of the most well-known causes is **insulinoma**, in which an insulin excess results from the presence of an insulin producing tumor of the pancreatic beta-cells. Liver disease, alcoholism, and some nonpancreatic tumors that produce an insulin-like substance can also result in fasting hypoglycemia. A fasting glucose < 50 mg/dL with symptoms that are alleviated by restoring the glucose level to normal is diagnostic of fasting hypoglycemia. Measuring serum insulin levels in conjunction with glucose levels facilitates the differentiation of causes of fasting hypoglycemia—excessive insulin or inappropriate mobilization of glucose. Insulin levels should decrease as the glucose level falls. When insulin levels do not decline as expected, the presence of an insulin producing tumor should be suspected. Because of other conditions (Cushing syndrome, chronic renal failure, and others) that may also produce insulin levels higher than expected based on serum glucose level, some clinicians prefer the use of a ratio of "immunoreactive" insulin to glucose (IRI:G). Some investigators find this ratio, or some variant of it, to be more sensitive and reliable in indicating the presence of insulinoma. *C-peptide,* which is a by-product of insulin production, can also be used to evaluate insulin production. The C-peptide level is increased in insulinoma when glucose levels are < 40 mg/dL. The 5-hour GTT commonly used in the past for detecting insulinoma is now rarely used for this purpose because a notable number of patients with insulinoma do not demonstrate the characteristic curve for the condition (normal or low fasting; normal sharp increase; slow fall to hypoglycemic level without return to normal). "Flat" GTT curves, a diabetic-like curve, or even a normal GTT curve have been reported in insulinoma.

Post-prandial, or **reactive**, **hypoglycemia** may be seen as a result of some gastrointestinal disorders and in early NIDDM, and in many cases is idiopathic.

Gastrointestinal postprandial hypoglycemia may be seen in patients who have undergone procedures such as pyloroplasty or gastrectomy. It results from rapid gastric emptying and duodenal absorption of carbohydrates, which results in a significantly elevated blood glucose level. The body responds with a swift, excessive increase in the production of insulin, creating an insulinemia that remains after carbohydrates are no longer being absorbed. This results in a temporary hypoglycemia about 1 to 3 hours after a meal. In early diabetes, NIDDM patients may experience hypoglycemia 3 to 5 hours after glucose ingestion. This type of postprandial hypoglycemia results from an inadequate early insulin response that allows blood glucose levels to rise unduly. An excessive, prolonged insulin response follows and produces hypoglycemia. In functional or idiopathic hypoglycemia, which includes the majority of hypoglycemia cases, decreased glucose levels are seen about 2 to 5 hours after a meal without a preceding hyperglycemia and without a recognized physiologic explanation. Symptoms in functional hypoglycemia are often corrected even without carbohydrate ingestion. In many cases symptomatic episodes do not correlate well with blood glucose levels, with symptoms either occurring at relatively normal glucose levels or not occurring in the presence of significantly decreased glucose levels. This type of hypoglycemia is perhaps the most controversial in terms of diagnosis. Prior to classifying cases of hypoglycemia as post-prandial it is important to first rule out fasting hypoglycemia, particularly in those patients in whom symptoms are noted several hours following a meal.

The conventional approach to the diagnosis of post-prandial hypoglycemia is the oral GTT. Although not absolute and as clear cut as one might desire, general GTT patterns expected in the various types of post-prandial hypoglycemia are presented in Table 6–8. A 5-hour tolerance is used because the hypoglycemia will often not be seen until after a 3-hour tolerance test has ended. It is imperative that patients in whom hypoglycemia is suspected be carefully monitored throughout the test period, as the high glucose challenge dose can provoke precipitous drops in blood glucose with the potential for loss of consciousness or shock. Patients should be instructed to notify staff members immediately of any symptoms. When symptoms are reported, a sample should be collected for testing in order to allow correlation

TABLE 6–8. Five-Hour Oral GTT Patterns in Postprandial Hypoglycemia

Sample	Gastrointestinal	Early Diabetes	Functional
Fasting	N	N or SL ↑	N
Peak	↑	N or ↑	N
2 hour	N or ↓*	↑	N
3 to 5 hours	↓*	↓**	↓***

*Peak followed by rapid fall in glucose reaching hypoglycemic level in 1 to 3 hours; **In early diabetes, hypoglycemia levels occur during 3 to5 hour interval; ***Hypoglycemia occurs in 2 to 4 hour intervals; N = normal and refers to the reference range for that particular sample type; ↑ = increased; ↓ = decreased.

Adapted from Ravel R. *Clinical Laboratory Medicine: Clinical Application of Laboratory Data,* 6th ed. St Louis, Mosby, 1995 of symptoms with glucose levels. In the presence of severe symptoms it is still important to determine the glucose level at that time, but discontinuation of the procedure is warranted and glucose should be administered.

Measuring insulin and cortisol levels for correlation with blood glucose levels can provide further useful information and provide additional means of distinguishing the various types of post-prandial hypoglycemia. Increased insulin secretion will be evident in the early diabetes form of hypoglycemia, but insulin levels in functional hypoglycemia will correlate appropriately with changes in glucose levels.

Another somewhat surprising but noteworthy cause of hypoglycemia may present an initial diagnostic challenge for the clinician. In hypoglycemia of this classification, patients may have significant observable symptoms and, when possible to do so, specimens collected at the time of symptoms are likely to reveal a decreased glucose level. However, no consistent relationship between the time of meals and the occurrence of symptoms can be demonstrated and supervised GTT results produce a normal curve with no hypoglycemic "dip." Surreptitiously injected insulin gives rise to this clinical picture, which is called **factitious hypoglycemia**. As extraordinary as it may seem, factitious hypoglycemia occurs at a frequency sufficient to be an issue of note in the evaluation of hypoglycemia. A clinical picture consistent with that described in a patient with access to insulin and syringes (eg, a family member of IDDM patient or employee in a medical setting) should raise the possibility of secretly administered insulin. One of the most important uses of C-peptide measurements is in the diagnosis of this condition. When a precursor of insulin called proinsulin is split by enzyme action in the pancreatic cells to form insulin, the amino acid C-peptide is produced. When insulin is prepared for injection the C-peptide is removed, so while factitious hypoglycemia will reveal elevated serum insulin levels, C-peptide levels will be low. Note that this differs from the results obtained in insulinoma, in that both the serum insulin and C-peptide levels will be elevated in insulinoma.

■ SPECIAL CONSIDERATIONS IN PREGNANCY

Pregnant diabetic patients require meticulous monitoring to ensure that glucose levels (serum or whole blood levels; monitoring urinary glucose is not sufficient) are maintained as close to normal as possible. This may require administration of insulin (oral hypoglycemics are not recommended during pregnancy according to guidelines of the ADA) to NIDDM patients during pregnancy, as poor glycemic control produces significant risk of complications to both the mother and her unborn child. A number of women who have had no symptoms of diabetes develop abnormalities of glucose metabolism during pregnancy. The term **gestational diabetes** is applied to such cases. It is important to evaluate glucose metabolism in pregnant women with glycosuria, those with significant family history of diabetes, and those who have previously given birth to large babies. Many clinicians follow ADA recommendations to screen pregnant women between 24 and 28 weeks' gestation by administering a 50 g oral glucose challenge and analyzing the glucose level 1 hour later. Patients need not be fasting prior to administration of the glucose dose.

One-hour levels exceeding 140 mg/dL require further investigation with a 3-hour oral GTT test. Although there is disagreement regarding cutoff points (some studies appear to indicate that lower cutoffs should be used), ADA criteria for the diagnosis of gestational diabetes require **two** elevated values on the GTT following administration of a 100 g glucose dose. The ADA cutoff values are as follows:

fasting:	≥105 mg/dL
1 hour:	≥190 mg/dL
2 hour:	≥165 mg/dL
3 hour:	≥145 mg/dL

Patients diagnosed with gestational diabetes should be tested again after pregnancy. Because women with gestational diabetes are at an increased risk for subsequent development of diabetes, education regarding nutrition, physical activity, and maintenance of appropriate body weight is important, along with regular follow-up.

6. SELF TEST

Choose the best response by circling the appropriate letter. The answer key may be found in the appendices.

1. **Glucose is stored in the liver in the form of**
   A. glycogen
   B. monosaccharides
   C. disaccharides
   D. fatty acids

2. **The pancreatic hormone that lowers glucose levels by increasing transport to tissues is**
   A. somatostatin
   B. glucagon
   C. insulin
   D. cortisol

3. **A temporary increase in blood glucose is called**
   A. persistent hyperglycemia
   B. transient hyperglycemia
   C. diabetes mellitus
   D. hypoglycemia

4. *Gluconeogenesis* **is the term applied to the**
   A. conversion of glucose to glycogen
   B. conversion of glycogen to glucose
   C. synthesis of proinsulin molecules
   D. synthesis of glucose from fatty acids

5. **The most specific methods for the assay of serum glucose levels are**
   A. chromatography methods
   B. reducing substance methods
   C. enzymatic methods

6. **Which set of results from an oral GTT would be diagnostic of diabetes mellitus on a nonpregnant adult using ADA criteria? Values are given in milligrams per dealiter.**
   A. fasting = 110; 1 hour = 220; 2 hour = 160; 3 hour = 120
   B. fasting = 90; 1 hour = 180; 2 hour = 130; 3 hour = 95
   C. fasting = 125; 1 hour = 230; 2 hour = 190; 3 hour = 160
   D. fasting = 130; 1 hour = 275; 2 hour = 210; 3 hour = 145

7. **Long-term blood glucose control is best evaluated by**
   A. hemoglobin A_{1C}
   B. C-peptide
   C. fructosamine
   D. home glucose monitoring

8. **Which of the following sets of laboratory data is most consistent with DKA?**
   A. serum and urine glucose elevated; blood pH = 7.43; increased serum osmolality and bicarbonate
   B. serum glucose and osmolality elevated; blood pH = 7.34; glucose and ketones in urine
   C. ketones in urine; blood pH = 7.36; normal serum osmolality and glucose

9. **Which of the following sets of laboratory data is most consistent with insulinoma?**
   A. low fasting glucose; decreased serum insulin and C-peptide levels
   B. high fasting glucose; increased serum insulin and C-peptide levels
   C. low fasting glucose; increased serum insulin and C-peptide levels
   D. low fasting glucose; increased serum insulin; decreased C-peptide level

10. **Which of the following sets of laboratory data is most consistent with factitious hypoglycemia?**
    A. low fasting glucose; decreased serum insulin and C-peptide levels
    B. low fasting glucose; decreased serum insulin; increased C-peptide levels
    C. low fasting glucose; increased serum insulin and C-peptide levels
    D. low fasting glucose; increased serum insulin; decreased C-peptide level

11. **The type of reactive, or post-prandial, hypoglycemia characterized by a normal fasting glucose level, an elevated peak level following a glucose challenge dose, and rapidly falling glucose levels that reach hypoglycemic levels 1 to 3 hours after the challenge dose is**
    A. hypoglycemia of early diabetes
    B. hypoglycemia of gastrointestinal causes
    C. idiopathic or functional hypoglycemia

12. **Factitious hypoglycemia results from**
    A. gastrointestinal disorders
    B. a currently unknown cause
    C. insufficient carbohydrate intake
    D. secret self-administration of insulin

13. **Choose the oral GTT results that would be classified as gestational diabetes by ADA criteria.**
    A. fasting = 100; 1 hour = 240; 2 hour = 200; 3 hour = 138
    B. fasting = 108; 1 hour = 180; 2 hour = 140; 3 hour = 110
    C. fasting = 90; 1 hour = 195; 2 hour = 156; 3 hour = 140
    D. fasting = 110; 1 hour = 185; 2 hour = 164; 3 hour = 127

7. TESTS OF LIPID METABOLISM

The term *lipids* refers to a group of fats or fat-like substances that are *hydrophobic* (literally, "water fearing") and thus insoluble in water. Lipids may be categorized as:

- *Neutral fats:* fatty acids in the form of triglycerides (esters of three fatty acids and glycerol)
- *Conjugated lipids:* lipids joined to phosphate (phospholipid) or sugar (glycolipid)
- *Sterols:* fat-related alcohols that may be esterified with fatty acids

FUNCTION AND METABOLISM

This chapter will focus on the three major lipids of biologic consequence in the serum. **Triglycerides** are stored in fat tissue and are readily available when needed to provide fatty acids for gluconeogenesis (conversion of fatty acids to glucose) and energy production. **Cholesterol** is an important component in the structure of cell membranes and in the synthesis of bile acids and the steroid hormones. **Phospholipids** are essential components of cell walls and play a role in lowering the surface tension of fluids in the lung.

Because lipids are not water soluble, they require specialized protein transport in the blood. These specialized proteins, **apolipoproteins**, are very important in the metabolism of lipids in that they aid in their solubility, in their transport from the gastrointestinal tract to the liver, and in their clearance, as well as serving to activate or inhibit the enzymes involved in lipid metabolism. Lipids bound to these proteins are called *lipoproteins* and exist in the circulation as large, complicated particles. The different types of particles differ in the amount of cholesterol, triglycerides, and protein they contain, in size, and in density. The distinctive density of each of the various lipoproteins in serum is an important classifying characteristic as will be seen later in this chapter.

Cholesterol and triglycerides in the blood come from the diet (exogenous) and from synthesis within the body (endogenous). Phospholipids are synthesized primarily in the liver and in the intestine. Most of the body's cholesterol is produced by the liver, from which a portion is excreted in bile. Although cholesterol is also provided by dietary intake, the body appears to supply sufficient quantities for fundamental metabolic processes through synthesis and a subsequent breakdown and "salvage operation" in which cholesterol is recycled.

Circulating triglycerides derived from dietary neutral fat are broken down by the pancreatic enzyme lipase into free fatty acids and single monoglyceride molecules that are absorbed through the intestine along with cholesterol. In the intestine the free fatty acids and monoglycerides again form triglycerides and, along with small amounts of free cholesterol, phospholipids, and protein, form **chylomicrons**. When they reach the blood, circulating chylomicrons release triglycerides to the adipose tissue, where it is stored and available for the body's fatty acid needs. Enzyme action (lipoprotein lipase) breaks the chylomicrons into smaller particles with the liberation of free fatty acids. A portion of the free fatty acids is utilized for energy in muscle tissue, some is transported to the liver, and some is converted back to triglyceride and stored in adipose tissue. The fragments of broken down chylomicrons, or *chylomicron remnants,* are metabolized by the liver. These processes constitute the **exogenous (or dietary) lipid pathway**.

The **endogenous lipid pathway** results in the formation of **very low density lipoproteins (VLDL)** and **low density lipoproteins (LDL)** aided by the liver, enzyme actions, and **high density lipoproteins (HDL)**. Triglycerides and cholesterol are synthesized in the liver. VLDL is secreted in conjunction with this synthesis and is acted on by the enzyme lipoprotein lipase to produce a lipoprotein of intermediate density. This intermediate lipoprotein can be removed by the liver or forms LDL. LDL then goes to the tissues, where metabolism releases cholesterol (cholesterol is present in significant amounts in LDL) that can be used in cell membranes or in steroid synthesis, or may form deposits called **atheromas**.

MAJOR CLASSES OF LIPOPROTEINS

Size, density, chemical composition, flotation, and patterns in electrophoresis are used to identify the various lipoprotein classes. Chylomicrons, VLDL, LDL, and HDL, constituting the four major classes, will be described here.

■ CHYLOMICRONS

Chylomicrons are the largest of the four and the least dense. In fact, the density of water is notably higher than that of the chylomicrons, allowing them to float to the top of serum even without centrifugation. A high chylomicron content is responsible for the milky appearance of serum after meals, and if serum is allowed to stand for several hours, the chylomicrons float to the top, collecting to form a creamy layer. This finding in a fasting specimen is abnormal. Triglycerides constitute the major portion of chylomicrons, with cholesterol, phospholipids, and protein present in smaller quantities. This high ratio of lipid to protein is responsible for the low density of chylomicrons.

■ VERY LOW DENSITY LIPOPROTEINS

Very low density lipoproteins, similar in structure to chylomicrons, also have triglycerides as a major constituent, although to a lesser degree than in chylomicrons. They have a slightly higher density than chylomicrons because of the somewhat lower lipid to protein ratio and are smaller in size, though still large particles. Because they are still rather large particles and to some extent floatable, high concentrations of VLDL also cause alterations in the appearance of serum, producing visible turbidity.

■ LOW DENSITY LIPOPROTEINS

Of significantly smaller size and higher density, LDL do not result in visible turbidity of serum even in very high concentrations. Their higher density is a consequence of a lower lipid to protein ratio. LDL have a considerably lower triglyceride content than either chylomicrons or VLDL and a substantially higher protein content. The major protein in LDL particles is apolipoprotein B (ApoB); the major lipid component is cholesterol and cholesteryl esters. Based on their major role in cellular cholesterol supply, LDL are important contributors to the development of atherosclerosis. This association has resulted in application of the term *bad cholesterol* to describe LDL in some public educational efforts.

■ HIGH DENSITY LIPOPROTEINS

Although high density lipoproteins can be separated into two subclasses with differences in size, density, and chemical composition, HDL are discussed here as a single lipoprotein. HDL particles are the smallest and least dense of the four major lipoproteins, with a composition that is about half protein. The remainder of the lipoprotein is composed primarily of cholesterol and phospholipids with only a small amount of triglycerides. In addition to their role in helping to form LDL (which could contribute to the development of atheroclerosis), HDL appear to function in some manner to remove cholesterol from the tissues and transport it to the liver. This function, though neither clearly identified nor fully understood, implies that higher levels of HDL lower the risk of coronary artery disease by reducing cholesterol deposits. HDL are often referred to as *good cholesterol* in materials targeted to public awareness of the association between lipids and coronary artery disease.

LABORATORY MEASUREMENTS AND REFERENCE RANGES

Laboratory determinations of the previously discussed lipoproteins are often combined into lipid panels or profiles from which a risk level can be determined and a lipoprotein phenotype established. Lipid profiles may be requested following detection of elevations in total cholesterol and triglyceride, in the evaluation of new patients, and in the assessment of patients in whom other risk factors (obesity, hypertension, family history of heart disease, smoking, diabetes mellitus, etc.) are present. The National Cholesterol Education Program (NCEP) recommends a total cholesterol determination on all individuals more than 20 years old and fractionation for all those whose cholesterol level does not fall within the desirable range.

The determination of cholesterol reference ranges is somewhat different than that described for other analytes in Chapter 1. Instead of testing a population of apparently healthy individuals and statistically determining a 95% confidence range, desirable levels have been developed by the NCEP along with ranges constituting borderline and high risk. The use of the traditional normal population study would not be prudent in this case as it would likely produce an invalid range resulting from the inclusion of persons who would subsequently develop coronary artery disease. A notable percentage of any randomly selected group of Americans could be anticipated to have high lipid levels based on the high calorie, high cholesterol diet that is common in this country.

■ TOTAL CHOLESTEROL

Total cholesterol levels include the measurement of the cholesterol found in all the lipoproteins. Most measurements today employ **enzymatic methods** that have replaced previous colorimetric chemical methods. Although not exclusively specific for cholesterol (other sterols can interfere), enzymatic methods are significantly more specific than the older chemical methods, which were subject to interference by a variety of sterol and non-sterol substances. Enzymatic measurements involve a series of steps in which a hydrolase enzyme breaks cholesterol esters into cholesterol and fatty acids; cholesterol is oxidized by the cholesterol oxidase enzyme; and the resulting hydrogen peroxide is measured following reaction with peroxidase and a special dye compound, allowing absorbance to be measured at a defined wavelength (500 nm).

In response to the variability of cholesterol measurements among methods and laboratories, the NCEP's Laboratory Standardization Panel (LSP) issued a number of recommendations to achieve a greater level of standardization. Among these recommendations is the use of calibration standards that are traceable to the NRS/CHOL (National Reference System Cholesterol Standard) of the Centers for Disease Control (CDC) or the National Institute of Standards and Technology (NIST) and laboratory participation in proficiency testing programs that use materials also traceable to the NRS/CHOL (such as the CAP or AAB-American Association of Bioanalysts).

The LSP report also gives considerable attention to the **"desk top" analyzers** often used in large scale screenings (like health fairs) or in small laboratories in physician offices or clinics. Of particular concern to the LSP was the assurance that operators of these systems are properly trained in the use of the instrument as well as in the recognition of potential sources of error, instrument maintenance, quality control protocols, and external quality assurance programs. Because these analyzers are designed to be used largely by individuals other than laboratory scientists, appropriate training is imperative to avoid improper use and to ensure understanding and recognition of pre-analytical, analytical, and post-analytical sources of error. Selected LSP guidelines for manufacturers, summarized from NIH Publication No. 90-2964, and for physicians and instrument operators are provided in Table 7–1. For a complete discussion of these and other recommendations along with the rationale for such recommendations, the reader is referred to the aforementioned NIH publication entitled "Recommendations for Improving Cholesterol Measurement."

In addition to a certain amount of analytical variability, considerable **physiologic variability** in cholesterol occurs, making it somewhat difficult to determine an individual's usual cholesterol level. For example, in the same 24-hour period and in the same individual, cholesterol values vary an average of 8 % and from day to day in the same individual vary 10 % to 15 %, with up to 44 % variation documented in the literature (Ravel, 1995). To realize the impact of this variation, coupled with the variation inherent in any analytical system, consider a patient whose serum cholesterol yields a value of 300 mg/dL. Assuming a low analytical variation of 3 % and strictly controlled pre-analytical factors, another test performed the same day on this patient could yield a cholesterol level as low as 267 mg/dL or as high as 333 mg/dL, or another test performed the next day could yield a value as low as 246 mg/dL or as high as 354 mg/dL. A patient with a cholesterol of 235 mg/dL (borderline risk) could conceivably move to the desirable range

TABLE 7–1. LSP Recommendations for Desk Top Cholesterol Analyzers

Manufacturers	Physicians and Instrument Operators
Instruments should be easy to use, requiring minimal reagent and sample handling.	Develop and employ standardized procedures for patient preparation and sample collection (venous samples preferred).
Instruments should not require frequent calibration and calibration standards traceable to the NRS/CHOL should be provided.	Verify manufacturer's claims of accuracy using certified reference materials with accurate target values from NIST, CDC, or CAP.
Methods with high degree of accuracy (± 5% of reference value) and precision (overall CV ≤ 5%) should be employed if operated by nonlaboratorians.	Adhere to appropriate quality assurance and quality control programs and assure analyst's understanding of analytical bias with the ability to graph control results for the visual detection of trends before result validity is compromised.
Written materials accompanying the analyzer should be easily understood by operators lacking formal education and training in laboratory science; include instructions for use and maintenance; pre-analytical factors affecting cholesterol values; discussion of quality control and quality assurance programs; identification of procedural steps in which undetected error may be introduced; and description of troubleshooting support and service for addressing analytical problems.	Choose an instrument with high degree of precision; thorough training program; adequate support and instrument service; that is not highly operator dependent; with standardization process traceable to NRS/CHOL; and that is in compliance with all LSP recommendations for manufacturers.
	Use uniform cholesterol reporting method based on NCEP and perform at least two separate cholesterol determinations prior to making medical decisions regarding further actions (if results are not within 30 mg/dL of each other, perform third test).

(value of 193 mg/dL) or to the high risk category (value of 277 mg/dL) based on day to day variability even when testing is performed under strictly controlled and standardized conditions.

This variability has led to recommendations, the prudence of which is apparent in light of the foregoing examples. The NCEP recommends that **medical decisions not be based on single measurements of cholesterol**. Instead, an average of at least two values performed at least 1 week apart, but within 2 months, should be used (assuming analytical CV of ~ 5 %). Further, when treatment has been instituted to lower cholesterol levels, measurements should not be performed too frequently to detect true decreases. The cholesterol level should be retested 6 weeks after the institution of drug therapy (Stein, 1993).

The importance of controlling pre-analytical factors is demonstrated by the list of factors, besides diet, that can influence cholesterol levels shown in Table 7–2.

Interference with cholesterol assays (method dependent) may result from some medications (including oral contraceptives and estrogen), high serum levels of vitamin C, bilirubin, hemoglobin in hemolyzed specimens, and the presence of large, light scattering particles such as chylomicrons or VLDP.

With the foregoing discussion of the variability in cholesterol measurement and the factors influencing or interfering with cholesterol measurements, one might be understandably tempted to question the validity and usefulness of cholesterol as an indicator of coronary artery disease risk. However, a significant body of scientific studies have unequivocally linked elevated total cholesterol (and LDL) levels to the development of atherosclerotic cardiovascular disease. Further, a number of additional studies have provided incontrovertible evidence that lowering cholesterol levels improves the prognosis in cardiovascular disease. These studies indicate that a 1 % reduction in total serum cholesterol is associated with a 2 %

TABLE 7–2. Non-Dietary Factors Influencing Cholesterol Test Results

Factor	Type of Influence	Comments
Body position	Values can be as much as 10% lower when patient changes from erect to reclining position	Use sitting position to collect all samples; if necessary to collect in reclining position, use this position to collect subsequent samples
Prolonged tourniquet application	Applied too long for venipuncture can cause apparent increase	Remove tourniquet within 2 minutes, preferably 1 minute, if possible
Pregnancy	May increase	Retest 3 to 4 months after pregnancy
Acute myocardial infarction	Increase	Retest after 2 months
Surgery	Increase	Test prior to surgery or repeat 2 months after
Bacterial sepsis or viral infection	Decrease	Avoid testing during illness

decrease in non-fatal myocardial infarction and deaths from coronary artery disease (Stein, 1993). It is important to be aware of the potential for variability in order to implement standardized methods to limit variation and interference with testing. Variability becomes especially significant when the combined effect of a number of factors is involved (ie, poorly controlled pre-analytical factors combined with imprecise or non-standardized test methodology and the inherent physiologic variation of cholesterol values would produce highly variable, unreliable test results). Conversely, cholesterol results obtained from an accredited laboratory in good standing that employs qualified personnel and uses standardized methods with materials traceable to the NRS/CHOL can be considered reliable for use in diagnostic and treatment decisions.

REFERENCE RANGES. As explained earlier, traditional "normal" population studies with statistical derivation of a reference range are not appropriate in cholesterol analysis. NCEP risk criteria are commonly used, although some clinicians may use the NIH consensus criteria developed prior to NCEP criteria. These two sets of criteria are listed in Table 7–3. Compare the desirable cholesterol levels and those at which patients are considered "at risk" in this table with the values obtained by the traditional approach to establishing normal reference ranges found in Table 7–4. This comparison demonstrates the fallibility of using conventional reference range derivation methods in this case.

TABLE 7–3. NIH Consensus and NCEP Cholesterol Criteria for Coronary Heart Disease Risk

		Low Risk	Moderate Risk	High Risk
	Age (yr)	Total Cholesterol (mg/dL)	Total Cholesterol (mg/dL)	Total Cholesterol (mg/dL)
	2–19	≤170	170–185	>185
NIH	20–29	≤200	200–220	>220
	30–39	≤200	220–240	>240
	>40	≤240	240–260	>260
		Desirable	**Borderline** **High Risk**	**High Risk**
NCEP	(all ages)	<200	200–239	≥240

TABLE 7–4. Traditionally Derived Total Cholesterol Reference Range (Upper Normal Limit; in mg/dL)

		Age (yr)				
		10–19	20–29	30–39	40–49	50–59
Frederickson et al		230	240	270	310	330
Heiss et al	Male	200	234	267	275	276
	Female	200	222	251	267	296

Adapted from Ravel R. *Clinical Laboratory Medicine: Clinical Application of Laboratory Data,* 6th ed. St Louis, Mosby, 1995

Although most cholesterol measurements are aimed at detecting possible increases, **hypocholesterolemia** (low total serum cholesterol) may result from a variety of conditions, a number of which are inherited disorders. These are discussed later in this chapter.

■ TRIGLYCERIDES

As with cholesterol, **enzymatic methods** are generally used for the measurement of serum triglyceride levels, having replaced a variety of earlier chemical methods. A commonly employed method utilizes the enzyme **lipase** to break triglycerides into fatty acids and glycerol (hydrolysis). The action of other enzymes results in the formation of glycerophosphate, which, depending on the type of method and enzyme action used, can be measured spectrophotometrically based on either the formation of NADH, the production of hydrogen peroxide (H_2O_2), or the disappearance of NADH. Measurements are standardized using materials of defined composition.

Though fasting samples should be used for measurement of all lipids, it is of particular importance with triglycerides, and a minimum of 12 hours of fasting should be required. Both within day and day-to-day variation of triglyceride levels are quite high. In addition to increases seen with a high fat diet, levels may be increased with estrogen therapy, in acute myocardial infarction, trauma, and pregnancy, and with alcohol intake. A number of diseases also can result in increased triglyceride levels, including diabetes mellitus, nephrotic syndrome, uremia, and hypothyroidism. Elevated levels are also seen in acute pancreatitis. In fact, very high levels may be indicative of pancreatitis and occasional cases have been detected on this basis. Interference with some methodologies is seen with high levels of bilirubin or vitamin C. Triglyceride levels are affected in the same manner as cholesterol by erect to reclining posture changes (the decrease in triglyceride is greater than that in cholesterol) and by prolonged tourniquet application.

Though supported by some studies, triglyceride as an independent risk factor remains somewhat controversial. For this reason, one does not see triglyceride screenings at health fairs and shopping malls as became popular for cholesterol with the development of portable, relatively operator independent analyzers. Triglyceride measurements are included in lipid panels for the calculation of LDL, and this is perhaps its use of primary clinical importance.

REFERENCE RANGES. Reference ranges for triglycerides vary based on age and gender, but a general reference range of 10 to 190 mg/dL is common in the literature. With cholesterol levels in the desirable range, triglycerides up to 250 mg/dL are not generally considered to be associated with risk (Jacobs, 1990).

■ HDL/LDL/VLDL/CHYLOMICRONS

The individual lipoproteins can be separated based on their density using ultracentrifugation. Electrophoresis may also be used to identify and quantitate chylomicrons, VLDL, LDL, and HDL. More practical methods for use in routine clinical laboratory analysis involve the precipitation of all the lower density lipoproteins, leaving only HDL. The HDL cholesterol (HDL-C) can then be measured and used in conjunction with total cholesterol and triglyceride values to calculate the LDL concentration. LDL cholesterol (LDL-C) is determined using the formula:

$$\text{LDL-C} = (\text{total cholesterol}) - \frac{(\text{HDL-C}) - (\text{triglycerides})}{5}$$

The cholesterol content of VLDL has been determined to be one fifth of the fasting triglyceride level. Thus the formula above subtracts the directly measured HDL-C and the mathematically determined VLDL cholesterol from the total cholesterol value to obtain the LDL-C. This formula cannot be used with significantly elevated triglycerides, in which case ultracentrifugation may be used. (For most laboratories this means referral of the sample to a reference laboratory, as ultracentrifugation techniques are not generally available.) The formula for the estimation of LDL-C provided here is called the *Friedewald formula* after its developer. There are at least two other proposed formulas. One of these suggests that dividing triglyceride by 6 instead of 5 produces more accurate results (Ravel, 1995) and the other multiplies the triglyceride value by 0.16 (Sacher, 1991), suggesting the approximation obtained in this manner is more representative of population data. Both of these alternate methods yield similar results as can be seen by the following sample calculations using each of the three formulas and measured values of total cholesterol = 200, triglyceride = 100, and HDL-C = 40:

LDL-C = 200 – 40 – 100/5 → 60 – 20 = 40   **LDL-C = 40**
LDL-C = 200 – 40 – 100/6 → 60 – 17 = 43   **LDL-C = 43**
LDL-C = 200 – 40 – (100)(.16) → 60 – 16 = 44   **LDL-C = 44**

With measured values of total cholesterol = 280; HDL-C = 35; triglyceride = 260:

LDL-C = 280 – 35 – 260/5 → 245 – 52 = 193   **LDL-C = 193**
LDL-C = 280 – 35 – 260/6 → 245 – 43 = 202   **LDL-C = 202**
LDL-C = 280 – 35 – (260)(.16) → 245 – 42 = 203   **LDL-C = 203**

The NCEP criteria for risk associated with LDL-C is provided in Table 7–5.

TABLE 7–5. NCEP Criteria for LDL-C

Category	LCL-C (mg/dL)
Desirable	<130
Borderline high risk	130–159
High risk	≥160

In the examples used previously to calculate LDL-C, a patient with the first set of results is in the desirable category and one with the second set of results falls into the high risk category.

High HDL-C levels have a negative association with cardiovascular disease; that is, the higher the HDL-C, the lower the level of risk. In terms of association with risk, HDL-C also appears to be an independent factor, meaning that significant increases lower the risk level independently of other risk factors and that significant decreases in HDL-C increase the risk of cardiovascular disease irregardless of other lipid values. Some clinicians use a **ratio of the total serum cholesterol to the HDL-C** as an indicator of risk, with a ratio of 5 representing average risk, 10 indicating a risk double the normal, and 20 denoting a triple risk. Not only is this ratio a convenient and simply calculated parameter (total cholesterol divided by HDL-C), but it is held by some to be the best single indicator of risk. This ratio would be 5 (normal risk) using the first data set and 8 (risk nearly double the normal risk) with the second set. It is worth noting that only one of the HDL fractions (HDL$_2$) is responsible for the association of higher HDL levels with reduced risk of cardiovascular disease. This is the fraction responsible for the increases seen in response to exercise. The other fraction (HDL$_3$) however, is elevated in heavy alcohol consumption, which is not associated with risk reduction. Thus an increased HDL-C resulting from a significant elevation in the HDL$_3$ fraction could falsely contribute to the impression of lowered risk, because routine clinical assays cannot distinguish the two fractions. Neither NIH nor NCEP have currently provided specific HDL levels deemed desirable or constituting specific categories of risk. However, levels < 35 mg/dL are almost always associated with increased risk. Reference levels are dependent on age and separate ranges are generally provided for males and females. Because black Americans have been shown to have higher HDL levels than white Americans, some sources also provide different ranges based on race as well. The levels in Table 7–6 are differentiated on gender only.

TABLE 7–6. HDL-C Association with Coronary Artery Disease Risk

HDL-C	Risk (× average)	
(mg/dL)	Male	Female
25	2.0	
30	1.8	
35	1.5	
40	1.2	1.9
45	Average	1.6
50	0.8	1.3
55	0.7	Average
60	0.6	0.8
65	0.5	0.6
70		0.5

Adapted from Jacobs DS, et al. *Laboratory Test Handbook,* 2nd ed. Cleveland, LexiComp Inc, 1990

High density lipoprotein levels are not reliable in thyroid disease because hyperthyroidism decreases the level and hypothyroidism increases the level. Levels are decreased with some hypertensive agents, including beta blockers and thiazides, and are temporarily decreased following acute myocardial infarction.

Assays for the specific apolipoproteins, though available, are not commonly used and are not discussed in this text.

 TIME FOR REVIEW. After studying the preceding sections, you should be able to respond correctly to the following:

■ Lipids require special transport because they are not_____.

■ Specialized proteins that transport lipids and are important in lipid metabolism are called _____ .

■ Of the four major classes of lipoproteins in the serum, choose the one best described below. Same classes may be used more than once.

composed of triglyceride and small amounts of cholesterol, phospholipid, and protein; largest and least dense of the four classes: _____

sometimes referred to as good cholesterol: _____

produce turbid serum in high concentrations; higher density than chylomicrons: _____

smallest and least dense of the four; about 50% protein: _____

play major role in supplying cholesterol to cells; sometimes called bad cholesterol: _____

form a creamy layer on top of serum; abnormal to find in fasting specimens: _____

higher levels imply lower risk of coronary artery disease: _____

does not cause visible turbidity of serum; major lipid component cholesterol/cholesterol esters: _____

triglycerides are major lipid component; particles in this class are smaller than chylomicrons: _____

■ List and briefly explain at least six non-dietary factors that can lead to variability in cholesterol measurements or interfere with methods of analysis.

■ Explain why cholesterol reference ranges are not derived in the traditional method.

■ Based on NCEP criteria, cholesterol levels should ideally be < _____
_____ mg/dL.

■ An individual would be classified as "high risk" (NCEP) with a cholesterol level > _____ mg/dL.

■ In routine clinical laboratory settings, which parameters are directly measured (denote as M) and which are derived by calculation (denote as C)?

_____ Total cholesterol

_____ HDL-C

_____ LDL-C

_____ Triglyceride

_____ VLDL

■ An LDL-C of 145 mg/dL would be in which NCEP risk category?

■ Based on Table 7–6, list the average HDL-C levels for men and for women.

■ A convenient, simply calculated risk indicator believed by some to represent the best single risk predictor for cardiovascular disease is the _____ ratio.

■ Very high triglyceride levels preclude calculation of which parameter? What technique may be used in such cases?

■ Remember to review all the tables presented in this section.

Check your responses by reviewing the preceding sections.

■ LIPOPROTEIN PHENOTYPES

In the mid-1960s a system for classifying lipoprotein disorders into six distinct types (originally five types, but type II later divided into two sub-types) was developed by Frederickson, Levy, and Lees. They called these classifications, based primarily on electrophoresis, *phenotypes*. This system has been used for many years, with institution of a specific type of therapy more frequently based on phenotypic patterns over the years. With an increased understanding of the inherited and acquired metabolism disorders, this classification is not as useful as it was in the past. However, the system is still useful in occasional situations to aid in the differentiation of some disorders of lipid metabolism. The various phenotypes remain a convenient and common system for referring to the various kinds of lipoprotein elevations found in hyperlipoproteinemia. Table 7–7 provides a description of the six lipoprotein phenotypes.

Observation of serum that has been refrigerated undisturbed overnight or for several hours allows visual determination of the presence of chylomicrons, which appear as a creamy layer on top of the serum. The presence of this **chylomicron layer with clear serum** underneath is suggestive of phenotype I (chylomicrons present, VLDL concentration not sufficient to produce turbidity). On the other hand, if **chylomicrons are observed on top of turbid serum**, type V is suggested (may also be seen in type III, but this type is not common and chylomicrons may or may not be noted). **Turbid serum without an upper layer of chylomicrons** is suggestive of type IV, a very common phenotype, but is also noted in type IIb and sometimes in type III—significant triglyceride elevation and normal or slightly increased cholesterol, type IV is more likely; conversely, with significant cholesterol elevation and normal or slightly increased triglyceride is suggestive of type IIb; elevations in both triglyceride and cholesterol is more suggestive of type III.

TABLE 7-7. Lipoprotein Phenotypes Based on Electrophoresis

Type	Disorder	Incidence	Laboratory Findings								Additional Information		Comments
			tot chol	trig	HDL-C	LDL-C	VLDL	chylo	turbid serum	early cad	xanthomas	pancreatitis	
I	Lipoprotein lipase is defective, deficient, or absent; apolipoprotein C-II deficient	Very rare	N or ↑	↑↑↑	↓	↓	↑	↑↑↑	No	No	Yes eruptive	Yes	Lipemia retinalis found in inherited disorder: may occur secondary to IDDM or lupus erythematosus
IIa	Familial combined hyperlipidemia or hypercholesterolemia	Common	↑↑	N	N	↑↑	N	0	No	Yes	Yes prominent	Rarely	Early vascular disease severe; may occur secondary to hypothyroidism, high cholesterol diet, nephrotic syndrome, obstructive liver disease, porphyria
IIb	Familial combined hyperlipidemia and occasionally familial hypercholesterolemia	Common	↑↑	↑	N	↑↑	↑↑	0	Yes	Occ	Yes prominent	Rarely	
III	Dysbetalipoproteinemia	Uncommon	↑↑	↑↑ or ↑↑↑	N	*	*	0 or ↑	Yes	Yes	Yes & palmar yellowing	No	Elevated uric acid; may occur secondary to uncontrolled diabetes, hypothyroidism; diet and drug therapy very effective
IV	Familial combined hyperlipidemia, increased apolipoprotein; familial hypertriglyceridemia	Very common	N or ↑	↑↑ or ↑↑↑	N or ↓	N or ↑	↑↑↑	0	Yes	Yes	No	No	Elevated uric acid; may occur secondary to diabetes, high alcohol consumption, obesity, oral contraceptives, glycogen storage disorders; weight loss effective in lowering VLDL; high fat diet may result in conversion to type V
V	Deficient apolipoprotein C-II, hyperlipoproteinemia, familial combined hyperlipidemia (rarely), familial (occ)	Rare	↑↑	↑↑↑	N or ↓	N or ↓	↑↑	↑↑	Yes	Poss	Yes eruptive	Yes	VLDL now lowered by weight loss; may occur secondary to diabetes, nephrotic syndrome, hypercalemia, high alcohol consumption

[1]These two bands merge on electrophoresis.

Based on electrophoretic migration patterns, VLDL is also referred to as pre-beta lipoproteins; LDL as beta-lipoproteins; and HDL as alpha-lipoproteins.

Table developed based on information from Henry JB. *Clinical Diagnosis and Management by Laboratory Methods*, 19th ed. Philadelphia, Saunders, 1996; Jacobs DS, et al. *Laboratory Test Handbook*, 2nd ed. Cleveland, LexiComp Inc, 1990; Kee JLeF. *Laboratory and Diagnostic Tests with Nursing Implications*, 4th ed. Stamford, CT, Appleton and Lange, 1995; Ravel R. *Clinical Laboratory Medicine: Clinical Application of Laboratory Data*, 6th ed. St Louis, Mosby, 1995; and Sacher RA, McPherson RA. *Widmann's Clinical Interpretation of Laboratory Tests*, 10th ed. Philadelphia, FA Davis, 1991

Most hyperlipoproteinemias fall into the type II and IV phenotype classifications, with type IV being the most common and most cases representing an acquired, rather than an inherited, disorder. A number of factors affect the phenotypic classifications, including those listed previously as affecting the individual tests used to determine phenotype. Further, phenotypic classification decisions may be unwittingly influenced by the particular laboratory's reference ranges depending upon how the ranges were derived (ie, based on general population study, national guidelines used, etc).

The disorders of lipid and lipoprotein metabolism that give rise to these phenotypic descriptions are now more often the focus than is the use of classification into phenotypes. Some of these disorders are described briefly in the following section.

■ DISORDERS OF METABOLISM

Abnormalities may be inherited in the endogenous or the exogenous pathways of lipid metabolism, and some disorders involve combined abnormalities of both pathways. Other inherited disorders result from abnormalities in the reverse cholesterol transport pathway. Reverse cholesterol transport involves the removal of excess cholesterol from tissues with transport back to the liver for recycling or excretion in bile. Examples of abnormalities in each pathway are described in Table 7–8.

■ OTHER RISK FACTORS AND TREATMENT DECISIONS

A variety of factors contribute to the risk of developing coronary artery disease (CAD) in addition to those resulting from abnormalities in lipid metabolism:

- obesity ($\geq 30\%$ above desirable weight)
- diabetes mellitus
- male sex (CAD 3 to 4 times more common in middle-aged males than females)
- age: male ≥ 45 years; female ≥ 55 years
- current smoking ($>$ 10 cigarettes per day)
- hypertension (indicated by BP $\geq 140/90$ mmHg or on antihypertensive medication)
- family history of early CAD
- definitive history of peripheral vascular disease or cerebrovascular disease

The **treatment** of patients with hyperlipidemia is aimed at reducing the likelihood of developing atherosclerotic cardiovascular disease and, in those disorders resulting in the development of pancreatitis and xanthomas, to prevent development of these conditions. As noted earlier in the chapter, Frederickson's phenotypic classifications are no longer the primary basis for determining therapeutic

TABLE 7–8. Inherited Disorders of Lipid/Lipoprotein Metabolism

Pathway	Disorder	Description
Endogenous	Familial hypercholesterolemia (FH)	Autosomal dominant trait; "dosage effect"—homozygotes more severely affected with total chol. and LDL-C levels 5-6 × normal & MI common in 2nd decade of life, xanthomas develop early and may be present at birth; 50% of heterozygote males have CAD by age 50, females by age 60; caused by defective LDL receptor gene; usually gives phenotype IIa, sometimes IIb
	Familial combined hyperlipidemia (FCHL)	Genetic defect unknown; number of variants, including: (1) overproduction of apolipoprotein B, VLDL and sometimes LDL, (2) hyperbetalipoproteinemia, (3) familial dyslipidemic hypertension and others; depending on variant, produces phenotypes IV, IIa, IIb, and rarely V; cardiovascular-vascular may appear as early as childhood or adolescence
	Increased triglyceride-rich VLDL	Liver overproduces triglyceride, but not ApoB, so VLDL has excessive triglycerides making it difficult for LPL to hydrolyze; cardiovascular disease not as common as in FCHL type IV patients with VLDL increases; adults often have peripheral vascular disease
	Defective Apolipoprotein B	Inherited defect resulting from amino acid substitution in ApoB that prevents normal binding of LDL receptor (LDL receptor is normal), which can result in increased LDL; xanthomas present; produces either normal or type IIa phenotype; causes only small percentage of CAD; need not distinguish from FH for treatment purposes
Exogenous	Abnormalities in lipoprotein lipase	Rare disorder from homozygous inheritance of a mutation on the LPL gene; LPL may be defective or missing; results in ineffective clearance of dietary fat, producing enormous increases in chylomicrons and extremely high triglycerides in homozygotes; usually presents by age 10 with initial symptom of abdominal pain; produces type I pattern; does not result in atherosclerosis (suggests that chylomicron remnants are atherogenic, not chylomicrons themselves—Henry); heterozygotes (carriers) may have mild dyslipidemia
	Apolipoprotein C-II deficiency	Rare autosomal recessive trait caused by genetic deletions or mutations in ApoC, an LDL cofactor; very high triglycerides and chylomicron content; type I or V phenotype; generally presents in adulthood, but may be seen earlier; pancreatitis is usual presenting condition
	Dysbetalipo-proteinemia	Significant elevations in both cholesterol and triglyceride resulting from genetic defect in an apolipoprotein that causes delayed clearance; produced type III pattern; usually not clinically evident before adulthood; premature atherosclerosis very common
Endogenous and exogenous	Abetalipo-proteinemia	Rare autosomal recessive disorder expressed in childhood; chylomicrons, VLDL, and LDL absent; fat malabsorption; large fat particles deposited in jejunum seen on biopsy; most dietary fat excreted in stool; causes deficiencies in vitamins A, E, K and sometimes D (fat soluble vitamins) with vitamin E deficiencies most clinically significant and responsible for major symptoms involving the retina and the nervous system
	Hypobetalipo-proteinemia	Similar to abeta-, except quantities reduced not absent; very low LDL, low total chol, low or normal VLDL and triglycerides; autosomal dominant trait may be heterozygous or homozygous; fat soluble vitamins low in homozygotes
	Hyperlipo-proteinemia type V	Genetic defect unknown, may be autosomal dominant; triglycerides very high because of increases in VLDL and chylomicrons from either increased synthesis, decreased clearance, or both; expression is delayed and premature CAD may occur, but is not as common as in some other disorders; phenotype V

TABLE 7–8. (*Cont.*)

Pathway	Disorder	Description
	Apolipoprotein B deficiency	Group of several unusual genetic defects in ApoB that impact both pathways and result in hypolipidemia
Reverse cholesterol transport	Hypo-alpha-lipoproteinemia	Group of conditions characterized by decreased HDL; may be due to decreased synthesis caused by defects in an apolipoprotein gene complex, to increased catabolism caused by ApoA-I variants, or to a deficiency in the enzyme system (LCAT, or lecithin:cholesterol acyltransferase) that catalyzes esterification of cholesterol
	Hyper-alpha-lipoproteinemia	A desirable "disorder" in which individuals have HDL levels above the 95th percentile associated with long life and decreased risk of CAD; total chol. is elevated as a result of increased HDL, LDL usually normal, triglycerides normal or low; a genetic defect prevalent in Japanese and leading to increased HDL has been identified, but other genetic defects not yet known

CAD = coronary artery disease.

Table developed primarily on description of disorders in Henry JB. *Clinical Diagnosis and Management by Laboratory Methods,* 19th ed. Philadelphia, Saunders, 1996; with additional information from Sacher RA, McPherson RA. *Widmann's Clinical Interpretation of Laboratory Tests,* 10th ed. Philadelphia, FA Davis, 1991; and Ravel R. *Clinical Laboratory Medicine: Clinical Application of Laboratory Data,* 6th ed. St Louis, Mosby, 1995.

regimens. The NCEP, through an expert panel, lists the major goal of treatment as lowering the LDL-C, thus the LDL level is important in the consideration of therapeutic regimens along with the total cholesterol. (Recall from an earlier discussion that LDL plays a major role in supplying cholesterol to tissues and is considered an important contributor to the development of atherosclerosis.) Also of significance, is the presence of additional risk factors and the interaction between risk factors.

Treatment may include a prescribed diet and exercise regimen, treatment of underlying secondary causes, and drug intervention. Drug therapy is usually instituted only after diet and exercise have failed to reduce the LDL to an acceptable level, or with very high LDL levels. Drug therapy may also be prudent in some cases with additional risk factors and when CAD is already present. Stein recommends consideration of drug therapy when diet and exercise have not reduced LDL levels sufficiently after 3 to 6 months. Because risk levels rise rapidly with increasing levels of total and LDL-C (patients with LDL of 160 and total cholesterol of 240 have double the risk of patients with LDL of 130 and total cholesterol of 200) and risk is increased further in the presence of other predisposing factors, drug intervention may be the initial treatment of choice in some cases, particularly if CAD is already present. Clinicians must base treatment decisions on a variety of factors, including those discussed, the patient's medical history, other clinical and laboratory findings, potential side effects of drug therapy, and generally accepted standards of practice. Patients with a history of cardiovascular disease require special consideration because the likelihood of a repeat incident is greater at any given level than for a person without such history at the same level of hypercholesteremia. Table 7–9 provides guidelines for treatment decisions. Figure 7–1 provides a practical screening and therapeutic approach consistent with NCEP guidelines for patients *without* CAD. A different approach is appropriate for patients with a history of CAD. The information offered in this flow chart (developed using NCEP guidelines, [Henry,1996; Stein, 1993]) is intended to supplement, not replace, the medical judgment of the physician. Because patients in whom CAD has already developed are at greater risk, a lipid profile is recommended upon initial evaluation of these individuals. Treatment should be directed at achieving and maintaining an LDL-C level < 100 mg/dL. This level may be attained primarily through dietary interventions or may require drug therapy, particularly if the LDL is > 130 mg/dL.

Regardless of the treatment instituted, it is important for the patient to have a clear understanding of lifestyle implications (smoking, diet, activity levels) and of the potential consequences of failure to adhere to the prescribed treatment regimen. Consistent monitoring for the evaluation of compliance and for the effectiveness of the instituted therapy is a vital part of the overall treatment. Repeat assays should not be performed too early to detect responses to therapy. However, timely follow-up can be quite beneficial in providing positive feedback to compliant patients in whom desired responses are achieved.

TABLE 7–9. Treatment Decisions Using LDL-C Levels

		Diet Therapy		Drug Therapy	
	Risk Factors	*Initiate at*	*LDL Goal*	*Consider at*	*LDL Goal*
With heart disease	N/A	>100 mg/dL	≤100 mg/dL	≥130 mg/dL	≤100 mg/dL
Without heart disease	2	≥160 mg/dL	<160 mg/dL	≥190 mg/dL	<160 mg/dL
	≥ 2	≥130 mg/dL	<130 mg/dL	≥160 mg/dL	<130 mg/dL

Adapted from Henry JB. *Clinical Diagnosis and Management by Laboratory Methods,* 19th ed. Philadelphia, Saunders, 1996.

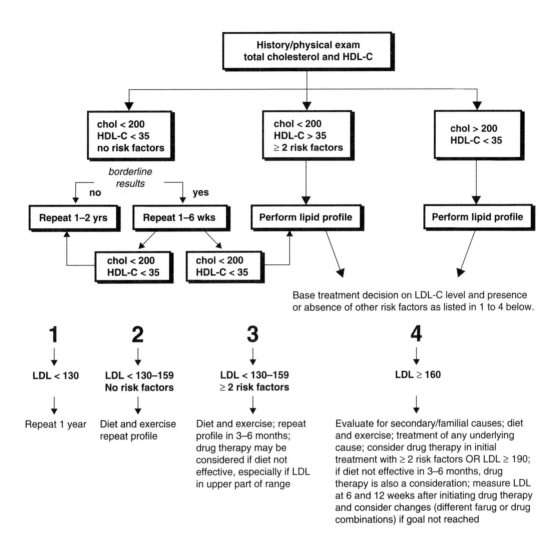

FIGURE 7–1. Screening and therapeutic approach for patients *without* CAD

7. SELF TEST

Choose the best response by circling the appropriate letter. The answer key may be found in the appendices.

1. **The specialized proteins that transport lipids and are important in lipid metabolism are**
    A. phospholipids
    B. cholesterol esters
    C. apolipoproteins
    D. immune complex proteins

2. **The lipids that are essential cell wall components and play a role in lowering the surface tension of fluids in the lung are called**
    A. phospholipids
    B. chylomicrons
    C. LDL-C
    D. HDL-C

3. **The lipid that is important in cell membrane structure, in synthesis of bile acids, and the formation of steroid hormones is**
    A. triglyceride
    B. cholesterol
    C. phospholipid
    D. lipoprotein

4. **The lipid stored in fat tissue to provide fatty acids for gluconeogenesis is**
    A. triglyceride
    B. cholesterol
    C. phospholipid
    D. lipoprotein

5. **A lipoprotein that plays a major role in the supply of cholesterol to cells and sometimes referred to as "bad cholesterol" is**
    A. chylomicrons
    B. LDL-C
    C. HDL-C
    D. VLDL

6. The lipoprotein demonstrating an inverse association to the risk of CAD in that higher levels of the lipoprotein are associated with reduced risk is
   A. chylomicrons
   B. LDL-C
   C. HDL-C
   D. VLDL

7. The abnormal finding of a "creamy" layer on the top of fasting serum allowed to stand undisturbed results from these large, low density lipoproteins.
   A. chylomicrons
   B. LDL-C
   C. HDL-C
   D. VLDL

8. NCEP guidelines establish a desirable total cholesterol level as one that is
   A. < 240 mg/dL
   B. < 200 mg/dL
   C. < 220 mg/dL
   D. < 230 mg/dL

9. NCEP guidelines establish a desirable LDL cholesterol level as one that is
   A. < 160 mg/dL
   B. < 150 mg/dL
   C. < 140 mg/dL
   D. < 130 mg/dL

10. An HDL-C < _____ is almost always associated with CAD risk.
    A. 65 mg/dL
    B. 35 mg/dL
    C. 70 mg/dL
    D. 50 mg/dL

11. The lipid profile parameters derived by calculation from measured analytes are
    A. LDL-C and VLDL
    B. LDL-C and HDL-C
    C. HDL-C and triglyceride
    D. VLDL and total cholesterol

12. **Which of the following sets of results would place an individual in a "high risk" category?**
    A. total cholesterol: 220; LDL-C: 140; HDL-C: 40
    B. total cholesterol: 180; LDL-C: 120; HDL-C: 50
    C. total cholesterol: 235; LDL-C: 155; HDL-C: 45
    D. total cholesterol: 250; LDL-C: 165; HDL-C: 30

13. **Which of the following sets of results would place an individual in a "desirable" category?**
    A. total cholesterol: 220; LDL-C: 140; HDL-C: 40
    B. total cholesterol: 180; LDL-C: 120; HDL-C: 50
    C. total cholesterol: 235; LDL-C: 155; HDL-C: 45
    D. total cholesterol: 250; LDL-C: 165; HDL-C: 30

14. **The results provided below are typical of the most common lipoprotein phenotype. This phenotype is type _____ (total cholesterol: 210 mg/dL; triglyceride: 300 mg/dL; chylomicrons absent; LDL-C: 140 mg/dL; turbid serum from significantly increased VLDL).**
    A. V
    B. IV
    C. III
    D. IIa

15. **This is an inherited disorder of endogenous lipid metabolism caused by a defective LDL receptor gene, inherited as an autosomal dominant trait. Total cholesterol and LDL-C levels are extremely elevated in homozygotes and myocardial infarction is common when such individuals are in their twenties.**
    A. familial hypercholesterolemia
    B. defective apolipoprotein B
    C. increased triglyceride-rich VLDL
    D. dysbetalipoproteinemia

16. **For which patient below would drug therapy most likely be considered for initial treatment?**
    A. 40-year-old female; non-smoker; no CAD; LDL-C: 150 mg/dL; no other risk factors
    B. 50-year-old male diabetic smoker on anti-hypertensives; LDL-C: 180 mg/dL
    C. 60-year-old female smoker; LDL-C: 145 mg/dL; family history of CAD
    D. 45-year-old male; non-smoker; BP 145/90; LDL-C: 135 mg/dL

8. TESTS OF ELECTROLYTE BALANCE

The term *electrolytes* is used to refer to a number of ions found in the body. As you will recall, **ions** are atoms (or groups of atoms) that have either a positive or a negative charge determined by the number of electrons orbiting the atomic nucleus. Ions with a positive charge are called **cations** and those with a negative charge are referred to as **anions**. Important cations in the body include sodium (Na^+), potassium (K^+), calcium (Ca^+), magnesium (Mg^+), and phosphorus in the form of phosphates (PO_4^+). Frequently measured anions include chloride (Cl^-) and bicarbonate (HCO_3^-), often replaced by measurement of CO_2. Electrolytes may be requested singly or as a panel or profile that typically includes Na^+, K^+, and Cl^-, with CO_2 often included. Measurement of these four electrolytes generally provides adequate information for the clinician to evaluate electrolyte and water balance. Concentrations of these electrolytes are also closely associated with acid-base balance and can provide an indication of acid-base status, with the more detailed information provided by arterial blood gas analysis used for a more comprehensive determination of status. Measurement also provides data useful in the evaluation of dehydration, ketoacidosis, alcoholism, toxicity, and other disorders. Discussions in this chapter will be based on these four primary electrolytes and on the anion gap. Calcium, magnesium, and phosphorous are included in Chapter 9.

ELECTROLYTE PHYSIOLOGY

An understanding of the basic principles of how the electrolytes function in the body, how their concentrations are regulated, and the maintenance of fluid or water balance is important to understanding the implications of abnormal electrolyte levels and the clinical conditions in which such abnormalities are found. The role of the kidney in electrolyte physiology and water balance is a crucial component of such understanding because many electrolyte disorders are associated with alterations in normal renal function.

Electrolytes are present both in the extracellular fluid (ECF) and in the intracellular fluid (ICF), with the concentration of electrolytes in both the ECF and ICF constituting a "true" total concentration. However, measurement of these "true" or *total body* concentrations does not lend itself well to analysis in the clinical laboratory because a practical means of determining ICF concentration is not available. Thus the concentrations typically reported reflect the concentrations found in the ECF of the blood—serum or plasma. Although not always the case, serum concentrations often mirror the concentrations in the intracellular compartments and in interstitial fluid because electrolytes pass back and forth from the different areas to some degree by the process of diffusion (from high concentrations to lower).

Recall from Chapter 2 that ultrafiltration and tubular reabsorption, secretion, and concentration result in urine formation and are important not only in the elimination of waste, but also in maintaining acid-base balance. In the proximal convoluted tubules sodium, chloride, and water are reabsorbed (water passively, sodium and chloride, as NaCl, actively). When the filtrate reaches the loop of Henle and is exposed to the higher salt concentration of the medulla, water is removed by osmosis in the descending loop and sodium and potassium are reabsorbed in the ascending loop. Because the ascending loop is not water permeable, excessive reabsorption of water is prevented. In the distal tubule, antidiuretic hormone (ADH) and aldosterone alter the permeability of the tubule walls to control the amount of reabsorption. Here sodium and water can be reabsorbed under the control of aldosterone, and potassium, hydrogen ions, and ammonia are secreted under the control of ADH. Bicarbonate may also be reabsorbed in the distal tubules. In the collecting tubules, where ADH also controls the permeability of tubular walls, reabsorption of water, sodium, and potassium may also take place in addition to the further secretion of hydrogen ions. Similarly, the kidney plays a crucial role in the control of water balance both in terms of the reabsorption of water (under the control of ADH) and by the influence of the renin-angiotensin and aldosterone feedback mechanism in the glomerular filtration process (see Chap. 2).

CATIONS

As a brief reminder of some basic chemistry principles, recall that the nucleus of atoms contains particles with a positive charge (called *protons*) and that negatively charged particles (called *electrons*) orbit the nucleus. When atoms have the same number of negatively charged electrons and positively charged protons, the net result is electrical neutrality. Atoms that carry an electrical charge are called *ions*. Positive ions (*cations*) have fewer electrons; negative ions (*anions*) have more electrons. The two cations of primary physiologic importance that are monitored by the clinical laboratory are sodium and potassium.

■ SODIUM

Sodium is the major extracellular cation and, as the cation present in the largest quantity in the extracellular fluid, it plays a vital role in maintaining neutrality of electrical charges in the body. Abnormalities of serum sodium concentration,

hypernatremia (increased serum sodium concentration) and particularly decreased serum sodium levels (**hyponatremia**), are commonly detected electrolyte disorders.

Methods of Measurement

Laboratory measurement of sodium is commonly performed using an *ion selective electrode* (ISE), usually made of a special type of glass with a selective permeability to the sodium ion. Flame emission photometry was the primary method of electrolyte analysis for many years and although it may still be used in some laboratories, this method has been almost completely replaced by the ISE methodology. Flame photometry used an internal standard of an alkali metal such as lithium with a controlled flame to "excite" the cations and quantitatively measure emissions. Results from ISE methodology give sodium results about 2% higher (Ravel, 1995) than those obtained with flame photometry, but this difference is not sufficient to alter clinical judgments.

Ion selective electrode methods are not only simpler from a technical standpoint than flame photometry, but also are less likely to demonstrate sodium decreases because of the effect of other substances in the serum. A high concentration of serum protein such as may be seen in multiple myeloma and a high concentration of serum lipids can result in decreased sodium levels by flame photometry, but direct ISE methods are not affected. By either method hyperglycemia may lead to decreased serum sodium levels, as large amounts of glucose cause intracellular fluids to move into the extracellular fluid by osmosis. This results in a dilutional effect in which the sodium level is low in relation to the ECF volume. Note that this phenomenon is not an "interference" in the truest sense of the word because the sodium concentration is actually reduced in regard to the ECF volume. In such cases, a sodium measurement performed on a sample collected subsequent to correction of the hyperglycemia would be expected to yield a normal value. A typical **reference range** for serum sodium is 135 to 145 mEq/L.

Hyponatremia

Sodium depletion leading to hyponatremia may result from a variety of causes and may be manifested as an acute or chronic condition. Although patients with either form may be symptomatic (usually when sodium levels fall to 120 to 125 mEq/L), acute hyponatremia is more likely to produce **symptoms** than chronic hyponatremia (Stein, 1993). Depending upon the degree of sodium depletion, patients may present with drowsiness, lethargy, muscle weakness or cramps, or nausea and vomiting, or with more pronounced symptoms of confusion, seizures, or stupor. Significant depletion may also result in coma. Tachycardia and hypotension may also be seen in hyponatremia.

Hyponatremia may result from a **loss of sodium** (both sodium and water are lost, but the sodium loss is excessive relative to the water loss) or from an **excess water volume**. As previously noted, many electrolyte imbalances are related to renal function disorders or are secondary to renal disease. In the case of hyponatremia, **renal abnormalities** may underlie either sodium loss or excessive water volume, but a number of **non-renal conditions** may also be responsible. This text will classify hyponatremia based on etiologic considerations. Other methods of classification may be used, including one based on serum osmolality findings and fluid volume such as that used by Stein (1993). This system classifies hyponatremia into two categories: one with normal or elevated serum osmolality and the other with decreased serum osmolality with subcategories defined on the basis of ECF volume. Hyponatremic patients may have a normal extracellular fluid volume (*euvolemia*), decreased ECF (*hypovolemia*), or an increase in ECF (*hypervolemia*). When the concentration of sodium in the extracellular fluid changes, serum osmolality and subsequently, water distribution, are influenced. Most "true" hyponatremias result in a decreased serum osmolality, because by definition, the sodium portion of the solute is decreased. Recall from Chapter 2 that osmolality is a measure of the concentration of solute (dissolved substances, in this case sodium) in a particular fluid (in this case serum or plasma). In hyponatremia the concentration of the sodium ion (Na^+) is decreased, producing, in most cases, a corresponding decrease in serum osmolality. Patients may become hyponatremic as the result of the effects of physician prescribed treatment for other conditions (**iatrogenic hyponatremia**) such as diuretic therapy or some instances of IV administration. This is not an uncommon occurrence, but is more likely to result in the presence of an underlying condition or other contributing factors that may induce hyponatremia. Similarly, home remedies, like using sugar water to replace significant fluid losses in severe diarrhea, can lead to hyponatremia. Table 8–1 summarizes a number of causes of hyponatremia and selected conditions from the table are further described in the text following.

Vomiting and/or diarrhea that is severe or of prolonged duration may lead to hyponatremia, particularly if replacement therapy is not instituted or is inadequate. Both fluid and electrolytes are lost in these conditions. The resultant

TABLE 8–1. Causes of Hyponatremia

	Sodium Loss	Water Excess	Pseudohyponatremia
Renal	"Salt-losing" nephropathy Bicarbonaturia Ketonuria Osmotic diuresis (glucose, urea…) Adrenal insufficiency Diuretic therapy	Acute or chronic renal failure Nephrotic syndrome	
Non-Renal	Vomiting Diarrhea "Third spacing" (severe burns, peritonitis) Hypothyroidism Glucocorticoid deficiency Inappropriate ADH secretion (SIADH) Reset osmostat	Congestive heart failure Cirrhosis	Hyperlipidemia Hyperglycemia Hyperproteinemia

decrease in fluid volume, though counteracted in part by an increase in the secretion of ADH to aid in fluid retention, may lead to dehydration. If the level of dehydration is severe enough and fluid replacement is not adequate, hypernatremia may result as a consequence of the significant fluid depletion. On the other hand, replacement therapy with fluids lacking in sodium or with insufficient sodium concentration will likely promote the development of, or the severity of, hyponatremia. Etiologically, the hyponatremia seen in severe or prolonged vomiting and diarrhea is the result of nonrenal sodium loss (*deficit hyponatremia*). In terms of serum osmolality and volume classifications, it is a *hypovolemic hyponatremia with decreased serum osmolality.* Findings similar to those produced with severe vomiting and diarrhea may be seen as a result of constant gastric tube suction that continues over a 24-hour period (Ravel, 1995). Fluid sequestration, or *third spacing* is another example of a nonrenal sodium loss, hypovolemic hyponatremia with decreased serum osmolality. Severe burns are an example of this type of hyponatremia, in which ECF and electrolytes are lost as a result of leakage into damaged areas. Renal sodium loss resulting in hypovolemic hyponatremia with decreased serum osmolality may also result from diuretics (particularly if the patient is also on a low salt diet), diabetic acidosis, bicarbonaturia, and salt losing nephropathy.

Hypervolemic hyponatremia, or *dilutional hyponatremia,* may occur secondary to an impaired renal ability to maintain appropriate water balance in such disorders as nephrotic syndrome and renal failure. In such conditions, the kidney's ability to appropriately regulate electrolytes is diminished. The serum osmolality is decreased in such cases and in the non-renal hypervolemic hyponatremias that can be seen in congestive heart failure and liver cirrhosis.

Hyponatremia with decreased serum osmolality in the presence of normal fluid volume, *euvolemic hyponatremia,* may be seen in a variety of conditions, including hypothyroidism, glucocorticoid deficiency, secondary to some drugs, and in the syndrome of inappropriate ADH secretion (SIADH). Endocrine disorders may also lead to hyponatremia, particularly dysfunctions involving the adrenal cortex in terms of the hormones it secretes or lack of ACTH (which stimulates the adrenal cortex) secretion by the pituitary gland. The adrenal cortex secretes a number of hormones, including aldosterone and cortisol (hydrocortisone). *Aldosterone* is a powerful hormone with the primary function of controlling sodium and potassium concentrations in the blood. *Cortisol* is involved in water metabolism. In *Addison's disease,* an idiopathic progressive destruction of the adrenal cortex occurs to varying degrees, often with subsequent chronic infections (tuberculosis, histoplasmosis and other fungal infections) in the damaged organ. The ensuing deficiency of both aldosterone and cortisol results in a marked decrease in renal salt retention abilities. Although quite responsive to treatment with adrenocortical hormones, the disease progression may include life threatening crisis points during which there is a devastating renal loss of both fluid and salt requiring immediate intervention.

In SIADH secretion of ADH is persistent even under conditions in which its secretion would normally be halted (ie, decreased serum osmolality and normal or increased fluid volume). Sodium excretion is also increased, likely as a result of suppressed sodium reabsorption (Ravel, 1995). SIADH is associated with a wide variety of conditions, perhaps induced in some manner by such conditions, including varied malignancies, some types of pulmonary infections, a number of central nervous system disorders (ie, trauma, infections, seizures), certain drugs (antineoplastics, oral antidiabetics, hypnotics [Ravel, 1995]), and in some endocrinopathies. The syndrome has also been demonstrated in individuals under extreme emotional stress and in those suffering significant pain or physical trauma including surgery (Henry, 1996; Ravel, 1995). A definitive diagnosis of SIADH rests partly in the exclusion of other disorders including renal disease with resulting sodium loss, Addison's disease, and urine sodium loss that is induced by the use of diuretics. Further, other conditions may mimic SIADH, presenting similar features in the absence of classic SIADH (refractory dilutional syndrome and reset osmostat syndrome [Ravel, 1995]). In addition to the obvious low serum sodium concentration, the following set of diagnostic criteria for the syndrome have been offered (Ravel, 1995):

- continued renal sodium excretion with low serum sodium
- decreased serum osmolality
- urine osmolality showing high concentration (would expect highly dilute urine)
- no blood volume depletion
- normal renal and adrenal function

Pseudohyponatremia may be seen as a result of high serum lipid, protein, or glucose concentrations as discussed in the Methods of Measurement section of this chapter. In addition, infusion of isotonic or hypertonic solutions containing mannitol, glycine, or glucose can result in low serum sodium concentrations by the mechanism previously described for high serum glucose concentrations. The serum osmolality is normal or increased in cases of pseudohyponatremia. Because serum osmolality is low (occasionally low normal or normal) in "true" hyponatremia, a finding of elevated serum osmolality in the follow-up of low serum sodium concentration is suggestive of a pseudohyponatremia and warrants evaluation of this possibility.

Hypernatremia

High serum sodium concentration, or hypernatremia (usually defined as serum sodium > 150 mEq/L [Stein, 1993]), is not seen as commonly as is hyponatremia. It may be seen as a consequence of dehydration, resulting from deficient fluid intake or excessive fluid loss. Hypernatremia may occur as a result of water loss (renal or non-renal) that is excessive in relation to the amount of sodium loss and when total body sodium levels are elevated; following as a result of excessive water loss alone; in Cushing syndrome; and occasionally following as a result of excessive sodium intake. As with hyponatremia, hypernatremia may be classified in terms of etiology and by volume status (ie, hypovolemic, hypervolemic, euvolemic). **Symptoms** are more severe in acute hypernatremia than in chronic conditions and include restlessness, twitching, ataxia, muscle spasms, and seizures. With serum sodium concentrations > 160 mEq/L, high mortality rates are seen in the elderly and in infants (Stein, 1993). These groups, along with incapacitated patients, are also at higher risk of developing a hypernatremic state. Because the body's thirst mechanism promotes adequate fluid intake and replacement, this greater likelihood results from a reduced, or lack of, access to water.

Laboratory findings in hypernatremia, in addition to the increased serum sodium concentration, include an increased serum osmolality. With an excessive renal loss of water in relation to the amount of sodium loss that results in dehydration and hypernatremia, additional laboratory findings include a low urine specific gravity and osmolality, a urine sodium concentration > 20 mEq/L, and an increased urine volume. On the other hand, with dehydration resulting from nonrenal water loss or water deprivation the urine volume is decreased and the specific gravity and osmolality of the urine is increased. These hypernatremias are hypovolemic.

Hypernatremia as a consequence of water loss alone (ie, without an accompanying sodium loss), can be seen in nephrogenic diabetes insipidus and in central diabetes insipidus. The water loss is caused by an ineffective response of the renal tubules to ADH in nephrogenic diabetes insipidus. Impairment of renal tubular response may be due to renal damage or it may be idiopathic with no discernible cause. Central diabetes insipidus, in which there is an impairment in the secretion of ADH by the pituitary, may result from head trauma or tumors that damage the pituitary, but often occurs without known cause. Diabetes insipidus produces euvolemic hypernatremia in most patients as a result of the thirst mechanism and appropriate water replacement.

Hypernatremia as a result of excessive sodium intake is uncommon, but may be seen in some instances (eg, from sodium bicarbonate administration in cardiac arrest; hypertonic saline administration; hypertonic feedings and is usually iatrogenic). Total body sodium is also increased in Cushing syndrome, an adrenal cortex or pituitary tumor disorder in which there is excessive secretion of glucocorticoids, leading to an increase in the reabsorption of sodium by the renal tubules. Both of these etiologies, excessive sodium intake and Cushing symdrome, result in a hypervolemic hypernatremia (Stein, 1993).

TABLE 8–2. Causes of Hypernatremia

	Water Loss Exceeds Sodium Loss	Excess Water Loss Only	Increased Total Body Sodium
Renal	Diuretics (including osmotic diuretics like glucose) Renal disease Diarrhea Vomiting	Impaired response to ADH Impaired release of ADH	Hypertonic saline administration Bicarbonate administration
Non-Renal	Profuse sweating Burns		Hypertonic feedings Cushing syndrome

■ POTASSIUM

Potassium is the major intracellular cation, with only about 2% (Henry, 1996; Stein, 1993) of the total body potassium stores found in extracellular fluid. **Hyperkalemia** refers to an increased serum potassium concentration, and **hypokalemia** to a decreased serum concentration. A number of conditions producing potassium abnormalities also produce sodium abnormalities. Similarities between abnormalities of these two electrolytes will be apparent upon comparison of the previously discussed sodium abnormalities and the following discussion of potassium abnormalities. Significant abnormalities of potassium concentration, whether low or high, can produce devastating consequences and may be lethal in the absence of immediate and effective intervention.

The intracellular storage of potassium assists in maintaining appropriate serum levels. The high concentration of potassium in intracellular spaces aids in protecting the body from clinically significant potassium loss, and excess extracellular potassium can also be taken up by the cells when concentrations become too high. Serum potassium levels are closely associated with hydrogen ion concentration and thus pH levels and are not always indicative of total body potassium. An excess of hydrogen ions (H^+), as occurs in *acidosis* (low pH), allows the exchange of intracellular potassium ions (K^+) for H^+. In this case, serum potassium levels could be increased even with depleted intracellular body stores. On the other hand, when potassium is lost and intracellular potassium depleted, H^+ replaces the intracellular K^+ resulting in extracellular *alkalosis* (low H^+ concentration/high pH).

Methods of Measurement

As with laboratory analysis of sodium, flame photometry measurements have essentially been replaced with ISE technology. In the case of potassium, the electrode is made selective for potassium with an antibiotic (valinomycin) coated membrane. The molecules of the antibiotic used provide an opening of a size to exclude all cations except potassium. A typical **reference range** for serum potassium is 3.5 to 5.0 mEq/L with values < 2.5 mEq/L or > 6.5 mEq/L considered *critical* and warranting immediate intervention. Reference values for newborns are generally higher than those for adults and concentrations may not be considered critical until > 8 mEq/L (Jacobs, 1990). Surgeons and anesthesiologists often establish a minimum potassium concentration required prior to administration of general anesthesia because of the potential for life-threatening arrhythmias. In view of the high intracellular concentration of potassium, any degree of hemolysis will elevate the potassium level. Use of hemolyzed specimens should be avoided, particularly with moderate or marked hemolysis, as results will not be representative of the true serum potassium level and will not provide clinically useful information. When it is necessary to analyze specimens with a slight degree of hemolysis (as may be the case with pediatric and newborn specimens, as well as some other instances of difficult venipuncture), this observation will be clearly indicated on the laboratory report by laboratorians practicing good laboratory science. Very high platelet counts or white cell counts may also falsely elevate potassium levels. In such cases, a plasma potassium level will be more valid than a serum potassium level.

Hypokalemia

Serum potassium concentrations < 3.5 mEq/L (Stein, 1993) are classified as hypokalemic. Low serum potassium levels may result from a variety of mechanisms (Table 8–3):

- decreased dietary intake
- loss through gastrointestinal tract
- renal loss
- intracellular shift
- endocrinopathies

A deficient intake of potassium is not a common cause of hypokalemia, but may be seen in anorexia nervosa, in alcoholics with poor nutritional status, in severe illness producing a lack of appetite, in starvation, or in syndromes in which potassium absorption is inadequate. Gastrointestinal loss of potassium may result in hypokalemia in severe diarrhea, laxative abuse, prolonged vomiting, and gastrointestinal drainage.

Without an excretion limiting renal threshold for potassium, urinary excretion continues to some degree even in the presence of depleted body stores. In normal

TABLE 8–3. Etiologic Classification of Hypokalemia

Etiology	Causes
Inadequate intake	Anorexia Severe illnesses Malabsorption Starvation Alcoholism with poor nutritional status
Renal loss	Diuretics Sodium penicillins and carbenicillin Renal disease
Gastrointestinal loss	Prolonged diarrhea and/or vomiting Laxative abuse GI drainage
Intracellular shift	Alkalosis Osmotic diuresis Insulin therapy
Endocrinopathies	Aldosteronism Cushing syndrome Congenital adrenal hyperplasia

subjects the daily excretion of potassium is about 30 to 90 mEq/L; however, because excretion continues even in depleted states and effective renal potassium conservation may take as much as 3 weeks (Henry, 1996), urinary potassium rarely falls to < 5 to 10 mEq/L. Renal mechanisms for the conservation of sodium are more effective and timely than for conservation of potassium. Further, one mechanism for renal sodium conservation involves the excretion of K^+ in exchange for reabsorbed Na^+.

Renal potassium loss is most often the result of diuretics and may be seen in patients as a result of treatment for hypertension or other conditions requiring the use of diuretics. Renal loss may also be seen as a consequence of treatment with sodium penicillins and carbenicillin (Stein, 1993) as these medications, after metabolism by the body, result in excretion of anions in the urine. These anions (negatively charged ions) cannot be reabsorbed by the renal tubules and thus a "wasting" of potassium occurs as additional K^+ is excreted into the urine to off-set the negatively charged ions. Although rare, renal loss may also occur in salt-wasting nephropathies and interstitial nephritis (Stein, 1993). Renal potassium loss is also involved in primary aldosteronism, which is discussed with endocrinopathies that may result in hypokalemia.

Intracellular potassium shift refers to the movement of potassium from the extra-cellular fluid into the intracellular fluid. This phenomenon may be seen in the presence of alkalosis or with insulin therapy. As previously noted, potassium concentration is closely associated with hydrogen ion concentration. When the hydrogen ion concentration of the ECF is decreased (high pH; alkalosis), hydrogen ions from intracellular sources will be drawn into the ECF in an attempt to compensate for the deficit. This then leads to an intracellular deficit, including inadequate hydrogen ions for exchange with sodium ions in the renal tubules. Recall that the kidneys are better able to conserve sodium than potassium and that potassium will be excreted in exchange for the reabsorption of sodium ions. Continuation of this potassium excretion without intervention leads to eventual hypokalemia. Not only does alkalosis produce hypokalemia, but the reverse may also be seen in that the presence of hypokalemia may lead to alkalosis. An intracellular potassium deficit can produce alkalosis in the ECF as hydrogen ions move into cells in an attempt to offset the cation deficiency within the cells because extracellular potassium is not available for this purpose. Hydrogen ions are also excreted into the urine in exchange for sodium ions as would occur with potassium were it not depleted. This leads to an interesting laboratory finding that might initially appear discrepant and inconsistent with other findings. In alkalosis (discussed in more detail in Chapter 11), expected laboratory findings include an increased pH (decreased hydrogen concentration) on arterial blood gas analysis and an alkaline urine. However, when alkalosis occurs as a result of hyponatremia, the latter is not true. Although blood gas findings are consistent with alkalosis, urinary pH will be decreased instead of increased as expected. This results from the increased hydrogen ion excretion by the renal tubules in order to conserve sodium; thus, the urine is acidic with the higher hydrogen ion concentration.

Insulin therapy also produces an intracellular potassium shift. Because potassium can also be lost from the ECF by osmotic diuresis in the presence of hyperglycemia, one might expect hypokalemia in diabetic ketoacidosis. However, dehydration disguises these losses and unless fluid therapy is potassium deficient, the majority of patients will have normal or elevated serum potassium levels (Ravel, 1995) despite a total body potassium deficit.

Hypokalemia may also be seen in certain endocrinopathies, particularly in primary aldosteronism (also called *Conn syndrome*). Recall from Chapter 2 that aldosterone controls the reabsorption of sodium in the distal tubule. The high levels of aldosterone produced in primary aldosteronism lead to excessive reabsorption of sodium, and consequently, excessive urinary excretion of potassium and development of alkalosis. Patients with secondary aldosteronism in volume depleted states such as cirrhosis, congestive heart failure, and nephrotic syndrome are prone to the development of hypokalemia as well. Cirrhosis patients may have a greater likelihood of developing hypokalemia because of the presence of other predisposing factors such as poor nutritional status with inadequate potassium intake. Cushing syndrome, in which there is hypersecretion of the adrenal cortex, and congenital adrenal hyperplasia are also associated with hypokalemia in some patients.

Although a diagnosis of hypokalemia may be made based upon the presence of a low serum potassium level, additional laboratory studies (particularly evaluation of acid-base status) are important to the appropriate treatment of the patient who may be complicated by other abnormalities. Further, the assumption that serum potassium concentrations reflect total body potassium cannot be made, particularly in metabolic acidosis or with dehydration. Hypokalemia can be masked by dehydration even with significant intracellular depletion and in severe metabolic acidosis with normal renal function, patients may have normal to low normal serum potassium concentrations although intracellular depletion is severe. In such cases, correction of acidosis before potassium replacement can result in hypokalemia at a level that is life threatening (Stein, 1993).

Laboratory studies that evaluate acid-base status and renal function are important in the evaluation of hypokalemia. Measurement of urine potassium can be beneficial in determining the etiology of hypokalemia. A random urinary potassium > 20 mEq/L in a hypokalemic individual suggests renal potassium loss or acute hypokalemia (refer to the previous discussion of potassium excretion and time required for effective renal potassium conservation) and a concentration < 20 mEq/L is suggestive of chronic hypokalemia of several weeks' duration, with the major potassium loss occurring by non-renal mechanisms (Henry, 1996).

Symptoms of hypokalemia include muscle weakness and spasms, decreased reflexes, drowsiness, lethargy, nausea, confusion, and cardiac arrhythmia. Significant hypokalemia may lead to respiratory paralysis or cardiac arrest. Hypokalemia is associated with digitalis toxicity at doses usually considered non-toxic.

Hyperkalemia

Serum potassium levels > 6.0 mEq/L (Stein, 1993) are classified as hyperkalemic. Hyperkalemia is less common than hypokalemia and is associated with few disease processes by comparison. Because 80% to 90% of ingested potassium is excreted in the urine with normal renal status, impairment of renal function is the most prevalent cause of hyperkalemia, with renal failure heading the list of such disorders. Other causes of hyperkalemia include increased intake (exogenous or endogenous) and a shift of potassium from the intracellular fluid to the extracellular fluid. Table 8–4 lists some of the causes of elevated serum potassium levels and provides an etiologic classification of hyperkalemia.

As previously noted, hypernatremia is most often the result of impairment of renal function. Because the normal kidney excretes such a large percentage of ingested potassium, mild renal tubular impairment does not necessarily result in the development of hyperkalemia, particularly if dietary intake is restricted. However, with inappropriate dietary intake, patients with impaired renal tubular excretion are likely to develop potassium excesses. Some drugs are implicated in a decreased excretion of potassium. These drugs include potassium sparing diuretics like spronolactone and triamterene, non-steroidal anti-inflammatory agents such as ibuprofen and indomethacin, heparin therapy (heparin therapy suppresses aldosterone release [Jacobs, 1990]), and immunosuppressant therapy with cyclosporine (Ravel, 1995).

Increased potassium intake may result from either exogenous or endogenous sources. Exogenous sources include salt substitutes (eg, potassium chloride [KCl] substituted for sodium chloride [NaCl]), which, in some cases, contain notable potassium concentrations; potassium replacement by IV infusion or oral potassium supplements; and medications such as some penicillins that contain potassium. Depending upon the age of transfused red cells and the number of units

TABLE 8–4. Causes of Hyperkalemia

Classification	Causes
Decreased excretion	Renal failure (acute or chronic) Renal tubular disorders or renal insufficiency Addison's disease
Increased intake	IV administration Certain drugs Blood transfusions Tumor lysis Burns
Shift from ICF to ECF	Acidemia Cellular damage/tissue necrosis Insulin deficit Digoxin overdose Certain drugs
Artifactual	Hemolysis Markedly increased platelet and/or white cell counts Prolonged tourniquet application Increased muscle activity Contamination with potassium containing anticoagulant

infused, blood transfusion may also result in hyperkalemia as a result of excessive exogenous intake of potassium. (Although preserved with special anticoagulants and additives and maintained under strictly controlled conditions, some hemolysis of red cells occurs in stored blood, raising the potassium concentration of infused units.) Endogenous potassium sources involve tissue destruction such as that seen as a result of burns, tumor lysis, crush injuries, and conditions resulting in significant *in vivo* hemolysis (eg, severe hemolytic anemia).

A redistribution of intracellular potassium to the extracellular fluid may also result in hyperkalemia. The increased H^+ concentration in acidemia may result in such a shift. ICF potassium may also be released into the ECF in the presence of insulin deficiency and with a variety of medications and therapies. These include beta androgenic blockers (propranolol and pindolol), digoxin overdose, and infusion of hyperosmotic glucose solutions (Ravel, 1995). In addition, some anesthetic agents, such as succinylcholine (a muscle relaxant), cause leakage of potassium from ICF to ECF, resulting in a temporary hyperkalemic state that returns to normal after a short period of time (Ravel, 1995; Stein, 1993).

Artifactual hyperkalemia (also called *spurious hyperkalemia* or *pseudohyperkalemia*) may be seen as a result of hemolysis as discussed in the Methods of Measurement section. The release of intraplatelet potassium during the clotting process may lead to elevations in serum potassium levels when platelet counts are very high. Artifactual hyperkalemia may also result from prolonged tourniquet application that causes cellular damage and a subsequent release of intracellular potassium (Henry, 1996). Increased muscle activity and significant leukocytosis may also result in an increased serum potassium concentration. When collecting a sample for potassium analysis, it is important to avoid contamination of the specimen with potassium containing anticoagulants such as K^+ EDTA (Henry, 1996). Those completing phlebotomy training may recall instructions regarding the "order of draw" for collection of samples requiring multiple collection tubes. Observing such guidelines and collecting the sample for potassium prior to collection of the CBC sample (collected in an EDTA-containing collection tube) prevents contamination of this kind.

Tests of renal function and evaluation of acid-base balance may be included in the laboratory evaluation of hyperkalemia. In the presence of significant thrombocytosis, it may be beneficial to repeat the potassium analysis on a plasma sample (if the initial measurement was performed on serum) to rule out artifactual hyperkalemia resulting from potassium released from platelets in the clotting process. An electrocardiogram should be obtained on hyperkalemic patients (Stein, 1993).

Symptoms of hyperkalemia are similar to those listed previously for hypokalemia, particularly in terms of the effects on the neuromuscular system. Significant hyperkalemia is toxic to the heart, resulting in cardiac abnormalities present the most critical complications of elevated potassium. Cardiac manifestations of potassium toxicity produces characteristic electrocardiographic changes and may lead to ventricular fibrillation, complete heart block, and asystole (Stein, 1993). Acute hyperkalemia is life threatening, requiring immediate intervention. Treatment includes calcium administration to block the effects of potassium on the heart and infusion of substances (sodium bicarbonate, insulin, glucose) to promote the movement of potassium in the ECF into the intracellular areas. Excess potassium can be removed by means of a potassium binding agent (cation exchange resin; eg, Kayexalate) and administration of diuretics (Henry, 1996; Stein, 1993). When more conservative methods fail to produce the desired potassium reduction, dialysis may be used with hemodialysis, producing results superior to peritoneal dialysis (Stein, 1993). Chronic hyperkalemia may be treated by withdrawing contributing medications, reducing dietary intake, diuretics, or oral administration of potassium binding agent (Henry, 1996; Stein, 1993).

 TIME FOR REVIEW. After studying the preceding sections, you should be able to respond correctly to the following:

■ Define the following terms:

ion:

cation:

anion:

electrolytes:

■ Laboratory electrolyte measurements typically reflect concentrations found in _____ (intracellular fluid/extracellular fluid/both).

■ In the proximal convoluted tubules sodium, chloride, and water are _____ (reabsorbed/secreted).

■ In the distal tubule _____ and _____ alter the permeability of the tubular walls.

■ The two cations of primary physiologic importance are _____ and _____.

■ The cation present in the largest quantity in the extracellular fluid is _____.

■ The method most commonly used for sodium and potassium measurement is _____.

■ List one or more examples of situations in which the following may be encountered:

hyponatremia due to renal sodium loss:

hyponatremia due to renal fluid excess:

hyponatremia due to non-renal sodium loss:

hyponatremia due to non-renal fluid excess:

hypernatremia due to renal fluid loss that exceeds sodium loss:

hypernatremia with an increased total body sodium:

hypokalemia due to "intracellular shift":

decreased potassium excretion:

■ Renal potassium loss is most often the result of _____.

■ How would a hemolyzed specimen be expected to affect the results of potassium testing? Why?

■ A finding of an elevated serum osmolality in the presence of a low serum sodium concentration is suggestive of _____ .

■ Define iatrogenic hyponatremia:

Check your responses by reviewing the preceding sections.

ANIONS

The two major extracellular anions (negatively charged ions) are chloride (Cl⁻) and bicarbonate HCO_3^-. Measurement of these electrolytes as single analytes is not common, but they are often included on electrolyte "panels" along with sodium and potassium. Many clinicians use sodium and potassium measurements routinely and request serum anion measurements only when specifically indicated.

■ CHLORIDE

Chloride is the extracellular anion present in the highest concentration and is generally affected by the same conditions affecting sodium concentrations and in the same manner (recall that sodium is the most abundant extracellular cation). For instance, conditions that result in increased sodium concentrations usually also produce an elevation in serum chloride (**hyperchloridemia**) and those conditions resulting in hyponatremia generally produce **hypochloridemia** as well. The degree of change in chloride concentration is also similar in most cases—more significant hypochloridemia is ordinarily seen with marked hyponatremia and a lesser hypochloridemia would be expected when sodium concentrations are not as markedly decreased. Although sodium concentration can serve as a predictor of chloride concentration in the majority of clinical situations, as with most "rules of thumb," there are exceptions, such as the hyperchloremic alkalosis of protracted vomiting (Ravel, 1995). Chloride is important, in conjunction with sodium, in maintaining the appropriate osmotic pressure of serum. Of the chloride that is ingested (often ingested in combination with sodium [ie, NaCl]), most is absorbed with excesses excreted in the urine. Selective renal secretion of chloride (and bicarbonate) ions helps to maintain acid-base balance.

Methods of Measurement

Methods for the laboratory analysis of serum chloride levels include mercurimetric titration, colorimetry, and ISE (Henry, 1996). Mercurimetric titration (a method using mercury [Hg^{+2}] to form mercuric chloride [$HgCl_2$], with excess Hg^{+2} combining with a special dye) is no longer in common use. Colorimetric methods are based on the addition of a special compound to the sample that will dissociate and form a new compound with Cl⁻ allowing the free ions remaining from the original compound to react with a dye that can be measured photometrically. Silver chloride (AgCl⁻) membranes are used in electrode measurements of chloride concentration. Although all methods produce similar results (Henry, 1996), ISE measurements are the most precise. Bromide interferes (Henry, 1996; Jacobs, 1990) with chloride measurements (would be measured along with chloride) and could result in elevated chloride levels. A typical reference range for serum chloride is 98 to 106 mEq/L. Chloride may also be measured in urine and measurements of the chloride concentration in sweat (sweat chloride) are useful in the diagnosis of cystic fibrosis. Special methodologies that require small sample sizes are employed for the determination of chloride concentration in sweat. These methods and the implications of test results are not discussed in this text.

Hypochloridemia (Hypochloremia)

A low serum concentration of chloride may result from excessive loss or from intracellular shift and increased renal excretion. It is also seen in conjunction with the hyponatremia of chronic diseases. Although dietary restriction of sodium may also result in a decreased intake of chloride (the two are often found in combination in food), this should not result in an inadequate level of serum chloride (Corbett, 1993).

Excessive loss of chloride may be seen as a result of

- gastrointestinal loss: vomiting, gastric suction (through the loss of HCl)
- diabetic ketoacidosis (refer to hyponatremia discussion)
- renal disease (salt losing nephropathies)
- diarrhea
- diuretics
- syndrome of inappropriate ADH secretion
- severe burns

Chloride is not, of course, the only electrolyte lost and its loss only reflects part of a larger problem. Sodium, potassium, and hydrogen ions are generally lost as well.

Low serum chloride concentrations may also be seen **in response to high serum bicarbonate concentrations** such as that seen in metabolic alkalosis and in compensated respiratory acidosis. In response to the increase in bicarbonate in alkalosis, there will be an intracellular shift and increased renal excretion of Cl^- to reduce the concentration of negatively charged extracellular ions. In conditions of alkalosis bicarbonate is increased by definition, but it may seem confusing to think of compensated respiratory *acidosis* in terms of elevated serum bicarbonate levels. The bicarbonate buffer system (explained in the bicarbonate section) and compensation for respiratory acidosis (refer to Chap. 9) provide the basis for understanding. Chronic lung disease produces an elevated pCO_2 level and a decreased pH (high H^+ concentration) as a result of ventilatory insufficiency. Although buffer systems in the blood and respiratory compensation play vital roles in compensating for acid-base disturbances and in the overall maintenance of acid-base balance, the regulation of acid-base balance is ultimately a renal function. The renal tubules respond to chronic respiratory acidosis by reabsorbing HCO_3^- to compensate. The chronic increase in this anion results in a decrease in the other major anion, chloride. Conversely, an excessive chloride loss can *produce* an alkalotic state. When serum chloride concentrations are significantly decreased, more HCO_3^- must be retained to maintain an appropriate level of negative ions in the serum. Note the *inverse relationship* between HCO_3^- and Cl^-: high HCO_3^- in alkalosis results in decreased Cl^-; decreased Cl^- results in an increased HCO_3^- concentration, causing alkalosis.

Hyperchloridemia (Hyperchloremia)

Elevations in serum chloride may be seen as a result of excessive loss of HCO_3^-, excessive infusion of normal saline (Corbett, 1993; Jacobs, 1990), dehydration, and hyperparathyroidism, and, though uncommon, with administration of ammonium chloride or acidic salts of amino acids (Henry, 1996) during hyperalimentation. Hyperchloridemia is generally not the clinical focus of treatment; rather, the corresponding increased sodium concentration or decreased HCO_3^- concentration will most likely be the target of treatment, with serum chloride levels normalizing after effective treatment to bring sodium or HCO_3^- back to desirable ranges. The hyperchloridemia may be evaluated in terms of the relationship to hypernatremia or decreased HCO_3^- levels. Examples of these relationships are summarized in Table 8–5.

When the action of aldosterone on the renal tubules results in reabsorption and retention of excessive sodium and chloride, proportional water increased generally result in a "masking" of the increases of these electrolytes and serum levels will not reflect hypernatremia and hyperchloridemia. However, if there is a *fluid deficit* or a very high intake of sodium chloride in conjunction with retention of sodium and chloride ions, serum levels will be elevated. Although chloride increases are usually similar in degree to sodium increases, some exceptions are noteworthy. Chloride increases may exceed those of sodium when the kidneys are unable to appropriately excrete Cl^- ions, as is the case in some types of renal failure, resulting in renal hyperchloremia acidosis (Corbett, 1993). Chloride excess may also be greater than sodium excess in cases where 0.9% NaCl ("normal" saline) is infused in large quantities. Both increased sodium and chloride levels may occur in this instance, as the concentration of these electrolytes in the saline solution is higher than normal serum levels. This difference is not as pronounced in the case of sodium as it is for chloride because normal saline contains 154 mEq/L of both Na^+ and Cl^-. Normal serum levels of sodium are slightly below this level, at 135 to 145 mEq/L, but normal serum chloride levels of 98 to 106 mEq/L are significantly lower.

When acidosis results from an excessive loss of HCO_3^- as may occur as a result of gastrointestinal loss in diarrhea or in renal tubular acidosis, chloride ions are retained to replace the negative bicarbonate ions. Hyperchloridemia may be either

TABLE 8–5. Relationship of Hyperchloridemia to Hypernatremia and Decreased Bicarbonate

	Condition/Mechanism
Hypernatremia	Retention of sodium and chloride with coexistent fluid deficit Renal failure Infusion of large amounts of normal saline
Decreased HCO_3^-	Metabolic acidosis Gastrointestinal tract loss in diarrhea Renal tubular acidosis

a result or the cause of metabolic acidosis. Recall the body's "balancing act" in terms of the electrical charges of ions from previous discussions. Both chloride and bicarbonate are ions with a negative charge (anions). In order to maintain the appropriate level of anions in the body, when one increases the other must decrease. Therefore if bicarbonate decreases occur first, the retention of chloride ions must increase to maintain the appropriate level of negative ions. In this case, hyperchloridemia is the *result of acidosis* produced by bicarbonate deficiency. Conversely, with an initial elevation of chloride, bicarbonate ions will be reduced in order to maintain suitable anion levels. *Acidosis is produced as a consequence* of the bicarbonate deficiency.

■ BICARBONATE OR TOTAL CO$_2$

Bicarbonate levels may be included in electrolyte panels and are usually part of a blood gas analysis. Measurements of total CO$_2$ are often used as an indirect measure of serum bicarbonate because about 89% to 90% of the CO$_2$ liberated from serum is from bicarbonate (Henry, 1996). As is evident from the previous discussions of bicarbonate in relationship to other electrolytes, any change in bicarbonate levels signifies a change in acid-base balance. The bicarbonate buffer system (carbonic acid-bicarbonate buffer system), depicted below, is the body's major buffer system (see Chap. 9 for more detail). This system works to maintain pH levels within narrowly defined limits by "absorbing" or releasing hydrogen ions. Normal body functioning is dependent upon maintaining optimal pH levels. Even seemingly small deviations from the normal range are significant and greater deviations can produce catastrophic consequences. Measurements of CO$_2$, along with pH and pCO$_2$, are useful in the evaluation of acid-base balance and are discussed in more detail in Chapter 9. A typical reference range for total CO$_2$ in a *venous* sample is 23 to 30 mEq/L (arterial blood has a lower concentration than venous blood).

Bicarbonate Buffer System

$$H^+ + HCO_3^- \leftrightarrows H_2CO_3 \leftrightarrows CO_2 + H_2O$$

■ ANION GAP

Because the body balances positive and negative charges to maintain electrical neutrality, the concentration of anions and the concentration of cations should be equal. If Na$^+$ and K$^+$ constituted all of the cations in the body and Cl$^-$ and HCO$_3^-$ constituted all of the anions in the body, we would expect the sum of the sodium and potassium concentrations to equal the sum of the chloride and bicarbonate concentrations. However, not all of the anions or cations in the body are measured. There are more unmeasured anions than unmeasured cations, creating a "gap." Sodium is responsible for the majority of the measured cations, with a small contribution from potassium. The primary "unmeasured" cations are calcium and magnesium. Chloride ions are responsible for the majority of the measured anions, with bicarbonate (as total CO_2) responsible for the remainder. Unmeasured anions consist of sulfates and phosphates and the negative charges from proteins and organic acids (Henry, 1996). Unmeasured anions total about 24 mEq/L compared to a total concentration of unmeasured cations of about 7 mEq/L (Sacher and McPherson, 1991). The difference, or *anion gap,* is thus about 17 mEq/L. The anion gap is calculated mathematically by summing the sodium and potassium concentrations and subtracting the sum of the chloride and CO_2 concentrations. Reference ranges, though varying slightly among laboratories, may be reported as < 17 mEq/L (Henry, 1996) or as a range approximating 12 to 18 mEq/L (Sacher and McPherson, 1991). Some laboratories use only the sodium concentration because a relatively small portion of the cation concentration is provided by potassium. Reference ranges reflect the difference in methodology. Figure 8–1 provides a graphic representation of the anion gap.

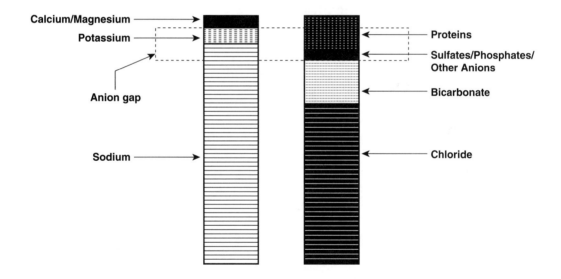

FIGURE 8–1. Anion gap.

(Adapted from Henry JB. *Clinical Diagnosis and Management by Laboratory Methods,* 19th ed. Philadelphia, Saunders, 1996).

An **increased anion gap** may be seen in a variety of conditions:

- uremia[1]: anion gap elevation due to retention of phosphates, sulfates
- non-ketotic hyperglycemic coma[1]
- lactic acidosis[1]
- ketotic states[1] (in diabetes, alcoholism, starvation)
- toxins[1] (methanol, ethylene glycol [antifreeze], salicylate)[2]
- increased plasma proteins (dehydration)

([1] = low pH [acidosis]; [2] = with normal osmolar gap in salicylate toxicity, increased osmolar gap with methanol and ethylene glycol).

A **decreased anion gap** results from either a decrease in unmeasured anions or an increase in unmeasured cations. A low anion gap resulting from increased unmeasured cations may be seen in IgG multiple myeloma, polyclonal gammopathy, lithium intoxication, polymyxin B therapy, severe hypermagnesemia, or marked hypercalcemia. Decreased unmeasured anions as a cause of a low anion gap may be seen in hypoalbuminemia and in hyponatremia with normal or increased ECF, as in SIADH (Henry, 1996). The most common cause of a low anion gap is hypoalbuminemia (Jacobs, 1990), such as that seen in nephrosis and cirrhosis.

Electrolyte disturbances do not necessarily result in an abnormal anion gap. As is evident in the preceding discussions of electrolytes, changes in one ion may result in a compensatory or "balancing" change in another. For instance, a fall in bicarbonate seen in metabolic acidosis may be balanced by a corresponding increase in chloride (both bicarbonate and chloride are anions). In such cases (hyperchloremic acidosis), the anion gap remains within normal range. The bicarbonate loss in these instances is through the gastrointestinal tract or the kidneys (diarrhea, renal tubular acidosis, hyperalimentation, as a result of certain drugs). Other causes of metabolic acidosis (lactic, diabetic, and uremic acidosis, and acidosis due to ingestion of foreign acids [Henry, 1996]), however, result in an increased anion gap. In these conditions, the chloride is only minimally increased, or may even be slightly decreased, in the presence of decreased bicarbonate, resulting in a greater anion gap. Thus the presence or absence of an increased anion gap can be useful in determining the underlying cause of metabolic acidosis.

 TIME FOR REVIEW. After studying the preceding sections, you should be able to respond correctly to the following:

■ The two anions of primary physiologic importance are _____ and _____.

■ The anion present in the largest concentration in the extracellular fluid is

_____.

■ In alkalotic states, an increased bicarbonate would generally produce a(n) _____ serum chloride.

■ What is the "anion gap" and how is it determined?

■ List conditions in which an abnormal anion gap might be seen. Would the anion gap be increased or decreased?

■ The _____ ion is generally affected by the same conditions and in the same manner as sodium concentration.

Check your responses by reviewing the preceding sections.

8. SELF TEST

Choose the best response by circling the appropriate letter. The answer key may be found in the appendices.

1. **The two cations of primary physiologic importance monitored in the clinical laboratory are**
   A. sodium and chloride
   B. potassium and chloride
   C. sodium and potassium
   D. chloride and bicarbonate

2. **The two anions of primary physiologic importance monitored in the clinical laboratory are**
   A. sodium and chloride
   B. potassium and chloride
   C. sodium and potassium
   D. chloride and bicarbonate

3. **Electrolyte measurements are most commonly performed in modern laboratories by**
   A. ion selective electrodes
   B. flame photometry
   C. colorimetry
   D. photometry

4. **The *cation* present in the largest concentration in extracellular fluid is**
   A. potassium
   B. chloride
   C. bicarbonate
   D. sodium

5. The *anion* present in the largest concentration in extracellular fluid is
    A. potassium
    B. chloride
    C. bicarbonate
    D. sodium

6. Hyponatremia attributable to renal sodium loss may be seen in
    A. prolonged vomiting
    B. cirrhosis
    C. diuretic therapy
    D. hypothyroidism

7. Hyponatremia attributable to renal water (fluid) excess may be seen in
    A. congestive heart failure
    B. diuretic therapy
    C. cirrhosis
    D. nephrotic syndrome

8. Hyponatremia attributable to non-renal sodium loss may be seen in
    A. protracted diarrhea
    B. "salt losing" nephropathy
    C. cirrhosis
    D. osmotic diuresis

9. Hyponatremia attributable to non-renal fluid excess may be seen in
    A. acute renal failure
    B. nephrotic syndrome
    C. congestive heart failure
    D. adrenal insufficiency

10. A finding of an elevated serum osmolality in the presence of a low serum sodium concentration is suggestive of
    A. iatrogenic hyponatremia
    B. pseudohyponatremia
    C. SIADH
    D. fluid sequestration ("third spacing")

11. **Hypernatremia resulting from excess renal loss of water alone may be seen in**
    A. impaired ADH release
    B. Cushing syndrome
    C. severe burns
    D. hypertonic saline administration

12. **Hypernatremia with an increased total body sodium is seen in**
    A. renal disease
    B. profuse sweating
    C. Cushing syndrome
    D. severe burns

13. **The hypernatremia that results from a renal fluid loss that exceeds sodium loss is seen in**
    A. impaired response to ADH
    B. prolonged vomiting
    C. hypertonic feedings
    D. renal disease

14. **A specimen with marked hemolysis**
    A. will result in a falsely decreased potassium concentration
    B. will result in a falsely increased potassium concentration
    C. will not affect potassium results

15. **Hypokalemia as a result of "intracellular shift" may be seen in**
    A. laxative abuse
    B. anorexia
    C. alkalosis
    D. malabsorption

16. **Renal potassium loss is most often the result of**
    A. deficient dietary intake
    B. aldosteronism
    C. alcoholism
    D. diuretics

17. **Hyperkalemia as a consequence of a shift from the ICF to the ECF may be seen in**
    A. IV administration
    B. acidemia
    C. chronic renal failure
    D. Addison's disease

18. **Decreased potassium excretion may result from**
    A. digoxin overdose
    B. markedly increased platelet counts
    C. insulin deficit
    D. renal insufficiency

19. **As the extracellular anion present in the highest concentration, this ion is generally affected by the same conditions and in the same manner as sodium concentration**
    A. bicarbonate
    B. potassium
    C. chloride
    D. sulfate

20. **In alkalotic states, an increased bicarbonate concentration would generally produce**
    A. a decreased serum chloride
    B. an increased serum chloride
    C. an unchanged serum chloride

21. **The anion gap is determined by**
    A. ion selective electrodes
    B. the sum of the measured anions
    C. the sum of the measured cations
    D. the difference between the measured cations and the measured anions

9. SCREENING WITH THE CHEMISTRY PROFILE

Chemistry profiles or panels (sometimes referred to as "general health profiles") include a number of analytes that allow the clinician to evaluate the status of multiple organ systems. The number of analytes included in chemistry profiles varies and institutions may have a variety of profiles or panels available. The advent of the multi-channel chemistry analyzer, making it possible for laboratorians to perform many different chemistry measurements on a single instrument, facilitated the rise in popularity of the multi-organ panel. Before such technology was available, performing such batteries of tests as a matter of routine would have been prohibitive not only in terms of cost and labor, but also in light of the amount of time required to complete testing. Other panels or profiles may be established for the evaluation of a particular organ or organ system or a certain disease or condition. Examples of such panels include a liver or hepatic function panel; arthritis profile; obstetric panel; thyroid profile; hepatitis profile; and anemia panel. In these cases, measurements specific to the evaluation of different aspects of the system or condition are grouped together as a battery of tests. The general chemistry panel differs from such panels in that it includes measurements that reflect the functioning of several organ systems rather than a specific target organ or system. Somewhat abbreviated panels may also be offered that are not targeted to a specific organ system or condition, yet do not include the large number of tests typically included in a general chemistry profile. A typical example of such a profile might include electrolytes along with glucose, BUN, and creatinine.

USE OF THE CHEMISTRY PROFILE

Chemistry profiles may be useful to the clinician in the evaluation of new patients and in other instances in which the survey of multiple organ systems is desirable. Collective review of the results of the variety of tests included on such panels not only allows the clinician to detect certain patterns of abnormalities, but is also beneficial in guiding the diagnostic work-up toward more definitive or confirmatory procedures (Table 9–1). It may, however, be difficult to establish the medical necessity of repeated profile testing. When an initial chemistry profile provides evidence of abnormality, the clinician will generally focus repeat and follow-up laboratory

TABLE 9–1. Common Chemistry Profile Analytes and General Organ/Condition Associations

Chemistry Analyte	May Also Be Requested As	General Organ/Organ System and Condition Association(s)[1]
Sodium[2]	Na or Na$^+$	Kidney; fluid/electrolyte balance
Potassium[2]	K or K$^+$	Kidney; fluid/electrolyte balance
Chloride[2]	Cl or Cl$^-$	Kidney; fluid/electrolyte balance
Carbon dioxide[2]	CO_2 (bicarb/bicarbonate)	Kidney; fluid/electrolyte balance; acid-base status
Glucose[3]	Gluc	Fluid/electrolyte balance; cardiac risk
Blood urea nitrogen[4]	Urea nitrogen	Kidney; liver; fluid/electrolyte balance
Creatinine[4]	Creat	Kidney; fluid/electrolyte balance
Uric acid[5]		Kidney
Calcium[5]	Ca or Ca$^+$	Bone; fluid/electrolyte balance
Phosphorus[5]	Phos or PO_4	Kidney; bone
Total protein[5]	T. Prot. or Tot. Prot.	Nutritional status; liver
Albumin[5]	Alb	Nutritional status; liver
Alkaline phosphatase[6]	AP or Alk Phos	Liver; bone
AST[6]	(formerly) SGOT	Liver; muscle
ALT[6]	(formerly) SGPT	Liver
LD[6]	LDH	Liver; muscle
Total bilirubin[6]	T. Bili or Tot. Bili	Liver
Cholesterol[7]	Chol	Nutritional status; cardiac risk
Triglyceride[7]	Trig	Nutritional status; cardiac risk
Anion gap[2,8]		Kidney; fluid/electrolyte balance
BUN:creat ratio[4,8]		Kidney; fluid electrolyte balance
Alb:glob ratio[5,8]	A/G ratio	Liver; nutritional status

[1]General associations only—more specific associations provided in discussions located elsewhere in text
[2]See Chapter 7
[3]See Chapter 5
[4]See Chapter 2
[5]See later section
[6]See Chapter 4
[7]See Chapter 6
[8]Calculated value

analyses on the areas of suspected abnormality by selecting only those laboratory measurements pertinent to the organ system or condition being evaluated. Chemistry panels are sometimes ordered routinely (or as a standing order) even after diagnosis has been made. Medical necessity probably does not exist in such cases and chemistry profiles should not be routinely requested following diagnosis without consideration of whether the patient's condition requires repeating all these measurements on a daily or other routinely scheduled basis. Such testing is not a cost-effective utilization of services when the repeated tests are not useful in clinical decision making. Further, reimbursement issues may arise when medical necessity is questioned by payors such as Medicare, Medicaid, and insurance companies. Many payors now have the capability to monitor the laboratory ordering patterns of physicians with computer software designed to alert them when a physician requests significant numbers of non-specific panel testing. Such "alerts" often trigger audits and investigation of ordering patterns and practices. It is thus prudent to limit the use of multi-organ panels to those situations in which the data are clinically useful and to employ more specific testing to monitor or evaluate established disease states and conditions.

Another argument against the routine use of chemistry profiles arises from the statistical probability of results on a "normal" individual falling outside the reference range in the absence of any condition of clinical significance. Recall from Chapter 1 that reference ranges are generally established using a 95 % confidence level. This means that the probability of a normal individual having a test within the established reference range is 95 % (or 0.95) and, conversely, that the probability of a normal individual having a test result outside this range is 5 % (or 0.05). The probability of an abnormal result increases as the number of simultaneously performed tests increases. The 5 % probability of a normal individual having a result outside of the established reference range is based on the performance of one test. When two tests are performed (reference ranges for each at 95 %), the probability of a healthy person having results within the reference range on each test is 0.95, but on both tests is just over 90 % ($0.95 \times 0.95 = 0.9025 = 90.25\%$). The probability that this individual will have a result outside the reference range in this case is nearly 10 % ($1 - 0.9025 = 0.0975 = 9.75\%$). Therefore when a battery of tests is performed, the likelihood of a result outside the reference range becomes more and more significant as the number of tests in the panel increases. For example, on a ten test panel, the likelihood of at least one result falling outside the reference range is more than 40 %. On a 20-test panel, the likelihood of "abnormal" results is extremely high, with the statistical probability of at least one abnormal result being slightly more than 64 % (probability 0.6415 [Sacher and McPherson, 1991]).

Recognition of patterns of abnormality is helpful in evaluating the results of a chemistry panel because the battery of tests is, in a sense, a combination of a number of different, sometimes overlapping, organ panels. Table 9–1 lists analytes commonly included in a chemistry panel and provides organ associations for selected analytes. Most of these analytes are discussed in other chapters of this text. The reader is referred to these chapters for more specific information. Those analytes listed and not discussed elsewhere are briefly discussed in later sections of this chapter.

COMMONLY INCLUDED ANALYTES

As noted previously, the measurements included on chemistry profiles vary widely among different institutions and each institution may offer a number of different profiles. The tests listed in Table 9–1 are often included in standard chemistry profiles and are used as the basis of discussion in this text.

■ URIC ACID

Uric acid is the major end product of purine metabolism. Purines are nitrogen containing compounds that result from the digestion of nucleoproteins. The uric acid found in the body (at the pH of body fluids, uric acid is present nearly exclusively in the form of urate ions [Henry, 1996]) may be derived from either endogenous or exogenous sources. Endogenous uric acid originates from the metabolism of nucleoproteins within the tissues or from direct transformation (Henry, 1996) of purine nucleotides in the body. *Exogenous uric acid* is a result of the metabolism of nucleotides from dietary consumption. Primary uric acid synthesis occurs in the liver, from which uric acid travels through the blood to the kidneys. The processes through which urate is handled by the kidneys are somewhat complex, but are easily summarized. Urate is freely filtered by the glomerulus and then largely reabsorbed by active transport in the proximal tubules. Tubule secretion of uric acid also occurs (some of this secreted uric acid is also reabsorbed by the proximal tubules) before final urinary excretion of uric acid. In a 24-hour period, average adults excrete about 400 to 800 mg (Henry, 1996) of uric acid in the urine. Additional excretion takes place via biliary, pancreatic, and gastrointestinal secretions with subsequent degradation of uric acid by bacteria found in the intestines. The body's "pool" of uric acid is largely (approximately 60% [Henry, 1996]) replaced on a daily basis as a result of excretion coupled with formation.

A variety of diseases and conditions are associated with increases or decreases in the urate concentration of serum, but **hyperuricemia** (increased concentration) is of greater clinical significance and is more frequent than **hypouricemia**. Serum urate levels are affected by both the amount produced and by the effectiveness of renal excretion. Common etiologies of abnormal concentrations are summarized in Table 9–2. Note that the causes of hypouricemia are relatively few in comparison with hyperuricemia.

Reference Range

Considerable variation in the reference ranges stated for serum uric acid levels are seen based on a variety of factors in addition to differences in methodology and ranges are typically relatively wide. Other factors are age, sex, race, and social and geographic factors (Henry, 1996). There may be significant day-to-day variation in levels, so it is not uncommon for clinicians to request repeat measurements over time. In addition, there remains controversy as to the level at which uric acid concentrations should be considered pathologic and the concentration used to define hyperuricemia. Because there is often overlap between normal individuals and those with clinical symptoms of hyperuricemic conditions, there is not a sharp defining line between what is abnormal and what is normal. To illustrate this quandary, typical reference ranges are provided below (from Henry, 1996). Although values > 7.0 mg/dL are sometimes considered to define hyperuricemia, both the male and female reference ranges below include values > 7.0 mg/dL.

> Male: 4.0 to 8.5 mg/dL
> Female: 2.7 to 7.3 mg/dL

TABLE 9–2. Etiologies of Hyperuricemia and Hypouricemia

	Etiology
	Decreased Renal Excretion:
	Renal failure
	Glomerulonephritis
	Polycystic kidney disease
	Diuretics (especially thiazides)
	Eclampsia/pre-eclampsia (reduced GFR)
	Ketoacidosis (diabetes and starvation)
	Lactic acidosis
	Lead poisoning
	Alcoholism
	Hypothyroidism
	Salicylate in low dosage (inhibits tubular secretion; not true of higher doses)
Hyperuricemia	
	Increased Production:
	Excessive dietary purines
	Malignancies
	Chemotherapy and radiation
	Polycythemia
	Sickle cell anemia
	Multiple myeloma
	Psoriasis
	Idiopathic mechanisms (associated with primary gout)
	Increased Excretion:
	Renal tubular reabsorption defects (congenital—Fanconi's; Wilson's or acquired)
	Salicylate (> 4 g/day)
	Corticosteroids
	Warfarin (Coumadin)
	Estrogens
Hypouricemia	
	Decreased Production:
	Severe liver disease
	Allopurinol
	Xanthinuria (xanthine oxidase deficiency; very rare)

Ranges for children may be somewhat narrower and have a lower upper limit. A marked rise in uric acid concentration may be seen in males between the ages of 12 and 14 coincident with puberty (Corbett, 1993), with a rise seen earlier in females.

Hyperuricemia

The ability of the body to break down uric acid is very limited and uric acid is not very soluble in water. Thus in the presence of high concentrations, urate crystals are readily formed. These crystals are often deposited in soft tissues, particularly in the joints, resulting in the condition known as **gout**. When these urate crystals precipitate from the urine, urate **kidney stones** may be produced.

More common in males than females, gout may result from either a disorder of purine metabolism or from ineffective renal excretion and is typified by

- hyperuricemia
- monosodium urate deposits throughout the body, but particularly in
    joints
    cartilage surrounding the joints
    bone
    bursae
    subcutaneous tissue
- recurrent attacks of arthritis
- nephropathy

When urate crystals are deposited in tissue, the body mounts an inflammatory response. This response results in tissue damage and the release of cellular substances that create an acidic environment facilitating the formation of additional urate crystals. Painful joint inflammation, usually involving specific small joints in the extremities, is the consequence of this repeated cycle. In about 75% of patients with gout, the metatarsal-phalangeal joint of the great toe is affected and 50% will have ankle and knee involvement (Ravel, 1995). In addition to joint manifestations, patients may also present with fever and leukocytosis. Interestingly, patients may present with symptoms of gout without elevations in serum uric acid levels and, conversely, may have elevated serum uric acid levels without symptomatic gout.

Increased uric acid concentrations are also seen in cases of abnormal cellular destruction and degradation of nucleic acids, as may be seen in malignancies. Treatment of malignant conditions with chemotherapy and radiation may result in markedly elevated uric acid levels that may persist for several days, also as a result of increased cellular destruction. Precautions may be necessary during this time to prevent the development of acute renal failure as a result of precipitated urates in the kidney (Sacher and McPherson, 1991).

An increased serum uric acid concentration may be seen with decreased urinary excretion consequential to various drugs or chemical substances, including low dose salicylates (< 2 g/day [Sacher and McPherson, 1991]), benzothiazide diuretics, and alcohol.

Hypouricemia

Although there are relatively few causes of hypouricemia, low serum uric acid concentrations may result from an increase in renal excretion or a decrease in production. Congenital or acquired defects in reabsorption of urates by the renal tubules may result in hypouricemia. Congenital reabsorption defects are seen in Fanconi syndrome and in Wilson's disease and acquired defects may result from toxic damage to the renal tubules (Henry, 1996). In some instances of severe liver disease, the conversion of xanthine to uric acid is impaired, resulting in low serum uric acid concentrations. A rare congenital condition, *xanthinuria,* results in a deficiency of xanthine oxidase used in the xanthine to uric acid conversion. Some drugs may lead to the development of hypouricemia by altering the excretion of urates (corticosteroids, ACTH, estrogens, warfarin, [Coumadin], salicylate > 4 g/day) or by decreasing production (allopurinol). Heavy metal poisoning, extremely low purine intake, Hodgkin's disease, multiple myeloma, bronchogenic carcinoma (Henry, 1996), and other rare congenital defects have also been implicated in hypouricemia.

 TIME FOR REVIEW. After studying the preceding sections, you should be able to respond correctly to the following:

- What impact does the number of tests included in a chemistry profile have on the likelihood of out-of-range results?

- Distinguish between endogenous uric acid and exogenous uric acid.

- Gout may result from a disorder of _____
  or from ineffective _____.

- Two mechanisms by which hyperuricemia may occur are decreased
  _____ and increased
  _____.

- Two mechanisms by which hypouricemia may occur are decreased
  _____ and increased
  _____.

- Provide two examples of each of the above mechanisms for hyperuricemia and for hypouricemia.

■ Abnormal cellular destruction is the mechanism for hyperuricemia in
_____.

Check your responses by reviewing the preceding sections.

■ CALCIUM

Calcium, the fifth most plentiful mineral element in the body (Henry, 1996), is found most abundantly (about 98 % of the body total) in the bones and teeth. The remaining calcium is found in the extracellular fluid and in skeletal muscle and other tissues. Very little calcium is present in intracellular fluid. Although the skeletal reservoir of calcium is great, only about 1 % (Henry, 1996) of this amount is available for ready exchange with the extracellular fluid. The calcium cation (Ca^{2+}) circulates in the bloodstream in three distinct forms:

- ionized ("free") state (approximately 50 %)
- bound to plasma proteins, especially albumin (approximately 45 %)
- in a complex with anions, especially phosphate and citrate (approximately 5 %)

In addition to its role in the mineralization of bone, calcium plays critical physiologic roles in a number of other functions:

- the coagulation process (see Chap. 11)
- transmission of nerve impulses
- maintaining normal tone in cardiac and skeletal muscle
- contraction of myocardium and skeletal muscle
- enzyme activity
- membrane permeability/integrity (especially transport of sodium and potassium ions across membranes)
- activity of exocrine and endocrine glands

Calcium balance is maintained by the three primary organs or systems (small intestine, kidneys, skeleton) and the action of a variety of hormones, particularly parathyroid hormone (PTH), hormones resulting from renal metabolism of vitamin D, and calcitonin. During gestation, the placenta and fetus become important in calcium homeostasis, as does the mammary gland during lactation. Calcium may be obtained from a variety of dietary sources and adult intake varies widely, but in healthy adults there is no persistent net gain or loss (Henry, 1996). It is absorbed by active transport in the small intestine. Vitamin D is required for the absorption process, which is also improved by dietary protein, growth hormone, and an acid environment in the intestines. The intestinal content of phosphorus, more specifically the ratio of intestinal calcium to phosphorus, is also important to the absorption of calcium. A ratio that is too high will inhibit absorption of calcium because of the formation of calcium phosphates that are not soluble. Just as an acidic intestinal environment promotes calcium absorption, an excessively alkaline environment has an inhibitory effect.

The hormones that are involved in regulating calcium homeostasis function predominantly by acting on the major organs involved in calcium metabolism. **Parathyroid hormone** (PTH; also called *parathormone*) acts to maintain adequate serum calcium concentrations by a number of mechanisms:

- acting on bone to induce the release of calcium into the bloodstream
- acting on the kidney to promote renal tubular absorption of calcium and reduced calcium excretion
- enhancing renal production of active vitamin D metabolites that increase intestinal absorption of calcium

Low serum calcium levels trigger the secretion of PTH by the parathyroid glands and high serum concentrations suppress secretion of the hormone.

Vitamin D refers to a group of fat soluble substances with numerical designations (ie, D_1, D_2, D_3, D_4, D_5) that enter the body in an inactive form, becoming biologically active as a result of renal metabolism. Ultraviolet rays, absorbed through the skin from sunlight, are necessary for the activation of some vitamin D precursors. In terms of calcium homeostasis, vitamin D_3 metabolites (the 1,25-dihydroxycholecalciferol hormones) are of particular importance. These hormones act on the small intestine and bone to increase the absorption of dietary calcium. They also enhance the action of PTH in promoting the release of calcium from bone into the bloodstream.

Although the role of **calcitonin** in the regulation of serum calcium concentrations is controversial (Henry, 1996), it may play a role in inhibiting the reabsorption of bone by osteoclasts, large cells formed in the bone marrow that absorb and remove tissue (Sacher and McPherson, 1991). High calcium levels trigger the production of calcitonin by the thyroid. Other hormones, including growth hormone, thyroid hormones, adrenal glucocorticoids, and gonadal steroids (Henry, 1996), play a lesser role in calcium metabolism.

Laboratory Measurement and Reference Ranges

Recall that calcium is present in ionized form or may be bound to proteins or complexed with other anions, such as phosphate. Laboratory measurements are available to measure the total calcium or ionized calcium only. Current methods for determining total calcium most commonly include the formation of a color complex between calcium and another substance. Spectrophotometric techniques are then employed to quantitate the resultant color complex. Depending on the substance used to form the color complex with calcium, magnesium may interfere with the reaction. Morning, fasting specimens are preferred for testing. Specimens should not be collected in tubes with oxalate or EDTA additives because EDTA chelates calcium and oxalates cause calcium to precipitate. Measurements may also be performed on urine samples.

Ionized calcium measurements determine the concentration of only the calcium circulating in the ionized form and are performed using an ion selective electrode. Sample collection is of particular importance to the validity of test results. Specimens should be collected exactly as directed and under anaerobic conditions (tube stopper must not be removed). The ionized calcium fraction is highly pH dependent with relatively small pH variations producing significant changes in the measured ionized calcium. For this reason, the patient's state of ventilation during sample collection is important.

Typical total serum calcium and ionized calcium reference ranges are provided below (Henry, 1996):

Total serum calcium:	9.2 to 11.0 mg/dL
Ionized calcium:	4.0 to 4.8 mg/dL (*or* 30% to 58% of total calcium)

Ranges are often somewhat higher in children and values fall gradually during pregnancy to a level about 10% lower than the concentration prior to pregnancy (Corbett, 1993).

TABLE 9–3. Selected Causes of Calcium Abnormalities

Hypercalcemia	Hypocalcemia
Primary hyperparathyroidism	Primary hypoparathyroidism
Malignancies	Pseudohypoparathyroidism
"Ectopic" PTH (neoplasm secretion of PTH-related protein)	Vitamin D deficiency
Renal hyperparathyroidism	Malabsorption syndromes (vitamin D, calcium, or both)
Thiazide diuretics	Unresponsiveness to vitamin D
Sarcoidosis	Acute pancreatitis
Hyperthyroidism	Massive blood transfusion
Vitamin D intoxication	Therapeutic hemapheresis
Lithium therapy	Alkalosis
Theophylline toxicity	Chronic alcoholism (vitamin D related)
Skeletal immobilization	Tumor lysis syndrome
Milk-alkali syndrome (excessive calcium intake)	Sepsis (vitamin D related)
Addison's disease	Drug induced (anticonvulsants, large doses of
Renal tubular necrosis (diuretic phase)	magnesium sulfate, gentamycin, cimetidine)
Idiopathic mechanisms	Idiopathic osteoporosis
Artifactual (dehydration, serum protein elevation)	Renal osteodystrophy
	Renal tubular acidosis

Table developed based on information from Henry JB. *Clinical Diagnosis and Management by Laboratory Methods,* 19th ed. Philadelphia, Saunders, 1996; Ravel R. *Clinical Laboratory Medicine: Clinical Application of Laboratory Data,* 6th ed. St Louis, Mosby, 1995; Sacher RA, McPherson RA. *Widmann's Clinical Interpretation of Laboratory Tests,* 10th ed. Philadelphia, FA Davis, 1991.

Hypercalcemia

Hypercalcemia may be seen in a variety of conditions, but is most commonly associated with primary hyperparathyroidism (PHPT) and malignancy. Other etiologies include thiazide diuretics, tertiary (renal) hyperparathyroidism, vitamin D intoxication, sarcoidosis, lithium therapy, immobilization, and hyperthyroidism (Table 9–3). Hypercalcemia may be asymptomatic or may produce a number of rather nonspecific symptoms, including vomiting, constipation, and polydipsia with polyuria. Renal calculi and calcification in soft tissues may develop and, in severe cases, mental confusion and coma may result. Peptic ulcers are a fairly common occurrence (Sacher and McPherson, 1991) as are bone lesions.

In PHPT, the parathyroid secretes excessive PTH even when no appropriate physiologic stimulus (ie, low serum calcium level) is present. This is often the result of a single adenoma, but may also result from parathyroid hyperplasia. PHPT is most commonly manifested by renal calculi. Malignancy, the cause of about 50 % of hypercalcemia cases detected on hospitalized patients (Ravel, 1995), may result in hypercalcemia by different mechanisms summarized in Table 9–4 in conjunction with the types of neoplasms resulting in hypercalcemia.

The differential diagnosis of hypercalcemia may be established based on laboratory measurements of serum calcium, serum phosphorus, serum alkaline phosphatase, PTH level, urine calcium, and urine phosphorus (Table 9–5). Ionized calcium measurements may also be useful.

TABLE 9–4. Malignancy-Associated Hypercalcemia

Mechanism	Associated Neoplasm(s)[1]	Average % of Cases Producing Hypercalcemia
Primary bone neoplasm	Myeloma (starts in bone marrow)	30
	Acute lymphocytic leukemia	5
Tumor production of PTH-like substance (ectopic PTH syndrome)	Lung carcinoma	25
	Breast	20
	Squamous non-pulmonary	19
	Renal cell carcinoma	8
Metastatic carcinoma to bone	(from primary sites of)[2]	
	Breast	15
	Lung	10
	Kidney	10

[1]Neoplasms are listed in descending order based on the approximate percentage of malignancy associated hypercalcemia cases linked to that site.

[2]Although bone metastasis occurs with prostatic carcinoma, the bone lesions are usually osteoblastic instead of osteolytic; thus, serum calcium is generally not elevated.

Data from Ravel R. *Clinical Laboratory Medicine: Clinical Application of Laboratory Data,* 6th ed. St Louis, Mosby, 1995.

Hypocalcemia

Hypocalcemia most often results from a deficiency in PTH or a deficiency or unresponsiveness to vitamin D. Other causes of hypocalcemia are presented in Table 9–4. Malabsorption syndromes can result in decreased serum calcium levels as a consequence of reduced intestinal absorption and are worsened by a decrease in absorption of vitamin D. Acute pancreatitis may result in hypocalcemia when fat necrosis traps calcium and causes a relative deficiency of PTH (Sacher and McPherson, 1991). Primary hypoparathyroidism is another cause of hypocalcemia and usually is seen as a consequence of the surgical removal of the hypothyroid glands. The surgical removal of the glands may be performed in the treatment of hyperparathyroidism or may be an unintended, inadvertent result of other surgical procedures such as thyroidectomy (Sacher and McPherson, 1991). Pseudohypoparathyroidism, an uncommon condition, results in low serum calcium levels caused by inadequate responsiveness to PTH. Hypocalcemia may also be seen in a variety of inherited disorders or subsequent to therapy with some drugs and is due to an alteration in the metabolism or responsiveness to vitamin D.

Symptoms of hypocalcemia include increased neuromuscular irritability with tingling that may progress to muscle cramps, twitching, and tetany. Mental changes and convulsions may occur and sustained or marked calcium deficiency can give rise to altered myocardial function.

Table 9–5 presents typical laboratory findings in some of the conditions affecting serum calcium and phosphorus concentrations. (As will be evident following the discussion of phosphorus, the metabolism and regulation of calcium and phosphorus are closely related.)

TABLE 9–5. Typical Laboratory Findings in Conditions Affecting Calcium and Phosphorus

Condition	Serum				Urine		
	CA	PHOS	ALK PHOS	PTH	CA	PHOS	c-AMP
Primary hyperparathyroidism	↑↑	↓	N/↑	↑↑	↑	↑	↑↑
Renal hyperparathyroidism[1]	↑	↑	↑	↑	↑	↓	↑
Renal tubular acidosis[1]	N/↓	N/↓	↑	N/↑	↑	↑	N/↑
Ectopic PTH syndrome	↑	↓	↑	↑	↑	N/↓	N
Metastatic neoplasm to bone	↑	N/↑	N/↑	N/↓	N/↑	N/↓	N
Vitamin D excess	↑	N/↑/↓	N	↓	↑	N/↑/↓	N
Vitamin D deficiency	N/↓	↓	↑	↑	N/↓	↑	N/↑
Primary hypoparathyroidism	↓	↑	N	↓	↓	↓	↓
Pseudohypoparathyroidism	↓	↑	N	↑	↓	↓	N/↑
Osteoporosis (idiopathic, senile)	N	N	N	N/↑	N/↑	N/↑	N
Paget's disease	N/↑	N	↑	N	N/↑	N/↑	N

[1]Acidosis present. c-AMP (cyclic adenosine monophosphate) is released into the urine as a result of the action of PTH on renal tubules.

Table based primarily on information from Henry JB. *Clinical Diagnosis and Management by Laboratory Methods,* 19th ed. Philadelphia, Saunders, 1996; Jacobs DS, et al. *Laboratory Test Handbook,* 2nd ed. Cleveland, LexiComp Inc. 1990; Ravel R. *Clinical Laboratory Medicine: Clinical Application of Laboratory Data,* 6th ed. St Louis, Mosby, 1995; Sacher RA, McPherson RA. *Widmann's Clinical Interpretation of Laboratory Tests,* 10th ed. Philadelphia, FA Davis, 1991.

■ PHOSPHORUS

Although the terms are often used interchangeably, *phosphates* and *phosphorus* are not one and the same. Phosphorus is one component of a group of phosphates. Most of the body's phosphorus is found in intracellular fluid, making it the most plentiful intracellular anion. It is found primarily in bone with about 10 % found in skeletal muscle (Ravel, 1995). It is an important component of cell membranes, energy storage compounds, nucleic acids, the compound that regulates the affinity of oxygen for hemoglobin molecules, a number of enzymes, and the urinary acid-base buffer system.

Phosphorus metabolism and regulation closely parallels that of calcium. As is the case with calcium, phosphorus is acquired through dietary sources and absorbed in the small intestine. The same principal organs and hormones contribute to the homeostasis of both minerals. When PTH acts on bone to cause release of calcium, phosphorus is also released. While promoting renal tubular reabsorption of calcium, PTH depresses the reabsorption of phosphates. Vitamin D metabolites contribute to the absorption of dietary phosphorus and enhance the mobilizing effect of PTH on skeletal phosphorus. Low serum levels stimulate the renal production of vitamin D metabolites. Most of the circulating phosphorus is reabsorbed in the renal proximal tubules.

Laboratory Measurement and Reference Ranges

Most laboratory assays of phosphorus involve the reaction of molybdates (a heavy metal substance) with phosphates to form a compound that can be quantitated. Although a number of techniques are available to quantify this complex, most involve photometric measurement of molybdium blue formed by the action of a reducing substance on phosphomolybdate (Henry, 1996). Serum phosphorus concentrations vary significantly throughout the day, with higher values noted on late afternoon and evening specimens than on morning specimens. Variation results from dietary influences, from shifts between the intracellular and extracellular fluids, and from changes in the excretion rate (Ravel, 1995). Hyperlipidemia and hemolysis can result in false elevations. Typical reference ranges for serum phosphorus are (Henry, 1996)

> Adult: 2.3 to 4.7 mg/dL
> Child: 4.0 to 7.0 mg/dL

Hypophosphatemia

Hypophosphatemia accounts for most of the significant phosphorus abnormalities. The symptoms of decreased serum phosphorus levels are similar to those of hyponatremia and include confusion, disorientation, and, in some cases, seizures. Weakness noted in the skeletal muscles may progress to myopathy and severe deficiencies may produce bone abnormalities and hematologic abnormalities involving oxygen delivery by red cells and altered white cell functions, making it more difficult to adequately protect against infection. Very mild decreases may produce no symptoms and are of little clinical significance. Hypophosphatemia may be seen as a result of

- insulin (causes shift from extracellular to intracellular fluid)
- antacid medications (antacid forms complex with phosphorus, preventing absorption)
- increased excretion (systemic acidosis; especially in diabetic acidosis when patient is also receiving insulin—additive effect of increased excretion and intracellular shift may lead to marked phosphorus depletion)
- alcohol abuse (reduced intestinal absorption, acidosis resulting from alcohol metabolism)
- renal tubular reabsorption disorders (in vitamin D deficiency, Fanconi syndrome, congenital disorders)
- alkaline intestinal contents (hampers absorption)

Decreased serum phosphorus concentrations may also be seen as a result of nasogastric suction, glucose administration, parenteral hyperalimentation, primary hyperthyroidism, acute respiratory failure with mechanical ventilation, and therapy of acute severe asthma, and in gram negative sepsis (Ravel, 1995).

Hyperphosphatemia

Hyperphosphatemia is most commonly caused by renal failure, but may also be seen as a result of severe muscle injury, phosphate containing antacids, hypoparathyroidism, and tumor lysis syndrome (Ravel, 1995). Measurement of calcium concentration is important in cases of hyperphosphatemia as elevated phosphorus concentrations can lead to hypocalcemia.

 TIME FOR REVIEW. After studying the preceding sections, you should be able to respond correctly to the following:

■ What hormone acts on the bone to release calcium and phosphorus?

■ Hypercalcemia is most commonly associated with _____ .

■ Hypocalcemia is most frequently caused by _____ .

■ Explain how the following can result in hypophosphatemia:

    Antacids:

    Insulin:

■ Review the tables provided in this chapter.

Check your responses by reviewing the preceding sections.

9. SELF TEST

1. **The number of tests on a profile**
   - **A.** has no impact on the likelihood of out-of-range results
   - **B.** increases the likelihood of out-of-range results
   - **C.** decreases the likelihood of out-of-range results

2. **Alkaline phosphatase is generally associated with**
   - **A.** liver and bone
   - **B.** cardiac risk and kidney
   - **C.** nutritional status and electrolyte balance

3. **Phosphorus is generally associated with**
   - **A.** liver and kidney
   - **B.** muscle and cardiac risk
   - **C.** bone and kidney

4. **Calcium is generally associated with**
   - **A.** bone and fluid/electrolyte balance
   - **B.** liver and muscle
   - **C.** bone and kidney

5. **Cholesterol is generally associated with**
   - **A.** nutritional status and liver
   - **B.** cardiac risk and nutritional status
   - **C.** liver and muscle

6. **LD is generally associated with**
   - **A.** nutritional status and liver
   - **B.** cardiac risk and nutritional status
   - **C.** liver and muscle

7. **A disorder of purine metabolism or ineffective renal excretion typified by an elevated uric acid is**
   - **A.** Fanconi syndrome
   - **B.** gout
   - **C.** xanthinuria

8. **Hyperuricemia would be an expected laboratory finding in all the following *except***
    A. renal failure
    B. severe liver disease
    C. chemotherapy and radiation

9. **Abnormal cellular destruction is the mechanism for hyperuricemia in**
    A. diuretic therapy
    B. polycystic kidney disease
    C. malignancy

10. **Corticosteroid therapy may lead to hypouricemia as a result of**
    A. decreased production
    B. increased production
    C. increased excretion

11. **The hormone(s) that act(s) on the bone to release calcium and phosphorus is/are**
    A. calcitonin hormone
    B. parathyroid hormone
    C. vitamin D metabolite hormones

12. **The hormone(s) that act(s) on the kidney to promote renal tubular absorption of calcium and reduced calcium excretion is/are**
    A. calcitonin hormone
    B. parathyroid hormone
    C. vitamin D metabolite hormones

13. **The hormone(s) that act(s) on the small intestine and bone to increase the absorption of dietary is/are**
    A. calcitonin hormone
    B. parathyroid hormone
    C. vitamin D metabolite hormones

14. **Hypercalcemia is most commonly associated with**
    A. PHPT and malignancy
    B. ectopic PTH and hyperthyroidism
    C. PTH deficiency or vitamin D deficiency/unresponsiveness

15. **Hypocalcemia most frequently results from**
    A. PHPT and malignancy
    B. ectopic PTH and hyperthyroidism
    C. PTH deficiency or vitamin D deficiency/unresponsiveness

16. **Increased serum calcium, phosphorus, alkaline phosphatase, and PTH in conjunction with decreased urine phosphorus and an increase in urinary calcium and cyclic AMP is most indicative of**
    A. primary hyperparathyroidism
    B. renal hyperparathyroidism
    C. primary hypoparathyroidism

17. **Antacid medications may result in hypophosphatemia by**
    A. preventing phosphorus absorption
    B. causing intracellular shift
    C. increasing renal excretion

18. **Insulin may cause hypophosphatemia by**
    A. preventing phosphorus absorption
    B. causing intracellular shift
    C. increasing renal excretion

10.TESTS OF PANCREATIC FUNCTION

PANCREATIC ANATOMY AND PHYSIOLOGY

The pancreas extends from the duodenum to the spleen. This organ has important functions of both an endocrine and an exocrine nature, each independent of the other. Groups of specialized cells called **islet cells** (islets of Langerhans) throughout the pancreas are involved in the **endocrine functions** of the organ. These cells secrete the hormones **insulin** and **glucagon** essential to the regulation of blood glucose levels. The pancreas is also an important accessory gastrointestinal organ that secretes a variety of **digestive enzymes** in its **exocrine role**:

- amylase: digests starches
- lipase: digests fats
- trypsin: digests proteins
- elastase: digests proteins

Pancreatic enzymes are secreted through the pancreatic duct into the duodenum. In addition to these enzymes, the pancreas secretes **bicarbonate**, which serves to neutralize the acidic contents of the duodenum and jejunum to protect the lining of the small intestine.

Diseases of the pancreas may involve either its endocrine or exocrine functions. Endocrine disorders are discussed in Chapter 14. Important pancreatic diseases include acute and chronic pancreatitis and pancreatic carcinoma. Obstruction of the pancreatic duct or bile ducts and disease in surrounding areas (eg, the gallbladder) can produce pancreatic abnormalities. This chapter presents a brief description of pancreatic diseases and a summary of the laboratory tests related to these conditions.

PANCREATIC DISEASES

Pancreatic diseases may be difficult to evaluate, particularly in chronic forms, because of the anatomy and location of the pancreas and the complexity of its physiologic functioning. The major diseases encountered are acute and chronic pancreatitis. Clinical presentation of the two forms may overlap as with an acute relapse in chronic pancreatitis.

Acute pancreatitis produces a sudden onset of constant, severe mid-epigastric pain in most patients. The pain often radiates to the back and is frequently associated with nausea and vomiting, abdominal tenderness and distension, and fever. Jaundice may be present in up to 30% of cases (Ravel, 1995). Abdominal fluid sequestration may result in volume depletion of varying degrees and may lead to the development of hypotension and shock. Hypoxemia (usually mild) and hypocalcemia are common findings (Stein, 1993). The diagnosis of classic, severe acute pancreatitis is rarely difficult, but many symptoms are also associated with other conditions making diagnosis of mild, moderate, or intermittent conditions more problematic. Diseases that may be clinically confused with acute pancreatitis include perforated peptic ulcer, biliary tract inflammation, biliary tract stones, intestinal infarction, and intra-abdominal hemorrhage (Ravel, 1995). More than 80% of patients with pancreatitis will either have gallstone disease or have a history of alcohol abuse (Henry, 1996).

Chronic pancreatitis may be more difficult to diagnose, especially when it develops slowly over a long period of time. It is typically associated with chronic, severe abdominal pain, fatty stools (steattorrhea), weight loss, and glucose intolerance. Pancreatic calcification noted on abdominal x-ray films is diagnostic of chronic pancreatitis and is seen in about 30% of cases (Stein, 1993). Chronic pancreatitis is most commonly the result of alcohol abuse, but may also occur as a result of hemochromatosis, hereditary pancreatitis, cystic fibrosis, pancreatic trauma, and other conditions.

Cystic fibrosis produces pancreatic disease as a result of its effect on the mucous glands of the pancreas. Pancreatic secretions are thickened and may block pancreatic ducts, causing atrophy of pancreatic cells, similar to the disease's characteristic effects on the lungs.

LABORATORY TESTS

Although somewhat non-specific, laboratory measurements of amylase and lipase have long been employed in the diagnosis of both acute and chronic pancreatitis. These pancreatic enzymes are found in the blood and urine in increased concentrations in pancreatitis.

■ AMYLASE

Amylase, specifically alpha-amylase, is the laboratory assay most commonly used when acute pancreatitis is suspected. It is also useful in chronic pancreatitis, but is a less reliable indicator in chronic cases, with levels often normal or only slightly elevated. Most amylase is cleared from the blood by glomerular filtration. Alpha-amylase (hereafter referred to simply as amylase) has a variety of isoenzymes of both pancreatic and salivary origin that may be separated electrophoretically or by selective inhibition techniques.

In acute pancreatitis elevated levels are seen within 24 hours in most patients, but may be seen as early as 2 hours after onset (Ravel, 1995). Elevations of 3 to 4 times the upper limit of the reference range are highly suggestive of acute pancreatitis. The degree of amylase elevation does not necessarily reflect the severity of disease. Levels typically return to normal within 3 to 5 days, with persistent elevations indicating continued destruction of pancreatic cells or possible pseudocyst formation.

Amylase (both serum and urine) is measured by a variety of methods with very different reference ranges, often making a comparison of results from one testing facility to another quite difficult. Different methods use different units to express the values. As a result of these factors and substrates that may not be well defined, conversion of values among different units is difficult to impossible. Even though use of International Units has been recommended to reduce confusion, reagent manufacturers seldom use them (Henry, 1996). When amylase results must be compared from differing methodologies, a comparison of the relative degree of elevation above the corresponding reference ranges is more practical. Results obtained on CAP proficiency testing (refer to Chap. 1) for amylase provides an illustration of the high degree of variability in amylase measurement. Table 10–1 summarizes results from 43 different methods used on a 1994 survey as reported by Henry (1996).

This means that a specimen tested at laboratories using a particular amylase method produced results averaging about 208 IU/L, while the same specimen tested at laboratories using a different amylase method produced results averaging about 506 IU/L (and 37 vs. 86; 167 vs. 373; etc). Note that the units of measure (IU/L) are the same for these methods.

Methods of measurement for amylase include those based on chromogenic reactions, coupled-enzyme kinetic methods, and turbidometric methods or nephelometry (a measure of light scatter).

Elevated serum amylase concentrations are seen in a variety of pancreatic and non-pancreatic disorders (Table 10–2). The increased levels may be the results of either increased amounts of amylase entering the bloodstream (ie, as in pancreatic duct obstruction) or of a reduction in the rate of amylase clearance as seen with impaired renal function. Levels are typically normal in pancreatic carcinoma. Elevations are seen in some carcinoma patients, but occur too late in the course of the disease to be of any diagnostic value. In a few cases, acute pancreatitis may be present along with the malignancy (Ravel, 1995).

TABLE 10–1. Amylase Variability by Method on the CAP Survey

Specimen	Lowest Mean Value (IU/L)	Highest Mean Value (IU/L)
C-06	37.2	86.2
C-07	166.7	372.5
C-08	64.8	152.5
C-09	208.2	506.2
C-10	210.6	506.7

Results from the 1994 CAP Chemistry Survey as reported in Henry JB. *Clinical Diagnosis and Management by Laboratory Methods,* 19th ed. Philadelphia, Saunders, 1996.

TABLE 10–2. Causes of Elevated Serum Amylase

Condition	Related to
Acute pancreatitis, primary Chronic relapsing pancreatitis	Alcohol abuse; trauma; certain drug sensitivities (thiazides, tetracycline, valproic acid, oral contraceptives, and others); viral hepatitis; idiopathic mechanisms
Biliary tract disease	Cholecystitis; tumor; after biliary tract cannulation
Intra-abdominal disease	Peptic ulcer; intestinal obstruction; intraabdominal hemorrhage; peritonitis; recent surgery
Other	Acute salivary gland disease; macroamylasemia (see later discussion); renal insufficiency; diabetic ketoacidosis; cardiac circulatory failure; extensive burns; renal transplant; pregnancy; ruptured ectopic pregnancy; cholecystography using contrast media

Falsely decreased or falsely normal serum amylase concentrations may occur as a result of the administration of glucose. For this reason, specimens collected during IV therapy with fluids containing glucose may not produce reliable results. Because blood glucose concentrations rise after meals, specimen collection should be delayed for at least 1 to 2 hours (Ravel, 1995) after patients have eaten. *Lipemic serum,* which is not uncommon in acute pancreatitis, may interfere with many test methods, yielding normal or decreased values in the presence of true elevations. In rare cases of massive pancreatic cell destruction levels may be falsely low as a result of an inability of the pancreatic cells to produce the enzyme.

Urine amylase measurements may be of benefit in the diagnosis of pancreatitis, particularly in cases with normal or only slightly elevated serum amylase values. Urine levels begin to rise several hours after serum amylase levels and remain elevated for 7 to 10 days (Ravel, 1995) after serum levels return to normal. Specimens for urine amylase assay should be collected over a defined time period (ie, 2 hours; 12 hours; 24 hours) so the values can be reported in units per hour to account for the influence of fluctuating urine volume. Although an increase in both serum and urine amylase concentrations is seen in most cases of acute pancreatitis, some patients may have only an elevated urine level. Reported diagnostic sensitivity and specificity levels are somewhat higher for urine amylase than serum amylase (Henry, 1996) in the detection of acute pancreatitis.

The adequacy of renal function is an important consideration in the evaluation of both urine and serum amylase values. Sufficiently impaired renal function produces a reduction in the clearance of amylase with a consequent decrease in urinary concentration and an elevation (mild to moderate [Ravel, 1995]) in serum concentration. Renal clearance of amylase typically correlates with creatinine clearance (see Chap. 2), but patients with acute pancreatitis often have increased rates of amylase excretion. This increased rate results in an increased ratio (> 4 % and often 7 % to 15 %; normal 1 % to 4 % [Henry, 1996]) of amylase clearance to creatinine clearance. Determination of the amylase clearance:creatinine clearance ratio requires collection of both a serum specimen and a urine specimen (timed collection not required), with creatinine and amylase measurements performed on both specimens. The ratio is then calculated using the formula:

$$\text{Amy CL:Creat CL (\%)} \ = \ \frac{\text{U Amy}}{\text{S Amy}} \ \times \ \frac{\text{S Creat}}{\text{U Creat}} \ \times \ 100$$

where Amy is amylase, Creat is Creatinine, S is serum, U is urine, and CL is clearance.

While this ratio may have diagnostic benefit, it is important to note that significant numbers of patients with acute pancreatitis have normal ratios and that elevated ratios may be seen in a number of other conditions, including diabetic ketoacidosis, severe burns, heart disease, and other conditions.

Urine amylase and amylase:creatinine clearance ratios may also be beneficial in distinguishing macroamylasemia from pancreatic disorders. The term **macroamylasemia** is used to describe a relatively uncommon, benign condition in which serum amylase levels persist at elevated concentrations in the absence of clinical findings consistent with a pancreatic disorder. In this condition, normal circulating amylase is bound to immunoglobulins or, less frequently, to a polysaccharide. The resultant complex, called **macroamylase**, is too large to pass through the glomerular filter for excretion in the urine. Consequently, serum amylase levels become elevated. Routine laboratory determinations do not distinguish between bound and unbound amylase, but specialized methods are available for the detection of macroamylase. Elevated serum amylase levels accompanied by a very low amylase:creatinine clearance ratio, normal renal function, normal serum lipase, and the absence of clinical symptoms of pancreatic disease is suggestive of macroamylasemia. A definitive diagnosis can be established only by demonstrating the presence of the macroamylase complex by direct test methods.

■ SERUM LIPASE

Serum lipase levels rise at about the same time as amylase levels and typically remain elevated longer. Lipase measurements are more specific for acute pancreatitis disease than amylase assays (lipase is not produced by the salivary glands), but are generally less sensitive (Ravel, 1995) except for methods employing a lipase cofactor (colipase) in which the diagnostic sensitivity is significantly improved (Henry, 1996; Ravel, 1995). Like amylase, lipase is filtered through the glomerulus, so impaired renal function can produce elevated serum values. Elevated lipase concentrations may also be seen in many of the same non-pancreatic disorders that produce elevations in serum amylase concentration (ie, acute cholecystitis, peptic ulcer, intestinal obstruction, recent surgery, etc). Lipemic serum may cause falsely decreased values by some methods.

■ TRYPSIN

Trypsin, a proteolytic enzyme produced exclusively by the pancreas, can now be measured in plasma with newly developed radioimmunoassay (RIA) methods. Much of the circulating trypsin is bound to inhibitors, including alpha-1-antitrypsin and, to a lesser degree, alpha-2-macroglobulin, with serum activity normally attributed to the trypsin precursor, trypsinogen. In acute pancreatitis the precursor is activated to form trypsin (Ravel, 1995). RIA methods differ in terms of whether trypsinogen and trypsin bound to alpha-1-antitrypsin are measured. (Current methods do not measure trypsin bound to alpha-2-macroglobulin [Ravel, 1995].) Serum immunoreactive trypsin (SIT) measurement by RIA is believed to be a reliable and specific indicator of the exocrine function of the pancreas (Henry, 1996), but the data evaluating SIT in non-pancreatic disorders are conflicting and insufficient to draw conclusions regarding expected values (Ravel, 1995). This test is generally available only through reference laboratories or in large medical centers and therefore may not be practical for routine diagnostic use.

■ ELASTASE

Elastase, another proteolytic pancreatic enzyme, appears to show great promise in the diagnosis of pancreatic disease, showing 100% sensitivity for the diagnosis of acute pancreatitis in some studies. RIA methods for measurement of this enzyme have only recently been developed and are not yet routinely available in most clinical settings.

Serum lipase and serum amylase assays remain the most useful and practical laboratory tools for the routine diagnosis of acute pancreatitis, acute relapse of chronic pancreatitis, and cystic complications of chronic pancreatitis. The assay of pancreatic enzymes is a less useful tool for detection of pancreatic carcinoma. Unfortunately, there are also no identified tumor markers specific for the early detection of pancreatic tumors despite evaluation of a number of tumor antigens. Other procedures, besides laboratory assays, may be useful in assessing pancreatic function and are summarized briefly in Table 10–3.

TABLE 10–3. Other Procedures for Evaluation of Pancreatic Function

Procedure	Comments
Endoscopic retrograde cholangiopancreatography (ECRP)	Involves insertion of fiberoptic scope and injection of contrast medium into common bile duct, pancreatic duct, or both; morphologic alterations seen on x-ray can detect acute pancreatitis, chronic pancreatitis, pancreatic carcinoma, and pancreatic cyst; clear distinction of conditions not always possible; insensitive to minimal or mild disease; not always successful, but is sensitive and reliable procedure for detection of significant pancreatic dysfunction; requires substantial expertise
Computerized tomography (CT) and ultrasound	Detect pancreatic abnormality in 80% to 85% (Ravel, 1995) of patients; CT usually easier to interpret, but ultrasound better for diagnosis of pancreatic pseudocyst; both may miss small tumors or mild generalized disease
Pancreatic stimulation	Collection of pancreatic fluid by duodenal drainage for direct assay before and after injection of pancreatic stimulating hormone, secretin; before ecrp, this was important diagnostic test for chronic pancreatitis and may still be useful; not abnormal until ~75% of exocrine function lost

Data from Ravel R. *Clinical Laboratory Medicine: Clinical Application of Laboratory Data*, 6th ed. St Louis, Mosby, 1995.

10. SELF TEST

Choose the most appropriate response for each item. The answer key may be found in the appendices.

1. The specialized islet cells of the pancreas are involved in the _____ function of the organ and secrete _____.
   - **A.** endocrine; amylase and lipase
   - **B.** endocrine; insulin and glucagon
   - **C.** exocrine; amylase and lipase
   - **D.** exocrine; insulin and glucagon

2. This pancreatic enzyme digests starches.
   - **A.** amylase
   - **B.** lipase
   - **C.** trypsin
   - **D.** elastase

3. This pancreatic enzyme digests fats.
   - **A.** amylase
   - **B.** lipase
   - **C.** trypsin
   - **D.** elastase

4. This proteolytic pancreatic enzyme is produced exclusively by the pancreas and is predominately bound to inhibitors in the blood.
   - **A.** amylase
   - **B.** lipase
   - **C.** trypsin
   - **D.** elastase

5. Significant impairment of renal function could produce
   - **A.** elevated urine amylase
   - **B.** decreased serum amylase
   - **C.** elevated serum amylase

6. **Serum amylase elevations of 3 to 4 times the upper limit of the reference range are highly suggestive of**
   A. pancreatic carcinoma
   B. increased renal clearance of amylase
   C. chronic pancreatitis
   D. acute pancreatitis

7. **Falsely decreased or falsely normal serum amylase concentrations may be the result of**
   A. glucose administration
   B. recent abdominal surgery
   C. acute salivary gland disease
   D. macroamylasemia

8. **Urine amylase levels are elevated**
   A. only in very severe, chronic pancreatitis
   B. longer than serum levels
   C. when renal function is impaired
   D. in all of the above cases

9. **Choose the findings most consistent with macroamylasemia.**
   A. elevated serum amylase and lipase; normal amylase:creatinine clearance ratio; impaired renal function; no clinical symptoms
   B. elevated serum amylase; normal serum lipase; very low amylase:creatinine clearance ratio; normal renal function; severe mid-epigastric pain
   C. normal serum amylase and lipase; elevated amylase:creatinine clearance ratio; normal renal function; no clinical symptoms
   D. elevated serum amylase; normal serum lipase; very low amylase:creatinine clearance ratio; normal renal function; no clinical symptoms

10. **Both the pancreas and the salivary glands secrete this enzyme.**
    A. amylase
    B. lipase
    C. trypsin
    D. elastase

11. **The size of the macroamylase complex results in**
    A. increased renal clearance
    B. decreased renal clearance
    C. increased serum and urine amylase levels
    D. decreased serum and urine amylase levels

11. ARTERIAL BLOOD GASES AND ACID-BASE BALANCE

The focus of this chapter is on the use of arterial blood gas determinations as a tool in the assessment of pulmonary function. Although an important part of the diagnostic process, blood gases are not sufficient alone to diagnose specific diseases. They may, however, provide valuable information regarding the presence of abnormalities in function, progression or improvement in the patient's status, and the effectiveness of treatment. Discussions of acid-base balance and of abnormal blood gas patterns in specific diseases are included to aid in the evaluation of blood gas results.

ANATOMY AND PHYSIOLOGY OF THE RESPIRATORY TRACT

Knowledge of the respiratory system's anatomy and physiologic function is necessary in order to assess the lungs and evaluate the laboratory findings in arterial blood gas studies. The basic structure and function of the respiratory system is included here to provide a basis for subsequent discussions of blood gas results, abnormalities, and disease processes.

■ BASIC STRUCTURE

A passageway for air is provided by the upper airway (nose and nasopharynx, mouth and oropharynx, and larynx) and the lower airway (trachea, main stem bronchi, bronchioles, and alveolar ducts leading to the alveoli). In addition to providing a passage for inspired air, the airway serves to filter, warm, and humidify the air. Filtering is accomplished by several mechanisms, including the secretion of mucus by cells in the epithelial layer of the airways. The mucus lines the airway and traps foreign particles, such as dust and bacteria, which are then propelled up into the pharynx by cilia. The foreign material can then be expelled by sneezing or coughing. The rich capillary blood supply in the airways makes the warming and humidifying functions possible. The inspired air is heated to body temperature and its humidity is raised to at least 80 %, a process that uses up to a liter of water a day. Some of the water is reabsorbed on expiration to conserve fluid.

The lungs lie in the thoracic cavity, surrounded by the sternum and ribs anteriorly and the ribs, scapulae, and vertebral column posteriorly. This cavity also provides protection to the lungs. The apices of the lungs lie just above the clavicles anteriorly and extend to the eleventh or twelfth rib posteriorly. The thoracic cavity is lined with the pleura, a continuous membrane that lines the rib cage with one surface and covers the lungs with its other surface.

The lungs are divided into lobes, with the right lung consisting of upper, middle and lower lobes and the left lung having only upper and lower lobes. Lobar bronchi branch off the main stem bronchus and conduct air to each lobe.

Alveoli, very small sacs arising from the alveolar duct, are the basic unit of gas exchange in the respiratory system and number over 300 million in a healthy adult. The smooth muscle of the alveolar ducts is capable of expanding and contracting. The alveolus is a layer of squamous epithelium and an elastic basement membrane. Gas exchange takes place between these two layers and the corresponding two layers of the adjoining capillary (across the alveolar–capillary interface) (Figs. 11–1 and 11–2).

■ PULMONARY VENTILATION, RESPIRATION, AND GAS EXCHANGE

The primary function of the lungs is that of gas exchange, and in order for gas exchange to be a continuous process, alveolar air must constantly be exchanged with environmental air. This is *pulmonary ventilation*—the act of breathing. Air moves in and out of the lungs because gases will move from an area of greater pressure to an area of lower pressure. Atmospheric air pressure is greater than that of the alveoli at the start of inspiration. When alveolar pressure exceeds atmospheric pressure, expiration occurs. The pressure gradient is established by changes in the size of thoracic cavity (ie, size is increased by contractions of the diaphragm; decreased from elastic recoil of the lungs and thoracic muscle).

Breathing is an *automatic process* that may be controlled to some extent (ie, breathing slower or faster). The automatic control of respiration is centered in the medulla and pons (responsible for rhythmicity). Primary control of the respiratory center in the medulla is maintained by the carbon dioxide tension (pCO_2), oxygen tension (pO_2), and the pH of arterial blood. A rise in pCO_2 or a fall in pO_2 or pH is detected by chemoreceptors and leads to an increase in respiratory rate. Other factors, of course, influence respiration, including pain, emotions, and stimulation of the pharynx or larynx.

As previously noted, the alveolus is the basic gas exchange unit in the lungs. Because the partial pressure (tension) of oxygen in the alveolus is greater than that of venous blood, oxygen diffuses across the alveolar–capillary membrane into the blood. The partial pressure of carbon dioxide in the alveolus is less than that of venous blood, so carbon dioxide diffuses in the opposite direction. Carbon dioxide diffuses more easily than oxygen and the diffusion capacity of oxygen can be reduced in high altitudes (lower pO_2 of atmospheric air), by decreased surface area in the alveoli, or by a decreased amount of oxygen reaching the alveoli.

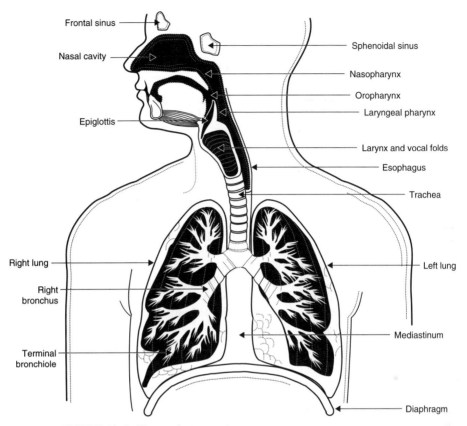

FIGURE 11–1. The respiratory system.

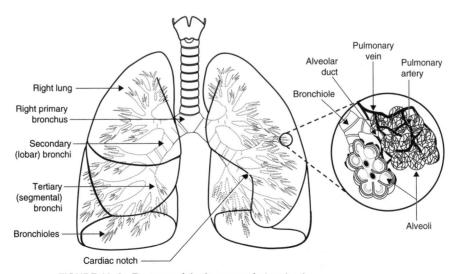

FIGURE 11–2. Features of the lower respiratory tract.

USE OF ARTERIAL BLOOD GASES

Arterial blood gas studies (ABGs) are an excellent indicator of overall pulmonary function and have become a common tool in the diagnosis and management of patients. However, as previously noted, ABGs are not of themselves sufficient to diagnose a specific disease. Before presenting a more detailed discussion of ABGs, it may be beneficial to look at what ABGs *cannot* do. ABGs

- cannot give a specific diagnosis: asthmatics may have values similar to those found in pneumonia and patients with chronic obstructive pulmonary disease (COPD) and respiratory failure may have the same values as a cardiac patient with pulmonary edema.
- do not indicate how much the patient is suffering from an abnormality detected: low pO_2 does not necessarily indicate tissue hypoxia, nor does a normal pO_2 ensure adequate oxygenation; cardiac output, regional blood flow, affinity of hemoglobin for oxygen, capillary perfusion, and tissue oxygen consumption are also important in oxygen utilization.
- are not a screening test to exclude pulmonary disease: although ABGs are an excellent indicator of overall pulmonary function, as with other organ systems, considerable disease may be present before system fails.

On the other hand, ABGs *can*

- assist in determining whether gas exchange is defective: based on pO_2 in conjunction with other variables.
- reflect the state of the ventilatory control system: determined by pCO_2 and consideration of the acid-base state.
- reveal the state of acid-base balance.

MEASUREMENT OF BLOOD GAS PARAMETERS

Blood gas studies include the measurement of the partial pressures of oxygen and carbon dioxide, and the pH. From these measured parameters along with the actual barometric pressure, hemoglobin value, patient temperature, and forced inspiratory oxygen level, the oxyhemoglobin (% oxygen saturation), base excess, total carbon dioxide, bicarbonate, oxygen content, and other parameters are calculated.

WHAT THE PARAMETERS MEAN

The oxygen and carbon dioxide are reported in terms of *partial pressure*. The partial pressure of a gas in liquid (in this case blood) is the partial pressure of that gas with which the liquid is in equilibrium, or that part of the total pressure exerted by a specific gas. For example, assuming a barometric pressure of 760 mm Hg, the partial pressure of oxygen in room air is approximately 21%, and 21% of 760 is about 160 mm Hg. A glass of water in that room is at equilibrium with the room air, so the pO_2 in the water is also 160 mm Hg. Although they are directly proportional, the *amount* of a gas is not the same as the partial pressure of the gas. Continuing the example just used, an open tube of blood beside the glass of water (never, of course, actually occurring in the world of infectious diseases!) is also in equilibrium with the room air and thus the oxygen in the tube of blood would also have a partial pressure of 160 mm Hg. However, the *quantity* of oxygen in blood is considerably greater than that in water. The amount of a gas in a liquid depends not only on the partial pressure of the gas, but also on the solubility of the gas in that liquid. The partial pressure, on the other hand, depends only on the gas with which the liquid is in equilibrium (room air in our example).

Oxygen saturation (SaO_2) refers to the oxygen carried by the hemoglobin. The *quantity* of oxygen in the blood is expressed as a percentage. This is the amount of oxygen in the blood that is combined with hemoglobin compared to the total amount of oxygen that *could* combine with the hemoglobin in that blood. The oxygen capacity depends on the amount and type of hemoglobin in the blood. (For this reason, the patient's actual hemoglobin should always be used, when possible, in the determination of oxygen saturation.) The oxygen content is related linearly to the SaO_2 through the oxygen capacity (ie, SaO_2 = oxygen content/oxygen capacity).

The amount of oxygen combined with hemoglobin is related to the pO_2 by the *oxyhemoglobin dissociation curve*. It is important to understand this relationship in order to assess the adequacy of tissue oxygenation. The sigmoid curve seen in Figure 11–3 represents the saturation percentages at various pO_2 values. Many factors affect the affinity of the heme molecule for oxygen, the most significant of which is the pO_2. In the upper portion of the oxyhemoglobin dissociation curve, hemoglobin has an increased affinity for oxygen. This means that changes in pO_2 will have a lesser effect on the SaO_2—large changes in pO_2 can be tolerated without significant change to SaO_2. At a pO_2 of 100 mm Hg, SaO_2 is about 97%. Even if the pO_2 falls to 70 mm Hg, the SaO_2 only drops to about 94%. This is a protective mechanism that serves to ensure adequate oxygenation of the tissues even in the presence of mild hypoxemia. The opposite is true for the lower part of the curve. Once the pO_2 falls below 60 mm Hg, the SaO_2 saturation decreases sharply, significantly reducing the ability of the hemoglobin to carry oxygen to the tissues.

The oxygen affinity of hemoglobin is influenced by other factors as well:

- temperature: the patient's temperature is used in this calculation to provide more accurate results; if unavailable, 37°C is used—if the patient's actual temperature differs significantly, results will not be accurate
- pCO_2
- pH

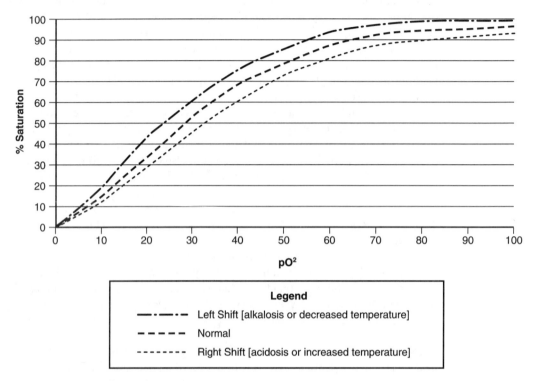

FIGURE 11–3. Oxyhemoglobin dissociation curve. Not drawn to scale and is intended to be representative only.

The oxyhemoglobin dissociation curve shifts to the right at higher temperatures, increased pCO_2 (*hypercapnia*), and decreased pH (*acidosis*); therefore, the hemoglobin has a lesser affinity for oxygen and lower SaO_2 will result at any given pO_2. With decreased temperature, decreased pCO_2 (*hypocapnia*), and increased pH (*alkalosis*), the curve shifts to the left, meaning a higher affinity for oxygen and higher SaO_2.

The pCO_2 measurement is the best clinical guide to the effectiveness of ventilation and the functional integrity of the ventilatory control system. Normally this control system maintains pCO_2 levels within narrow limits. Both the amount of carbon dioxide produced by the body and the ability of the lungs to eliminate it affect this value. Either hypocapnia or hypercapnia indicates a serious defect in ventilatory control.

The pH is a measure of hydrogen ion concentration or the level of acidity in the blood. The pH is expressed as a negative logarithm, so as the concentration of hydrogen ions in the blood increases the pH decreases (more acidic), and as the concentration of hydrogen ions decreases the pH increases (more alkaline).

Base excess (also called *delta base*) is a measure representing the difference from normal buffer base used to describe situations with metabolic imbalance. It is the difference of the concentration of strong base in whole blood and the concentration of the same blood titrated to pH 7.40 with either a strong acid or strong base at standard conditions of pCO_2 = 40 mm Hg and temperature of 37°C. The value is calculated using a standard nomogram. Base excess is used to assess abnormalities of metabolic acidosis or alkalosis. Values more negative than the reference value indicate a deficiency of fixed base or an excess of acid (metabolic acidosis); values more positive than the upper limit of the reference range indicate excess fixed base or non-volatile acid deficit (metabolic alkalosis).

The *bicarbonate* (HCO_3) level is a measurement in acid-base balance used in evaluation of fixed base. It is calculated using the Henderson–Hasselbalch equation

$$pH = pK_a + \log \frac{(HCO_3^-)}{H_2CO_3}$$

and the measured values of pH and pCO_2. The value is *increased* with metabolic alkalosis and with compensated respiratory acidosis and is *decreased* in metabolic acidosis or in compensated respiratory alkalosis (low in ketoacidosis).

The CO_2 *content* refers to CO_2 in solution or bound to protein and equals carbonic acid (H_2CO_3) plus bicarbonate (HCO_3^-).

REFERENCE RANGES

pH: 7.350 to 7.450
pO_2: 72 to 108 mm Hg
pCO_2: 35 to 45 mm Hg
SaO_2: 95 % to 99 %

 TIME FOR REVIEW. After studying the preceding sections, you should be able to respond correctly to the following:

■ The basic unit of gas exchange in the respiratory system is the

_____ .

■ The primary function of the lungs is _____ .

■ Oxygen and carbon dioxide are reported in terms of

_____ .

■ The quantity of oxygen carried by hemoglobin is referred to as

_____ .

■ Oxygen saturation drops most rapidly at (high/low) _____ levels of pO_2.

■ In addition to the oxygen dissociation curve, the oxygen affinity of hemoglobin is influenced by what three factors?

■ With higher temperature, increased CO_2, and decreased pH, hemoglobin has a (lesser/greater) _____ affinity for oxygen.

■ With a decreased temperature, decreased CO_2, and an increased pH, hemoglobin has a (lesser/greater) _____ affinity for oxygen.

■ _____ is a measure of hydrogen ion concentration.

■ The measure of the difference from normal buffer base is the _____.

Check your responses by reviewing the preceding pages.

ABNORMALITIES IN OXYGEN AND CARBON DIOXIDE

This section will deal only with hypoxemia and with hypocapnia and hypercapnia. Following a later discussion of acid-base balance, blood gas patterns seen in specific diseases will be provided.

■ HYPOXEMIA

Oxygen is unlike the other substances obtained from the environment and used by the body in that the body's stores of oxygen are virtually non-existent. Thus complete oxygen deprivation results in death within a matter of minutes. For this reason, any level of hypoxemia is cause for concern. However, as long as a continuous supply of oxygen is available, the defense mechanisms of the body can compensate for surprising levels of hypoxemia. The shape of the dissociation curve provides one important line of defense. Recall that significant reductions in oxygen's partial pressure from normal result in much smaller decreases in oxygen saturation until a level of about 60 mm Hg.

An oxygen deficit (and carbon dioxide excess) can be caused by a variety of conditions that interfere with either ventilation, diffusion, or perfusion (Table 11–1). Anemia may also lead to an oxygen deficit as the amount of hemoglobin available to transport oxygen to the tissues for cellular metabolism is reduced. The arterial oxygen content is only one of the factors involved in the delivery of oxygen to the cells. Other factors that play a role in this vital process include cardiac output, regional blood flow, oxygen extraction, position of the dissociation curve, and hemoglobin concentration.

The early signs of inadequate oxygenation may include restlessness, dyspnea, tachycardia, and confusion. Cyanosis is a classic sign of hypoxia, but is not a reliable indicator because it does not occur until there are 5g or more of reduced hemoglobin in the blood and because cyanosis (even severe cyanosis) may be seen even when the arterial oxygen level is adequate (Phipps et al, 1983), as in polycythemia.

It is difficult to predict, in any individual case, the level of hypoxemia that presents a life threatening situation (survival has been reported in instances with pO_2 levels as low as 7.5 mm Hg.). The presence or absence of other conditions or factors may be decisive. For instance, hypoxemia increases susceptibility to cardiac glycoside intoxication and may cause intractable arrhythmias in patients with severe pre-existing cardiac or pulmonary disease (Phipps et al, 1983). Because oxygen delivery is a product of cardiac output and arterial oxygen content, the combination of hypoxemia and a low cardiac output is especially dangerous.

■ HYPERCAPNIA AND HYPOCAPNIA

As noted earlier, pCO_2 is the best clinical guide to the effectiveness of ventilation and the functional integrity of the ventilatory system. It is rigidly controlled and maintained within narrow limits, therefore, any abnormal pCO_2 value is cause for concern.

Recognition of **hypercapnia** is more important in terms of what it indicates about underlying pathophysiology than in regard to harmful effects of increased pCO_2 levels (as opposed to oxygen, for which the harmful effects of decreased levels are of significant concern). The level of hypercapnia indicating a rapidly dete-

TABLE 11–1. Oxygen Deficit and Carbon Dioxide Excess: Causes from Interference with Ventilation, Perfusion, and Diffusion

Ventilation	Perfusion	Diffusion
Inhibition of thorax or lung (bronchioles, alveoli) expansion Decrease in elastic recoil	Circulatory collapse, shock Blockage of pulmonary capillaries (emboli) Vasoconstriction from alveolar hypoxia Decrease in blood pH Destruction or compression of pulmonary capillary bed	Decrease in alveolar surface area Thickening of alveolar membrane Increase in fluid/secretions in interstitial space or alveoli

riorating disease and requiring immediate action depends on the nature of the disease. With previously normal pulmonary function, any level of hypercapnia is of great significance. In an acute bronchial asthma attack in a patient known to have normal pCO_2 levels between attacks, mild hypercapnia is cause for concern and moderate to severe hypercapnia is often an indication for intubation and assisted ventilation (Phipps et al, 1983). On the other hand, patients with COPD in acute episodes of respiratory failure can often be managed without assisted ventilation even with severe elevations in pCO_2 levels.

The harmful effects of hypercapnia are difficult to separate from those of hypoxemia and acidosis which often accompany hypercapnia. Further, the effects do not correlate well with the pCO_2 level. One study showed no significant abnormalities in mental state if pCO_2 was below 90 mm Hg and the pH above 7.25 and that coma or semi-coma was always seen with pCO_2 above 130 mm Hg and pH below 7.14 (Phipps et al, 1983). However, within these limits great variability was noted.

Many critically ill patients have spontaneous hyperventilation resulting in **hypocapnia**. The left shift in the oxygen dissociation curve would be expected to interfere with oxygen utilization. Because these patients are critically ill, it is difficult to assign particular harmful effects to either the hypocapnia or the accompanying alkalosis. However, hypocapnia and respiratory alkalosis resulting from assisted ventilation can cause cardiac arrhythmias until the respiratory alkalosis is corrected. No convincing evidence indicates that spontaneously occurring hypocapnia has significant harmful effects. In general, it is not wise to attempt to treat the hyperventilation itself, but rather attention should be focused on the underlying cause (Phipps et al, 1983).

ACID-BASE BALANCE

This section is not intended to be a comprehensive discussion of the complex process of acid-base balance, but rather a general discussion to add to the understanding of ABGs and the respiratory system.

Both the respiratory system and the renal system are involved in maintaining acid-base balance. A normal diet results in the ingestion of a large quantity of acid on a daily basis. Acids are also produced endogenously as a result of metabolism. The acids are of two basic types:

1. those that can be converted to carbon dioxide (**volatile acids**)
2. those that cannot be converted to a gaseous state (**non-volatile acids**)

The respiratory system assists in the elimination of acid by excreting carbon dioxide. The non-volatile acids are excreted in the urine.

The pH of both intracellular and extracellular fluids in the body must be maintained within narrow limits because many metabolic reactions are catalyzed by enzymes that will only function at an optimal pH level. The body possesses efficient mechanisms for pH maintenance, including buffering the blood, respiration, and renal mechanisms.

A *buffer* is a substance that tends to preserve the original hydrogen ion concentration of its solution (a weak acid in solution with its conjugate base which is in the form of a salt) upon the addition of an acid or a base. Buffering action serves to neutralize excess acid or base to prevent change in the pH of the solution or to result in a smaller change. The body's extracellular buffers, which account for a little less than half of the systemic buffering capacity, are (in descending order of capacity) *bicarbonate/carbonic acid, hemoglobin, plasma proteins,* and *erythrocyte and plasma phosphate* (Henry, 1996).

The specific mechanisms and chemical reactions involved in the actions of these buffers cannot be dealt with fully here. However, the equilibrium equation for the bicarbonate/carbonic acid buffer system is expressed as $H_2O + CO_2 \rightleftharpoons H_2CO_3 \rightleftharpoons H^+ + HCO_3^-$. This is an extremely effective buffer system because the ratio of base to acid is finely regulated by respiration (excretion of CO_2) . The second most important buffer in the blood is hemoglobin. Each hemoglobin molecule contains 38 histidine (an amino acid from tissue proteins) residues that can bind with hydrogen ions (H^+) to lower the pH. The plasma proteins have free carboxyl and amino acid groups that can also bind with hydrogen ions.

The action of the blood buffers to minimize pH changes is immediate, but the capacity of the buffers to minimize the change is limited. Compensation by the respiratory system is prompt, but the ultimate regulation of acid-base balance and regeneration of free buffers is accomplished by the renal system (Henry 1996). Compensation by the renal system is more gradual and takes place over a 3-to 4-day period following an acid-base imbalance.

As is evident from this discussion, adequate respiration is necessary not only for appropriate oxygenation, but also to maintain acid-base balance by the elimination of volatile acid through excretion of CO_2. The level of CO_2 and thus the level of H^+ (see above equilibrium equation) is decreased in conditions leading to hyperventilation and leads to *respiratory alkalosis* (lower H^+ concentration = higher pH). In diseases in which CO_2 is trapped in the alveoli, the levels of CO_2 and H^+ are increased result in *respiratory acidosis.* The respiratory system also functions as a compensatory mechanism for metabolic acid-base imbalances. When metabolic acidosis exists, the respiratory system can excrete higher amounts of H^+ in the form of carbon dioxide with deep, rapid respiration. Hydrogen ions are conserved in metabolic alkalosis with slow, shallow respiration.

ACID-BASE IMBALANCES

Four general classifications of imbalances will be defined: alkalemia, acidemia, mixed imbalances, and renal tubular acidosis.

Acidemia

pH < 7.35. Acidemia can result from an accumulation of CO_2 in the body (respiratory acidosis) or from an accumulation of fixed acids or loss in HCO_3^- (*metabolic acidosis*). Respiratory acidosis results from hypoventilation or ventilation/perfusion inequalities. The kidneys are able to compensate by reabsorbing HCO_3^-. The degree of compensation possible is dependent on the chronicity of the ventilatory insufficiency and on the capacity of the renal tubules.

Metabolic acidosis may be further divided into two types. One, acidemia with increased anion gap, may be seen as a result of uremia with retention of fixed acids; ketotic states (such as in diabetes, starvation, and alcoholism); lactic acidosis as in shock; and with increased plasma proteins in dehydration. The second, acidemia with normal anion gap, is associated with loss of HCO_3^- through the gastrointestinal tract or kidneys.

Alkalemia

pH > 7.45. Alkalemia may occur from decreased pCO_2 concentrations in the blood (*respiratory alkalosis*) or from a loss of fixed acids or an increase in blood alkalis such as HCO_3^- (*metabolic alkalosis*). Respiratory alkalosis is secondary to hyperventilation. The kidneys compensate by decreasing the absorption of HCO_3^-. Metabolic alkalosis as a result of a loss of fixed acids is most often due to prolonged vomiting or nasogastric suctioning. Excess alkali may also result from excessive ingestion of basic substances such as antacids. Metabolic alkalosis may be seen in disease states in which too much H^+ leaves the extracellular spaces or is excreted in the urine, such as Cushing syndrome, prolonged administration of corticosteroids, and hypokalemia (extreme potassium depletion).

Mixed Imbalances

Mixed imbalances are often seen because respiratory disturbances are often accompanied by metabolic ones. The history and setting of the patient are often clues to the possibility of a mixed imbalance as can be seen from the examples that follow. In addition, laboratory data may be beneficial—in some cases an increased anion gap is the only clue. Mixed imbalances may also be detected if the compensatory response falls short of or exceeds the expected response (adequacy of response is assessed using either mathematical equations or an "acid-base map"). Mixed imbalances and an example of each are listed below.

- *Respiratory acidosis and metabolic acidosis:* acute pulmonary edema and cardiopulmonary arrest causing both poor tissue perfusion (lactic acidosis) and pulmonary edema (poor alveolar ventilation)
- *Respiratory alkalosis and metabolic alkalosis:* patient with cirrhosis given diuretics
- *Respiratory acidosis and metabolic alkalosis:* COPD patient receiving diuretics
- *Respiratory alkalosis and metabolic acidosis:* patient with chronic renal failure and hyperventilation
- *Metabolic acidosis and metabolic alkalosis:* patient with chronic renal failure complicated by severe vomiting

Renal Tubular Acidosis

Renal tubular acidosis (RTA) may be of two types. Type 1 results from impaired excretion of hydrogen ions giving a high urine pH even in the presence of acidemia due to a distal tubular defect. Secondary causes of type 1 RTA include cirrhosis, nephrotoxic drugs, kidney transplant rejection, and diseases with hypergamma-globulinemia. Type 2 RTA results from a reduction in the reabsorption of HCO_3^- by the proximal tubules. Secondary causes of type 2 RTA include multiple myeloma, cystic renal diseases, diseases of inborn metabolism errors, and drugs and toxins. Both types may occur together (type 3 RTA).

EVALUATING ACID-BASE DATA

Although many uncomplicated cases may be interpreted and diagnosed with relative ease, interpretation of acid-base data is often a complicated process and one of the more difficult aspects of laboratory medicine. A relatively simple approach to the initial evaluation of data is to first look at the arterial pH value:

$$\uparrow pH = \textbf{alkalosis}$$
$$\downarrow pH = \textbf{acidosis}$$

Next, look at the arterial pCO_2 level and note the direction of change (from normal). If the change in pCO_2 is in the *same direction* as the change in pH (eg, increased pH and increased pCO_2), the primary disorder is *metabolic*. Conversely, if the pCO_2 change is in the opposite direction of that of the pH change (eg, pH increased, but pCO_2 decreased), the primary disorder is *respiratory*. Combining these two steps to classify primary, uncomplicated disorders provides the following guide:

$$\uparrow pH \text{ and } \uparrow pCO_2 = \text{metabolic alkalosis}$$
$$\uparrow pH \text{ and } \downarrow pCO_2 = \text{respiratory alkalosis}$$
$$\downarrow pH \text{ and } \downarrow pCO_2 = \text{metabolic acidosis}$$
$$\downarrow pH \text{ and } \uparrow pCO_2 = \text{respiratory acidosis}$$

Another approach that may be useful is to begin the evaluation with the arterial pCO_2 level, because the primary respiratory imbalances result from hyperventilation or hypoventilation and produce changes in the arterial pCO_2. Using this approach, with **decreased pCO_2 consider** (as primary disorder)

- **Respiratory alkalosis:** resulting from hyperventilation (anxiety, pain, fever, hypoxia, improper ventilator setting). The respiratory alkalosis may be an acute, uncompensated disorder (increased pH; also increased in partial compensation). In compensated respiratory alkalosis, the pH may be within the reference range—perhaps on the upper end of the range.

- **Metabolic acidosis:** pH decreased in partial compensation and within reference range with full compensation (may be on low end of range).

With **increased pCO$_2$ consider** (as primary disorder)

- **Respiratory acidosis:** from hypoventilation as seen in chronic lung disease. Acute, uncompensated, pH is decreased; if fully compensated, pH is within reference, but may be on lower end.
- **Metabolic alkalosis:** with pH increased in partial compensation and within the reference range with full compensation (may be on upper end of range).

The base excess is usually negative (–2 or less) in both metabolic acidosis and respiratory alkalosis (to a lesser extent) and positive (+ 2 or more) in metabolic alkalosis and respiratory acidosis (to a lesser extent).

When metabolic acidosis is detected, the anion gap may be useful in determination of the cause. As you will recall from the discussion of electrolytes in Chapter 7, the anion gap is the difference between the major cations and the major anions. It is calculated by the formula:

$$(Na^+ + K^+) - (Cl^- + HCO_3^-) = \text{anion gap}$$
$$or$$
$$Na^+ - (Cl^- + HCO_3^-) = \text{anion gap}$$

An increased anion gap (especially more than 10 mEq/L above the reference range [Ravel, 1995]) in metabolic acidosis may be indicative of

- excessive endogenous production of fixed acids (ketone bodies, lactic acid)
- inadequate renal excretion of fixed acids (uremia, renal failure)
- ingestion of exogenous acids or acid producing substances (alcohol, salicylate overdose, ethylene glycol poisoning)

These methods of evaluation are useful in evaluating acid-base imbalance resulting from a single primary abnormality. Mixed imbalances and ABG measurements following institution of therapy are more complicated. In cases of mixed imbalances, it is important to diagnose from the first set of ABGs with subsequent measurements used to evaluate the response to therapy. In order to evaluate and interpret acid-base data in mixed imbalances, it is important to determine any significant condition (such as diabetic acidosis, renal failure, or chronic lung disease) that affect acid-base balance. Other considerations that may change the acid-base balance in a particular direction must also be evaluated (ie, is the patient vomiting, on diuretic therapy, etc). Tables 11–2 and 11–3 provide additional aids in evaluating acid-base imbalances.

TABLE 11-2. Summary of Findings in Primary Acid-Base Imbalance Categories

Imbalance	Clinical Observations[1]	Common Causes[2]	PH	PCO_2	HCO_3^-	BE
Metabolic acidosis	Kussmaul respirations— faster/deeper than norm; shock; coma	Excess acid (ketones in diabetic acidosis or lactic acid in cardiac arrest); HCO_3^- loss thru intestines; increased Cl—-renal failure	↓	N (uncomp) ↓ (comp)	↓	↓ (neg)
Metabolic alkalosis	Parethesias, tetany, weakness	Vomiting/gastric suction (loss of H^+, Cl^-, K^+); ingestion or infusion of sodium bicarbonate	↑	N (uncomp) ↑ (comp)	↑	↑ (pos)
Respiratory acidosis	Acute: air hunger, disorientation Chronic: hypoventilation, hypoxia, cyanosis	Hypoventilation—chronic lung disease causing CO_2 retention; respiratory depression from drugs or anesthesia	↓	↑	N (uncomp) ↑ (comp)	N/↑
Respiratory alkalosis	Acute: hyperventilation, parethesia, light-headedness Chronic: hyperventilation, latent tetany	Hyperventilation—anxiety, pain, fever, hypoxia, improper ventilator adjustment	↑	↓	N (uncomp) ↓ (comp)	N/↓

"neg" refers to –2 or more negative numbers; "pos" refers to +2 or more positive numbers.

[1]Data from Sacher RA, McPherson RA. *Widmann's Clinical Interpretation of Laboratory Tests,* 10th ed. Philadelphia, FA Davis, 1991.

[2]Data from Corbett JV. *Laboratory Tests and Diagnostic Procedures with Nursing Diagnoses,* 3rd ed. Norwalk, CT, Appleton and Lange, 1992.

TABLE 11-3. Summary of Compensation in Acid-Base Imbalances

Imbalance	Type of Compensation	Limits of Expected Compensation[1]
Metabolic acidosis	Respiratory; reduction of pCO_2	pCO_2 ↓ of 1.0 – 1.3 mm Hg for each mEq/L ↓ in HCO_3^- pCO_2 should be 1.5 x (HCO_3^-) + 8 pCO_2 should equal last two digits of pH (pH = 7.21 and pCO_2 = 21) last two pH digits should equal HCO_3^- concentration + 15 (eg, HCO_3^- of 16, pH should be 7.31)
Metabolic alkalosis	Respiratory; slight increase in CO_2	pCO_2 ↑ of 6 mm Hg for each 10 mEq/L ↓ in HCO_3^- last two pH digits should equal HCO_3^- concentration + 15
Acute respiratory acidosis Chronic respiratory acidosis	Renal; kidneys will retain more HCO_3^- over time	HCO_3^- ↑ of 1 mEq/L for each 10 mm Hg ↑ in pCO_2 pH disturbance more pronounced than change in HCO_3^- HCO_3^- ↑ of 3.5 mEq/L for each 10 mm Hg ↑ in pCO_2
Acute respiratory alkalosis Chronic respiratory alkalosis	Renal; kidneys will excrete more HCO_3^- over time	HCO_3^- ↓ of 2 mEq/L for each 10 mm Hg ↓ in pCO_2 HCO_3^- ↓ of 5 mEq/L for each 10 mm Hg ↓ in pCO_2

[1]Compensation limits from Sacher RA, McPherson RA. *Widmann's Clinical Interpretation of Laboratory Tests,* 10th ed. Philadelphia, FA Davis, 1991.

When evaluating measures of acid-base balance it is essential to keep in mind that more than one process may be occurring at the same time. Using the two primary indicators of pH and pCO_2 as discussed previously, evaluating the magnitude of the abnormality, evaluating the HCO_3^- level, and determining what, if any, other abnormalities are present (serum sodium, potassium, chloride, etc) can assist in determining whether the results are produced from a single disorder or a combination of different processes occurring simultaneously. A mixed disorder should be suspected when significant abnormality of pCO_2 or HCO_3^- is accompanied by a normal pH (Sacher and McPherson, 1991). A mixed alkalosis and acidosis in which the opposing influences nullify any change in measured pH level could produce such results.

EXPECTED COMPENSATORY CHANGES

When disorders of acid-base balance occur, the body's regulatory mechanisms attempt to correct or compensate for the abnormal state. These regulatory mechanisms include buffer systems, and the functions of the lungs and kidneys. Understanding the expected compensatory changes in these disorders can be beneficial to the evaluation of acid-base laboratory data.

Metabolic Acidosis

In metabolic acidosis there is a deficit of HCO_3^- that results in a decreased pH and a decreased CO_2 content. Metabolic acidosis may result in several situations:

- *Acid gain:* The HCO_3^- deficit is due to its use in the effort to buffer H^+. Acid is gained by

  - excess endogenous production (metabolic), as in ketoacidosis and starvation
  - direct administration or ingestion (ammonium chloride administration, salicylate poisoning)

- *Base loss:* direct loss of HCO_3^- from intestine, as in severe, prolonged diarrhea
- *Renal acidosis:* inability of renal tubules to adequately excrete H^+ from metabolic acids; results in H^+ buildup in the bloodstream; much of the HCO_3^- is used in an attempt to buffer.

Regardless of the etiology of the metabolic acidosis, the body's initial compensatory attempt is the conversion of bicarbonate to carbon dioxide to buffer the excess hydrogen ions. The carbon dioxide is then "blown off" through the lungs. The compensatory result as indicated by ABG results is a reduction in both the HCO_3^- and the pCO_2.

Metabolic Alkalosis

In metabolic alkalosis, an excess of bicarbonate produces an increased pH. The excess HCO_3^- may be a consequence of either excess generation or abnormal retention. The alkalosis may also result from a loss of H^+.

- *Bicarbonate excess:* Bicarbonate will increase when kidneys are stimulated to retain sodium; if the kidneys are stimulated (by aldosterone) to retain sodium (Na^+) and excrete potassium (K^+), but insufficient K^+ is available, the kidneys will increase generation of H^+ and a subsequent increase in HCO_3^- occurs. Bicarbonate concentration may also increase with diuretic use. Diuretics can cause a decrease in blood volume, which can stimulate the renin/angiotensin/aldosterone system resulting in an increase in the exchange between Na^+ and K^+ or H^+ at the distal tubule. The resultant increase in bicarbonate concentration produces alkalosis.
- *Hydrogen loss:* Hydrogen ions may be lost as a result of severe vomiting, which causes a depletion in the body stores of H^+ and Cl^-. Greater excretion of H^+ may occur in response to the body's efforts to conserve sodium (H^+ is the cation excreted in place of sodium).

With most etiologies of metabolic alkalosis, decreased levels of Na^+, K^+, and Cl^- are seen along with the increase in HCO_3^-. The compensatory attempt is respiratory, but only slight compensation is generally possible. Complete compensation would require depression of ventilation to a degree appreciable enough to raise the pCO_2 to a level that would re-establish a normal buffer proportion. This is rarely achieved because of the overriding need for ventilatory maintenance of an adequate pO_2.

Respiratory Acidosis

An accumulation of carbon dioxide (hypercapnia) occurs in respiratory acidosis and raises the pCO_2 and lowers the pH. This condition may be either acute or chronic.

- *Acute respiratory acidosis:* seen with sudden airway obstruction, damaged respiratory muscles from chest trauma, acute paralysis or depression of CNS respiratory centers. In such instances the immediate response required is treatment of the problem producing the respiratory acidosis or ventilatory assistance rather than laboratory evaluation of imbalance (Sacher and McPherson, 1991).
- *Chronic respiratory acidosis:* occurs more frequently and is more difficult to treat than acute. Results from chronic obstructive pulmonary diseases such as chronic bronchitis, emphysema, and pulmonary fibrosis. Excretion of CO_2 is impaired.

The compensatory response in acute respiratory acidosis begins with protein buffers followed by the HCO_3^- buffering system. Acute hypercapnia also provides a powerful respiratory stimulus, resulting in obvious "air hunger" and a corresponding ventilatory effort. In acute conditions this takes place before impaired oxygen exchange has an impact on respiration (Sacher and McPherson, 1991). In chronic conditions, the protracted accumulation of CO_2 causes a continued increase in the generation of HCO_3^- as well as augmented renal excretion of H^+. A compensatory decrease in Cl^- concentration may result from the climbing levels of bicarbonate and serum Na^+ and K^+ levels may be mildly elevated (Sacher and McPherson, 1991).

Respiratory Alkalosis

Respiratory alkalosis results from hyperventilation (overbreathing), which produces excessive CO_2 excretion.

Compensation in acute cases, as with acute respiratory acidosis, begins with protein buffers followed by the HCO_3^- buffer system. If hyperventilation continues to the point of loss of consciousness, it is reversed by slowed respiration (from CNS depression) that allows accumulation of CO_2. Hyperventilation as a result of excessive mechanical ventilation is more dangerous (Sacher and McPherson, 1991) because the respiratory rate cannot automatically correct itself.

A summary of the physiologic changes seen in compensation for "simple" acid-base disturbances is provided in Table 11–4.

TABLE 11–4. Compensatory Physiologic Changes in Simple Acid-Base Disorders

Imbalance	Physiologic Changes
Metabolic acidosis	HCO_3^- is consumed to buffer organic acids pCO_2 drops as respiration increases
Metabolic alkalosis	Excess HCO_3^- is generated pCO_2 rises as respiration is suppressed (limited mechanism)
Respiratory acidosis	CO_2 is retained in response to impaired ventilation HCO_3^- rises; acute changes are buffered by hemoglobin and other proteins; bicarbonate buffer system produces changes after several minutes; later kidney excretes H^+ and retains Na^+ and HCO_3^-
Respiratory alkalosis	Too much CO_2 is blown off during hyperventilation HCO_3^- falls initially as intracellular buffers remove HCO_3^- later sustained fall occurs with renal H^+ retention and HCO_3^- excretion

Adapted from Sacher RA, McPherson RA. *Widmann's Clinical Interpretation of Laboratory Tests,* 10th ed. Philadelphia, FA Davis, 1991

BLOOD GAS ABNORMALITIES IN SPECIFIC DISEASES

General patterns of abnormalities in ABGs may be noted in a variety of diseases. As with all laboratory data, interpretation and evaluation should be made in conjunction with all other available information.

Chronic Obstructive Pulmonary Disease

Because COPD is a group of diseases, a variety of patterns may be seen in this category. In type A (emphysematous, or "pink puffer"), the most common pattern is a normal pCO_2 and a normal or slightly decreased pO_2. The pO_2 may fall further during exercise. In type B (bronchitic or "blue bloater"), more severe hypoxemia is seen along with hypercapnia as a general rule. In both groups, ventilation/perfusion inequalities are the primary cause of hypoxemia.

Bronchial Asthma

Normal patterns are seen in symptom free periods. The usual pattern in a moderately severe attack is hypoxemia with a normal or low pCO_2. Hypercapnia may be present during a severe attack and is indicative of a rapidly deteriorating condition that may require intubation and assisted ventilation.

Pulmonary Edema

Usually moderate to severe hypoxemia with a normal or low pCO_2. A combination of respiratory and metabolic acidosis may also be seen.

Pulmonary Embolism

Hypoxemia is the rule, with pO_2 values above 80 mm Hg seen occasionally. The usual acid-base imbalance seen is respiratory alkalosis.

Myocardial Infarction

Mild hypoxemia may be seen in patients without complications. If other conditions exist, such as pulmonary edema, shock, or pulmonary embolism, that condition will dominate the blood gas picture.

Adult Respiratory Distress Syndrome

In the early stages, blood gases show mild hypoxemia, hypocapnia, and a mixed respiratory and metabolic alkalosis. In later stages, more severe hypoxemia occurs as a result of shunting and an extreme reduction in diffusing capacity. In terminal stages, metabolic and respiratory acidosis are seen.

Aspirin Intoxication

Respiratory alkalosis is seen within the first few hours in response to a direct effect on the CNS. Metabolic acidosis follows (especially in infants and young children) as a result of a defect in intermediary metabolism. A low pCO_2 with a normal pH on a young child may indicate the possibility of aspirin intoxication.

EXERCISE AND BLOOD GASES

The impact of exercise on the results of ABG studies is dependent upon the subject's health status and any existing disease conditions. In normal and cardiac patients, the pO_2 is generally normal even at the "breaking point" of exercise and is higher than the resting level. Patients with type A emphysema (pink puffers) have a decrease in pO_2 with severe exercise, whereas type B patients (blue bloaters) usually show a slight rise, probably the result of more uniform blood flow and ventilation during exercise (Phipps et al, 1983).

Normal individuals at the breaking point of severe exercise almost always exhibit a metabolic acidosis, often uncompensated. Respiratory alkalosis seen at the breaking point of exercise usually indicates a hyperventilation syndrome.

SAMPLES FOR ANALYSIS

The sample most commonly used for blood gas analysis is arterial, but venous and capillary specimens may also be utilized. Reference ranges vary according to the source. Whole blood is analyzed and the proper amount of heparin must be used to prevent clotting. After collecting a syringe sample, any air bubbles must be removed immediately. Blood gases and pH values will change because of metabolism of the red cells if the sample remains at room temperature for more than 5 to 10 minutes, so samples should be placed on ice upon collection. Changes may also occur, although less rapidly, at reduced temperatures. For this reason, it is generally recommended that analysis be completed within 30 minutes of collection to ensure more accurate results.

 TIME FOR REVIEW. After studying the preceding sections, you should be able to respond correctly to the following:

■ Oxygen deficit can be caused by conditions interfering with

   _____ .

■ The best clinical guide to the effectiveness of ventilation and the functional integrity of the ventilatory system is _____ .

■ The respiratory system assists in the elimination of acids by excreting

   _____ .

■ Acidemia results from _____ .

■ Alkalemia results from _____ .

■ Type 1 renal tubular acidosis results from _____ .

■ In evaluating ABG results, a decreased pH and an increased pCO_2 is indicative of _____ .

■ Why is complete respiratory compensation rarely possible in metabolic alkalosis?

■ The compensatory mechanism in metabolic acidosis is _____ .

■ List three general causes of metabolic acidosis.

■ List the typical blood gas pattern for

    COPD type A:

    COPD type B:

    Bronchial asthma:

    Pulmonary edema:

Pulmonary embolism:

Adult respiratory distress syndrome:

■ Review the tables presented in this chapter.

Check your responses by reviewing the preceding sections.

11. SELF TEST

Choose the best response by circling the appropriate letter. The answer key may be found in the appendices.

1. **The primary unit of gas exchange in the respiratory system is the:**
   A. trachea
   B. right main bronchus
   C. alveoli
   D. pleura

2. **Oxygen and carbon dioxide are reported on a blood gas analysis in terms of:**
   A. excreted quantities
   B. partial pressure
   C. mg/dL
   D. measured mass

3. **The quantity of oxygen carried by hemoglobin is referred to as:**
   A. oxygen saturation
   B. base excess
   C. pO_2
   D. bicarbonate

4. **At which pO_2 level will the oxygen saturation drop most rapidly?**
   A. 85 mm Hg
   B. 75 mm Hg
   C. 65 mm Hg
   D. 55 mm Hg

5. **What impact would the following results have on the hemoglobin's affinity for oxygen? Temperature: 102° F; pCO_2: 60 mm Hg; pH: 7.30**
   A. no impact
   B. decreased affinity
   C. increased affinity

6. **The measure of the difference from normal buffer base is the:**
    A. oxygen saturation
    B. base excess
    C. pO_2
    D. bicarbonate

7. **The best clinical guide to the effectiveness of ventilation and the functional integrity of the ventilatory system is:**
    A. oxygen saturation
    B. base excess
    C. pCO_2
    D. bicarbonate

8. **Acidemia results from**
    A. deficient levels of CO_2 or fixed acids
    B. accumulation of CO_2 or fixed acids
    C. elevated pH levels
    D. increase in bicarbonate

9. **The blood gas results most typical of a patient with a moderately severe bronchial asthma attack are:**
    A. pO_2: 55 mm Hg; pCO_2: 33 mm Hg
    B. pO_2: 85 mm Hg; pCO_2: 33 mm Hg
    C. pO_2: 95 mm Hg; pCO_2: 40 mm Hg
    D. pO_2: 100 mm Hg; pCO_2: 30 mm Hg

10. **The blood gas results most typical of a patient in the early stages of adult respiratory distress syndrome are:**
    A. pO_2: 90 mm Hg; pCO_2: 39 mm Hg
    B. pO_2: 85 mm Hg; pCO_2: 33 mm Hg
    C. pO_2: 60 mm Hg; pCO_2: 42 mm Hg
    D. pO_2: 63 mm Hg; pCO_2: 30 mm Hg

11. **Pulmonary edema may result in:**
    A. normal oxygen levels with hypocapnia and acidosis
    B. hypoxemia with low/normal carbon dioxide and low pH
    C. hypoxemia with hypercapnia and alkalosis
    D. normal oxygen level with hypocapnia and elevated pH

12. **Type 1 renal tubular acidosis results from:**
   A. inborn metabolism disorders
   B. accelerated absorption of hydrogen ions due to damaged glomerular membrane
   C. impaired excretion of hydrogen ions due to a distal tube defect
   D. increased reabsorption of bicarbonate

13. **Assuming the results are produced by a single uncompensated disorder, an increased pH and a decreased pCO_2 is indicative of:**
   A. metabolic alkalosis
   B. metabolic acidosis
   C. respiratory alkalosis
   D. respiratory acidosis

14. **Assuming the results are produced by a single uncompensated disorder, a decreased pH and a decreased pCO_2 is indicative of:**
   A. metabolic alkalosis
   B. metabolic acidosis
   C. respiratory alkalosis
   D. respiratory acidosis

15. **A very anxious patient who is hyperventilating would be expected to have ABG results consistent with:**
   A. metabolic alkalosis
   B. metabolic acidosis
   C. respiratory alkalosis
   D. respiratory acidosis

16. **Metabolic acidosis with an elevated anion gap may be the result of:**
   A. renal failure
   B. prolonged severe vomiting
   C. respiratory depression from anesthesia
   D. infusion of sodium bicarbonate

17. **Complete compensation by respiratory mechanisms (depression of ventilation) is not possible in this disorder because of the need for ventilatory maintenance of adequate pO_2.**
   A. metabolic alkalosis
   B. metabolic acidosis
   C. respiratory alkalosis
   D. respiratory acidosis

12. LABORATORY CONFIRMATION OF ACUTE MYOCARDIAL INFARCTION

Laboratory testing is only one of a variety of factors that play a role in the diagnosis of acute myocardial infarction (MI). The importance of clinical signs and symptoms in the initial suspicion of MI, as well as in the diagnostic process, is considerable. Particularly noteworthy is the type and duration of pain, its location and distribution, and the response to nitroglycerin (Stein, 1993; Ravel, 1995). In many cases patients may present with quite characteristic severe, prolonged chest pain that is unresponsive to nitroglycerin. It may be difficult to distinguish acute MI pain from that of angina in other cases and in 25 % (Stein, 1993) or more acute MI episodes patients may report no chest pain at all (this is particularly true of diabetics). The electrocardiogram (ECG) is a simple, effective, and direct assessment that often shows unequivocal changes (50 % of acute MI's on first ECG [Ravel, 1995]). The ECG may also show abnormalities or irregularities that are not considered diagnostic or, in about 20 % of cases (Ravel, 1995), may show no significant abnormality.

Early recognition of MI is essential because approximately one third (Stein, 1993) of acute MI patients die within the first few hours following the onset of pain. Further, earlier institution of newer therapies to remove coronary obstruction improves the outcome for those surviving the infarct. Because patients may not seek medical attention immediately with the onset of pain, the time factor becomes even more critical. Therefore, when diagnosis is virtually certain based on the clinical picture, laboratory studies play a confirmatory role. Newer laboratory test techniques provide the clinician with data more rapidly and thus earlier confirmation of the acute MI. In patients presenting with more anomalous symptoms, particularly when the ECG pattern is also not diagnostic for acute MI, the value of confirmatory—perhaps diagnostic—laboratory data becomes even more important. Subsequent laboratory monitoring is useful to assess the effectiveness of therapy, particularly the success of coronary artery reperfusion. The information presented in this chapter is limited to a discussion of laboratory analyses that are of benefit in the diagnosis, confirmation, or monitoring of acute MI and should not be construed to represent a diagnostic or treatment approach for myocardial infarction.

A variety of substances, including creatine kinase, lactic dehydrogenase, aspartate transaminase, myoglobin, and troponin, are released when myocardial injury occurs. Laboratorians are able to detect acute MI by testing the blood for the presence and quantity of these substances released from the damaged heart muscle. By the same token, serial measurements of some substances can be beneficial in assessing the effectiveness of therapy and the success of reperfusion. A number of factors must be considered in the evaluation of laboratory measurements of these substances, particularly:

- **Time of release:** substances with smaller molecular size are released sooner than larger ones and thus can be detected earlier following the onset of pain.
- **Time to peak:** substances reach their highest concentration at varying times
- **Time to clear:** some substances remain detectable in the blood for a longer period; others are more rapidly cleared.
- **Specificity to myocardium:** certain substances are released from other tissues in addition to myocardium, so elevations are not specific for damaged heart muscle. In some cases, the substances can be separated into component fractions that have more specific sites of origin.

CARDIAC ENZYMES

Enzymes, a special type of protein, serve as *catalysts* for specific chemical reactions. (A catalyst is a substance that speeds up a chemical reaction. The catalyst is not altered or used up in the reaction.) Enzymes are important in nearly every cellular function and are generally found within the cell. Injury to the cell causes the enzyme to be released into the circulation where detection of elevated amounts indicates damage to the tissue(s) for which the enzyme has specificity. The enzyme is subsequently cleared from the blood by normal body processes, because it has no function to fulfill in the circulation.

Enzymes are often divided into component parts or fractions called isoenzymes. **Isoenzymes** are the different forms of the enzyme in various tissues. All of the isoenzymes together constitute measurement of the enzyme's total activity and behave similarly in terms of their catalytic functions. Each fraction, however, possesses certain distinguishing characteristics that allow it to be separated from the other isoenzymes. Examples of identifying characteristics include:

- how the particular fraction behaves when migrating in an electrical field in electrophoresis studies (ie, fractions may travel at differing speeds, appear at different locations, produce different patterns, etc)
- how the fractions respond to temperature changes (ie, some fractions may be destroyed by heat while others remain stable)

The three enzymes are released from myocardium as a result of tissue necrosis:

1. Aspartate aminotransferase (AST), formerly called *serum oxaloacetic transaminase* and abbreviated SGOT: elevated at some point in 90 % to 95 % (Ravel, 1995) of acute MI patients
2. Creatine kinase (CK); also referred to as *creatine phosphokinase* and abbreviated CPK: elevated at some point in 90 % to 93 % (Ravel, 1995) of acute MI patients
3. Lactic dehydrogenase (LD or LDH): elevated at some point in 92 % to 95 % (Ravel, 1995) of acute MI patients

Figure 12–1 illustrates the typical time for rise and fall and the amount of elevation of each of these cardiac enzymes.

■ CREATINE KINASE

Creatine kinase (CK) is an enzyme that catalyzes a reversible chemical reaction in which a phosphate group is transferred between creatine phosphate and adenosine diphosphate (ADP). The reaction results in the products creatine (reused by cell) and adenosine triphosphate (ATP): used in energy requiring cellular functions. CK is found not only in **heart muscle**, but also in **skeletal muscle** and in the **brain**. Elevations of serum CK may be found in virtually any muscle injury, in inflammation, or with significant muscle exertion. Importantly, CK levels are *not increased as a result of liver damage* (both LD and AST may be elevated in cer-

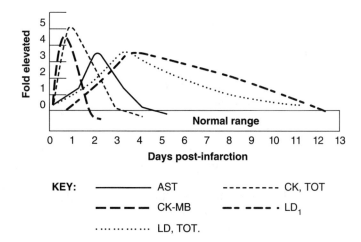

FIGURE 12–1. Rise and fall of cardiac enzymes. (Figure compiled based on data from Henry, 1996; Ravel, 1995; and Sacher & McPherson, 1991.)

tain hepatic conditions). Because the CK enzyme can be broken down into three major components (isoenzymes or fractions), elevated total CK levels alone do not pinpoint the area of tissue injury. An elevation in total CK may result from the elevation of one or more of its component fractions. Total CK elevations may be seen in response to a myriad of conditions besides MI:

- muscular dystrophy
- surgery
- childbirth
- muscle trauma from various causes, such as auto accidents
- intramuscular injections
- myositis
- moderate/severe exercise (especially long distance running)
- delirium tremens
- convulsions
- hypothyroidism
- severe hypokalemia (due to changes caused to skeletal muscle)
- after heavy drinking episode (alcohol effect on skeletal muscle)
- agitated psychoses (especially schizophrenia)
- electrocution
- brain surgery/trauma
- bacterial meningitis[1]
- encephalitis[1]
- cerebrovascular accident[1]

Despite the number of conditions in which total CK levels may be elevated, the *primary clinical use of CK is the detection of acute myocardial injury.* The various other conditions become important principally in terms of ensuring that such conditions are not responsible for CK elevations detected in the investigation of a possible acute MI. (Isoenzyme measurement is useful in determining the source of elevation as will be detailed in a subsequent section of this chapter.)

Total CK in Acute Myocardial Infarction

Of the three cardiac enzymes (CK, LD, AST), CK is the first to rise in acute MI and the first to return to normal range following acute MI (see Figure 12–1). Serum levels begin to rise within 4 to 6 hours after infarction and reach high peak levels at about 24 hours (level may peak as early as 12 hours [Ravel, 1995; Stein,1993] or as late as 36 hours [Ravel, 1995]). Values will generally return to normal within 2 to 4 days (ranges from 1.5 to 10 days reported [Ravel, 1995]). Because an individual's baseline CK may be unknown, it is possible for a total CK to be within the established reference range with acute MI, particularly prior to

---

[1] Presence and degree of elevation in conditions affecting the brain are quite variable because of poor perfusion of swollen brain tissue (Ravel, 1995; Sacher & McPherson, 1991).

reaching peak and in individuals with a very low baseline total. However, measurement of CK-MB (see section on CK isoenzymes) would reveal an elevation of this fraction. Normal CK values may also be detected in acute MI when testing is performed very early after the infarction and before values begin to rise. Measurement of CK and CK-MB on samples collected every 6 to 8 hours (Stein, 1993; some sources suggest 12-hour intervals) after the onset of chest pain for a total of three samples should detect an increase if acute MI is present. After an initial elevation is detected, clinicians often request collection of samples at 12-hour intervals for a total of three samples with additional samples requested in some cases. Serial sampling, depending on when the patient first seeks medical attention, often allows detection of the initial rise in serum levels as well as the peak level and declining levels that return to baseline. Measurement of total CK alone can not establish or confirm the presence of acute MI. Total CK measurements are more likely to be misleading in the elderly or in others with small muscle mass. *Measurement of isoenzymes is necessary to demonstrate the origin of CK.* Isoenzyme measurement is generally performed as a matter of routine when total CK is significantly elevated. However, measurement of the CK-MB fraction may be indicated whether or not total CK values show an abnormality, particularly in the presence of clinical findings suggestive of myocardial infarction.

METHODS OF TOTAL CK MEASUREMENT. The laboratory determination of total CK activity is based on the principle of "coupled reactions" and the chemical reaction catalyzed by CK in the body, as shown in the equations below. The NADPH is measured photometrically for calculation of CK activity. Note that the activity of the CK enzyme was determined by measuring an end product of a chemical reaction in which CK participates. Higher levels of CK in the sample produce greater concentrations of end products.

$$\text{Creatine phosphate} + \text{ADP} \underset{\rightleftarrows}{\text{CK}} \text{Creatine} + \text{ATP}$$

$$\text{ATP} + \text{Glucose} \underset{\rightleftarrows}{\text{HK}} \text{G-6-P} + \text{ADP}$$

$$\text{G-6-P} + \text{NAD} \underset{\rightleftarrows}{\text{GP6A}} \text{NADH}$$

REFERENCE RANGE. Although reference ranges may vary among laboratories, most will have a relatively low upper limit (usually no more than 22 U/L) in order to avoid missing a mild, acute elevation. Because most CK is found in skeletal muscle, CK levels in healthy adults are highly dependent on muscle mass and baseline levels vary significantly among individuals. Very thin, inactive individuals may have CK levels significantly lower than muscular, athletic individuals. By the same token, men generally have higher CK levels than women. Muscular persons exercising a great deal may have "normal" CK levels ranging from 500 to 1000 U/L and marathon runners generally have levels above 1000 U/L (Sacher & McPherson, 1991). Ranges are provided from the work of Henry (1996) for testing at 37°C.

Male: 55 to 170 U/L
Female: 30 to 135 U/L

CK Isoenzymes

Creatine kinase is a dimer with two monomeric chains, M and B. There are three possible combinations of the M (originally labeled "M" for muscle) and B (originally called "B" for brain) chains: MM; BB; and MB. Thus total CK can be divided into three major fractions that have distinctive characteristics allowing them to be identified. (Although subtypes of these major fractions have been identified, methods for detecting and quantifying them are not routinely available.) CK isoenzymes are **BB**, **MB**, **and MM** (also referred to as **CK1**, **CK2**, and **CK3**, respectively) (Table 12–1). Isoenzyme analysis provides a means of determining the contribution of myocardial damage to elevated CK levels with minimal "interference" from skeletal muscle CK.

BB (CK$_1$) is found primarily in the brain and in the lung. Elevations may be seen after head injuries, brain surgery or trauma, and crushing chest injuries (Henry, 1996; Sacher & McPherson, 1991). The BB fraction has also been detected in individuals with certain carcinomas, particularly of the lung and prostate, and has been reported in carcinoma of the colon, intestines, bladder and esophagus (Henry, 1996; Sacher & McPherson, 1991). Levels seen with such tumors are fairly constant as opposed to the rapid rise and subsequent return to normal seen in acute injuries. *The MM fraction (CK$_3$) comprises nearly 99% of the total CK in skeletal muscle and about 20% of the CK in the myocardium.* Because there is so much more skeletal muscle in the body than heart muscle, most elevations of the MM fraction result from some sort of skeletal muscle injury. Many of the conditions listed previously as causing an elevated total CK result from predominantly MM elevations. Elevations of this fraction are seen in various traumas, including surgery, with moderate to severe exercise, and with intramuscular injections, muscle hypoxia, convulsions, muscular dystrophy, and a variety of other conditions.

CK$_2$, the MB fraction, is of primary interest in the detection of acute MI. Most of the CK-MB in the body is found in the myocardium. MB is found in trace amounts in skeletal muscle, but comprises 20% of the total CK in the heart muscle. CK-MB levels begin to rise as early as 2 hours after an infarction, peak at about 18 hours, and return to normal in approximately 2 days (but can persist as long as 72 hours [Henry, 1996]). Because myocardium also contains significant quantities of MM, this fraction will also be increased. In fact most of the total CK increase in MI will

TABLE 12–1. Tissue Distribution of CK Isoenzymes

CK Fraction	Predominant Tissue of Origin
BB (CK$_1$)	Brain and lung
MB (CK$_2$)	Myocardium
MM (CK$_3$)	Skeletal muscle and myocardium

be from the MM fraction, but the source of origin (skeletal vs myocardial) for MM cannot be differentiated. Although elevated MB is indicative of myocardial damage, the elevation never exceeds 40 % of the total CK (Henry, 1996) with the remaining 60 % attributable to the MM fraction. Elevations of the MM fraction persist longer (4-5 days after onset of pain) than elevations of MB, isoenzyme studies performed more than 4 days post-infarct will not reveal MB elevations, even with an elevated total CK (Henry, 1996). The fraction detected at this point will be MM, the origin of which cannot be ascertained. Although the MB fraction can also be increased above normal in skeletal muscle injury (overall, skeletal muscle contains only very small amounts of MB, but particular skeletal muscles may contain as much as 5 %), the MM fraction would generally be increased as well, and to a much greater degree (Ravel, 1995). In such cases, using a *relative index* method of reporting CK-MB is of benefit. The relative index depicts the MB fraction as a percentage relative to the total CK value. Instances in which concurrent skeletal muscle injury and acute MI exist (eg, MI in an auto accident victim) can present difficulties in interpretation even with the relative index method of reporting. It is important that each laboratory determine their own MB relative index because total CK and CK-MB methodologies vary considerably.

METHODS OF MEASUREMENT FOR CK ISOENZYMES. The three major CK fractions may be separated and quantitated by *electrophoresis*. CK_1 (BB fraction) migrates most anodally (to the negative pole) and CK_3 (MM fraction) migrates the most cathodally (toward the positive pole). CK_2 (MB fraction) migrates between the two. The quantity of each fraction is generally reported as an absolute value (actual amount present) and as a percentage (relative to the total CK value). Quantities reported relative to the total CK are more meaningful than are absolute values. Other techniques have been developed for the direct measurement of the MB fraction. An *immunoassay method* using a monoclonal antibody specific for CK-MB allows rapid direct measurement of this fraction, making it a much more useful analysis than the lengthy time consuming process of electrophoresis. Results from either method should be reported as a percentage of the total CK or as a relative index in order to provide meaningful data.

Some patients have a variant isoenzyme called *macro-CK* that may erroneously be included with the MB isoenzyme in some situations. This aberrant isoenzyme is actually a variant of the BB isoenzyme that is complexed to gamma globulin. On electrophoresis, it migrates between the MM and MB isoenzymes rather than in the usual BB location. Careful visual inspection of the electrophoretic pattern by a knowledgeable technologist prior to quantitation is necessary to avoid reporting falsely elevated MB fractions in these situations. When fractions are quantitated by automated analysis, macro-CK may be included in the MB fraction. However, visual careful inspection of the electrophoretic pattern on patients with abnormal MB fractions may alert the technologist to the presence of macro-CK and the need for manual quantitation.

REFERENCE RANGES. It is important that each laboratory establish a reference range for CK-MB based upon the methodologies employed for total CK measurement and CK-MB measurement. In terms of CK-MB, instead of an actual range within which "normal" results should fall, laboratories provide a cut-off value above which the MB fraction is considered significant. As previously noted, the reported MB value (and, of course, the cut-off value) should be provided in relative terms as compared to the total CK activity. The following example illustrates the importance of reporting in relative or percentage terms. If significant skeletal muscle injury results in a total CK of 10,000 U/L and MB accounts for 1% of the CK in skeletal muscle, the absolute CK-MB value would be significantly elevated at 100 U/L. However, as a percentage of the total CK, the MB fraction is not significant at 1%. Although **cut-off values** for CK-MB vary among laboratories, most **fall between 3% and 5%**.

LACTIC DEHYDROGENASE

Lactic dehydrogenase (LD or LDH) is an enzyme that catalyzes the oxidation reaction in which lactate is converted to pyruvate with oxidation of NADH to NAD. LD is distributed widely throughout body tissues, including heart, liver, skeletal muscle, red blood cells, lungs, kidneys, and lymphocytes, and is present in neoplasia. With such extensive distribution, virtually any condition resulting in cellular damage can be expected to produce an elevation in total serum LD values. The enzyme is particularly abundant in heart muscle, liver, kidney, and skeletal muscle. Its primary diagnostic use is the diagnosis and monitoring of hepatic dysfunction and the diagnosis of myocardial infarction. Table 12–2 lists a variety of conditions in which elevations of total LD may be present classified by approximate degree of elevation.

TABLE 12–2. Degrees of Total LD Elevations in Various Conditions

Degree of Elevation	Conditions
Up to 3 times normal	Various liver diseases Nephrotic syndrome Hypothyroidism Cholangitis
3 to 5 times normal	Myocardial infarction Pulmonary infarction Hemolytic disorders Leukemias Infectious mononucleosis Delirium tremens Muscular dystrophy
≥ 5 times normal	Megaloblastic anemia Widespread carcinomatosis (esp. Hepatic metastases) Systemic shock and hypoxia Hepatitis Renal infarction

Adapted from Sacher RA, McPherson RA. *Widmann's Clinical Interpretation of Laboratory Tests,* 10th ed. Philadelphia, FA Davis, 1991.

Methods of Total LD Measurement

The chemical reaction employed to determine total LD activity is a reversible one (depicted below), depending on test conditions, so that methods may be based upon either the appearance or the disappearance of NADH. In either case, the rate of change in the concentration of NADH is determined by spectrophotometric means. Colorimetric and fluorometric methods (Henry, 1996) are also available for determination of total LD.

Pyruvate + NADH → lactate + NAD   (disappearance of NADH measured)
Lactate + NAD → pyruvate + NADH   (appearance of NADH measured)

LD Isoenzymes

As is the case with CK, the LD enzyme can be separated into different components. In the case of LD, a tetrameric molecule, four subunits of two forms (H and M) result in **five isoenzymes** that can be measured by electrophoresis. These tissue specific isoenzymes are designated **LD_1, LD_2, LD_3, LD_4,** and **LD_5** based on their electrophoretic mobility (1 is the most anodic and 5 is the least anodic). Measurement of isoenzymes is useful in determining the origin of the enzyme. Table 12–3 depicts the tissue source and relative content of the LD isoenzymes. Note that *LD_1 and LD_2 are the isoenzymes present in the greatest concentration in the myocardium.*

An elevation in total serum LD without benefit of isoenzyme measurement and/or other diagnostic assays does not provide specific evidence of organ source. It is, however, a rather sensitive indication of the presence of a pathologic process, the nature of which can be ascertained more reliably with additional testing. Isoenzyme measurement may also be indicated in some situations even though the total LD activity does not show significant abnormality. Because of the relatively wide reference range for total serum LD activity, it is possible for an abnormal elevation of one of the LD isoenzymes to occur in the absence of an elevated total activity (Ravel, 1995).

TABLE 12–3. Tissue Source and Relative Content of LD Isoenzymes

Isoenzyme Fraction	Monomer Composition	Relative Isoenzyme Content					
		Myocardium	Liver	Skeletal Muscle	Brain	Kidney	RBCs
LD_1	HHHH	++++	±	±	++	+	+++
LD_2	HHHM	+++	±	±	++	+	+++
LD_3	HHMM	+	+	+	++	++	+
LD_4	HMMM	±	++	++	++	++	±
LD_5	MMMM	±	++++	++++	±	++	±

Adapted from Henry JB. *Clinical Diagnosis and Management by Laboratory Methods,* 19th ed. Philadelphia, Saunders, 1996.

Total LD and LD Isoenzymes in Myocardial Infarction

Elevations in total serum LD are seen in most patients 24 to 48 hours after MI. As depicted in Figure 12–1, total LD begins to rise later than does CK and remains elevated after the CK has returned to normal. This characteristic can be particularly useful in aiding the confirmation of MI when CK has returned to normal or yield equivocal results.

Measurement of LD isoenzymes, most commonly by electrophoresis, is necessary to determine the source of elevation. The five isoenzymes produce characteristic electrophoretic patterns that are generally representative of the source or etiology of the enzyme elevation. The characteristic pattern associated with MI derives from the relationship between the LD_1 and LD_2 isoenzymes. Although the myocardium is rich in both LD_1 and LD_2, LD_1 is present in higher concentration. As a result, *damage to the myocardium leads to an inverted LD_1:LD_2 ratio frequently referred to as a "flip."* This LD_1:LD_2 flip remains detectable for several days. It is *critical to avoid testing hemolyzed samples* (any degree of hemolysis) for determination of total LD and for measurement of isoenzymes. Red cells contain significant quantities of LD and have a LD_1:LD_2 ratio similar to that of myocardium. Thus, *testing on a hemolyzed sample could produce results suggestive of myocardial damage* when no such damage has occurred. Conditions that lead to *in vivo* hemolysis (eg, hemolytic anemias) also produce elevations, making diagnosis more difficult. Multi-organ disease can produce electrophoretic LD isoenzyme patterns that are quite troublesome to interpret. Table 12–4 describes some characteristic LD isoenzyme abnormalities and the condition(s) with which the pattern is typically associated. These patterns are representative only.

Newer methods allow *measurement of LD_1 alone using an immunoassay method* similar to that used for measurement of CK-MB. Some evidence indicates that immunoassay methods for the detection of LD_1 are more sensitive than the traditional LD_1:LD_2 flip, however, this increase in sensitivity should be weighed against the possible loss of specificity seen with this method.

REFERENCE RANGES. Reference ranges may vary significantly based on methodology (Henry, 1996). The isoenzyme percentages below indicate percentage of total LD.

Total LD:	90 to 190 U/L	LD_3:	18% to 25%
LD_1:	17% to 27%	LD_4:	3% to 8%
LD_2:	27% to 37%	LD_5:	0% to 5%

TABLE 12–4. Representative LD Isoenzyme Abnormalities and Associated Conditions

LD Isoenzyme Electrophoretic Abnormality					
LD_1	LD_2	LD_3	LD_4	LD_5	**Associated Conditions**
↑ and > LD_2	May be ↑, but < LD_1				Acute MI Artifactual hemolysis Renal cortex infarct
↑ may be > LD_2	↑ may be < LD_1				Hemolytic anemia Megaloblastic anemia Artifactual hemolysis
↑	↑		↓	↓	Muscular dystrophy (increase in 1 and 2 is relative only due to depression of 4 and 5)
			May be ↑ in acute hepatitis	↑	Acute hepatitis (and other conditions producing acute hepatocellular injury) Acute skeletal muscle damage
	↑	↑			Conditions producing pulmonary hypoxia Pulmonary congestion Granulocytic leukemia Extensive carcinomatosis Pancreatitis
			↑	↑	Viral and toxic hepatitis Cirrhosis Congestive heart failure Pulmonary infarction (LD_3 may also be elevated)
	↑	↑	↑	↑	Both lung and liver abnormality
↑	↑	↑	↑	↑	Multi-organ hypoxia (with or without MI) Malignancy

(All fractions elevated, but with normal relative relationships—see Figure 12–2; LD_5 may be disproportionately increased in some cases.) Adapted from Ravel R. *Clinical Laboratory Medicine: Clinical Application of Laboratory Data,* 6th ed. St Louis, Mosby, 1995.

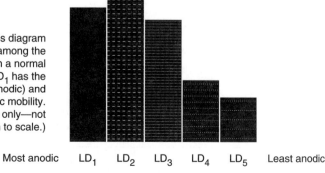

The shaded bars in this diagram represent the relationship among the isoenzyme fractions of LD in a normal electrophoretic pattern. LD_1 has the greatest mobility (most anodic) and LD_5 has the least anodic mobility. (Representative only—not drawn to scale.)

Most anodic LD_1 LD_2 LD_3 LD_4 LD_5 Least anodic

FIGURE 12–2. Isoenzyme relationships in normal pattern.

TIME FOR REVIEW. After studying the preceding sections, you should be able to respond correctly to the following:

■ List and briefly describe four factors that must be considered in the evaluation of laboratory measurements of substances that are released in myocardial injury.

■ The first cardiac enzyme to rise following MI is _____.

■ The cardiac enzyme that remains elevated for the longest period following MI is _____.

■ CK is found in _____ muscle, in _____ muscle, and in the _____.

■ List five conditions, excluding MI, in which total CK may be increased.

■ List and briefly describe the three components of CK.

■ Explain the importance of reporting CK-MB in relative terms.

■ LD is widely distributed throughout the body, but is particularly rich in _____, _____, _____, and _____.

■ List and briefly describe the five LD isoenzymes.

■ Describe the LD isoenzyme pattern most consistent with MI.

■ Describe the effect that hemolyzed specimens may have on total LD and LD isoenzyme analysis.

■ The CK isoenzyme most indicative of myocardial damage is

_____.

■ The variant CK that may be erroneously included in CK-MB by electrophoresis is _____.

Check your responses by reviewing the preceding sections.

■ ASPARTATE AMINOTRANSFERASE

Aspartate aminotransferase (AST, formerly called SGOT) is an aminotransferase (or transaminase; see Chapter 4) that catalyzes the transfer of an amino group between an amino acid and an alpha-keto acid. Although the transaminases are found in a number of areas of the body, they are most predominant in the liver. AST is also found in the myocardium and in skeletal muscle. Serum elevations of AST may be seen as soon as 6 hours after an MI and return to normal in about 3 to 4 days (peak occurs within about 24 to 48 hours). Although this is a simple and readily available test, it is not as helpful to the clinician in confirming acute MI as are the other enzymes (CK and LD). CK levels generally rise sooner and fall more rapidly than do AST levels and thus are more useful early in the diagnostic process. On the other hand, LD is more useful for late diagnosis of acute MI because it stays in the circulation longer. Further, elevations of AST may be seen in a variety of conditions unrelated to acute MI and in some conditions that may be confused with or with acute MI or may be present as a complicating or co-existing condition. Elevated serum AST may originate from a variety of sources, as listed in Table 12–5.

TABLE 12–5. Causes of AST Elevations

Site of Origin	Condition
Liver	Viral infections: hepatitis, CMV; EBV Active cirrhosis Liver hypoxia or congestion Alcohol or drug induced liver dysfunction Early extrahepatic biliary obstruction Tumors
Heart	Acute myocardial infarction Cardiac arrhythmias/ischemia not progressing to infarct (Sacher, 1991) Some cases of pericarditis (Ravel, 1995)
Skeletal muscle	Acute muscle injury Active muscular dystrophy Delerium tremens Surgery
Other	Circulatory collapse (shock) Pulmonary infarction Cerebrovascular accident Acute pancreatitis Intestinal infarction

REFERENCE RANGE. Typical adult reference ranges for AST have a lower limit between 5 and 8 U/L and an upper limit between 35 and 45 U/L. Newborn levels are significantly higher and values in the elderly may be slightly higher.

■ COMBINED ISOENZYME ANALYSIS

Henry (1996) offers the criteria summarized in Table 12–6 for diagnosis of acute MI within the initial 48 hours of onset of suspected ischemic heart disease. If both criteria are met, the diagnosis is validated and repeat determinations are not necessary. CK-MB determinations may be used to estimate the size of the infarct or to detect re-infarction. If criteria are not met in 48 hours, the presumptive diagnosis is not acute MI; however, MI is not ruled out with the same degree of certainty using these criteria after 48 hours.

TABLE 12–6. Combined Isoenzyme Analysis to Rule Out Acute MI (during acute 48-hour period)

CK-MB Absent	CK-MB Present/Usual LD	CK-MB Present/Flipped LD
100% predictive value of no MI	Both MI and non-MI cases	100% predictive value for MI

Adapted from Henry JB. *Clinical Diagnosis and Management by Laboratory Methods,* 19th ed. Philadelphia, Saunders, 1996.

OTHER MEASURES OF CARDIAC DAMAGE

■ MYOGLOBIN

Myoglobin is a protein found in muscle tissues (smooth, cardiac, and skeletal) and serves as an oxygen carrier. Serum concentrations of myoglobin are elevated in conditions that result in the destruction of muscle tissue and begin to rise in about 3 hours (as little as 1.5 hours) following onset of MI. By 4 hours after onset 50% to 60% of MI patients will have an elevated myoglobin level and by 6 hours 85% to 95% will have elevated values.

Although an elevation in serum myoglobin is not specific for acute MI (because it is found in other muscle tissue as well) and despite a significant false positive rate, myoglobin measurement has gained popularity with some clinicians as a useful early screening tool in symptomatic patients. Its primary advantage is that it is elevated in a considerably higher percentage of patients than is the case with CK-MB during the 6 hours following MI onset during which thrombolytic therapy is most effective. The false positive rate in patients who exhibit chest pain, but do not clinically present as strongly suspicious for acute MI, ranges from 0% to 50% (Ravel, 1995) and may reduce the impact of early detection. Further, because myoglobin is excreted by the kidneys, deficient renal function can result in elevated serum levels.

Elevations of myoglobin may be detected in the serum or in urine in a variety of conditions besides damage to cardiac muscle (thus the low degree of specificity), with skeletal muscle damage presenting the most common etiology. Some examples of conditions leading to myoglobinemia and myoglobinuria are listed below.

- Acute MI
- Surgical procedures
- Crushing muscle trauma
- Burns and electrical shock
- Alcoholic myopathy
- Hypothermia
- Convulsions and delirium tremens
- Severe exercise
- Muscular dystrophy
- Myositis
- Tetanus
- Renal failure

REFERENCE RANGE. The reference ranges for myoglobin are given in Table 12–7.

TABLE 12–7. Myoglobin Reference Ranges

Sample Type	Range
Serum	< 90 µg/L
Urine, random sample	Negative
Urine, 24-hour sample	< 4 mg/L

■ TROPONIN

Troponin is a regulatory protein made up of three components that regulate the interaction of the contractile proteins (myosin and actin) in muscle tissue:

- Troponin T: binds the myosin/actin complex
- Troponin C: binds calcium to initiate muscle contraction
- Troponin I: blocks muscle contraction in absence of calcium

Troponin T

Troponin T is found in both skeletal and cardiac muscle and is released when the muscle tissue is damaged. The troponin T found in each type of muscle tissue is immunochemically distinct; thus, cardiac troponin T can be detected by using an antibody specific for the form released in myocardial muscle injury. As a result, the specificity of cardiac troponin T is nearly 100%. In terms of time to release and time to peak following the onset of MI, cardiac troponin T responds much like CK-MB with increases seen in 4 to 6 hours and a peak at about 11 hours. The level of increase in troponin T levels is much greater (up to 80 times the upper normal limit [Henry, 1996]) than that seen with CK-MB. Cardiac troponin T remains elevated longer than CK-MB, requiring 10 days or more to return to normal levels. Elevations of cardiac troponin T levels can therefore be detected for several days after CK-MB levels have returned to normal. Sensitivity levels for troponin T and CK-MB are initially similar, but 96 hours after onset cardiac troponin T is significantly more sensitive (93% vs about 10% for CK-MB [Henry, 1996]). Following the initial rapid rise, troponin T begins to decline and then increases again as bound troponin is released from necrotic myocardial cells about 4 days later (Henry, 1996).

Reference Range: 0 to 0.1 ng/ml (Henry, 1996)

Troponin I

Troponin I is also specific for myocardial injury and has a response similar to that of troponin T. However, troponin I returns to normal levels sooner. Troponin I is also similar to CK-MB in its response to acute MI.

SUMMARY

The laboratory tests discussed in this chapter are summarized in Table 12–8 in terms of response to acute MI.

TABLE 12–8. Laboratory Tests in Acute MI

Test	Elevation Begins	Peak Reached	Return to Normal
AST	8 hours	24–48 hours	4 days
CK, total	4–6 hours	24 hours	3–4 days
CK-MB (CK_2)	4 hours	18 hours	2 days
LD, total	24 hours	3 days	8–9 days
LD_1	24 hours	3 days	12 days
Myoglobin	3 hours	9 hours	30 hours
Troponin T	4–6 hours	11 hours	$\geq$10 days
Troponin I	4–6 hours	11 hours	4 days

Average response times; literature ranges for response times are significantly broader as typified by total CK: rises 2 to 8 hours, peaks: 12 to 36 hours, returns to normal 1.5 to 10 days.

Data from Ravel R. *Clinical Laboratory Medicine: Clinical Application of Laboratory Data,* 6th ed. St Louis, Mosby, 1995.

12. SELF TEST

Choose the best response by circling the appropriate letter. The answer key may be found in the appendices.

1. **The first cardiac enzyme to become elevated following myocardial infarction is**
   A. AST
   B. LD
   C. CK

2. **The CK isoenzyme most indicative of myocardial damage is**
   A. BB
   B. MB
   C. MM
   D. Macro-CK

3. **CK-MB results are most meaningful when reported as**
   A. a percentage or relative value in terms of total CK
   B. an absolute concentration of MB fraction
   C. relative to the MM fraction

4. **The cardiac enzyme that becomes elevated last in response to myocardial damage and remains elevated for the longest period of time is**
   A. AST
   B. LD
   C. CK

5. **The LD isoenzyme pattern most indicative of acute MI is**
   A. elevation in L_4 and L_5 only
   B. elevation in L_2 with L_2 greater than L_1
   C. elevation in L_2 and L_3 with L_3 greater than L_2
   D. elevation in L_1 with L_1 greater than L_2

6. **During the initial 48 hours following onset of acute MI, the presence of CK-MB and an LD "flip" are**
   A. seen in both MI and non-MI cases
   B. a 100% predictive value for MI
   C. suggestive of MI, but require confirmation by repeat determination after 48 hours

7. The group of test results most likely to be present in a patient 6 hours after onset of MI is
   A. elevated AST, CK, LD, myoglobin, troponin T, CK-MB, and LD flip present
   B. elevated AST, CK, myoglobin, troponin T, CK-MB, and LD flip present
   C. elevated CK, CK-MB, myoglobin, troponin T
   D. elevated CK, LD, troponin T, CK-MB, and LD flip present

8. The group of test results most likely to be present in a patient 36 hours after onset of MI is
   A. elevated AST, CK, LD, myoglobin, troponin T, CK-MB, and LD flip present
   B. elevated AST, CK, LD, troponin T, CK-MB, and LD flip present
   C. elevated CK, CK-MB, myoglobin, troponin T
   D. elevated CK, LD, troponin T, CK-MB, and LD flip present

9. The group of test results most likely to be present in a patient 60 hours after onset of MI is
   A. elevated CK, CK-MB, myoglobin, troponin T
   B. elevated AST, CK, LD, myoglobin, troponin T, CK-MB, and LD flip present
   C. elevated AST, CK, LD, troponin T, and LD flip present
   D. elevated CK, LD, troponin T, CK-MB, and LD flip present

10. Testing for the presence of myocardial damage using a hemolyzed sample may produce
    A. false positive troponin and myoglobin results
    B. significantly decreased total CK and CK-MB values
    C. LD result suggestive of MI
    D. false negative troponin results

11. The cardiac troponin T protein
    A. is less specific for myocardial damage than cardiac enzymes
    B. returns to normal levels before CK-MB
    C. is more sensitive for late detection of MI than CK-MB
    D. all of the above

13. TESTS OF THYROID FUNCTION

The thyroid gland is composed of two oblong lateral lobes connected by an isthmus. It is located in the base of the neck at the lower part of the larynx and lateral to the upper part of the trachea. The two lobes can usually be palpated at the level of the second and third tracheal rings. When any significant enlargement of the gland is present, one or both lobes can generally be seen upon visual examination. Small **parathyroid glands** are found on the back of the thyroid gland and at the lower edge (Figs. 13–1, 13–2).

In a process composed of several steps, the thyroid gland synthesizes hormones from iodine and *tyrosine,* an essential amino acid. Most of the iodine utilized in production of thyroid hormones is obtained from dietary iodide that is extracted from the blood by the thyroid cells and then converted to organic iodine. A single iodine atom joins with tyrosine to form *monoiodotyrosine* and attachment of an additional iodine atom results in the formation of *diiodotyrosine.* When a monoiodotyrosine molecule and a diiodotyrosine molecule combine on the thyroglobulin molecule, *triiodotyrosine*—T_3—is formed. The combination of two diiodotyrosine molecules results in the formation of *tetraiodotyrosine* (thyroxine), or T_4. Within the thyroid follicles, a large number of closed vesicles, is a substance called *colloid.* **Thyroglobulin** is the principal component of colloid and is the storage site for the thyroid hormones, which are reconstituted and released when needed. Although T_3 is more physiologically significant, most of the thyroid hormone released into the circulation under normal circumstances is T_4 with only about 7% (Ravel, 1995) being T_3. Most of the T_3 and T_4 in the circulation are bound to the serum proteins **thyroxine binding globulin** (TBG), **prealbumin**, and **albumin**. The significant majority (> 99%) of both T_3 and T_4 are bound to TBG (80% to 85% of T_4 and 70% of T_3 [Ravel, 1995]). Most of the remaining T_3 is bound to albumin and the remaining T_4 is bound to prealbumin and albumin (10% to 15% and 5%, respectively [Ravel, 1995]). Because protein-bound thyroid hormones are not metabolically active, < 1% of the circulating thyroid hormone (the "free" or unbound portion) is responsible for physiologic hormonal activity. Because it is more tightly bound to TBG, T_4 has a longer circulating half-life (about 1 week [Sacher & McPherson, 1991]) than T_3 (about one day [Sacher & McPherson, 1991]).

Most of the daily production of T_3 results from the deiodination of free T_4 within the hepatocytes, with the kidney also playing an important role in this conversion. In another transformation, some of the T_4 is converted into a biologically inactive compound called *reverse T_3.* In a somewhat intricate stimulation and negative feedback process (depicted in the flow chart in Figure 13–3), the thyroid stimulating hormone (TSH; also called *thyrotropin*) stimulates the synthesis and release of the thyroid hormones from thyroglobulin. Secretion of TSH by the anterior pituitary results from pituitary stimulation by thyrotropin releasing hormone (TRH) from the hypothalamus. The hypothalamic TRH is responsive to the levels of free T_3 and T_4 in the peripheral circulation as blood passes through the hypothalamus. Low levels of circulating free T_3 and T_4 results in TRH stimulating secretion of TSH, whereas high levels directly inhibit pituitary TSH secretion and TRH production by the hypothalamus via a negative feedback mechanism.

The thyroid hormones have important roles in a variety of **physiologic functions**, including the control of oxygen consumption, protein and carbohydrate metabolism, electrolyte mobilization, and the carotene-to-vitamin-A conversion (Sacher, 1991). By mechanisms as yet unknown, the thyroid hormones are also vital to the development of the central nervous system as is evident in the irreversible damage seen in thyroid deficient newborns. On the other hand, the central nervous system (CNS) manifestations of thyroid deficiency in adults are reversible with appropriate hormone replacement therapy.

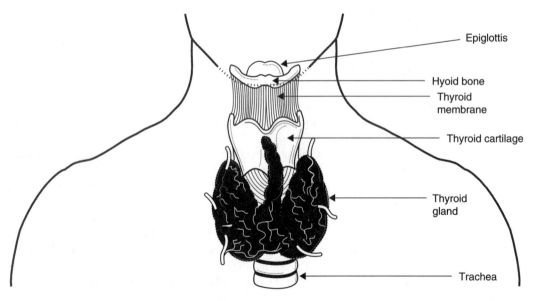

FIGURE 13–1. Anterior view.

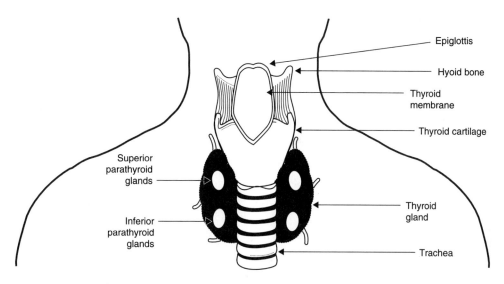

FIGURE 13–2. Posterior view.

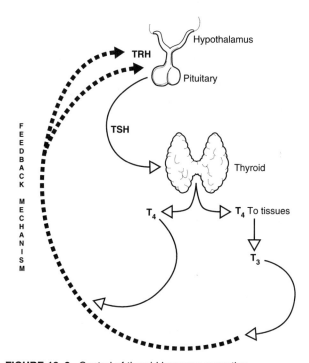

FIGURE 13–3. Control of thyroid hormone secretion.

Although a variety of factors can influence thyroid activity, most irregularities in thyroid function beyond the newborn period are the result of an underlying ailment of the thyroid itself. Autoimmune disorders, such as Graves' disease and Hashimoto's thyroiditis, are the most common causes of abnormal thyroid function and occur much more frequently in patients with a history of other types of autoimmune disorders. Thyroid disorders are also seen more frequently in females than in males. Thyroid dysfunction resulting from a disorder of the thyroid itself in terms of hormone secretion are referred to as **primary disorders**, while dysfunctions related to the secretion of TSH or TRH are considered **secondary disorders**.

Thyroid function may be generally classified as:

- *hyperthyroid:* hyperactivity of the thyroid; excessive thyroid hormone secretion
- *hypothyroid:* hypoactivity of the thyroid; deficient thyroid hormone secretion
- *euthyroid:* normal activity of the thyroid; normal thyroid hormone secretion

Signs and symptoms of abnormal thyroid function are quite non-specific and may occur in a variety of other conditions. Conversely, a number of non-thyroid conditions can mimic the presence of a thyroid disorder. Although certain symptoms are considered "classic" findings in some thyroid diseases, disease may be present without observation of some or all of the expected manifestations and clinical presentation with the classic set of symptoms does not unequivocally indicate the presence of a thyroid disorder. The two general classifications of thyroid dysfunction are briefly described in this chapter, with the majority of the text devoted to a discussion of the various thyroid tests, evaluation and implications of test results, and selection of appropriate tests for various aspects of thyroid function.

THYROID DISORDERS

■ HYPERTHYROIDISM

Hyperthyroidism refers to an excessive secretion of the thyroid hormones. The heightened secretion may be produced from localized areas of hyperfunctioning thyroid tissue (eg, nodular areas: adenoma, toxic nodular goiter) or from overall thyroid hyperactivity as is seen in Graves' disease and in diffuse toxic goiter. Hyperthyroidism most commonly results from an autoimmune disorder (Graves' disease) in which antibodies are directed against the TSH receptor (Henry, 1996). Other disorders leading to hyperthyroidism include toxic multi-nodal goiter, toxic adenoma, thyroid carcinoma, and pituitary adenoma secretion of TSH (Henry, 1996). Symptoms of thyroid disease in general and hyperthyroidism in particular are fairly non-specific. However, signs and symptoms of hyperthyroidism typically include nervousness, weight loss, weakness, emotional lability, heat intolerance, tachycardia, tremor, and increased sweating—all symptoms of abnormally increased metabolic activity. *Exophthalmus* (abnormal prominence of the eyes) may be seen in Graves' disease along with a widening of the opening between the eyelids.

A **"thyroid storm"** (thyrotoxic crisis) refers to the most severe presentation of hyperthyroidism and is a medical emergency requiring immediate intervention. Thyroid storms most often develop in Graves' disease and are generally precipitated by factors such as stress, infections, or surgical emergencies (Stein, 1993). Although measurement of total serum T_3 and T_4 levels are usually not significantly higher than those for other thyrotoxic patients, clinical presentation includes climbing fever with diarrhea, CNS abnormalities, and hypermetabolism (Stein, 1993).

■ HYPOTHYROIDISM

A deficiency of thyroid hormones results in hypothyroidism (also called *myxedema*), which produces general symptoms of an abnormally slow metabolism such as lethargy, bradycardia, muscle weakness, dry skin, and constipation. Other signs of hypothyroidism include slowed reflexes, facial puffiness, impaired memory, and slowed speech and motor activity (Sacher & McPherson, 1991). Congenital hypothyroidism (*cretinism*), if not promptly treated, leads to irreversible, severe mental retardation and characteristic changes in facial features and stature. Fortunately, modern medicine allows complete prevention of such cases by screening all newborn infants for hypothyroidism. When hypothyroidism is detected and confirmed, lifelong administration of thyroid hormone prevents the development of the characteristic features of cretinism.

LABORATORY TESTS OF THYROID DISEASE

A number of laboratory assays are available to detect and evaluate thyroid disease. Tests may be basic tests of thyroid function, confirmatory tests, tests of etiology, or specialized tests used to answer a specific question regarding the thyroid disease. In choosing and evaluating the results of thyroid tests, it is important to understand exactly what is measured by each particular analysis and how the measured substance affects thyroid activity. It some cases, it may also benefit the clinician to be aware of the particular methodology employed by the laboratory for a particular analyte. Table 13–1 provides a summary of many of the tests related to thyroid function, most of which are discussed in detail following this summary. Other procedures related to the thyroid include diagnostic imaging procedures that produce a scan of the thyroid using small amounts of radioactive isotopes.

■ THYROXINE ASSAYS

Total serum levels of thyroxine (T_4) are commonly determined by direct measurement using **radioimmunoassay** (RIA) or **enzyme-linked immunoassay** (ELISA) techniques. The RIA techniques allow measurement of circulating T_4

TABLE 13–1. Laboratory Thyroid Tests

Test Category	Test	Abbrev.	Comments
Thyroxine tests	Thyroxine	T_4	Measures total circulating T_4; often used in screening
direct measures	Free thyroxine assay	FT_4	Measures unbound, biologically active T_4; good indicator of thyroid status with TSH
	Free thyroxine index	$FT_4 I$ (prev. T_7)	Calculated estimate of free T_4
indirect measures	Triiodothyronine uptake	T_3U	Measures % of T_3 that does not bind to TBG in test serum; provides info about free binding sites on TBG
	Reverse triiodothyronine	rT_3	Aids in evaluating tissue utilization of T_4
Triiodothyronine tests	Triiodothyronine by RIA	T_3-RIA	Measures circulating T_3
	Free triiodothyronine	Free T_3	Useful in confirming hyperthyroidism or in diagnosis of T_3 thyrotoxicosis
	Triiodothyronine uptake ratio	T_3UR	Compares T_3 in test serum to T_3 in pooled normal sera
Pituitary and hypothalamic function	Thyroid stimulating hormone	TSH	Provides info about pituitary secretion; good indicator of thyroid status, especially with FT_4
	Thyrotropin releasing hormone	TRH	Measures TRH stimulation of TSH; TSH levels measured pre- and post-stimulation; not frequently used
Thyroid uptake of iodine	Radioactive iodine uptake	RAIU	Based on need of iodine for thyroid hormones; is an indirect estimate of thyroid hormone production
Stimulation and suppression tests	Thyrotropin stimulation test		Assists in distinguishing primary thyroid disorder from disorders secondary to pituitary deficiency
	Triiodiothyronine withdrawal	T_3 withdrawal	Aids confirmation of borderline hyperthyroidism
	Thyrotropin releasing hormone	TRH	See previous listing under pituitary and hypothalamic tests
Other thyroid tests	Thyroglobulin		Primarily used to follow PTS with papillary and follicular carcinoma after total thyroidectomy
	Thyroid autoantibodies		Detects/quantitates autoantibodies to thyroglobulin or thyroid microsomes; antibody to TSH receptor
	Thyroxine binding globulin	TBG	Aids in assessment of free T_4

levels by providing a radioactive-labeled thyroxine that competes with the patient's thyroxine for a hormone binder. The amount of patient T_4 determines how much of the labeled T_4 will be bound. After the patient and labeled T_4 have reacted with the binder, the bound and unbound portions are separated and the radioactivity in one of the fractions is counted. Total thyroxine may also be directly measured using an antibody specific for T_4. Methods employing such antibodies require that T_4 first be released from endogenous proteins, accomplished by an extraction step. (RIA methods do not require this step.) Total T_4 assays measure both bound (metabolically inactive) and unbound (free; active) circulating T_4.

T_4 is a frequently used "first round" screening test for detecting the presence of thyroid abnormalities. The test is generally relatively inexpensive and easily performed by automated methods. Although once the primary diagnostic test for suspected cases of hyperthyroidism and hypothyroidism, newer highly sensitive TSH assays are rapidly superseding T_4 assays in diagnostic importance.

The specificity of total T_4 assay is reduced when changes occur in the thyroxine binding proteins or in the binding characteristics of these proteins resulting in levels that do not accurately reflect the true clinical state of the patient. In fact, more thyroxine results fall outside the reference range because of altered protein binding characteristics than from true thyroid dysfunction (Henry, 1996).

Free thyroxine (FT_4) assays do not have this limitation because such assays measure only unbound T_4. Original methods for determination of free T_4 employed a dialysis solution and membrane to separate the free T_4 from protein bound T_4. Enhancements to the original method improved sensitivity and specificity, but remained time consuming and relatively expensive. Further, such methods must be performed manually. Consequently, most laboratories use immunoassay techniques that do not require dialysis for direct measurement of free T_4, or employ indirect methods for the estimation of free T_4. A typical commercially available test method for direct measurement employs a synthetic material that is similar to T_4, but will not bind with TBG. This synthetic material is referred to as a "T_4 analog" and competes with free T_4 for binding with an anti-T_4 antibody. The amount of the analog that binds with the antibody is proportional to the amount of free thyroxine available in the patient's serum. The bound analog is "labeled" by enzymes or isotopes in order to provide a means of detection and quantitation. A frequently used, low-cost method of estimating free T_4 is the **free thyroxine index**, referred to as FTI or T_7 (the American Thyroid Association recommends the designation FT_4I). This index is a calculation employing the results of a total thyroxine assay and a T_3 uptake (T_3U; now referred to as thyroid hormone binding ratio, or THBR, by the American Thyroid Association). The total T_4 multiplied by the uptake result provides the FT_4I. This calculation was developed to correct the T_4 assay for alterations in thyroxine binding proteins. (Table 13-2 provides some of the causes of abnormal protein binding.) It takes advantage of the fact that T_4 values and T_3U values will move in opposite directions from normal in the presence of altered thyroid binding proteins or with alterations in the binding characteristics of these proteins, but will move in the same direction in the absence of such alterations, with the only variable being the

T$_4$ concentration (Ravel, 1995). While the FT$_4$I generally provides an acceptable estimate of free T$_4$, there are limitations; notably the validity of the index is dependent on the validity of the two measurements (T$_4$ and T$_3$U) used in its calculation. Table 13-3 lists a variety of causes for abnormal thyroxine or free thyroxine values and Table 13-4 presents typical T$_4$ and free T$_4$ test results in various disease states.

Typical **reference ranges,** from Henry (1996), are **total T$_4$** = 5.5 to 12.5 µg/dL and **free T$_4$** = 0.9 to 2.3 ng/dL.

Severe, non-thyroid diseases are a frequent cause of "false" abnormalities in T$_4$ test results. The impact of such illnesses, when severe, is generally to produce a decreased T$_4$; however, the result may occasionally be an elevated T$_4$. Reports have indicated that 20% to 30% of cases of severe non-thyroid illness result in decreased T$_4$ values. Severe non-thyroid illnesses may also affect other tests of thyroid status:

- free thyroxine: affect of illness is dependent on test method
- T$_3$: many severe non-thyroid illnesses cause decreased values
- reverse T$_3$: severe non-thyroid illness may cause increased values
- TSH: depends on stage of illness; initially decreases along with T$_4$, but to a lesser degree; in recovery phase may increase before T$_4$ and, in some cases, may be elevated
- T$_3$ uptake (THBR): usually normal to mildly increased; may be decreased, especially in acute viral hepatitis (Henry, 1996).

TABLE 13-2. Abnormal Protein Binding Capacity

Protein	Increased Capacity	Decreased Capacity
TBG (thyroxine binding globulin)	estrogens oral contraceptives pregnancy endocrine secreting tumors hepatic disease acute intermittent porphyrias genetic factors hypothyroidism	prednisone phenytoin active acromegaly androgens hepatic disease nephrotic syndrome severe illness/surgical stress thyrotoxicosis
TBPA (thyroxine binding pre-albumin)	active acromegaly prednisone androgens	severe illness/surgical stress thyrotoxicosis salicylates

Adapted from Henry JB. *Clinical Diagnosis and Management by Laboratory Methods,* 19th ed. Philadelphia, Saunders, 1996 with information from Ravel R. *Clinical Laboratory Medicine: Clinical Application of Laboratory Data,* 6th ed. St Louis, Mosby, 1995 and Sacher RA, McPherson RA. *Widmann's Clinical Interpretation of Laboratory Tests,* 10th ed. Philadelphia, FA Davis, 1991.

TABLE 13-3. Causes of Abnormal Thyroxine and Free Thyroxine Results

Decreased Values	Increased Values
Primary hypothyroidism	Primary hyperthyroidism
Secondary hypothyroidism	Familial dysalbuminemic hyperthyroxinemia
Moderate to severe iodine deficiency	Familial euthyroid thyroxine excess
Cushing syndrome	Factitious hyperthyroidism
Pituitary insufficiency	Iodine-induced hyperthyroidism (JOD-basedow)
Addison's disease (30% of patients ([Ravel, 1995])	Sample drawn too soon (2-4 hours) after synthroid dose
Some drugs (phenytoin, depakene,	Excess therapy for hypothyroidism
high dose salicylates)[1]	Post-partum transient toxicosis
Severe TBG or albumin decrease[1]	Hyperemesis gravidarum (50% of patients ([Ravel, 1995])
Severe non-thyroid illness[1] (see Table 13-5)	Active thyroiditis (some patients)
	TSH secreting pituitary tumor
	Severe non-thyroid illness[1] (see Table 13–5)
	Struma ovarii (ovarian congenital tumor—teratoma; mass
	has typical colloid filled thyroid follicles)

[1]T_4 more affected than FT_4.

TABLE 13-4. Typical Thyroid Function Test Results in Selected Conditions

Condition	T_4	$F\,T_4$
Hyperthyroidism	↑	↑
factitious (T_3)	↓	↓
factitious (T_4)	↑	↑
Hypothyroidism		
primary	↓	↓
secondary, pituitary/hypothalamic	↓	↓
secondary, selective deficiency	↓	↓
Peripheral hormone resistance	↑	↑
Familial dysalbuminemica hyperthyroxinemia (FDH)	↑	N
TBG deficiency	↓	N
FDH with TGB deficiency	N	N

N = normal; ↑ = elevated; ↓ = decreased; factitious = artifically produced.

Henry JB. *Clinical Diagnosis and Management by Laboratory Methods,* 19th ed. Philadelphia, Saunders, 1996.

TABLE 13-5. Non-thyroid Conditions Affecting Thyroid Results

Cirrhosis or severe hepatitis
Renal failure
Cancer
Chemotherapy
Severe infection or inflammation
Trauma
Post-surgical conditions
Extensive burns
Starvation or malnutrition
Acute psychiatric illness

From Ravel R. *Clinical Laboratory Medicine: Clinical Application of Laboratory Data,* 6th ed. St Louis, Mosby, 1995.

Table 13-5 lists examples of some of these conditions.

Conversely, thyroid disorders often result in abnormal test results for non-thyroid parameters (Table 13-6).

TABLE 13-6. Effect of Thyroid Disorders on Non-thyroid Laboratory Assays

Hypothyroidism	Hyperthyroidism
Increased cholesterol and triglycerides	Increased aminotransferases
Increased CK, AST, LD (muscle fractions)	Increased alkaline phosphatase
Increased prolactin	Decreased cholesterol and triglycerides
Normochromic anemia (slight)	Altered glucose-insulin relationship
Increased CSF protein	Increased % of lymphocytes on WBS differential
Increased carotene (yellow skin color)	Increased urinary calcium excretion
Decreased excretion of 17-ketosteroids	

Adapted from Sacher RA, McPherson RA. *Widmann's Clinical Interpretation of Laboratory Tests,* 10th ed. Philadelphia, FA Davis, 1991.

■ TRIIODOTHYRONINE ASSAYS

Serum levels of T_3 are generally measured using immunoassay techniques that utilize a very specific antibody to T_3. Many of these methods also use a blocking agent to liberate T_3 bound to endogenous proteins, allowing quantitation of **total T_3** concentrations (bound and unbound). In the same manner as thyroxine assays, but to a lesser degree, T_3 assays are affected by changes in binding proteins. It is important to remember that total serum T_3 or T_3 by RIA is *not* the same as the T_3U (THBR). Unfortunately, it has not been uncommon in the past to refer to T_3U simply as a "T_3," adding to the confusion of which test is requested and/or is being performed. Despite the test's name, **T_3U** is not a measure of T_3 and was initially developed as an alternative for *direct T_4* measurement. The test actually provides an estimate of the unsaturated thyroid binding sites (sites not occupied) on serum proteins. (The American Thyroid Association recommends the test be renamed "thyroid hormone binding ratio" or THBR.) **Free T$_3$** measurements are performed using methods similar to those for free T$_4$. Because T$_3$ is not as tightly bound to serum proteins as T$_4$, more T$_3$ is found in the free condition.

Serum T$_3$ is elevated along with T$_4$ levels in most patients with hyperthyroidism and has its greatest diagnostic importance in cases of T$_3$ thyrotoxicosis. Levels are also helpful in assessing the severity and recovery from hyperthyroidism. Because T$_3$ levels are generally within the reference range except in the most severe cases of hypothyroidism, its measurement is not as beneficial in diagnosing this condition. A typical **reference range** for serum **T$_3$** is 60 to 160 ng/dL or 0.92 to 2.46 nmol/L, and for **T$_3$U** (resin uptake method) is 25 to 38 relative % uptake (Henry, 1996).

 TIME FOR REVIEW. After studying the preceding sections, you should be able to respond correctly to the following:

■ The thyroid gland synthesizes hormones from _____ and _____.

■ _____ is the principal component of colloid and the storage site for the thyroid hormones.

■ Most circulating T$_3$ and T$_4$ are found in the _____ (bound/free) state. In which state are they metabolically active?

■ List the three serum proteins to which T$_3$ and T$_4$ are bound and indicate which of the three is bound to the significant majority of these hormones.

■ Briefly describe the location and anatomy of the thyroid.

■ Most of the daily production of T$_3$ takes place in the _____ from deiodination of free T$_4$.

■ The hormone that stimulates the synthesis and release of the thyroid hormones from thyroglobulin is _____, also called _____.

■ TSH is secreted by the _____.

■ A hormone secreted by the hypothalamus called
_____ stimulates TSH secretion.

■ Describe the effect of T_3 and T_4 levels on TSH and TRH levels in the following cases:

    Low circulating levels:

    High circulating levels:

■ Distinguish between primary and secondary thyroid disorders.

■ Briefly explain why symptoms (or lack of symptoms) can be misleading in thyroid abnormalities.

■ Heightened secretion of the thyroid hormones can be produced from
_____ areas of hyperfunctioning thyroid tissue or
from _____.

■ Hyperthyroidism most commonly results from an
_____ disorder.

■ List additional disorder that may result in hyperthyroidism.

■ Though non-specific, symptoms of hyperthyroidism typically include:

■ Symptoms of hypothyroidism include:

■ Hypothyroidism is also sometimes called _____.

■ Untreated congenital hypothyroidism or cretinism results in:

■ Distinguish between total thyroxine and free thyroxine.

■ Which thyroid test provides information about the number of free binding sites on TBG?

■ How is the free thyroxine index determined?

■ Both total T_3 and T_4 assays may be affected by changes in _____.

■ Review the tables provided in this section.

Check your responses by reviewing the preceding sections.

■ REVERSE TRIIODOTHYRONINE ASSAY

Measurement of reverse T_3 (rT_3) is not often used in the evaluation of thyroid function because it has little or no apparent metabolic activity. It can, however, be used as an indication of tissue utilization of T_4 because it is a major metabolite of thyroxine. Reverse T_3 assay can also be useful in the evaluation of peripheral resistance to thyroid hormones (rT_3 is normal with an elevated T_4 and a normal TSH [Henry, 1996]) and in determining whether other thyroid function test results are due to a non-thyroidal illness or are indicative of hypothyroidism. Reverse T_3 assays are performed using RIA methods with a typical reference range of 10 to 50 ng/dL (Henry, 1996).

■ THYROTROPIN (THYROID STIMULATING HORMONE) ASSAY

Measurement of thyroid stimulating hormone (TSH) has become one of the most useful tests of thyroid function due, in large part, to the significant improvement in the assay. Further, TSH assays provide the clinician with information about not only thyroid function, but about pituitary function as well. In fact one of the greatest values of the TSH is its use in distinguishing a primary thyroid deficiency from secondary hypothyroidism as a result of pituitary dysfunction. Levels are also helpful in separately functional euthyroid conditions with low thyroid hormones from true hypothyroidism. Currently available methods of measurement are exceptionally specific for TSH because of the use of monoclonal antibody technology. The new techniques are also adaptable to automated analyzers allowing the test to be performed with relative ease and improved speed compared to methods employed only a few years ago.

Currently available assays also boast increased levels of sensitivity (third and fourth generation assays, generally marketed as "sensitive," "highly sensitive" or "ultra-sensitive" TSH assays). Better sensitivity, or how close the lower limit of detection of the assay is to zero, allows better differentiation of hyperthyroidism and other causes of decreased TSH levels. Evaluation of TSH test results as compared to the reported reference range specific for the assay is essential, because reference ranges, as well as lower detection limits, vary considerably among the various "generations" of assays. Using the sensitive or ultra-sensitive TSH assays, results that fall within the established reference range can generally be considered to exclude the presence of abnormal thyroid function (Henry, 1996). Abnormal levels, however, do not necessarily indicate the presence of thyroid disease without confirmation by additional test procedures and clinical evaluation. Time of specimen collection should be noted when evaluating the results of a TSH assay because notable diurnal variation is seen, with values highest about 10 to 11 PM and lowest about 10 AM (Ravel, 1995). **Reference ranges** for TSH are method dependent, but usually have an upper limit of < 10 μIU/mL. Two examples of ranges are 0.5 to 5.0 μIU/mL (Henry, 1996) and 1.5 to 9.0 μIU/mL (Ravel, 1995). Table 13-7 lists some conditions that may produce abnormal TSH levels.

TABLE 13-7. Causes of Abnormal TSH Values (High Sensitivity Assay)

Increased Values	Decreased Values
Primary hypothyroidism	T_4/T_3 Toxicosis (diffuse or nodular etiology)
Addison's disease	T_3 Toxicosis
Pituitary TSH secreting tumor	Excessive therapy for hypothyroidism
Synthroid therapy, insufficient dose (some cases)	Active thyroiditis (subacute, painless or early active Hashimoto's;
Later stage of Hashimoto's thyroiditis (some cases)	some cases)
Moderate to severe iodine deficiency	Severe non-thyroidal illness (esp. acute trauma, dopamine or
Severe non-thyroid illness, recovery phase (some	glucocorticoid; some cases)
cases)	Pituitary insufficiency
Some drugs (amphetamines, lithium; some cases)	Cushing syndrome
X-ray contrast media (telepaque/iopanic acid and	Jod-basedow hyperthyroidism (iodine induced)
oragrafin/ipodate; some cases)	Post-partum transient toxicosis
Acute psychiatric illness (few patients)	Factitious hyperthyroidism
Large doses of inorganic iodide	Struma ovarii
Antibodies that interfere with test method (HAMA	Hyperemesis gravidarum
[human anti-mouse antibody])	Specimen drawn 2 to 4 hours after synthroid dose (some
Evening specimen collection (diurnal variation)	cases)
Therapy for hypothyroidism, 1 to 8 weeks after therapy	Radioimmunoassay, surgery, anti-thyroid drug therapy
initiated or longer when pretherapy TSH >100	for hyperthyroidism, ~4 to 6 weeks post-therapy (up to 2 years)
High altitudes (some cases)	Interleukin-2 drugs or alpha-interferon therapy
	(small percentage of cases)

Testing errors may result in either increased or decreased results, as with most assays.

Adapted from Ravel R. *Clinical Laboratory Medicine: Clinical Application of Laboratory Data,* 6th ed. St Louis, Mosby, 1995.

■ THYROXINE BINDING GLOBULIN ASSAYS

Recall that most of the circulating T_3 and T_4 are bound to thyroxine binding globulin (TBG) as a carrier protein. The capacity of TBG to bind with thyroxine can be measured using immunoassay and electrophoretic methods. Although not frequently indicated in the evaluation of thyroid function, this measure can be of benefit when a patient's T_3 levels do not agree with other measures of thyroid function or with clinical findings. A number of factors can influence the capacity of TBG to bind thyroxine as listed in Table 13-2.

■ THYROGLOBULIN ASSAYS

The primary use of thyroglobulin assays is in monitoring patients with papillary and follicular carcinoma after total thyroidectomy (Henry, 1996). It can also be used to identify factitious (artificially induced) thyrotoxicosis, because thyroglobulin levels are undetectable in such patients, but are elevated in hyperthyroidism of most other etiologies. Thyroglobulin levels, which are normally about 30 to 40 ng/mL, are increased with goiters, thyroiditis, adenomas, and some nonthyroid malignancies (Henry, 1996). The most common method employed for measurement is immunoassay.

■ STIMULATION AND SUPPRESSION TESTS

This group of tests, though not frequently employed in the evaluation of thyroid function, can provide useful information in certain situations, particularly in the confirmation or differentiation of questionable diagnoses. Each of the tests described here involves administration of a substance to stimulate or suppress a specific function and then measuring the response by measuring the affected parameters.

In the **thyrotropin stimulation test**, the substance administered is TSH (bovine TSH) and the parameters to be subsequently measured are T_4 and/or RAIU. This test may be used when initial testing indicates a thyroid dysfunction, but etiology in terms of primary disease or secondary abnormality consequent to pituitary deficiency is uncertain. Baseline levels must be obtained prior to administration of TSH in order to provide a basis for evaluation of later results. Administration of TSH is expected to more than double the baseline values for T_4 and radioactive iodine uptake (RAIU). If these values fail to increase following TSH stimulation, primary thyroid dysfunction is strongly suggested. Conversely, a normal response suggests that the original test results occurred as a result of a pituitary or hypothalamic disorder or from some artifactual abnormality (Ravel, 1995). Other uses for this procedure, as outlined by Ravel (1995) include

- confirmation of primary hypothyroidism (thyroid does not respond to TSH stimulation)
- evaluating patients on long-term therapy for hypothyroidism to confirm the appropriateness of the original diagnosis (TSH stimulation can be performed without termination of therapy as opposed to ceasing therapy and waiting several weeks for the thyroid and pituitary to return to "pretherapy equilibrium")
- to determine whether areas of the thyroid that are non-functional on a thyroid scan are capable of function (ie, is the area non-functional as a result of an inability to function or as a result of suppression from other areas of hypersecretion)

A number of issues, in addition to lack of clinical indication, contribute to the rare use of this test procedure. Because bovine TSH is administered and the introduction of "foreign" substances carries the risk of antibody development, patients subjected to this procedure may develop anti-TSH antibodies. The presence of such antibodies in the circulation could be problematic in future TSH assays or, particularly noteworthy, could produce an allergic response if the TSH stimulation test were to be used again on the patient. Another limitation of the procedure involves the effect of iodine levels on RAIU response to TSH (iodine overload decreases the RAIU response [Ravel, 1995]). Clinicians may prefer to use the T_3 withdrawal test (discussed below) in place of TSH stimulation.

Another rarely used is test is the **triiodothyronine withdrawal test**, used for the same general purposes as the TSH stimulation test. When initial testing indicates the need for a T_3 withdrawal test, the patient is placed on T_3 therapy for a 1-month period after which medication is withdrawn. Ten days following withdrawal of T_3 therapy a TSH sample is collected. Elevated TSH levels at this time are indicative of primary hypothyroidism while normal or decreased levels are seen with secondary hypothyroidism or in euthyroid conditions. While T_4 therapy could be used in the same manner, it takes longer (about 4 weeks versus 10 days [Ravel, 1995]) following cessation of therapy to re-establish equilibrium of the thyroid-pituitary-hypothalamic feedback system.

The **thyroid releasing hormone stimulation test** is useful in the confirmation of equivocal cases of hyperthyroidism and in distinguishing forms of hypothyroidism. This was the primary method for the confirmation of hyperthyroidism prior to development of the more sensitive TSH assays capable of measuring suppressed levels of TSH. Results using these assays correlate well with TRH stimulation test results provided the hypothalamic-pituitary axis is intact (Henry, 1996). In this test, a synthetic TRH (Thypinone, Protirelin) is administered after a baseline sample has been drawn and the TSH response (amount of increase above baseline) is evaluated. Although a number of procedural variations exist, the TRH is generally administered by a single IV bolus of 100 to 500 µg (some studies indicate that 400 µg is needed to achieve full TRH effect [Ravel, 1995]). Samples for TSH assay are collected at defined intervals following administration (20, 30, or 60 minutes [Henry, 1996]; 15, 30, and 60 [Stein, 1993]). TSH levels may begin to rise as soon as 5 minutes following administration (Henry, 1996), peak by 30 minutes ([Ravel, 1995]; 20 to 30 minutes [Henry, 1996]), and return to baseline levels in 2 to 4 hours. The level of increase in TSH values is proportional to the baseline measurement. The "fold" (ie, twofold, threefold) increase in the TSH above baseline is a better measure of the TSH response to stimulation than the absolute increase (ie, increase of 12 µU/mL). A graphic representation of the rise and fall of TSH levels following TRH stimulation is provided in Figure 13-4. A TSH increase of ≥ 6 µU/mL in males and females under the age of 40 and increases of ≥ 2 µg/mL in men over 40 is generally considered to be a normal response (Stein, 1993), but limits above which the response is considered exaggerated vary from 20 to 40 µU/mL (range from Ravel [1995], who suggests 25 µU/mL as the limit). Because pituitary secretion of TSH is suppressed in response to high circulating levels of T_3 and T_4, significant increases following TRH stimulation are not expected in hyperthyroidism. The TSH response in primary hypothyroidism is generally exaggerated. In secondary hypothyroidism (pituitary disease), post-stimulation TSH values should not show a significant increase, and in tertiary hypothyroidism (hypothalamic dysfunction) the TSH increase is usually normal in degree but delayed for about 30 minutes (Ravel, 1995). A "flat curve" of TSH response to TRH is suggestive of thyrotoxicosis. Interpretation of TRH stimulation results is dependent on whether the patient has indications of hyperthyroidism or hypothyroidism and upon the level of TSH increase above baseline one defines as "exaggerated" (Ravel, 1995). Table 13-8 provides guidelines for the interpretation of TRH stimulation results.

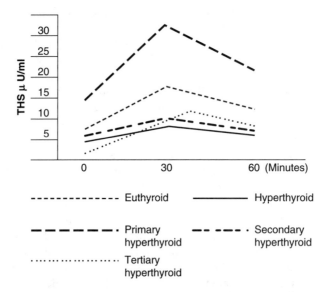

FIGURE 13-4. Typical TSH responses to TRH stimulation (500 μg TRH; presented for illustration purposes only). Note the similarities in results for hyperthyroid patients and for patients with secondary hypothyroidism. This is a good illustration of the previous comment that interpretation of results is dependent on whether the patient exhibits evidence of hyperthyroidism or of hypothyroidism. The results of the TRH stimulation test must consequently be interpreted in light of initial tests that indicated thyroid abnormality as well as the presence of any nonthyroid illness that may impact thyroid test results.

TABLE 13-8. Interpretation of TRH Stimulation Test Results[1]

Thyroid Status	Baseline TSH μU/mL	TSH (μU/mL) Increase at 30 min
Euthyroid	≤ 10 (usually ≤ 6)	≥ 2 (usually 6 to 30)
Hyperthyroid	≤ 10 (usually ≤ 4)	< 2
Hypothyroid, primary	>10	≥ 2 (usually ≥ 20)
Hypothyroid, secondary	≤ 10 (usually ≤ 6)	< 2 (60%)
Hypothyroid, tertiary	≤ 10 (often < 2)	≥ 2 (95%)

[1]500 μg of TRH administered IV.

Adapted from Ravel R. *Clinical Laboratory Medicine: Clinical Application of Laboratory Data,* 6th ed. St Louis, Mosby, 1995.

While not usually measured as a part of the test, increases in T_3 and T_4 are also seen in euthyroid patients, with T_3 increasing to approximately 70% above baseline in 1 to 4 hours following TRH administration (Henry, 1996). T_4 increases are not as great. Secretion of prolactin is also usually stimulated as is growth hormone in conditions such as acromegaly (Henry, 1996). Prolactin and growth hormone measurements are not part of the standard test procedure.

Although reported evidence is conflicting, severe non-thyroid illness may affect TRH results (based on some data), causing a "blunted" response in euthyroid patients with decreased T_4 levels as a result of non-thyroid disease and in some hypothyroid patients (Ravel, 1995). If present, such effects would make evaluation of TRH stimulation results in terms of the diagnosis of hypothyroidism and differentiation of primary and secondary hypothyroidism much more complex. TSH responses may be impaired (similar to hyperthyroid response) in some conditions, including certain psychiatric disorders (unipolar depression), fasting of 48 hours or more, renal failure, multi-nodular goiter, Cushing syndrome, high-dose aspirin therapy, levodopa use, or adrenocorticosteroids use (Henry, 1996; Ravel, 1995). Graves' disease patients who are euthyroid following therapy may also have an impaired response (Henry, 1996). Thyroid therapy must be discontinued for a significant time period (2 to 5 weeks [Ravel, 1995]) before performing the TRH stimulation test.

The **T_3 suppression test** (also called the *thyroid suppression test*) is rarely used; the TRH stimulation test is often used instead. Briefly, this test employs the administration of standard T_3 doses for a week and then measurement of the thyroid response. (Note that although the test is often referred to as a *thyroid* suppression test, it is actually the *pituitary* that is directly suppressed with thyroid suppression being secondary.) Administration of additional T_3 in conjunction with the T_3 and T_4 already in the circulation is expected to suppress the secretion of TSH by the pituitary and, consequently, the production of thyroid hormone. In hyperthyroidism, the thyroid continues hormone production despite the absence of pituitary stimulation. Uses of this test include confirmation of borderline hyperthyroidism and demonstration (in conjunction with a thyroid scan) of nodule autonomy (Ravel, 1995). Cautious use of the procedure is necessary in elderly patients and in those with cardiac disease (Ravel, 1995).

Numerous drawbacks to the procedure and the availability of other test methods have significantly reduced the use of the **radioactive iodine uptake (RAIU) test**. The procedure involves administration of a small dose of radioactive iodine. About 24 hours after the dose the amount of radiation detectable in the thyroid is measured. This provides an indirect estimate of thyroid hormone production, because iodine is needed for this process. The thyroid's need for iodine is also dependent on the rate of hormone synthesis (Ravel, 1995). Although perhaps of value in some situations, the value of the RAIU test is questionable because of a number of factors (Ravel, 1995):

- false normals in up to 80% of patients with hyperthyroidism resulting from toxic nodules

- the effects of numerous medications
- uncertainty of normal values
- poor separation of normal and hypothyroid patients
- the large number of factors (besides destruction of thyroid tissue) resulting in decreased values

Further, two patient visits and two days are needed to complete the procedure and small amounts of radioactivity are administered.

■ AUTOIMMUNE ANTIBODY ASSAYS

A number of autoantibodies directed against thyroid tissue have been identified and associated with various thyroid conditions. Thyroid antibodies include:

- TSH receptor antibody: autoantibody against the TSH receptor; previously known as thyroid stimulating immunoglobulin (TSIg) or long acting thyroid stimulator (LATS)
- Anti-TPO: autoantibody to thyroid peroxidase (TPO; previously known as antibody to thyroid microsomal antigen); antibodies may be referred to as anti-microsomal antibodies
- Thyroglobulin antibody: autoantibody directed against the binding protein, thyroglobulin, and abbreviated TgAb
- Thyrotropin-binding inhibitor immunoglobulin (TBII)

The **antibodies to thyroglobulin and to TPO or the microsomal antigen** are more frequently measured and one or both are found in virtually all cases of chronic thyroiditis. Microsomal/TPO antibodies are found more often in these cases than TgAb (Ravel, 1995). Significant titers are generally found, but high titers of these antibodies are not specific for chronic thyroiditis (Table 13-9). When titers are normal or show only mild elevation, chronic thyroiditis is less likely to be the diagnosis. Results for these antibodies in selected conditions are shown in Table 13-9.

TABLE 13-9. Thyroglobulin and Microsomal Antibodies in Selected Conditions

	Hashimoto's	Graves'	Hyperthyroidism, Primary	Nontoxic Nodular Goiter	Thyroid Carcinoma	Normal Male	Normal Female
Thyroglobulin, % abnormal[1]	70 (50–86)	55 (29–65)	55 (50–64)	(5–50)	20	(0–2)	(2–20)
Microsomal, % abnormal[1]	97 (92–100)	75 (71–86)	75 (67–86)	27	20[2]	(0–3)	15[2]

[1]Expected percentage of cases in which antibody is present, numbers in parentheses are ranges in literature.
[2]Based on immunofluorescence method; all other on hemagglutination methods.

Adapted from Ravel R. *Clinical Laboratory Medicine: Clinical Application of Laboratory Data,* 6th ed. St Louis, Mosby, 1995.

Thyroid stimulating hormone receptor antibodies block the binding of TSH to the TSH receptor and can stimulate cyclic AMP, which causes T_3 and T_4 to be released, and may result in hyperthyroidism. These antibodies are present in Graves' disease and have been used to predict the outcome for Graves' disease patients treated with drug therapy. (Detectable levels after therapy is predictive of a relapse of thyrotoxicosis [Henry, 1996]). The test is also used with patients who have borderline or conflicting evidence of Graves' disease (Ravel, 1995) and as a predictor of thyroid dysfunction in newborns born to mothers with Graves' disease (Henry, 1996). (Graves' disease, named for an Irish physician, refers to an exopthalmic goiter/thyrotoxicosis; it is characterized by abnormally protruding eyes, an enlarged thyroid gland, nervous symptoms, loss of weight, and increased basal metabolism.) These patients may also have the blocking antibody **TBII**, which generally does not produce symptoms but may lead to hypothyroidism in some cases (Henry, 1996). Monitoring levels of this antibody, along with antibodies to the TSH receptor, is useful in preventing overtreatment with antithyroid drugs (Henry, 1996).

Methods used to detect and quantitate the autoimmune thyroid antibodies include immunofluorescence, hemagglutination, and RIA. Latex agglutination methods are also available for TgAb (Ravel, 1995). Although somewhat more sensitive and becoming more widely used, RIA and immunofluorescence are not as widely available as hemagglutination methods (Ravel, 1995).

TEST SELECTION AND RESULTS IN SELECTED CONDITIONS

Initial test selection is dependent on a number of variables, including whether testing is being performed for screening purposes, to exclude disease, or because disease is suspected based on symptoms and clinical findings, the degree of sensitivity and specificity desired, test availability, and principles of cost containment. Follow-up and confirmatory test selection decisions are based on some of the same factors (particularly test sensitivity/specificity, test availability, and cost containment), but are guided in large part by the results of initial testing. Table 13-10 provides some general test selections for initial and confirmatory testing. The test selections indicated cannot be assumed to be appropriate in all instances nor to be a substitute for the clinician's judgment. Each particular patient may present with a number of variables that must be considered and with varying patterns on initial testing. Table 13-11 presents thyroid test results in selected conditions.

Some clinicians may prefer to screen using a single test assay, in which case the ultra-sensitive TSH is a good screening choice (as the best *single* screening tool). However, if clinicians intend to use only TSH measurement for routine screening purposes, it would be prudent to ensure that the laboratory performing the testing uses an ultra-sensitive TSH method with reproducible detectability to 0.01 μIU/mL. (Previous generation TSH methods are not as suitable for single assay screening and not all ultra-sensitive TSH methods are equal in terms of performance characteristics.) Other clinicians may choose to screen using both the TSH and the T_4 (or free T_4). This screening approach is particu-

TABLE 13-10. General Test Selection

Test Purpose /Test Type	Initial Testing			Follow-Up/Confirmatory/Differentiation Testing							
	T_4, Tot	FT_4	TSH^1	T_3-RIA or FT_3	T_3U	TRH Stim	ANTI-TPO	TGAb	T_3 Suppress	RAIU	Thyroid Scan
Screening[2]	✓	✓	✓	Dependent on results of initial testing							
Suspected hyperthyroidism	✓	✓	✓	✓	✓	✓			✓	✓	✓
Suspected hypothyroidism	✓	✓	✓		~✓	✓					
Differentiation of hypothyroidism	NA	NA	NA			✓					
Thyroiditis	✓	✓	✓			✓	✓	✓		✓	✓
Monitoring replacement therapy	✓[3]		✓[3]	✓[3]							

[1]ultra-sensitive method; [2]healthy population assumed; [3]o distinction between screening and confirmatory tests in this instance, only one of the three indicated tests is necessary and sources vary as to preferred test. Clinician should be aware of the test characteristics and responses to replacement therapy prior to selecting preferred monitoring test. KEY: ✓ preferred (screening) or required (confirmatory); ✓ may be used instead of or in addition to preferred test (screening) or may also provide additional useful information (confirmatory); ~somewhat useful; NA—not applicable.

TABLE 13-11. Thyroid Test Results in Selected Conditions

Condition	T₄, TOT	FT₄	TSH[1]	T₃-RIA or FT₃	T₃U	TRH STIM	ANTI-TPO[2]	TgAb	T₃ Suppress	RAIU	Notes
Hyperthyroidism	↑	↑↑	↓	↑	↑	No signif response			No suppression		
T₃ toxicosis	N	N	N/↑	↑	Usually N					N	
Factitious T₃	↓	↓	↓	↑							
Factitious T₄	↓	↓	↑↑	N/↓	↓						
Primary hypothyroidism	↓	↓	↑↑	N/↓	↓	Exag response					
Secondary hypothyroidism	↓	↓	↑/N	↓		No signif response					
Tertiary hypothyroidism	↓	↓	↓	↓		N, but response delayed					
Graves' disease	↑	↑	↓	↑	↑		↑	↑ (60%)			Most patients also have TSH receptor antibody
Hashimoto's thyroiditis[3]	N (50%) or ↓	↓	↑	↓	↓		↑	↑ (80% of pts >1:1000)		N/↑	
Subacute thyroiditis	↑	↑	↓	↑	↑					↓	Painful, tender enlarged thyroid; scan shows patchy isotope conc or very little uptake; ESR signif ↑
Painless (silent) thyroiditis	↑	↑	↓	↑	↑					↓	Differs from subacute in lack of pain and norm ESR
Postpartum transient thyroiditis	↑	↑	↓	↑	↑		↑	↑		↓	In previously euthyroid women; may/may not be symptomatic; may be followed by transient hypothyroidism
Peripheral hormone resistance	↑	↑	N	↑							

[1]Highly sensitive TSH method assumed.

[2]Must be differentiated from anti-microsomal AB if course granular cytoplasmic staining is noted.

[3]Hashimoto's has slow progression to hypothyroid state; anti-TPO and TgAb most important for diagnosis.

From Henry JB. *Clinical Diagnosis and Management by Laboratory Methods*, 19th ed. Philadelphia, Saunders, 1996.

larly suitable if the clinician is unsure of the TSH methodology used in the laboratory that will perform testing. Clinicians may also prefer two assay screening for the additional information provided in the event abnormalities are detected and for the added reassurance of the absence of disease when both tests are normal. A list of some of the possible causes for nine T_4/TSH test patterns is given in Table 13-12 because this test combination is frequently employed for screening purposes.

Congenital hypothyroidism screening is employed in the neonatal period to identify the one infant in 3500 to 4000 live births (range from Henry [1996]; other sources differ: 1 in 6000 with literature range of 3000 to 10,000 [Ravel, 1995]) that will have this condition. Early detection is essential because promptly instituted therapy prevents the irreversible severe mental retardation and characteristic changes in facial features and stature that occur if the condition is not treated. The vast majority of detected cases result from agenesis of the thyroid gland, but about 10 % are due to defective enzymes in thyroid synthesis with the remaining cases secondary to pituitary or hypothalamic dysfunction (Ravel, 1995). Although a small percentage of cases are transient in nature, nearly 90 % (Henry, 1996) of detected cases are permanent conditions requiring life-long therapy. (Low levels of T_4 are also seen in premature infants and in infants with a congenital deficiency of TBG [Henry, 1996].) There is a strong correlation between birth weight and T_4 levels (Ravel, 1995).

Even though screening programs may vary somewhat, the most commonly used approach is an initial measurement of T_4 with TSH follow-up for any results that fall below an established level. This is used as the initial test because it is usually less expensive to perform, it is less likely to give false negative results when subjected to adverse storage or transport conditions (Ravel, 1995), and because the TSH would not detect cases secondary to hypothalamic dysfunction. Blood collected by heel puncture onto filter paper is used in most screening programs (cord blood could be used, but presents difficulties in proper storage and transport to the testing facility). Exact adherence to the collection protocol established by the testing facility is crucial to obtaining a specimen that is suitable for testing.

Neonatal reference ranges are *not* the same as those for adults. For example, TSH values in the neonate are about twice those seen in adults. Ranges provided by the testing laboratory must be used for evaluating neonatal test results. It is also important to collect specimens within the time interval established by the testing laboratory when possible. However, it is often not possible to collect neonatal specimens at standardized times—particularly when the time of discharge may be dictated by the insurance carrier or other third party payer. Specimens for all neonatal screening tests should be obtained on all infants prior to discharge! T_4 levels increase about 30 % to 40 % after birth, with a plateau at 24 to 48 hours, and return to the levels at birth within about 5 days. The TSH value rapidly increases after birth (peaks in about 30 minutes) to 5 to 7 times (Ravel, 1995) the value at birth. The level then falls back to values that are about twice the birth value at 24 hours and is approximately equal to the birth level at 48 hours. When initial T_4 measurement indicates a potential abnormality, a second specimen should be provided for repeat T_4 testing and/or TSH assay.

TABLE 13-12. Evaluation of T_4 and TSH Patterns

	Decreased T_4			Normal T_4			Increased T_4		
	↓ TSH	N TSH	↑ TSH	↓ TSH	N TSH	↑ TSH	↓ TSH	N TSH	↑ TSH
Pituitary insufficiency		Severely ↓ TBG or albumin	Primary hyperthyroidism	T_3 toxicosis	Normal thyroid function	Mild hypothyroidism	1° hyperthyroidism	Increased TBG	TSH-secreting pituitary tumor
Severe nonthyroid illness		Severe nonthyroid illness	Large doses of ioraganic iodide	Mild hyperthyroid w/ decr. TBG, dilantin ther., or severe non-thyroid disease	Few cases of early hypothyroidism (only TRH reveals abnormality)	Hypothyroidism w/ increased TBG	Excess hypothyroid therapy	Acute psychiatric illness (some pts, esp paranoid schizophrenia)	Peripheral resistance to T_4 (some patients)
Cushing's syndrome		Dilantin or valproic acid	Lithium therapy (some patients)	Early hyperthyroid	Low T_4 and norm. TSH w/ heparin therapy	Hypothyroidism w/ sl inadequate therapy	Active thyroiditis (some patients)	T_4 sample drawn 2 to 4 hours after T_4 dose	Some x-ray contrast media
High dose glucocorticoid		High dose salicylates	Severe iodine deficiency	Increased TBG with pituitary insufficiency		Addison's disease (majority of cases)	Jod-Basedow hyperthyroidism	Peripheral resistance to T_4 (some patients)	Some patients on amiodarone therapy or amphetamines
T_3 toxicosis w/ dilantin ther.		Moderate iodine deficiency	Addison's disease (30% of patients)	Low T_4 and TSH with heparin therapy		TSH specimen collected in evening	Post-partum transient toxicosis	Some pts w/ pituitary TSH-secreting tumor if pretumor TSH was low normal	Acute psychiatric illness (few patients)
T_3 toxicosis w/ severe TBG deficiency		Some cases secondary hypothyroidism	Interleukin −2 therapy (15–26% of cases)	Multinodular goiter w/ area of autonomy (some patients)		Mild Hashimoto's (some patients)	Factitious hyperthyroidism	Acute porphyria	
				Synthroid therapy in slightly excess dose (some patients)		Acute psychiatric illness (few patients)	Struma ovarii	Some X-ray contrast media	
						Hypothyroidism with familial dysalbuminemic hyperthyroxinemia	Hyperemesis gravidarum		
						Low T_4 and ↑ TSH w/ heparin therapy			

High sensitivity TSH method assumed. Impact of heparin therapy depends on particular methods; 1° = primary.

Interpretations of test patterns used in table are from Ravel R. *Clinical Laboratory Medicine: Clinical Application of Laboratory Data*, 6th ed. St Louis, Mosby, 1995.

Misleading test results may be seen in a variety of situations, including the presence of other conditions/illnesses that impact thyroid results and laboratory error. Test patterns may seem to indicate T_3/T_4 hyperthyroidism, T_3 hyperthyroidism, or T_4 hyperthyroidism when the condition does not, in fact, exist, or may indicate a euthyroid state when hyperthyroidism does exist. Possible causes for misleading patterns of test results include:

- apparent T_3/T_4 hyperthyroidism: increased levels of TBG; thyroiditis (subacute, painless, and some cases of Hashimoto's [Ravel, 1995]); peripheral resistance to thyroid hormones; self-medication with thyroid hormones (factitious)
- apparent T_3 hyperthyroidism: increased TBG; specimen collected within 1 to 2 hours of T_3 dose or within several hours of dessicated thyroid (Ravel, 1995); severe iodine deficiency
- apparent T_4 hyperthyroidism: severe non-thyroid illness; increased TBG with decrease in T_3-RIA or with disproportionate T_4 increase relative to T_3-RIA (Ravel, 1995); specimen collected 1 to 4 hours after levothyroxine; some medications—including amphetamine abuse—and x-ray contrast media; some cases of acute psychiatric illness
- apparent euthyroidism in hyperthyroid state: decreased TBG; severe non-thyroid disease

When an unexpected pattern of test results is seen, one or all of the assays should be repeated. Confirmatory test procedures may also be of benefit in such cases.

 TIME FOR REVIEW. After studying the preceding sections, you should be able to respond correctly to the following:

■ TSH measurement provides information about thyroid function and about _____ function.

■ Though they are not frequently used, the assays below may be beneficial in some situations. Indicate one instance in which each may provide useful information.

Reverse T_3:

Thyroxine binding globulin:

■ The primary use of thyroglobulin measurements is to
_____.

■ List three instances in which the thyrotropin stimulation test is useful.

■ Administering TSH is expected to more than double baseline results for
_____ and _____.

■ List two drawbacks for use of the thyrotropin stimulation test.

■ TRH stimulation tests are useful in confirming _____
and in distinguishing forms of _____.

■ Briefly describe the expected TSH response to administration of TRH in the
following conditions:

Hyperthyroidism:

Primary hypothyroidism:

Secondary hypothyroidism:

Tertiary hypothyroidism:

Euthyroidism:

■ Briefly describe the T_3 suppression test.

■ List five drawbacks for the use of the RAIU test.

■ List four thyroid antibodies and indicate the two most frequently measured.

■ Which thyroid antibody, seen in Graves' disease, blocks binding of TSH and can stimulate cyclic AMP?

■ What antibody is found in nearly all cases of Hashimoto's thyroiditis?

■ The two antibodies most important in the diagnosis of Hashimoto's are _____ and _____.

■ If only one test is to be used for screening purposes, which test should be used? What particular information is important for the clinician to know about the methodology for this test?

■ List two reasons for using a two-assay screening approach.

■ Why is early detection of congenital hypothyroidism essential?

■ What is the most common screening approach for neonatal hypothyroidism?

■ How do neonatal TSH values compare to adult TSH values?

■ List two situations in which each of the following may be falsely indicated by laboratory results:

Apparent T_3/T_4 hyperthyroidism:

Apparent T_3 hyperthyroidism:

Apparent T_4 hyperthyroidism:

Apparent euthyroidism in hyperthyroid state:

Check your responses by reviewing the preceding sections.

13. SELF TEST

Choose the best response by circling the appropriate letter. The answer key may be found in the appendices.

1. **The thyroid gland synthesizes thyroid hormones from**
   A. iodine and thyroglobulin
   B. albumin and thyroglobulin
   C. iodine and tyrosine
   D. tyrosine and albumin

2. **Most circulating thyroid hormone is bound to**
   A. thyroxine binding globulin
   B. albumin
   C. prealbumin

3. **The principal component of colloid and the storage site for thyroid hormones is**
   A. thyroxine binding globulin
   B. thyroglobulin
   C. albumin
   D. tyrosine

4. **The hypothalamic hormone that is sensitive to circulating thyroid hormone levels and stimulates or suppresses TSH secretion based on these circulating levels is**
   A. thyroxine
   B. triiodothyronine
   C. thyrotropin releasing hormone
   D. thyroid stimulating hormone

5. **Hyperthyroidism most frequently results from**
   A. thyroid carcinoma
   B. multinodular goiter
   C. pituitary adenoma secretion of TSH
   D. autoimmune disorder

6. **Tertiary hypothyroidism is the result of**
   A. abnormality in the thyroid itself
   B. pituitary abnormality
   C. hypothalamic abnormality

7. **Which pair of thyroid measurements provides information about thyroxine from *direct* measurements?**
   A. total T_4 and free T_4 index
   B. total T_4 and T_3 uptake
   C. free T_4 and total T_4
   D. free T_4 and free T_4 index

8. **Two assays that provide information about thyroxine by indirect measure are**
   A. total T_4 and T_3 uptake
   B. T_3 uptake and free T_4 index
   C. free T_4 and free T_4 index
   D. total T_4 and free T_4 index

9. **Two measures of pituitary functionality and responsiveness are**
   A. TSH and TRH
   B. TRH and TgAb
   C. anti-TPO and TBG
   D. TBG and RAIU

10. **A common cause of reduced specificity in total thyroxine assays is**
   A. abnormal levels of iodine
   B. abnormalities of thyroid binding proteins
   C. abnormalities of tyrosine
   D. abnormal levels of microsomal antibodies

11. **Increased levels of total and free thyroxine are expected in all of the following *except***
   A. primary hyperthyroidism
   B. peripheral hormone resistance
   C. pituitary insufficiency
   D. factitious T_4 hyperthyroidism

12. **Increased TSH values may be seen in all of the following *except***
   A. pituitary insufficiency
   B. primary hypothyroidism
   C. TSH-secreting tumor
   D. Addison's disease

13. The thyroid status most likely to produce a baseline TSH of 15 μU/mL and a 30-minute TSH of 35 μU/mL in a TRH stimulation test is
    A. euthyroid
    B. hyperthyroid
    C. primary hypothyroid
    D. secondary hypothyroid

14. The two antibodies found in nearly all cases of chronic thyroiditis are
    A. anti-TPO and antibody to TSH receptor
    B. antibody to thyroglobulin and antibody to thyrotropin binding inhibitor
    C. antibody to thyroglobulin and antibody to TSH receptor
    D. anti-TPO and antibody to thyroglobulin

15. Differentiation of primary and secondary hypothyroidism is best established by
    A. thyroid scan
    B. TRH stimulation of TSH
    C. TSH stimulation of TRH
    D. detection of autoimmune antibodies

Match each test pattern provided with the condition most likely to produce this pattern by placing the appropriate letter in column 1. Assume high sensitivity TSH assay and valid results.

Condition	Question #	T_4, TOT	F T_4	TSH	T_3-RIA	T_3U	TRH Stimulation	Anti-TPO	TgAb	T_3 Suppression
	16.	↑	↑↑	↓	↑	↑	No signif. response			No suppression
	17.	↓	↓	↑↑	N/↓	↓	Exag response			
	18.	↓	↓	↑/N	↓		No signif. response			
	19.	N (50%) or ↓		↑	↓	↓		↑	↑ (80% >1:1000)	
	20.	↑	↑	N	↑					

A. primary hypothyroidism
B. secondary hypothyroidism
C. hyperthyroidism
D. peripheral hormone resistance
E. Hashimoto's thyroiditis

14. TESTS FOR ENDOCRINE DISORDERS

The endocrine system is composed of different **hormone secreting glands** located throughout the body. The various hormones from these glands are secreted directly into the blood and serve to elicit specific responses elsewhere in the body. Hormones act on specific targets either by binding to a specific receptor site on the cell's surface or by binding to a specific receptor molecule before traveling to the cell. Some hormones have the ability to stimulate the secretion of other hormones from certain endocrine glands. Hormones effect a wide variety of body processes, including growth, metabolism, and reproduction. They may be classified into a variety of categories based on chemical composition, but most are amino acid compounds. The hormones produced by the adrenal cortex and sex glands are steroids derived from lipids. The concentration of hormones is regulated by **continuous feedback mechanisms** that maintain each hormone at desired physiologic levels in the absence of disease. The diagnosis of endocrine disorders is made primarily by the direct measurement of specific hormone levels in the serum. Thyroid function is discussed in Chapter 13 and pancreatic endocrine function related to the regulation of blood glucose levels is discussed in Chapter 6. This chapter focuses on laboratory evaluation of disorders involving the pituitary and adrenal glands and on gonadal hormones.

THE PITUITARY GLAND

■ ANATOMY AND PHYSIOLOGY

The pituitary is a small, spherical gland with two physiologically distinct lobes: the **anterior lobe** and the **posterior lobe**. It is located just behind the point where the optic nerves cross and is connected to the brain by a short stalk. The body of the pituitary is contained within a small, bony structure called the *sella turcica*. Because of the number of hormones secreted by the pituitary and its effect on a number of other glands (ie, thyroid, adrenal, gonads), it is often referred to as the **master gland**.

■ PITUITARY HORMONES

Hormones secreted by the **anterior pituitary** (called the *adenohypophysis*) include those that stimulate endocrine secretion by the

- adrenal gland: **ACTH** (adrenocorticotropic hormone)
- thyroid gland: **TSH** (thyroid stimulating hormone)
- gonads: **FSH** (follicle stimulating hormone); **LH** (lutenizing hormone)
- mammary gland: **prolactin**

The anterior pituitary also secretes **growth hormone**, which affects skeletal growth, protein synthesis, and overall metabolism.

The **posterior pituitary** (neurohypophysis) secretes **ADH** (antidiuretic hormone or vasopressin) and **oxytocin** (stimulates smooth muscle contractions as in uterine contractions following childbirth). These hormones are only stored in the posterior pituitary after production in the hypothalamus.

■ FEEDBACK MECHANISMS

Release of hormones from both the anterior and posterior lobes of the pituitary is under the control of the hypothalamus, but is achieved by differing mechanisms. The release of hormones stored in the posterior pituitary, which is directly innervated by the hypothalamus, is controlled by **nerve impulses** traveling between the hypothalamus and the posterior pituitary. Hormones produced in the anterior pituitary are released when stimulated by **releasing hormones** from the hypothalamus. Feedback from target organs also serves to regulate the secretion of many hormones. Figure 14–1 illustrates the pituitary gland, pituitary hormones, and the relationship among the pituitary, hypothalamus, and feedback mechanisms.

PITUITARY HORMONES

Pituitary disorders may be **primary** (abnormality related to the pituitary gland itself) or **secondary** to a hypothalamic disorder or to target organ feedback mechanisms. The effect of disorders caused by tumors of the pituitary depends on the type of tumor present. Tumors may contain excessive numbers of cells that produce hormone or may destroy hormone-producing cells. Laboratory diagnosis or evaluation of pituitary disorders involves the measurement of the specific hormone levels in the blood. Although measurement of only a single hormone may be sufficient in some cases, measurement of additional hormone levels is often desirable in the determination of a disorder and is particularly helpful in establishing whether the disorder is primary or secondary. Most laboratory methods for the determination of hormone concentrations employ **immunoassay techniques** using monoclonal antibodies or enzyme labeling procedures. These methods are suitable for automated analyzers and provide results within a shorter time frame with greater ease of testing than radioimmunoassay methods. Testing for fre-

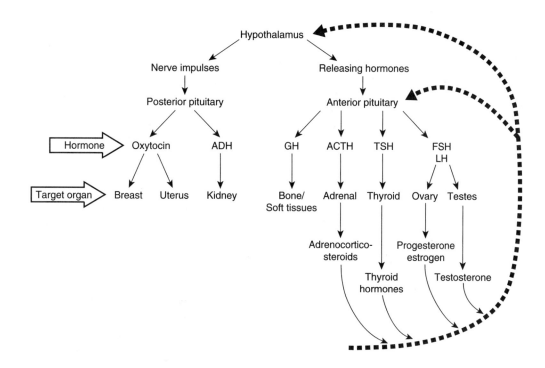

FIGURE 14-1. The pituitary hormones, target organs, and regulatory/feedback mechanisms.

quently requested hormone levels is available through most clinical laboratories, but those ordered less frequently may only be available through larger reference laboratories. Because of its anatomic location, pituitary disorders (especially those involving tumor or other enlargements of the gland) are often detected during evaluation of the optic chiasm. Other methods for evaluating the pituitary include x-ray examination of the skull, computed tomography (CT), and magnetic resonance imaging (MRI).

■ GROWTH HORMONE DISORDERS

Growth hormone (GH; also called *somatotropin*) is a peptide produced by the anterior pituitary. Two hypothalamic hormones regulate the release of growth hormone:

1. growth hormone releasing hormone (GHRH): stimulates the pituitary to release GH
2. growth hormone inhibiting hormone (GHIH; somatostatin): inhibits GH release

Although its principal effect is on bone and muscle development, GH has a general effect on most body tissues in terms of protein synthesis. It also mobilizes fatty acids for use by muscles during exercise and increases output of hepatic glucose. GH stimulates tissue to produce **somatomedins** (a group of growth factors), including somatomedin-C, which is produced by the liver and acts on cartilage. The somatomedins are an important component of the feedback mechanism. High concentrations of somatomedins directly inhibit pituitary release of GH and stimulate hypothalamic secretion of GHIH for further inhibition. A variety of other factors, including the level of some other hormones and the level of nutrients, also influence the production of GH. Secretion of GH occurs in short, irregular bursts primarily during sleep.

Growth hormone disorders may be seen in both children and adults, with symptoms of increased production evident in both groups. **Deficiencies of GH**, however, are more notable in children because the most noticeable physiologic effects of GH take place during infancy and childhood. Although a number of factors and hormones are necessary for appropriate growth and development, a deficiency of GH can produce profound clinical manifestations in children. GH deficiency may be suspected in children having very small stature or significantly retarded growth. Depending on the degree of deficiency, varying degrees of growth retardation are seen, with a total absence of GH producing growth rates as low as one-half that of normal (Henry, 1996). GH deficiency may occur alone or as part of a multihormonal dysfunction of the pituitary in which thyroid, adrenal, and gonadal development deficiencies are also present. The latter condition is referred to as **panhypopituitarism**. The pituitary dwarfism (very small stature with normal body proportions) produced by decreased GH levels is an uncommon condition and may be produced by

- pituitary tumors
- other types of pituitary damage
- isolated GH deficiency

In adults, a deficiency of GH alone does not produce a recognizable condition, with symptoms typically so vague as to remain undetected. A GH deficiency occurring with other pituitary hormone deficiencies produces symptoms related to those deficiencies (hypogonadism, hypothyroidism, hypoadrenalism). Pituitary tumors produce half of the pituitary deficiencies seen in adults, with most of the remainder resulting from idiopathic changes that develop gradually.

Excessive GH in actively growing children leads to **gigantism**, with abnormal elongation of the long bones. In adults, in whom an excess is more commonly seen, acromegaly is produced gradually. **Acromegaly** involves a thickening of the bones of the hands, feet, and skull—especially the bones of the forehead and lower jaw. Hypertrophy of the heart muscle and other internal organs is also seen and joint abnormalities may occur as a result of enlarged cartilage. Nerve compression may be seen as well.

Laboratory evaluation of growth hormone disorders involves direct measurement of GH, somatomedin-C assay, and GH stimulation tests. **Direct measurement of GH** is typically performed using immunoassay techniques (eg, radioimmunoassay) that measure the number of immunoreactive molecules of GH. Older bioassay methods measure biologic activity and modifications of these methods remain useful for assessment of functional activity of variant forms of GH (Henry, 1996). Assay of a single random specimen for GH can produce misleading results and is rarely clinically useful for a variety of reasons:

- variety of physiologic stimuli and inhibitors of GH secretion in addition to feedback mechanisms: stimuli include sleep, exercise, stress, hypoglycemia, various foods, and some pharmacologic agents; inhibitors include hyperglycemia and childhood emotional deprivation (Henry, 1996)
- circadian rhythm and sporadic secretion
- short half-life
- variations during menstrual cycle (highest during late follicular phase)
- clinical depression; clinically depressed patients secrete more GH than normal during waking hours (not during sleep) (Ravel, 1995)
- test method variations, including antibodies of varying specificities and measurement of different aspects of GH biochemistry

If a **single specimen** is to be used for screening purposes, it should be collected after an overnight fast and when the patient has awakened, but is not out of bed. Results that are at a level sufficient to rule out GH deficiency ($\geq$ 7 ng/ml [Ravel, 1995]) may be clinically useful. Any other result from a single specimen should not be relied upon for diagnostic purposes. More useful data are obtained by measuring GH in terms of 24-hour secretions and by GH stimulation tests. Other single specimen screening tests include collection of a sample 60 to 90 minutes after the patient enters deep sleep (determined by observation or by electroencephalographic stage 3 or 4). Approximately 70% of patients will have GH levels high enough to rule out GH deficiency (Ravel, 1995). Alternatively, a specimen may be collected following 20 to 30 minutes of vigorous exercise. Most normal children (75% to 92%) will have levels high enough to rule out GH deficiency (Ravel, 1995).

Determining **24-hour GH secretion** requires collection of specimens every 20 to 30 minutes. Although these measurements provide information regarding both 24-hour secretion and the diurnal pattern of secretion, other methods that are less time and labor intensive and require fewer specimens also provide meaningful data. Measurement of 24-hour secretion (some reports indicate measurement over 12 hours from 8 PM to 8 AM provides similar information [Ravel, 1995]) may be most useful when other tests produce equivocal findings.

Somatomedin C assay may be useful in the evaluation of GH disorders as well. Due to the relationship between the somatomedins and GH in terms of somatomedin mediation of GH activity and their role in feedback mechanisms, a normal somatomedin-C value suggests normal GH levels. Somatomedin-C levels are typically low in patients with isolated GH deficiency and in patients with pituitary insufficiency and elevated in acromegaly. Unlike direct GH measurement, somatomedin-C levels are not dependent on the time of day or on food intake. A number of non-pituitary conditions may produce low results, including a variety of severe chronic illnesses, malabsorption, malnutrition, hypothyroidism, and severe liver disease. Normal values are dependent on gender, age, and developmental stage. Unequivocally normal results are the most useful because low results should be confirmed by further testing.

Growth hormone stimulation tests are useful to confirm GH deficiency when results of previous testing are suggestive of deficiency or are low normal. Stimulation, or provocative, tests involve collection of a baseline sample followed by administration of a stimulus for GH secretion and subsequent sample collections. Because **insulin induced hypoglycemia** is a powerful stimulus for GH secretion, this is a frequently employed method, as is infusion of arginine. Induction of hypoglycemia with insulin requires a baseline glucose measurement (collected with the baseline GH specimen) followed by IV insulin administration until the serum glucose falls below a designated level (40 mg/dL [Henry, 1996]; 50 mg/dL [Sacher and McPherson, 1991]) or the patient is symptomatic of hypoglycemia. Samples are then collected at 30-minute intervals for 90 minutes (three samples). Glucose determinations may also be performed on these samples. Patients must be closely monitored for symptoms of severe hypoglycemia, and a failure to achieve sufficient GH increases in response to either insulin or arginine suggests GH deficiency, but does not differentiate between pituitary and hypothalamic etiologies. **L-dopa**, which stimulates hypothalamic release of GHRH, may be a useful stimulating agent in distinguishing the two. In addition to laboratory evaluation of GH, hand-wrist x-rays for bone maturation studies are important in the evaluation of suspected growth disorders.

■ PROLACTIN DISORDERS

Prolactin is a single chain polypeptide (recent evidence suggests a "family" of hormones of varying size and biochemical and physiologic properties [Henry, 1996]) hormone secreted by the anterior pituitary. In females, its primary role is the stimulation of lactation. Its role in the male, though less certain, may involve growth and development of the prostate (Henry, 1996). Prolactin may also have a role in immunoregulation in terms of lymphocyte actions (Henry, 1996; Sacher and McPherson, 1991). Physiologic regulation of prolactin levels is primarily through inhibition by PIF (prolactin inhibiting factor) rather than by positive stimulation of secretion. A specific prolactin stimulating factor has not been identified, but TRH (thyroid releasing hormone) stimulates hypothalamic release of prolactin in addition to TSH (Ravel, 1995). Prolactin is secreted in a **diurnal pattern** similar to that of GH, with the highest levels occurring during sleep. Serum prolactin levels increase in response to nursing, pregnancy, sexual intercourse, sleep, stress, exercise, hypoglycemia, anxiety, and a variety of medications. Pathologic increases in prolactin secretion are associated with hypogonadism and may result in suppression of ovulation in women and inhibited testosterone synthesis in men. Prolactin measurements are useful in the evaluation of amenorrhea and galactorrhea and in the diagnosis of prolactinomas, pituitary acidophil adenomas. Pathologic conditions associated with increased serum prolactin levels are listed in Table 14–1.

Although there is considerable overlap, very high prolactin levels are more likely to result from pituitary adenoma that other causes. Most (45% to 81%) pituitary adenomas produce prolactin levels > 1000 ng/mL (Ravel, 1995).

Laboratory assays for prolactin are available as immunoassays and as bioassays. Test methods that utilize monoclonal "sandwich" immunoassays calibrated against the same standard provide the least amount of interassay variability (Henry, 1996). Bioassay results are typically higher than immunoassay values (bioassay about 1.5 times higher than IRMA [immunoradiometric assay]; Henry, 1996), with some noteworthy exceptions. In some lactating women whose ovulation was not suppressed by elevated prolactin levels (by immunoassay), bioassay results were significantly lower, and breast cancer patients had a significantly higher ratio of bioassay to immunoassay prolactin results—breast cancer group 2.9; control group 1.3 (Henry, 1996). The cause for this difference is as yet unknown.

Autoantibodies directed against prolactin have been detected in the serum of some patients with elevated prolactin levels. These autoantibodies can interfere with immunoassay methods by competing with the reagent antibody, producing falsely decreased prolactin levels. Tests for the presence of these autoantibodies are available from reference laboratories. Falsely reduced levels can also be produced by the prozone effect with very high prolactin levels. Dilution of the sample overcomes the prozone effect.

Prolactin stimulation and suppression tests are available and may be useful in differentiating pituitary adenoma from other causes of elevated serum prolactin levels. Normally administration of TRH or chlorpromazine produces a significant increase (≥ two-fold increase [Ravel, 1995]) in serum prolactin levels and L-dopa

TABLE 14–1. Pathologic Increases in Serum Prolactin Levels

Pituitary adenoma
Hypothalamic lesions (space occupying; granulomatous; or destructive)
Primary hypothyroidism
Nelson's syndrome (see Addison's disease discussion)
Empty sella syndrome
Nonpituitary prolactin secreting neoplasms (ectopic prolactin secretion)
Polycystic ovary disease
Post-partum amenorrhea
Post-pill amenorrhea–galactorrhea syndrome
Chronic renal failure
Alcoholic cirrhosis

TABLE 14–2. Prolactin Stimulation/Suppression Test Results[1]

Condition	Response to		
	TRH	**Chlorpromazine**	**L-Dopa**
Pituitary adenoma	Blunted	Blunted	Normal
Pituitary insufficiency	None	None	None
Hypothalamic dysfunction	Normal	Little to none	Blunted

[1]Expected/typical results; overlap is seen between adenoma and nonadenoma responses; results of these tests alone may be diagnostically insufficient.

produces a decrease. Table 14–2 summarizes typical responses to these substances in selected conditions. Other factors that influence pituitary function or prolactin secretion can affect these results.

◼ ANTIDIURETIC HORMONE DISORDERS

Antidiuretic hormone (ADH; also called *arginine vasopressin* [AVP] or *vasopressin*) is synthesized in the hypothalamus and stored in the posterior pituitary. The antidiuretic effects of ADH result from its action on the distal convoluted tubule and the collecting ducts. ADH acts to increase cellular permeability to water allowing reabsorption of water from the renal tubules. It also promotes the reabsorption of sodium and chloride in the ascending loop of Henle. This hormone promotes the contraction of smooth arterial muscle as well. By virtue of its antidiuretic and vasopressor effects, ADH acts in conjunction with other mechanisms and the angiotensin-renin-aldosterone system to maintain blood pressure, volume, and tonicity at appropriate levels. ADH levels are influenced by several factors and physiologic stimuli:

- changes in blood volume: diminished volume ($\sim 10\%$ loss) directly provokes ADH release
- changes in serum osmolality: hypothalamus is responsive to changes as small as 1% and ADH is usually secreted when osmolality exceeds 285 mOsm (Sacher and McPherson, 1991)
- dehydration: results in ADH secretion to decrease water loss which, in conjunction with the thirst reflex, works to stabilize water status
- alcohol and phenytoin: inhibit ADH secretion
- morphine, barbiturates, and cholinergic drugs: stimulate release of ADH

The two major ADH abnormalities are **diabetes insipidus** and **the syndrome of inappropriate ADH secretion** (SIADH). Diabetes insipidus (DI) occurs when the production of or response to ADH is inadequate. Thirst and hypotonic polyuria with daily urinary excretion of 3 liters or more and urine specific gravity 1.010 or osmolality < 300 mOsm characterize this condition. Differing etiologies can produce DI:

- impaired hypothalamic production or pituitary release of ADH resulting from tissue destruction (trauma, neoplasm, inflammation, surgery); neurogenic
- impaired renal response to ADH; nephrogenic; may be congenital or acquired as a result of certain drugs or secondary to hypercalcemia, hypokalemia, or amyloidosis
- temporary overpowering of ADH system by abnormal fluid intake (psychogenic polydipsia or compulsive water drinking)
- idiopathic; no clearly defined etiology

Laboratory assays for the diagnosis of DI are usually based on determinations of responses to body fluid alterations. **Direct measurement of ADH** may be used in conjunction with water deprivation testing, but is often unnecessary. ADH is measured using radioimmunoassay (RIA) techniques. A variety of interfering substances make ADH values difficult to interpret and may obscure ADH, which is normally present in low concentration (normal values about 2.3 to 3.1 pg/ml [pg = picogram]; Sacher and McPherson, 1991). These assays are also generally expensive, technically difficult, and available only through some reference laboratories. Serum ADH levels may be undetectable in DI patients. ADH assays should never be used for diagnostic and treatment decisions without knowledge of the patient's serum and urine osmolality, intravascular volume status, and blood pressure (Henry, 1996). Direct measurements may be more useful when a renal function disorder coexists with ADH deficiency or with patients who are unable to tolerate physiologic testing.

The usual diagnostic procedure for DI is the **water deprivation test** (also called the *dehydration test*). Before this testing is initiated, preliminary testing to establish the presence of hypotonic polyuria and to rule out common causes of polyuria should be performed. A 24-hour urine specimen and a blood specimen should be collected and tested:

- urine volume measurement: quantity in excess of 2L/24h establishes polyuria
- urine osmolality: values < 300 mOsm are hypotonic
- serum osmolality
- serum sodium, potassium, calcium, glucose, BUN

Other tests may be warranted to rule out other suspected conditions. Water deprivation testing can be initiated if hypotonic polyuria is demonstrated and other causes (especially hyperglycemia, hypokalemia, hypercalcemia, uremia, excessive electrolyte or diuretic therapy, osmotic diuresis, severe chronic renal disease, acute tubular necrosis) have been ruled out. Other relatively common causes of polyuria include pregnancy and sickle cell disease. Any medications affecting ADH secretion should be stopped at least 24 hours prior to testing. Patients should refrain from using alcohol, caffeine, and tobacco 24 hours prior to and throughout testing and hypercalcemia or hypernatremia should be corrected before testing begins

(Ravel, 1995). Baseline urine and serum samples are collected for osmolality determinations. All fluids are then withheld for a period of 6 to 12 hours (or until concentration plateau is reached) with urine samples collected each hour for osmolality determinations. It is essential that patients are closely monitored throughout testing to avoid overdehydration, especially patients with severe polyuria (ie, the greater the urinary output, the greater the need for careful monitoring). Close monitoring also aids in preventing surreptitious fluid consumption, particularly in patients with psychogenic polydipsia. Patients may be weighed at the time of urine collection as an additional monitoring tool. A total weight loss exceeding 2 kilograms warrants termination of the procedure (Ravel, 1995).

As body water diminishes urine concentration increases until a plateau is reached at which no further concentration occurs. This plateau is demonstrated during testing by a stable urine osmolality for three consecutive hours. This concentration plateau usually occurs after 16 to 18 hours in normal individuals, but may occur after 4 to 8 hours in DI (Sacher and McPherson, 1991). Normal individuals will preserve serum osmolality and have urine osmolality values $\geq$ 800 mOsm following 8 to 12 hours of fluid deprivation. Urine osmolality in individuals with ADH deficiency does not rise above 300 mOsm. After the concentration plateau is reached, exogenous ADH administration (subcutaneous administration of 5 units of aqueous AVP [Henry, 1996; Ravel, 1995]) can provide additional diagnostic information and aid in determination of etiology. A serum osmolality should be performed before administration to assure a serum osmolality of $\geq$ 288 mOsm. A urine specimen for osmolality determination is collected 1 hour (Henry, 1996; 30 to 60 minutes according to Ravel [1995]) after administration. Table 14–3 summarizes the results of testing.

In **SIADH** (syndrome of inappropriate ADH secretion), as implied by the name, ADH secretion continues despite conditions in which ADH would not normally be secreted. The syndrome may result from a variety of causes:

- various malignancies (especially lung cancer)
- infections, trauma, or neoplasms of the central nervous system
- pulmonary infections
- secondary to several endocrinopathies (including Addison's disease)
- various medications (the antineoplastics vincristine and cyclophosphamide, the oral antidiabetic drugs chlorpropamide and tolbutamide; opiates; barbiturates; carbamazepine [Ravel, 1995])

Patients may present with lethargy, nausea, vomiting, muscle cramps, confusion, anorexia, coma, and seizures. SIADH is characterized by:

- significant hyponatremia with continued renal excretion of sodium (hyponatremia may be masked by dehydration)
- low serum osmolality
- urine osmolality inappropriately elevated for serum sodium and osmolality levels (hallmark finding)

TABLE 14–3. Water Deprivation and ADH Testing for Diabetes Insipidus

	Normal	Neurogenic DI	Nephrogenic DI	Primary Polydipsia	Osmotic Diuresis
Urine osmolality					
Baseline	N (avg 300-800 mOsm)	↓	↓	↓	↑
Plateau	↑ (≤ 1600 mOsm)	↓/N	↓/N	↓/(N (but > serum)	↑
Change post-AVP	little to none	increases (> 9%)	very little	very little	very little
Serum osmolality					
Baseline	N	N/↑	N/↑	N/↓	↑
Post-fluid depriv.	N	↑	↑	N	↑
Serum ADH					
Baseline	N	↓	N/↑	↓	
Post-fluid depriv.	↑	↓	↑	N/↑	
Urine sodium					
Baseline	N	↓	↓	↓	
Post-fluid depriv.	↑	↓/N	↓/N	N/↑	
Serum sodium					
Baseline	N	N/↑	N/↑	↓/N	
Post-fluid depriv.	N	↑	↑	N	

N = normal; ↓ = decreased; ↑ = increased; depriv. = deprivation.

Table compiled from data from Henry JB. *Clinical Diagnosis and Management by Laboratory Methods,* 19th ed. Philadelphia, Saunders, 1996; Ravel R. *Clinical Laboratory Medicine: Clinical Application of Laboratory Data,* 6th ed. St Louis, Mosby, 1995; and Sacher RA, McPherson RA. *Widmann's Clinical Interpretation of Laboratory Tests,* 10th ed. Philadelphia, FA Davis, 1991.

Measuring ADH levels is rarely necessary to make a diagnosis of SIADH. It is important to rule out other causes of hyponatremia including renal disease, adrenal dysfunction, and chronic gastrointestinal tract disease. The high blood volume, hyponatremic conditions of cirrhosis, and cardiac failure should also be ruled out (Sacher and McPherson, 1991).

The **water loading test** is used to assess the ability to suppress ADH secretion. The test is contraindicated for patients with renal or adrenal insufficiency and should not be initiated until other causes of hyponatremia have been ruled out and the serum sodium level is raised to a minimum level of 125 mEq/L (Henry, 1996; Sacher and McPherson, 1991). This test involves giving the patient a specified volume of water to drink (1 liter according to Sacher and McPherson, [1991]; 20 ml water per kilogram of body weight according to Henry [1996]) and collecting urine specimens for osmolality and volume determinations for 5 hours. Serum samples are also collected hourly for osmolality determinations. Baseline samples should be collected before water loading begins. The patient should drink the entire volume of water in < 30 minutes and should be lying down for the remainder of the test period. Table 14–4 summarizes the results of the water loading test in SIADH and in normal individuals.

If serum ADH is assayed, SIADH patients will have elevated values. Patients are treated with water restriction and may be given demeclocycline (600 to 1200 mg daily) to induce a nephrogenic diabetes insipidus (Stein, 1993). Demeclocycline is contraindicated in the presence of liver disease.

TABLE 14–4. Water Loading Test Results

	Normal	**SIADH**
Serum Osmolality		
Baseline	N	↓
Post-H_2O load	Falls	Falls
Urine Osmolality		
Baseline	N	N - ↑
Post-H_2O load	Falls	Remains higher than
	w/ lowest < 100 mOsm	serum osmolality
Water Excretion	> 60% of H_2O load at 4 hrs	< 60% of H_2O load at 4 hrs
	> 80% of H_2O load at 5 hrs	< 80% of H_2O load at 5 hrs

↑ = increased; ↓ = decreased; N = normal.

Table compiled from data from Henry JB. *Clinical Diagnosis and Management by Laboratory Methods,* 19th ed. Philadelphia, Saunders, 1996; Ravel R. *Clinical Laboratory Medicine: Clinical Application of Laboratory Data,* 6th ed. St Louis, Mosby, 1995; and Sacher RA, McPherson RA. *Widmann's Clinical Interpretation of Laboratory Tests,* 10th ed. Philadelphia, FA Davis, 1991.

 TIME FOR REVIEW. After studying the preceding sections, you should be able to respond correctly to the following:

■ List the hormones secreted by

the anterior pituitary:

the posterior pituitary:

■ Briefly describe the feedback mechanisms regulating pituitary hormone release.

■ Distinguish between primary and secondary pituitary disorders.

■ Growth hormone is also called _____.

■ Growth hormone release is stimulated by _____ and inhibited by _____.

■ Briefly describe the effects of growth hormone.

■ Growth hormone deficiencies may occur alone or as part of a multihormonal dysfunction of the pituitary called _____ .

■ List three causes of pituitary dwarfism.

■ Excessive growth hormone in adults produces a condition called _____. List symptoms of this disorder.

■ Laboratory evaluation of growth hormone disorders involves _____, _____, and _____.

■ Why is a single, random specimen for growth hormone generally not clinically useful?

■ Briefly describe the test for growth hormone stimulation including appropriate patient care precautions.

■ The stimulating agent that may be useful in distinguishing between pituitary and hypothalamic etiologies of growth hormone deficiency is

_____.

■ Prolactin levels are increased in response to a variety of factors, including

_____, _____,

_____, _____, and

_____.

■ Prolactin measurements are useful in the evaluation of

_____ and _____ and

in the diagnosis of _____.

■ List seven conditions associated with pathologic increases in prolactin levels.

■ Very high prolactin levels are more likely to result from

_____ than from other causes.

■ Briefly describe the typical responses to prolactin stimulation and suppression tests in

pituitary adenoma:

pituitary insufficiency:

hypothalamic dysfunction:

■ Briefly describe the actions of ADH.

■ The two major ADH abnormalities are _____ and
_____. Provide a brief description of each of these
abnormalities.

■ Describe the water deprivation test and its diagnostic usefulness.

■ Review Table 14–3.

■ Describe the water loading test and its application to the diagnosis of SIADH.

Check your responses by reviewing the preceding sections.

THE ADRENAL GLANDS

The adrenal glands are small, triangular endocrine glands consisting of an inner medulla and an outer cortex. One adrenal gland is located on the top of each kidney. These glands play an important role in:

- maintaining blood pressure
- maintaining appropriate electrolyte levels
- controlling renal function
- controlling overall body fluid concentration

■ ADRENAL HORMONES

The **adrenal hormones** include catecholamines, steroids, and androgens as summarized below.

- medulla: dopamine, epinephrine, and norepinephrine; involved in regulation of acute responses to environmental stimuli (eg, acutely stressful situations, "fight or flight" responses)
- cortex: three groups of hormones
  — glucocorticoids: involved in carbohydrate metabolism; needed in times of stress to help maintain glucose levels, prevent shock; cortisol is an important glucocorticoid
  — mineralcorticoids: aldosterone, which promotes reabsorption of salt and water in the kidney and cortisone
  — androgens: sex hormones important in growth and maturation

■ LABORATORY ASSAYS

Adrenal hormone deficiencies or excesses can be diagnosed by laboratory assay of the hormone or metabolites of the hormone. Table 14–5 lists some of the tests used in the evaluation of adrenal disorders. Although laboratory assays are discussed in terms of specific adrenal disorders in the subsequent sections, plasma cortisol is presented here in more detail as it is a widely used test and is affected by a variety of variables.

PLASMA CORTISOL. Direct measurement of total cortisol (ie, bound, physiologically inactive and unbound or free cortisol—10% of total) is available by a variety of immunoassay techniques including RIA and enzyme immunoassay (EIA). Older, less specific methods include colorimetric (Porter-Silber method) and fluorescent techniques. Table 14–6 summarizes factors important in the evaluation of plasma cortisol levels.

TABLE 14–5. Laboratory Assays Used in Evaluating Adrenal Disorders

Category	Test
Plasma tests	Cortisol
	Aldosterone
	17-hydroxyprogesterone
	11-deoxycortisol
	Renin
	ACTH
Urine tests	Free cortisol
	Aldosterone
	VMA
	Metanephrines and normetanephrines
	17-ketosteroids
	17-hydroxycorticoids
	ACTH
	Pregnanetriol
Suppression, stimulation, and other tests	Dexamethasone suppression
	ACTH stimulation
	CRH stimulation
	Metyrapone suppression
	Insulin tolerance test
	Cortrosyn response
	Vasopressin volume expansion
	Furosemide response
	Clonidine suppression

TABLE 14–6. Important Factors in Plasma Cortisol Evaluation

Factors Causing		Other Factors
Increased Values	Decreased Values	
Oral contraceptives (increases free and bound)	Increased androgens (affects bound only)	Diurnal variation: AM values are significantly higher than PM values; values peak about 8 AM (6 to 8 AM)
Hyperthryroidism (affects bound only)	Hypothyroidism (affects bound only)	Method variables: specificity interferences cross-reactivity with other steroids
Pregnancy (increases free and bound)	Markedly decreased serum albumin (affects bound only)	
False elevations caused by stress obesity severe liver disease severe renal disease	Dilantin (decreases binding proteins)	

ADRENAL DISORDERS

■ ADDISON'S DISEASE

Addison's disease, also called *chronic adrenal insufficiency* or *hypocortisolism,* occurs as a result of insufficient production of the glucocorticoid cortisol. Aldosterone is also deficient in some cases. In addition to its role in responses to stress, cortisol plays a role in the maintenance of blood pressure and cardiovascular function; assists in balancing insulin's effects; aids in the regulation of protein, carbohydrate, and fat metabolism; and assists in slowing inflammatory responses.

Symptoms of Addison's disease usually begin gradually and include fatigue, weight loss, muscle weakness, and hypotension worsening on standing. A craving for salty foods is common. Irritability, depression, irregular menstrual cycles, and hypoglycemia may also be present. Hyperpigmentation of the skin may be present and is most obvious on scars, elbows, knees and other pressure points, lips, and mucous membranes. Although symptom severity is typically sufficient to prompt the patient to seek medical attention, symptoms may be ignored in some cases until a stressful event precipitates an **addisonian crisis**, or acute worsening of symptoms. An addisonian crisis characteristically results in sudden pain in the lower back, abdomen, or legs, with severe vomiting and diarrhea leading to dehydration, low blood pressure, and eventual loss of consciousness. Without appropriate medical intervention, the crisis may be fatal.

Cortisol production occurs when the adrenal glands are stimulated by pituitary secretion of ACTH in response to hypothalamic release of corticotropin releasing hormone (CRH). Insufficient cortisol production, then, may be primary due to a disorder of the adrenal glands themselves or secondary as a result of inadequate pituitary secretion of ACTH. **Primary adrenal insufficiency** occurs as a result of damage to or destruction of the adrenal glands. Most cases (~ 70% according to NIH publication 90-3054) result from a gradual destruction of the adrenal cortex due to autoimmune processes. Mineralcorticoid hormones may also be deficient because adrenal insufficiency is evident only after significant destruction of the cortex occurs. The adrenal glands are the only affected gland in idiopathic adrenal insufficiency, but adrenal insufficiency also occurs in the polyendocrine deficiency syndrome. There are two types of this syndrome:

1. Type I, seen in children: adrenal insufficiency can be accompanied by hypoparathyroidism, slow sexual development, pernicious anemia, chronic candidiasis, chronic active hepatitis, or, rarely, hair loss (NIH publication 90-3054)

2. Type II, also called *Schmidt syndrome,* usually seen in young adults: features may include hypothryoidism, slow sexual development, and diabetes mellitus; patients may also have vitiglio (loss of pigmentation in some areas of the skin) (NIH publication 90-3054)

Primary adrenal insufficiency may also result from tuberculosis of the adrenal glands. Less common causes include chronic infections, metastatic carcinoma, amyloidosis, and surgical removal of the adrenal glands.

Secondary adrenal insufficiency occurs as a result of ACTH deficiency from a variety of causes, including:

- glucocorticoid hormone therapy (eg, prednisone); such therapy is used to treat inflammatory conditions and autoimmune disorders, and is included in some anticancer regimens and in immunosuppressive therapy; prednisone blocks the release of CRH and ACTH
- surgical removal of ACTH producing tumors of the pituitary (Cushing disease); replacement therapy allows normal ACTH production to resume
- pituitary tumors or infections
- surgical removal of portions of the pituitary or hypothalamus

Addison's disease patients typically have low plasma cortisol levels, low urinary free cortisol, and decreased levels of the urinary metabolites. Although single plasma cortisol samples have been used to screen for Addison's disease, this approach is generally considered to be unreliable. A specimen collected at 8:00 AM may, in some cases, be useful in excluding Addison's. A morning plasma cortisol level > 20 µg/dL is strong evidence against the presence of Addison's disease (Ravel, 1995). However, because stress and other factors can increase plasma cortisol levels, results must be evaluated cautiously. A more specific and diagnostically reliable test involves assessing the response to injection of synthetic ACTH (cosyntropin [Cortrosyn; Synacthen]). The test may be referred to as the *rapid ACTH stimulation test* or the *Cortrosyn response test*. In this procedure a baseline plasma cortisol sample is collected and 0.25 mg of Cortrosyn administered intramuscularly or intravenously (IM routinely used; IV preferred for severely ill or hypotensive patients to avoid absorption problems [Ravel, 1995]). Samples for plasma cortisol assay are collected at 30 minutes and at 60 minutes following Cortrosyn administration. (Some procedures eliminate collection of a 30-minute sample.) A doubling of the plasma cortisol level is considered to be a normal response, but other criteria may also be applied by some endocrinologists, as summarized in Table 14–7.

TABLE 14–7. Additional Criteria for Determination of Normal Rapid Cortrosyn Response Test

Criteria	Baseline	Amount Above Baseline		Peak	Comments
		30 MIN	*60 MIN*		
1[1]	5 µ/dL	≥ 7 µ/dL	≥ 11 µ/dL	—	Or 30 min sample > 18 µ/dL
2[2]	—	—	≥ 10 µ/dL	—	
3[3]	—	—	≥ 7 µ/dL	20 µ/dL	

From [1]Henry JB. *Clinical Diagnosis and Management by Laboratory Methods,* 19th ed. Philadelphia, Saunders, 1996; [2]Sacher RA, McPherson RA. *Widmann's Clinical Interpretation of Laboratory Tests,* 10th ed. Philadelphia, FA Davis, 1991; and [3]Ravel R. *Clinical Laboratory Medicine: Clinical Application of Laboratory Data,* 6th ed. St Louis, Mosby, 1995.

Patients with a primary adrenal insufficiency should have little to no response. Those with secondary adrenal insufficiency may or may not respond. Aldosterone levels can be measured along with cortisol levels to aid in distinguishing the two. Patients with pituitary insufficiency should have significant increases in aldosterone levels, while those with primary adrenal insufficiency have no significant increase. Confirmation of an abnormal rapid Cortrosyn response test and substantiation of a diagnosis of primary or secondary adrenal insufficiency is accomplished by using prolonged ACTH stimulation. In this procedure, synthetic ACTH is administered daily for 2 to 3 days (sources vary on how long the test should be: 2 days according to Henry [1996]; 3 to 5 days according to Sacher and McPherson [1991]; and 8-hour infusion for 1 day, 2 days if pituitary deficiency suspected, and 5 to 7 days if exogenous steroids have been taken for long periods according to Ravel [1995]). Samples for plasma cortisol assay and urine samples for 17-hydroxycorticoid assay are collected the day before testing begins and each day during the test. Results are summarized in Table 14–8.

Because long periods of glucocorticoid hormone therapy interfere with the pituitary-adrenal feedback system, the adrenal glands require longer periods of ACTH stimulation to achieve adequate responsiveness. Normal responses may not be achieved for as long as 5 to 7 days (Ravel, 1995). Rapid ACTH stimulation testing can be performed on patients in crisis if dexamethasone therapy is initiated to supply steroid treatment (Henry, 1996; Ravel, 1995; Stein, 1993; see Stein, 1993, for additional treatment information). Low doses of dexamethasone do not significantly interfere with cortisol assays (Ravel, 1995).

The **insulin tolerance test** (ITT), or insulin induced hypoglycemia test, is a reliable test for evaluation of the entire hypothalamic-pituitary-adrenal axis. After an overnight fast, baseline samples are collected for glucose and cortisol assay. An IV bolus of 0.10 units of regular insulin per kilogram of body weight (Stein, 1993) is administered and samples collected at 30, 60, and 90 minutes. Glucose levels should fall to 50% of the baseline measurement of to ≤ 40 mg/dL in order to produce an adequate stimulus. A plasma cortisol increase of at least 10 µ/dL above baseline or to at least 20 µ/dL total is considered a normal response. As noted in the previous discussion of this test for the stimulation of GH production, close observation of the patient is essential throughout the test because of the potential for development of severe hypoglycemia. Supplies should be readily available for reversal of the hypoglycemic state if warranted.

TABLE 14–8. Evaluation of Prolonged ACTH Stimulation Test

	Plasma Cortisol	**Urinary 17-Hydroxycorticoids**
Normal response	2-4 X baseline value	2-5 X baseline value
Primary Addison's	Little or no change from baseline	Little or no change from baseline
Secondary Addison's	Relatively small, gradual response with adequate response generally seen by day 2 or 3	Little or no change from baseline on day 1; slight increase on day 2; response usually adequate by day 3

Treatment for Addison's disease involves glucocorticoid replacement therapy. Those with primary adrenal insufficiency typically require mineralcorticoid therapy as well and an adequate salt intake (Stein, 1993).

■ CONGENITAL ADRENAL HYPERPLASIA

Congenital adrenal hyperplasia (CAH) is an autosomal recessive inherited disorder resulting from genetic defects in the genes that code for one of several enzymes involved in the chain of reactions leading to the production of adrenal hormones from precursor substances. The majority of CAH cases result from a deficiency of the enzyme 21-hydroxylase necessary for the effective production of cortisol and aldosterone. Although clinical and laboratory findings are dependent on which enzyme is deficient and thus which metabolic pathway and precursor substance is affected, all CAH variants affect the cortisol pathway to some extent. The following discussion focuses on CAH variants involving 21-hydroxylase deficiency.

In **21-hydroxylase CAH,** the precursor substances required for the formation of cortisol and aldosterone are still manufactured, but cannot be converted to these hormones because of the deficient enzyme. Feedback mechanisms, sensing the low cortisol levels, cause ACTH to be secreted at increased levels in an attempt to stimulate adrenal production of cortisol. The result is glandular hyperplasia with increasingly higher levels of the precursor substances. Most of the early cortisol precursors are also intermediate compounds in the production of androgens. Because normal production of cortisol is blocked, metabolic pathways shift to utilize excess precursors for the production of androgens resulting in abnormally high levels of testosterone.

Although CAH is an inherited disorder typically detected at birth or in early childhood, symptoms may manifest at any time. Symptoms are dependent on the degree of enzyme deficiency, which is impacted by heterozygous versus homozygous inheritance and by degrees of penetrance. In some cases of partial enzyme deficiency, hormones may be produced at or near normal levels. In other cases, patients may be symptomatic only in times of stress. Classic CAH-21-hydroxylase deficiency results in **deficient levels of both cortisol and aldosterone** with excessive androgen production beginning in utero. The impaired aldosterone production results in sodium loss causing salt losing crises similar to those seen in Addison's disease. Affected infants are predisposed to severe dehydration, shock, and, without proper diagnosis and treatment, death. The abnormally high levels of testosterone cause the clitoris of female infants to grow abnormally. Masculinization of the genitourinary structures results in pseudohermaphroditism, or ambiguous genitalia. Severely affected females may be identified as males at birth. Affected males typically have normal genitalia at birth, but will have unusually fast growth, early puberty, premature growth completion, and accentuation of the male genitalia.

Hormone measurements in conjunction with clinical evaluation have traditionally constituted the basis for diagnosis of CAH. Newer genetic testing techniques may be useful in the resolution of ambiguous hormone assays and in providing information to parents of CAH children as to their risk of having another affected infant. The genotypic sex of infants with ambiguous genitalia can be presumptively established by obtaining a buccal smear for the **Barr body examination**. In this procedure, a scraping of the oral mucosa is obtained and the epithelial cells examined for the presence or absence of Barr bodies. Barr bodies are stainable sex chromatin masses found in the nuclei of various cells. A Barr body is present for each X chromosome above one that the cell contains. Because the normal male genotype is XY, cells contain only one X chromosome and thus no Barr bodies. Normal females have two X chromosomes (XX), so cells have one Barr body. Barr bodies are only identifiable in about half of normal female cells (Ravel, 1995). This testing should not be performed until after the first week of life because the incidence of chromatin positive cells is lower during this period. **Chromosome karyotyping** (chromosome analysis) may be used as confirmation of Barr body results if indicated. To perform chromosome karyotyping, cell cultures are chemically treated to kill cells at the metaphase stage of mitosis, when chromosomes are organized and separated. The chromosomes are then photographed and the individual chromosomes separated and classified, and a chromosome chart is prepared and analyzed. Such studies require significant knowledge, expertise, and specialized equipment typically available only through reference laboratories. Chromosome karyotyping can be performed on a variety of specimen types including blood, bone marrow, and tissue. The laboratory should be contacted for specimen collection and transport instructions. Laboratory findings for hormone measurements in CAH-21-hydroxylase deficiency are summarized in Table 14–9 along with some other CAH variants.

TABLE 14–9. Laboratory Hormonal Findings in Selected CAH Enzyme Deficiencies

| Deficient Enzyme | Laboratory Findings | | Comments |
	Plasma/Serum	Urine	
21-Hydroxylase	↑ 17-Hydroxyprogesterone	↑ 17-Ketosteroids ↑ Pregnanetriol	Most common cause of CAH; deficient in CAH types I & II; adrenocorticoid insufficiency present in < 1/3; female virilized
11-Hydroxylase	↑ 11-Deoxycortisol	↑ 17-Hydroxycortico-steroids	Hypertension present in most cases; female virilized
17-Hydroxylase	—	↑ 17-Hydroxycortico-steroids ↑ 17-Ketosteroids ↑ Metabolites of corticosterone & 11-deoxycorticosterone	Absent secondary sex characteristics; hypertension present
20,22-Desmolase	All adrenal steroids ↓	All adrenal steroids ↓	Adrenocorticoid insufficiency present; lack of masculinization

Manifestation of virilism in females and excessive masculinization of males in later childhood or in adulthood may result from late manifestation of a congenital enzyme deficiency, from idiopathic hyperplasia of the adrenal cortex, or from adenoma or carcinoma of the adrenal cortex. **Carcinoma of the adrenal cortex** is the more common (Ravel, 1995; Sacher and McPherson, 1991) of these causes and results in increased levels of 17-hydroxycorticosteroids and 17-ketosteroids.

■ CUSHING SYNDROME

Cushing syndrome (also called *hypercortisolism*) is a relatively rare disorder resulting from the exposure of the body's tissues to excessive concentrations of cortisol or other adrenal glucocorticoids. Androgens may also be produced in excess. The condition may be the result of **adrenal cortex overproduction** or may be **secondary to glucocorticoid hormone therapy** (iatrogenic). Adrenal overproduction of cortisol, the form addressed in this section, may be seen as a consequence of:

- ACTH-secreting pituitary tumors: benign tumors of pituitary that secrete increased amounts of ACTH cause the most common form of Cushing syndrome called *Cushing disease;* affects women more frequently than men
- adenoma of the adrenal cortex: ademonas release excess cortisol; average age of onset is 40
- adrenocortical carcinoma: malignant cells secrete excess levels of several hormones including cortisol and androgens; very high hormone levels and rapid symptom development; least common cause of Cushing syndrome
- ectopic ACTH production: excess ACTH production from benign or malignant non-pituitary tumors; lungs are most common site

Symptoms of Cushing syndrome are variable but typically include upper body obesity, a rounded puffy face ("moon face"), increased fat deposits on the back of the neck ("buffalo hump"), and thinning of the extremities. The highest incidence of Cushing is in adults, but affected children tend to be obese and have slowed growth rates. Other symptoms include easy bruising; the appearance of striae on the abdomen, thighs, and other areas; osteoporosis; and severe fatigue. Affected individuals have a tendency to develop hypertension and hyperglycemia and may exhibit irritability, anxiety, and depression. Affected females (women are affected four times more often than men [Ravel, 1995]) typically have excess hair growth on the face, neck, chest, abdomen, and thighs and menstrual periods may become irregular or stop. Men exhibit diminished or absent sexual desire and decreased fertility.

Laboratory diagnosis includes measurement of **24-hour urinary free cortisol level**. Although this test is a relatively specific diagnostic screening test for Cushing syndrome, results may be affected by some of the same factors affecting plasma cortisol levels. Accurate collection of the 24-hour sample is essential for valid results. Levels are elevated in about 95 % of Cushing syndrome patients (Ravel, 1995). Single specimen plasma cortisol levels and measurement of urine 17-ketosteroids are not reliable screening tools for Cushing syndrome, but may provide useful information in some cases. Urine 17-ketosteroid measurement was one of the first tests used for diagnosing Cushing syndrome, but elevations are not seen in about half of Cushing patients and the incidence of false positive results is higher than that of urinary free cortisol assays. Results are more likely to be increased, and increased to greater levels, with adrenal carcinoma than with other etiologies. Plasma cortisol levels collected at 8 AM and again at 8 PM in Cushing syndrome patients do not show the normal diurnal variation in about 90 % of patients, but is not specific for Cushing syndrome because alteration of diurnal pattern can be seen in a variety of other conditions.

The **single dose dexamethasone suppression test** (rapid DST) is another reasonably reliable screening test. A baseline or pre-suppression plasma cortisol sample is collected followed by oral administration of a low dose of dexamethasone (a synthetic glucocorticoid) at 11 PM and collection of a plasma cortisol sample at 8 AM. In normal patients, dexamethosone suppresses pituitary production of ACTH, which leads to suppression of cortisol levels so that the normal AM peak of cortisol does not occur. The 8 AM cortisol level is typically < 50 % of the baseline sample in normal persons following dexamethosone suppression. In the majority of Cushing syndrome patients there is a failure to suppress cortisol levels. Other conditions may also produce a failure to adequately suppress cortisol production, including severe stress, clinical depression, acute alcoholism, renal failure, and some severe nonadrenal illnesses. The degree of suppression considered to be a normal response in the rapid DST varies among endocrinologists and other clinicians, with some considering use of the 50 % decrease from baseline insufficiently sensitive and using a fixed value for the AM cortisol sample (5μg/dL or 7 μg/dL [Ravel, 1995]). Although perhaps more sensitive in the detection of Cushing syndrome, use of a fixed value may present additional complications in the evaluation of test results, including method variability and the false appearance of a normal response caused by some drugs, including phenytoin and phenobarbital. A combined evaluation of urinary free cortisol levels, the rapid DST, and of the diurnal pattern of cortisol production provides greater, more reliable diagnostic evidence of Cushing syndrome.

Confirmatory testing and differentiation of etiologies is accomplished by stimulation or suppression of adrenal function. These tests are summarized in Table 14–10.

Serum ACTH measurements by immunoassay may also provide useful data in the diagnosis of Cushing disease and in the differentiation of etiologies. This test is typically available only through reference laboratories. ACTH has a diurnal pattern that corresponds to that of cortisol production with a peak between 8 and 10 AM and lowest values occurring around midnight (Ravel, 1995). Values are usually markedly increased in ectopic ACTH syndrome. In Cushing syndrome resulting from adrenal tumors, pituitary activity is suppressed by the cortisol produced by the tumor and ACTH values are significantly decreased.

TABLE 14–10. Stimulation and Suppression Tests in Cushing Syndrome

Test	Description	Results/Comments	
		Normal	*Cushing Syndrome*
Dexamethasone suppression	Same principle as rapid DST, but test continued for 4 days; DST administered every 6 hours with dose increasing last 2 days; 24-hour urine collection on day before test and each day of test for 17-OHCS measurement	17-OHCS < 50% of baseline	Little to no response at low dose for Cushing syndrome of any etiology; most pts. with adrenal hyperplasia due to increased pituitary ACTH respond (ie, 17-OHCS decreased) at higher doses
CRH Stimulation	CRH is administered to stimulate pituitary secretion of ACTH; plasma cortisol and ACTH measured baseline and after CRH administration; helps distinguish pituitary adenoma from ectopic ACTH tumors or adrenal tumors in those already diagnosed with Cushing syndrome	Increased cortisol and ACTH levels; normal results overlap with those seen in Cushing syndrome due to pituitary adenoma	Rise in cortisol of at least 20% above baseline and in ACTH of ≥ 50% of baseline in pituitary ACTH producing tumor; response is rarely seen in ectopic ACTH producing tumors and virtually never seen in cortisol secreting adrenal tumors; significant overlap between normal individuals and those with pituitary adenoma
Metyrapone suppression	Metyrapone blocks conversion of intermediate compound (compound S) to cortisol; administration should induce pituitary secretion of ACTH to stimulate cortisol production by adrenal glands; cortisol is measured baseline and after administration (some authorities recommend measurement of compound S as well [Ravel, 1995]); note that some cortisol assay methods include measurement of compound S; method should be chosen that does not measure this compound such as cortisol by RIA or fluorescent techniques	Reduced cortisol levels (using methods that do not include compound S measurement) and increased levels of compound S; cortisol methods that measure both cortisol and compound S will show an apparent increase in cortisol when cortisol is, in fact, decreased	Cushing syndrome due to adrenal tumors produces no significant change; decreased cortisol levels in pituitary-induced hyperplasia of the adrenal cortex (response seen in normal individuals; see cortisol methodology note in normal results discussion)
ACTH Stimulation	Injection of ACTH for direct stimulation of adrenal cortex and collection of 24-hour urine specimen day before, day of, and day after ACTH administration for measurement of 17-OHCS; test not frequently used; plasma cortisol and 17-OHCS may also be measured	Increased 17-OHCS on day of administration with return to normal day after	Increased plasma cortisol and plasma 17-OHCS in adrenal cortex hyperplasia and some adenomas; urine 17-OHCS shows significant increase day of and day after administration in these cases, but is not affected by carcinoma

Data for table from Ravel R. *Clinical Laboratory Medicine: Clinical Application of Laboratory Data*, 6th ed. St Louis, Mosby, 1995.

Diagnostic imaging studies (particularly CT and MRI) are important for determination of the presence and location of tumors after Cushing syndrome has been diagnosed. These studies are best used after the diagnosis is made rather than as a part of the diagnostic process, since benign tumors unrelated to Cushing syndrome and that do not produce hormones are not uncommon findings. On the other hand, up to 50% of patients who ultimately require surgery for pituitary tumors related to Cushing syndrome will not have the tumor detected by diagnostic imaging (NIH publication 96-3007, June, 1996).

Treatment for Cushing syndrome may include the use of cortisol-inhibiting drugs, surgery, radiation, or chemotherapy depending upon the underlying cause. When Cushing syndrome results from glucocorticoid hormone therapy to treat another disorder such as lupus or rheumatoid arthritis, the dosage is gradually reduced to the lowest dose effective for the disorder under treatment. When control is established, the dosage may be doubled and given on alternate days to lessen side effects (NIH publication 96-3007, June, 1996).

■ HYPERALDOSTERONISM

The secretion of aldosterone is regulated by the renin-angiotensin mechanism as well as by pituitary secretion of ACTH. **Renin** is a proteolytic enzyme stored in the kidneys and secreted in response to reduced blood volume or reduced blood flow in the renal arterioles. In the liver, renin causes the transformation of angiotensinogen (an angiotensin precursor) into angiotensin I, which is subsequently converted to angiotensin II, the polypeptide that causes aldosterone secretion. **Aldosterone** is the most potent of the mineralcorticoids produced by the adrenal glands and acts to retain sodium in exchange for potassium and hydrogen in the renal distal tubule.

Hyperaldosteronism may be primary as a consequence of adrenal adenoma, carcinoma, or hyperplasia; or secondary to stimuli originating outside the adrenal (eg, pathogenic changes in blood volume and electrolyte balance). **Primary aldosteronism** (Conn syndrome) is usually the result of a unilateral, benign adenoma of the adrenal cortex. Hypersecretion of aldosterone (either primary or secondary) is manifested by low serum potassium levels with increased urinary potassium secretion and hypertension. Serum sodium and chloride levels may be elevated as well and hypovolemia may be present. Hypokalemic alkalosis, if present, may result in episodic weakness with transient paralysis and tetany (Merck Manual, 1996–1997). Polyuria and polydipsia are common findings.

The **diagnosis of primary hyperaldosteronism** requires that both the presence of excess aldosterone and unresponsiveness of the renin-angiotensin mechanism be established. **Administration of spironolactone**, an aldosterone antagonist, can be used to confirm aldosterone excess. The response to spironolactone allows correction of serum potassium levels and a drop in urinary potassium excretion to < 20 mEq/24 h (Sacher and McPherson, 1991). Hypertension is also reversed within 5 to 8 weeks of daily oral administration of 200 to 400 mg of spironolactone (Merck Manual, 1996–1997). The appropriate response to spironolactone rules out renal dysfunction, diuretic excess, and systemic electrolyte imbalance resulting from abnormal potassium metabolism (Sacher and McPherson, 1991), but does not rule out other causes of hypertension unrelated to aldosterone (Merck Manual, 1996–1997). **Renin levels** are evaluated by collection of an AM specimen for plasma renin determination while the patient remains in the recumbent position (postural status can affect renin values). Oral administration of 80 mg (Sacher and McPherson, 1991; Merck Manual, 1996–1997) of furosemide follows and a second sample for renin is collected 3 hours later. The patient should remain in an upright position throughout this 3-hour period. Ideally, patients should not have taken diuretics for 3 weeks prior to the test or antihypertensives for 1 week prior. A marked increase in renin concentration is seen in the normal individual, but not in patients with hyperaldosteronism.

Secondary hyperaldosteronism may be seen in response to high renin levels resulting from renal vasoconstriction. It is related to hypertension and a variety of edematous disorders, including cardiac failure and nephrotic syndrome. Hypovolemia, common in edematous disorders, especially in conjunction with diuretic therapy, is a renin-angiotensin mechanism stimulant that results in increased aldosterone production. Table 14–11 summarizes some of the clinical features and laboratory findings in primary and secondary hyperaldosteronism.

TABLE 14–11. Clinical and Laboratory Findings in Primary and Secondary Hyperaldosteronism

Findings	Primary Hyperaldosteronism		Secondary Hyperaldosteronism	
	Adenoma	Hyperplasia	Edematous Disorders	Hypertension
Clinical				
Hypertension	↑↑	↑	↑/N	↑↑↑↑
Edema	Absent	Absent	Present	Present
Laboratory				
Serum Sodium	N / ↑	N	N / ↑	N / ↑
Serum Potassium	↓	N / ↓	↓	N / ↓
Plasma Renin	↓↓	N / ↑	↑↑	↑
Plasma Aldosterone	↑	↑	↑↑	↑
Vasopressin Volume Expansion	No effect or slight increase in serum Na		↓ renin ↓ aldosterone secretion[1]	
80 mg. Furosemide	Aldosterone remains high		Aldosterone secretion decreases	
Fluorocortisone acetate[2] or deoxycorticosterone administration	Aldosterone remains high		Aldosterone secretion decreases	

↑ = increased; ↑↑ = greatly increased; ↑↑↑↑ = markedly increased; ↓ = decreased; ↓↓ = greatly decreased; N = normal

[1]These results also seen in normal individuals in response to volume expansion by vasopressin; other responses include increased urine sodium and decreased serum sodium

[2]Reduces aldosterone stimulation resulting in ≥ 50% reduction in aldosterone secretion after 4 days of 400 mg three times per day if adrenal glands are normally responsive (Sacher and McPherson, 1991)

Table compiled based on information in Henry JB. *Clinical Diagnosis and Management by Laboratory Methods,* 19th ed. Philadelphia, Saunders, 1996; Merck Manual (on-line), Section 8. Endocrine Disorders, Merck & Co., Inc., Whitehouse Station, NJ, © 1996–1997; Ravel R. *Clinical Laboratory Medicine: Clinical Application of Laboratory Data,* 6th ed. St Louis, Mosby, 1995; and Sacher RA, McPherson RA. *Widmann's Clinical Interpretation of Laboratory Tests,* 10th ed. Philadelphia, FA Davis, 1991.

■ PHEOCHROMOCYTOMA

Pheochromocytomas are **catecholeamine secreting tumors** of the adrenal medulla. The adrenal medulla is the production site of epinephrine (adrenaline, the "fight or flight" hormone) and, to a lesser extent, of norepinephrine (noradrenaline). Most norepinephrine is produced by sympathetic nerve endings. Both epinephrine and norepinephrine, which are very similar chemical compounds, are synthesized from the amino acid tyrosine through the intermediate compounds dehydroxyphenylamine (DOPA) and dopamine. Catecholeamines are degraded to form the **metabolites metanephrine** (from epinephrine) and **normetanephrine** (from norepinephrine), with a final **common end product vanillymandelic acid** (VMA). These metabolic processes are dependent upon enzyme action, particularly that of **monoamine oxidase**, which acts on epinephrine, norepinephrine, and dopamine as well as a number of their metabolites, including metanephrines, normetanephrines, and 3-methyoxydopamine. (Note that pharmacologic agents that act by inhibiting the action of this enzyme—MAO inhibitors—have been used in the treatment of clinical depression. MAO inhibitors are rarely the drug of choice today because of their potential side effects—especially hypertensive crises resulting from catecholeamine excess—and the development of effective antidepressants with fewer or less serious side effects.) Another enzyme important in the metabolism of catecholeamines is **catechol-O-methyltransferase** (COMT), which acts on epinephrine, norepinephrine, dopamine, and some metabolites. Metabolites are excreted in the urine along with small amounts of epinephrine, norepinephrine, and dopamine.

Pheochromocytomas are typically benign (about 90%) and usually occur in only one adrenal gland. A few of these hormonally active tumors occur in nonadrenal sites, most often the abdomen (Ravel, 1995). Hypertension may be the most conspicuous manifestation of this disorder and may be continuous or paroxysmal (occurring in short episodes). Although pheochromocytoma is not a common cause of hypertension (0.5% of cases according to Sacher and McPherson [1991]; 0.1% of cases as reported by Henry [1996]), it should be considered as a possible etiology (especially in the young or middle aged with sudden onset, hypertension that is very difficult to control, family history of endocrine tumors, or strong clinical suspicion based on clinical presentation) because it is one of the few curable causes of hypertension. Early, accurate diagnosis can prevent some of the dire consequences associated with severe hypertension such as stroke, myocardial infarction, and renal failure. The signs and symptoms of pheochromocytomas are attributable to the excess of catecholeamines and, along with the hypertension seen in most cases, may include

- severe headaches
- tachycardia and palpitations
- excessive sweating
- anxiety or apprehension
- heat intolerance

- nausea (may or may not be accompanied by vomiting)
- abdominal or lower chest pain
- nervousness and tremors
- weight loss

When clinical suspicion of pheochromocytoma exists, **diagnosis** requires demonstration of excess catecholeamines and/or their metabolites. Provocative testing is rarely indicated and may be dangerous. Although epinephrine is the major adrenal catecholeamine and norepinephrine and dopamine are the predominant catecholeamines in the brain, norepinephrine is usually the catecholeamine secreted in greater concentration in pheochromocytoma. (In the few cases where epinephrine is predominantly secreted, diastolic hypertension may not be present [Henry, 1996].) In many cases confirmation of a clinical suspicion of pheochromocytoma is straightforward, particularly when hormone secretion is continuous, and accomplished by measuring catecholeamines or their metabolites in urine. Urine specimens may be collected for 24 hours, 12 hours (overnight), or randomly collected. Twenty-four-hour specimens provide a more complete picture of catecholeamine production. Randomly collected specimens are unlikely to produce valid data with episodic hormone production unless they are collected shortly after symptomatic attacks. Urinary assays that may be used are summarized in Table 14–12. Plasma catecholeamines may also be measured. They are most useful if hormone secretion is continuous or if collected immediately following a symptomatic attack (often not feasible). Plasma catecholeamine assay is generally considered to be a less sensitive indicator of pheochromocytoma than the testing of 24-hour urine specimens.

TABLE 14–12. Urinary Assays for Catecholeamines and Metabolites in Pheochromocytoma

Test	Comments
VMA	Final common metabolite for epinephrine and norepinephrine; good indicator of total catecholeamines, but does not distinguish between secretion of epinephrine vs norepinephrine
Metanephrine and normetanephrine	Probably best single assay for diagnosing or excluding pheochromocytoma
Total catecholeamines	May be useful, but wide reference range can make it difficult to detect a minimally secreting tumor
Free catecholeamines (total) or free epinephrine or free norepinephrine	Highly variable results in pediatric patients, but most pheochromocytomas occur in adults
Dopamine	Major intact catecholeamine in urine; usually increased in pheochromocytoma, but most useful along with normetanephrine, VMA, and HVA (homovanillyic acid, a dopamine metabolite) in diagnosing neuroblastoma, a neuroendocrine tumor and common malignancy of infancy

The **clonidine suppression test** may be useful in borderline cases. Clonidine suppresses sympathetic nervous system release of catecholeamines from post-ganglionic neurons in normal patients. This suppression does not occur in the presence of pheochromocytomas with autonomous catecholeamine production. In this test, a plasma epinephrine sample is collected before administration of 0.3 mg (Henry, 1996; Ravel, 1995; Sacher and McPherson, 1991) clonidine and again 3 hours after administration. Patients with pheochromocytoma typically show little change from the baseline sample, whereas normal individuals have values that are reduced by at least 50% ([Henry, 1996; Ravel, 1995]; Sacher [1991] states decrease of 25% for normal persons and for those in whom catecholeamines are increased as a result of stress).

Measurement of a substance produced in the adrenal medulla and secreted along with catecholeamines, **chromogranin A** (CgA), may also be beneficial in borderline cases (Henry, 1996; Ravel, 1995). It is measured in serum and has a high degree of specificity. Decline of serum CgA values may be useful after surgical resection to follow the response to treatment (Henry, 1996). Once diagnosed, pheochromocytomas are localized using diagnostic imaging techniques such as CT and MRI.

 TIME FOR REVIEW. After studying the preceding sections, you should be able to respond correctly to the following:

■ List the hormones of the adrenal medulla and the three groups of hormones of the adrenal cortex.

■ List two factors causing increased plasma cortisol values and two factors causing decreased values.

■ Addison's disease occurs as a result of insufficient production of

_____.

■ Distinguish between primary and secondary adrenal insufficiency.

■ Briefly describe the rapid Cortrosyn response test.

■ Confirmation of an abnormal Cortrosyn response can be accomplished by prolonged _____ stimulation.

■ The most common form of congenital adrenal hyperplasia (CAH) results from deficiency of the enzyme _____.

■ Classic CAH-21-hydroxylase deficiency results in deficient levels of both _____ and _____ and excessive production of _____.

■ Briefly describe the two procedures (one presumptive and one confirmatory) for determining the genotypic sex of CAH infants with ambiguous genitalia.

■ Cushing syndrome may result from _____ or may be secondary to _____.

■ The most common form of Cushing syndrome is called Cushing disease and results from _____.

■ Laboratory diagnosis of Cushing syndrome includes measurement of 24-hour urinary _____.

■ Describe the rapid dexamethasone suppression test as a screening test for Cushing syndrome.

■ Describe the stimulation and suppression tests used for confirmatory testing and differentiation of etiologies in Cushing syndrome.

■ Distinguish between primary and secondary hyperaldosteronism in terms of laboratory findings and etiology.

■ Pheochromocytomas are _____ secreting tumors of the adrenal medulla.

■ List two enzymes important in the metabolism of catecholeamines.

■ The final common metabolic end product of epinephrine and norepinephrine is _____.

■ An intermediate metabolite of epinephrine is _____ and of norepinephrine is _____.

■ Excess catecholeamines can be demonstrated by measuring catecholeamines or their _____ in _____.

■ The best single urinary assay for the diagnosis or exclusion of pheochromocytoma involves the measurement of _____ and _____.

■ List and briefly describe two tests that may be beneficial in diagnosing pheochromocytoma when initial findings are borderline or equivocal.

Check your responses by reviewing the preceding sections.

14. SELF TEST

Choose the best response by circling the appropriate letter. The answer key may be found in the appendices.

1. **The hormone produced by the anterior pituitary that has its principal effect on bone and muscle, but also has a general effect on most body tissues, is**
   A. growth hormone
   B. prolactin
   C. ADH

2. **When prolactin levels are increased as a result of pituitary adenoma, the response to**
   A. TRH and L-DOPA is normal with a blunted response to chlorpromazine
   B. TRH is normal with a blunted response to L-DOPA and chlorpromazine
   C. TRH and chlorpromazine is blunted with a normal response to L-DOPA
   D. TRH, chlorpromazine, and L-DOPA is blunted

3. **Excessive growth hormone in adults leads to the gradual development of**
   A. gigantism
   B. pituitary dwarfism
   C. panhypopituitarism
   D. acromegaly

4. **Somatomedin C assay may be useful in the evaluation of**
   A. prolactin disorders
   B. growth hormone disorders
   C. ADH abnormalities
   D. pheochromocytoma

5. **The insulin tolerance test (or insulin induced hypoglycemia) may be useful in the evaluation of**
   A. overproduction of ACTH and Addison's disease
   B. diabetes insipidus and diabetes mellitus
   C. growth hormone deficiency and Addison's disease
   D. SIADH and diabetes insipidus

6. **Pituitary and hypothalamic etiologies of growth hormone deficiency may be distinguished using stimulation with**
   A. L-DOPA
   B. insulin
   C. TRH
   D. dexamethasone

7. **Very high prolactin levels are more likely to result from this condition than any other cause**
   A. hypothalamic lesions
   B. ectopic prolactin secretion
   C. postpartum amenorrhea
   D. pituitary adenoma

8. **A low urine osmolality that increases after AVP administration and a serum ADH that is low and remains low after fluid deprivation is most indicative of**
   A. nephrogenic diabetes insipidus
   B. neurogenic diabetes insipidus
   C. primary polydipsia
   D. normal response

9. **The water loading test is used to assess the ability to suppress secretion of**
   A. ADH
   B. ACTH
   C. VMA
   D. epinephrine

10. **The water loading test results most consistent with a diagnosis of SIADH are**
    A. normal baseline serum osmolality that falls after water load; decreased urine osmolality that remains low after water load; and water excretion ≥ 80% of the water load at 5 hours
    B. elevated baseline serum osmolality that falls after water load; decreased urine osmolality that increases after water load; and water excretion < 80% of the water load at 5 hours
    C. decreased baseline serum osmolality that falls after water load; normal or increased urine osmolality that remains higher than serum osmolality after water load; and water excretion < 80% of the water load at 5 hours
    D. decreased baseline serum osmolality that increases after water load; normal or increased urine osmolality that remains higher than serum osmolality after water load; and water excretion > 60% of the water load at 5 hours

11. **All of the following factors result in increased plasma cortisol levels**
    except
    A. oral contraceptives
    B. hyperthyroidism
    C. pregnancy
    D. increased androgens

12. **In normal individuals, the AM cortisol level is**
    A. significantly lower than PM values
    B. significantly higher than PM values
    C. not significantly different from the PM value

13. **Addison's disease occurs as a result of insufficient production of the glucocorticoid**
    A. epinephrine
    B. cortisol
    C. prolactin
    D. ADH

14. **In the rapid Cortrosyn response test, the substance administered is**
    A. synthetic ACTH
    B. synthetic ADH
    C. insulin
    D. dexamethasone

15. **Patients with primary adrenal insufficiency respond to Cortrosyn administration with**
    A. peak cortisol levels exceeding 20 µg/dL
    B. 30-minute cortisol levels ≥ 18 µg/dL
    C. rapid doubling of the baseline cortisol level
    D. little or no change in cortisol level

16. **All CAH variants affect the metabolic pathway of _____ to some extent.**
    A. ACTH
    B. ADH
    C. epinephrine
    D. cortisol

17. **Classic CAH-21-hydroxylase deficiency results in**
   A. decreased aldosterone; increased cortisol; and decreased androgen production
   B. increased aldosterone; increased cortisol; and decreased androgen production
   C. decreased aldosterone; decreased cortisol; and increased androgen production
   D. increased aldosterone; decreased cortisol; and increased androgen production

18. **In most patients with Cushing syndrome cortisol levels**
   A. do not show normal diurnal variation
   B. show normal diurnal variation
   C. are not important to diagnosis or evaluation

19. **The single dose dexamethasone suppression test is used to test the ability**
   A. to suppress the production of ADH
   B. of pituitary ACTH suppression to suppress cortisol production
   C. of pituitary ACTH suppression to stimulate cortisol production
   D. to suppress catecholeamine production
   E. to suppress catecholeamine degradation

20. **Diagnosis of primary hyperaldosteronism requires demonstration of the presence of**
   A. excess aldosterone and a normally responsive renin-angiotensin mechanism
   B. decreased aldosterone and an unresponsive renin-angiotensin mechanism
   C. decreased aldosterone and a normally responsive renin-angiotensin mechanism
   D. excess aldosterone and an unresponsive renin-angiotensin mechanism

21. **When clinical suspicion of pheochromocytoma exists, laboratory diagnosis is best accomplished using**
   A. provocative testing
   B. testing for plasma cortisol concentrations
   C. urine tests for catecholeamines and/or their metabolites
   D. MRI

22. **The clonidine suppression test used produces**
   A. no suppression of catecholeamine release in the presence of pheochromocytoma
   B. significant suppression of catecholeamine release in the presence of pheochromocytoma
   C. increased catecholeamine release in the presence of pheochromocytoma

15. TESTING FOR COAGULATION AND FIBRINOLYTIC DEFECTS

An understanding of current concepts of blood coagulation and maintenance of normal hemostatic balance serves as a framework from which evaluation and interpretation of related laboratory data can be undertaken. Despite an initial appearance of simplicity—clotting to prevent excess blood loss and lysis to prevent intravascular clot formation—the mechanisms involved in achieving and maintaining hemostatic balance are intricate and complex.

OVERVIEW OF HEMOSTASIS

The term *hemostasis* is of Greek derivation and refers to the stoppage of blood flow. There are **three general components of hemostasis**:

- extravascular component: tissues that surround blood vessels and become involved when the vessel is injured
- vascular component: capillaries, arteries, and veins through which blood flows; vessel injury causes vasoconstriction and exposes a substance that promotes platelet adherence and initiates further coagulation phases
- intravascular component: platelets and a variety of plasma proteins (generally designated by Roman numerals) that interact to ensure clot formation to prevent blood loss and to prevent excessive clotting

These three components respond to vessel injuries (Figure 15–1 summarizes the processes initiated by injury to blood vessels) and act in concert to maintain a delicate, essential balance between **coagulation** (clot/thrombus formation) and **fibrinolysis** (dissolution of clots/thrombi), which are the two fundamental processes in hemostasis. Hemostasis occurs in primary and secondary phases. In the **primary phase**, blood vessels and platelets act in response to vessel injury. The various coagulation factors become involved in the response to the injury in the **secondary phase**.

Clotting mechanisms are activated along two different pathways that eventually come together in a third, common pathway. The **extrinsic pathway** is activat-

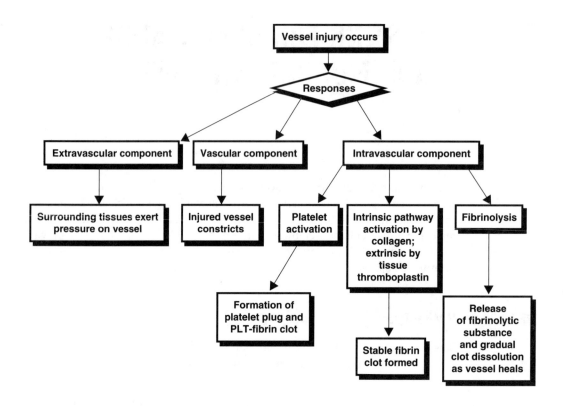

FIGURE 15–1. General responses to vessel injury.

ed when a substance called *tissue thromboplastin* is released in response to a vessel injury. Activation of the **intrinsic pathway** occurs when collagen and the subendothelial basement membrane are exposed as consequence of vessel injury. Following initial activation of these pathways, subsequent activation, release, and action of a variety of substances occur in a defined, step-wise fashion sometimes referred to as the *coagulation cascade.* The extrinsic and intrinsic pathways come together in the common pathway following activation of coagulation factor X by either of the pathways. The **common pathway** ends with the formation of a stable fibrin clot. Fibrinolysis then gradually dissolves the fibrin clot as the damaged vessel heals, so that a normal flow of blood can be restored in the affected vessel. These pathways will be discussed in more detail later in the chapter. However, because of the intricacies of the processes of hemostasis, much of the material can only be presented in a more general manner rather than detailing many of the system complexities.

Coagulation disorders can be classified into one of two general categories:

- hypocoagulation: failure to achieve adequate thrombus formation, as is typified by classic hemophilia that results from a deficiency of coagulation factor VIII
- hypercoagulation: inappropriate thrombus formation within blood vessels; results in occluded blood flow and can be life threatening depending upon the location and size of the occlusion; results from a defect in the fibrinolytic process

Laboratory assays are readily available to identify and assess either type of abnormality. Most assays are either partially or completely automated, allowing results to be available to the clinician much sooner. Some tests are general in nature and work well to indicate the presence of an abnormality. Subsequent, more specialized testing can then be performed in order to determine the particular nature of the abnormality and to quantitate deficiencies in coagulation factors. Subsequent sections of this chapter deal with laboratory measurements in detail.

SPECIMENS FOR TESTING

Valid results, as with all testing, are dependent on appropriate specimen collection. This is especially true for specimens that will be used to assess hemostasis. Standard collection procedures established by the testing laboratory should be followed exactly in terms of the type of anticoagulant used, methods of storage and/or transport, amount of specimen and size of collection tube, delivery time, and all other specifications. Failure to follow appropriate collection procedures virtually ensures that invalid data will be provided to the clinician. Invalid data may lead to harmful diagnostic and treatment decisions, thus good laboratory practice dictates the rejection of inappropriate specimens submitted for testing, and failure to do so is irresponsible. However, not all unsuitable specimens will be apparent by visual examination to the laboratorian; consequently collection personnel must ensure that an appropriate sample is collected and submitted for testing. Some of the common reasons for rejection of specimens submitted for coagulation testing include:

- improperly filled collection tubes: tubes must not be over- or underfilled; a standard blood-to-anticoagulant ratio is essential; this cannot be overemphasized
- collection in inappropriate anticoagulant: anticoagulant specified for each test is chosen to preserve the substance being measured and to minimize interferences; substitutions should *not* be made
- specimen submitted too long after collection: maximum time frames for delivery are established to ensure the substance(s) being measured are not depleted; some coagulation factors are quite labile and are rapidly depleted

- improper specimen storage or transport: specimens must be maintained at the specified temperature for the same reasons provided in regard to delivery time
- hemolysis: hemolysis interferes with a variety of measurements
- inadequately mixed specimens: evidenced by the presence of clots or small fibrin strands; some factors will be decreased or depleted as they are used in the *in vitro* clotting process; clots and fibrin strands also interfere with automated equipment function and, undetected, can lead to erroneous test values on testing performed subsequent to their entry into the system (not to mention requiring that time be taken by testing personnel to remove fibrin strands from the equipment!); specimens should be mixed thoroughly, but gently—tilted, not shaken

Good venipuncture technique is also important in coagulation testing. Traumatic venipuncture can lead to activation of the clotting process as a result of contamination of the specimen with tissue thromboplastin. Quick, clean puncture prevents such contamination. Activation can also occur as a result of inappropriate specimen containers, inappropriate temperatures, and the presence of hemolysis. In many instances, specimens for coagulation testing may be collected at the same time as specimens for other testing. The established order of collection must be followed in these instances. Particularly notable is the collection of complete blood count (CBC) specimens along with specimens for coagulation testing. CBC specimens are collected into test tubes containing the anticoagulant EDTA. This anticoagulant prevents the clotting process by chelating calcium, which, as will be evident following later discussions, is an important coagulation factor. When a CBC must be collected at the same time, the EDTA sample must be collected *after* the coagulation tubes to avoid contamination of the coagulation sample with EDTA. Prolonged tourniquet application should also be avoided because hemolysis of the sample can result from excessive stasis.

PRIMARY HEMOSTASIS

The primary phase of hemostasis involves the **vascular and platelet responses** to vessel injury. These responses are triggered when platelets are exposed to components within the subendothelial tissue of the blood vessel, especially collagen. The normal, intact endothelial lining of blood vessels provides a smooth surface which promotes unimpeded blood flow without inducing clot formation. Blood vessels are capable of both constriction and dilation by virtue of smooth muscle tissue in the vessel walls. These capabilities are important to control blood flow and blood pressure under normal circumstances. When a vessel is damaged, the **vascular response involves vasoconstriction** to restrict the amount of blood flow through the vessel. Vessel damage also interrupts the smooth surface of the endothelial lining, resulting in exposure of **collagen**, a fibrous and insoluble protein. Collagen causes platelets to adhere to the area of damage and leads to the activation of the intrinsic coagulation pathway. **Tissue thromboplastin**, a substance found in the tissue cells that accelerates clotting, is also released in response to injury and serves to activate the extrinsic coagulation pathway. In addition, the endothelial cells of blood vessels secrete a number of substances that affect platelets and the processes of coagulation and fibrinolysis. Four examples of such substances are

1. von Willebrand factor: necessary for platelets to adhere to the site of injury
2. adenosine: stimulates the vessel to constrict to reduce blood flow
3. prostacyclin: stimulates the vessel to dilate to increase blood flow; also limits activation of platelets
4. tissue plasminogen activator: prevents excessive clotting when vessel damage occurs and starts gradual dissolution of clot as the vessel heals

Platelets play several critical roles in hemostasis, including:

- adhering to the area of vessel injury and aggregating at the site of damage
- promoting coagulation on their surface
- releasing substances important to hemostasis (Table 15–1)
- instigating clot retraction

TABLE 15–1. Substances Released by Platelets

Secreted by	Substance	Role in Hemostasis/Primary Function
Alpha granules	Platelet factor 4	Facilitates platelet aggregation
	Thrombospondin	Facilitates platelet aggregation
	HMWK[1]	Contact activation of intrinsic pathway
	Fibrinogen	Forms fibrin for clot formation
	Factor V	Assists in fibrin clot formation
	Factor VIII:vWF	Assists platelet adhesion
	Plasminogen	Clot lysis (plasmin precursor; plasmin instigates clot lysis)
	Alpha-2-antiplasmin	Inhibition of clot lysis
	Platelet derived growth factor	Promotes vessel repair
	C_1 esterase inhibitor	Inhibition of complement system
Dense bodies	ADP	Facilitates platelet aggregation
	Calcium	Facilitates platelet aggregation
	Serotonin	Promotes vasoconstriction
Membrane phospholipids	Precursors to thromboxane A_2	Promotes vasoconstriction

[1]High molecular weight kininogen.

Adapted from Lotspeich-Steininger C, Stiene-Martin A, Koepke J. *Clinical Hematology: Principles, Procedures, Correlations.* Philadelphia, Lippincott, 1992.

Under normal conditions platelets do not adhere or "stick" to vessel walls. When exposed to collagen in a damaged vessel, platelets will **adhere** to the injured area in a response that is proportional to the degree of injury. The different levels of platelet response may be due to exposure to different types of collagen (types I, II, III, and IV) located at varying levels of the vessel wall—types I and III found in deeper regions (Lotspeich-Steininger, 1992). When stimuli for **aggregation** (clumping together of platelets) are present, platelets begin to change shape, form pseudopods, and clump together at the site of the injury. Following formation of a platelet and fibrin clot the platelets act to contract and stabilize the clot in a process referred to as **clot retraction.** Further, platelets furnish a surface phospholipid on which clotting factors can bind, interact with vitamin K dependent clotting factors in the coagulation process, and play a role in the prothrombin to thrombin conversion.

A variety of substances that play a role in hemostasis are secreted from miscellaneous structures within the platelet cytoplasm. Table 15–1 lists some of these substances by source of secretion and primary function or role in hemostasis.

SECONDARY HEMOSTASIS

Secondary hemostatic processes include a series of biochemical reactions along the extrinsic, intrinsic, and common pathways of coagulation. Considerable interaction occurs among the three pathways as plasma proteins, tissue factors, and calcium work together in a response to vessel damage. Before a discussion of the intricacies of these responses, a listing of coagulation factors with some of their characteristics is provided (Table 15–2) followed by a diagrammatic representation of the coagulation pathways (Fig. 15–2). The coagulation factors are often referred to by Roman numerals that were assigned to the factors as they were discovered. It is important to note that the order of discovery did not correspond with the sequence in which the factors react, therefore the Roman numeral designations serve only as a convenient means of identification, not as an indication of the order in which the factors participate in the coagulation pathways.

Activation of the extrinsic pathway begins with *tissue thromboplastin (factor III)* that, with the aid of calcium ions, *activates factor VII.* The resultant *factor VIIa* ("a" is used to indicate the active form of a factor), in a complex *with factor III* and calcium, *converts factor X* to its activated form (Xa). This conversion *begins the common pathway.* Platelet phospholipid, Xa, and Va act with calcium to *convert prothrombin (factor II)* to *thrombin (IIa). Thrombin* then *converts* soluble *fibrinogen* to insoluble *fibrin* monomers and converts (with calcium) *factor XIII to XIIIa.* The fibrin monomer becomes an insoluble polymer. *Factor XIIIa* assists in *stabilization of fibrin* to facilitate the formation of a stable, insoluble clot.

Exposure of collagen and the subendothelial basement membrane as a consequence of vessel damage activates the intrinsic pathway. The exposed *collagen acts in conjunction with kallikrein* (an enzyme that forms kinin) *to activate factor XII* to XIIa. The *activated factor XII* will, in turn, act with high molecular weight kininogen (HMWK) to *convert prekallikrein* to produce more kallikrein. *Factor XIIa also activates factor XI* and the activated *factor XI (XIa)* along with calcium *converts factor IX to IXa. Factor VIII, following activation by thrombin (IIa),* acts with platelet phospholipid, calcium, *and IXa to convert factor X to Xa beginning the common pathway* as previously described. The basic reactions in coagulation pathways are presented in Figure 15–3.

TABLE 15–2. Coagulation Factors

Roman Numeral	Name(s)	Vitamin K Dependent	Site of Production	Pathway	Half-Life (hrs)[1]	Comments
I	Fibrinogen		Liver	Common	90	Activity destroyed during coagulation Found in absorbed plasma
II	Prothrombin (prethrombin)	✔	Liver	Common	60	Consumed during coagulation
III	Tissue thromboplatin (tissue factor)		Present in most tissues	Activates extrinsic		
IV	Calcium			Required for several functions		
V	Proaccelerin (labile factor)		Liver	Common	12–36	Activity destroyed during coagulation Found in absorbed plasma
VI	Factor designated "VI" subsequently found to be activated form of factor V (Lotspeich-Steininger, 1992)					
VII	Proconvertin (stable factor)	✔	Liver	Extrinsic	4–6	Found in serum
VIII:C	Antihemophilic factor (AHF) or antihemophilic factor A		Endothelial cells (uncertain)	Intrinsic	12	Activity destroyed during coagulation Found in absorbed plasma
VIII:vWF	von Willebrand factor		Platelets and endothelial cells		12	
IX	Plasma thromboplastin component (PTC) or antihemophilic factor B or Christmas factor	✔	Liver	Intrinsic	24	Found in serum
X	Stuart-Prower factor	✔	Liver	Common	48–72	Found in serum
XI	Plasma thromboplastin antecedent		Liver	Intrinsic	48–84	Found in serum and absorbed plasma
XII	Hageman factor (glass or contact factor)		Liver	Intrinsic	48–52	Found in serum and absorbed plasma
XIII	Fibrin stabilizing factor (laki-lorand factor)		Liver or platelets	Common	3–5 days	Actively destroyed during coagulation Found in absorbed serum
NA	Prekallikrein		Liver	Intrinsic	35	
NA	HMWK		Liver	Intrinsic	6.5 days	

[1]In vivo half-life.

Adapted from Lotspeich-Steininger C, Stiene-Martin A, Koepke J. *Clinical Hematology: Principles, Procedures, Correlations.* Philadelphia, Lippincott, 1992.

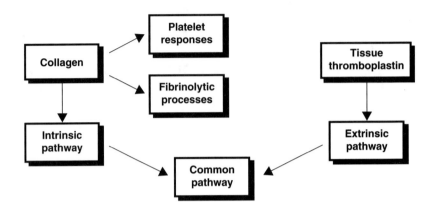

FIGURE 15–2. Coagulation pathways.

Intricately interwoven with clotting mechanisms is the process of **fibrinolysis**. The **fibrinolytic system**, composed of a variety of enzymes and the body's natural anticoagulants, is triggered by the same stimuli that activate clotting processes. This system is important in ensuring that clotting process remains localized to the area of injury and that the clots are dissolved when they are no longer needed. The end result of a sequence of biochemical reactions in the fibrinolytic system is the generation of **plasmin**. This activated substance functions to dissolve the fibrin clot by breaking it into smaller fragments (**fibrin degradation products**).

Simply stated, the fibrinolytic process involves specific activator substances that initiate the conversion of plasminogen to plasmin and another group of substances (**antiplasmins**) that inhibit the actions of plasmin. See Figure 15–4 for a basic graphical representation of the fibrinolytic system.

In the **degradation of fibrin** (and/or fibrinogen, because plasmin cannot distinguish the two), the fibrin polymer is split into smaller **fragments referred to as X, Y, D, and E** in a series of proteolytic steps. The X and Y fragments result from earlier proteolytic steps (first X, which is still clottable [Henry, 1996] and then Y) and are called *"early" degradation products*. D and E fragments result from further cleavage of the Y fragment and are classified as *"late" degradation products*. The fibrin degradation products (FDP) produced by the action of plasmin on fibrin can block the conversion of fibrinogen to fibrin by interfering with the action of thrombin. A number of actions are attributable to plasmin beyond the degradation of fibrin. These additional roles include destruction of factors V and VIII and activation of the complement system (Lotspeich-Steininger, 1992).

Plasminogen is a zymogen (a "proenzyme" or an inactive substance that becomes an enzyme upon activation) normally found in plasma. It can be **activated to form plasmin** by either endogenous or exogenous mechanisms. **Endogenous activation** of plasminogen can occur as a result of *intrinsic mechanisms* (by substances normally found in the plasma) or by *extrinsic mechanisms*

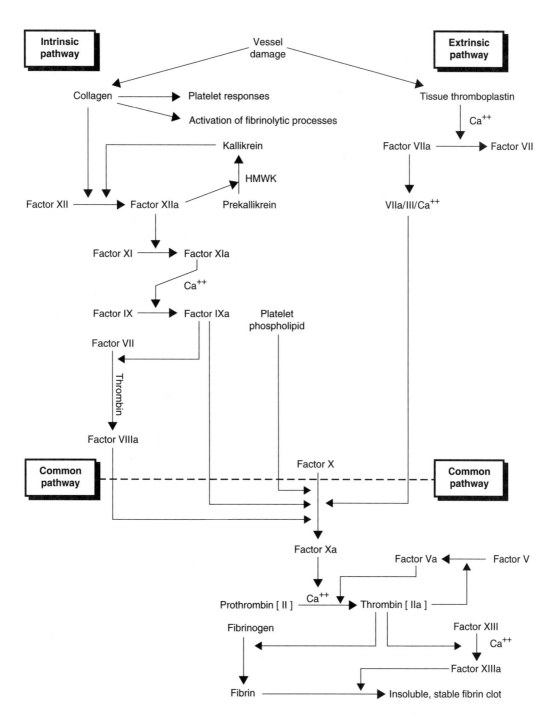

FIGURE 15–3. Basic reactions in coagulation pathways.

(by substances released into the plasma from organ tissues or the vascular endothelium). Perhaps the most important of the endogenous activators is **tissue plasminogen activator** (tPA). tPA is an extrinsic activator that is released at the site of vascular injury and requires the presence of fibrin to function effectively. As a result of this requirement for fibrin, tPA degradation of circulating fibrinogen (versus the degradation of fibrin in thrombi) is relatively minor (Henry, 1996). Another extrinsic endogenous activator results from the conversion of a single chain urokinase-like plasminogen activator (referred to as *scu-PA*) into urokinase. Intrinsic endogenous activation can occur via one or more pathways involving factor XIIa, kallikrein, HMWK, and a plasma protein "proactivator" activated during contact activation of coagulation (Lotspeich-Steininger, 1992). Exogenous plasminogen activation may be employed for the therapeutic dissolution of thrombi. Such therapeutic thrombolytic agents include

- streptokinase: a purified bacterial protein that binds to fibrin
- urokinase: a protease purified from urine
- TPA: a recombinant form of human tPA

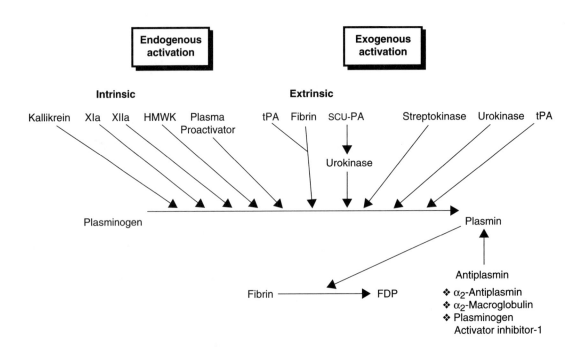

FIGURE 15–4. The fibrinolytic system.

Because inappropriate fibrinolysis is a damaging, often life threatening process, a number of naturally occurring inhibitors (antiplasmins) act to keep the actions of plasmin in appropriate balance. The primary inhibitor of plasmin is **alpha-2-antiplasmin**. Alpha–2-antiplasmin binds with free plasmin to prevent it from binding with fibrin and also inhibits the clot promoting activities of kallikrein and restrains the conversion of plasminogen to plasmin by inhibiting tPA activator (Lotspeich-Steininger, 1992). This and other naturally occurring inhibitors of both the fibrinolytic and the coagulation systems are summarized in Table 15–3.

TABLE 15–3. Natural Inhibitors of the Coagulation and Fibrinolytic Systems

Inhibitor	Inhibits	Action
Antithrombin III	Coagulation	Binds with activated forms of factors II, IX, X, XI XII (activated factor II is thrombin); actions enhanced by heparin
Protein C	Coagulation	Neutralizes active forms of factors V and VIII
Protein S	Coagulation	Serves as "cofactor" to accelerate activity of protein C
Tissue factor pathway inhibitor (TFPI)	Coagulation	Binds with Xa and VIIa to limit extrinsic pathway
Heparin cofactor II	Coagulation	Minor role in inhibiting thrombin
Alpha-2-antiplasmin	Fibrinolysis	Binds with plasmin to prevent binding with thrombin and premature clot dissolution; rapid action; principle plasmin inhibitor
Plasminogen activator inhibitor 1 (PAI-1)	Fibrinolysis	Forms complexes with either tPA or urokinase to prevent plasminogen activation
Alpha-2-macroglobulin	Fibrinolysis	Binds plasmin when alpha-2-antiplasmin depleted
	Coagulation	Inhibits activity of thrombin and kallikrein
Alpha-2-antitrypsin	Fibrinolysis	Binds plasmin after alpha-2-antiplasmin and alpha-2-macroglobulin
	Coagulation	Powerful inhibition of Xa; minor thrombin inhibition
C' 1 inactivator	Fibrinolysis	Inactivates plasmin
	Coagulation	Inactivates XIa, XIIa, and kallikrein

INHIBITORS OF THE COAGULATION AND FIBRINOLYTIC SYSTEMS

Both the coagulation system and the fibrinolytic system are regulated by naturally occurring substances. Nine of the coagulation factors require activation prior to participation in the coagulation cascade. Specific substances act to regulate these activated factors. Other "checks and balances" in both systems function to avoid inappropriate activation of either of the systems. Inhibitors work by a variety of mechanisms and by inhibiting a number of functions.

Alpha-2-antiplasmin and alpha-2-macroglobulin are two of the most important inhibitors of fibrinolysis. The primary inhibitor, **alpha-2-antiplasmin**, acts rapidly to bind with any free plasmin (plasmin not yet bound to fibrin). Plasmin bound to alpha-2-antiplasmin is not capable of binding with fibrin and thus, further fibrinolysis is precluded. A much larger molecule, **alpha-2-macroglobulin**, reacts more slowly than alpha-2-antiplasmin. Nonetheless, it effectively binds with plasmin to inhibit fibrinolysis, particularly when alpha-2-antiplasmin is depleted. It also has the capability to inhibit components of the coagulation system. Alpha-1-antitrypsin is another inhibitor of fibrinolysis that inactivates plasmin after both alpha-2-antiplasmin and alpha-2-macroglobulin have been consumed (Lotspeich-Steininger, 1992). It is also an important inhibitor in the coagulation system.

Of the naturally occurring inhibitors of the coagulation system (natural anticoagulants), **antithrombin III** (ATIII) is of primary significance. Antithrombin III is a selective serine protease inhibitor that is produced in the liver. (Most of the coagulation factors—II, VII, IX, X, XI, and XII, as well as prekallikrein and HMWK—are serine proteases in their activated form.) Principal targets for the neutralizing action of ATIII are thrombin (factor IIa) and factor Xa. The ability of ATIII to inhibit factors IXa, XIa, and XIIa has also been shown (Henry, 1996, Sacher and McPherson, 1991). The activity of antithrombin III is remarkably enhanced by heparin (ATIII was formerly referred to as the *heparin cofactor*), which substantially intensifies the affinity of ATIII for the serine proteases. Heparin and ATIII form a complex that rapidly inactivates thrombin as it is generated by the coagulation cascade.

Protein C is a polypeptide made in the liver and, like some coagulation factors (II, VII, IX, and X), is dependent on vitamin K. This protein circulates in an inactive form, but converts (under regulation of a protein called *thrombomodulin*) to an active form (protein C$_a$) in response to coagulation activities (specifically the prothrombin to thrombin conversion [Sacher and McPherson, 1991]). The activity of the activated forms of factors VIII and V is neutralized by protein C$_a$. **Protein S**, a similar protein that is also synthesized in the liver and dependent on vitamin K, acts to expedite protein C's neutralization of factors VIII and V. Some evidence indicates that protein C is capable of activating the fibrinolytic system through an interrelated pathway (Sacher and McPherson, 1991).

These natural inhibitors to the activities of the coagulation system and to the fibrinolytic system play crucial roles in maintaining normal hemostasis. The number of intricately interwoven and interrelated activities within the coagulation pathways serves to make the study of hemostasis an interesting one despite the level of complexity encountered as a result. The nature of these processes also provides a backdrop for intriguing "detective" work in detecting and identifying hemostatic defects.

TIME FOR REVIEW. After studying the preceding sections, you should be able to respond correctly to the following:

■ List and briefly describe the three general components of hemostasis.

■ In primary hemostasis, _____ and _____ respond to vessel injury.

■ In secondary hemostasis, the _____ become involved in the response to the injury.

■ List and briefly describe two general categories used to classify coagulation disorders.

■ List five common reasons for rejection of specimens submitted for coagulation testing.

■ Traumatic venipuncture can contaminate specimens with _____.

■ CBC samples should be collected after samples for coagulation tests in order to avoid contamination with _____.

■ Indicate the end result of the response to vessel injury by each component listed.

   Extravascular component: _____

   Vascular component: _____

Intravascular component: _____

platelet activation: _____

intrinsic/extrinsic coagulation pathways: _____

fibrinolysis: _____

■ List four hemostatic roles of platelets.

■ _____ causes platelets to adhere to the area of damage and leads to activation of the intrinsic coagulation pathway.

■ Provide the role or primary function of each of the following substances released by platelets.

Platelet factor 4:

Factor VIII:vWF:

Plasminogen:

Platelet derived growth factor:

ADP:

Calcium:

Serotonin:

■ List the vitamin K dependent coagulation factors.

■ List the coagulation factors that are destroyed during the coagulation process.

■ Outline the sequence of reactions in the coagulation pathways (intrinsic, extrinsic, common).

■ The activated form of factor _____ functions to stabilize the fibrin clot.

■ Thrombin is the activated form of factor _____ called _____ (factor name).

■ Activated factor _____ from the intrinsic pathway serves to activate factor X.

■ A series of biochemical reactions in the fibrinolytic system results in the generation of a substance called _____ that acts to dissolve fibrin clots.

■ The two fragments of early fibrin degredation are _____ and _____; late degradation products are _____ and _____ fragments.

■ Distinguish between intrinsic and extrinsic mechanisms of endogenous plasminogen activation and list substances involved in each.

■ List three substances used for exogenous plasminogen activation for therapeutic clot dissolution.

■ List two natural substances that inhibit coagulation and briefly state the action of each.

■ List two natural substances that inhibit fibrinolysis and briefly state the action of each.

■ The primary inhibitor of fibrinolysis is _____.

■ The activity of the natural anticoagulant _____ is significantly enhanced by heparin.

■ List three substances that can inhibit both the coagulation and fibrinolytic systems.

Check your responses by reviewing the preceding sections.

LABORATORY ASSAYS AND DEFECTS OF HEMOSTASIS

Laboratory assays are available to evaluate aspects of both primary and secondary hemostasis and to assess the coagulation and fibrinolytic systems. Laboratory measurements may be employed for a variety of purposes, including

- screening for coagulation defects
- detecting specific factor deficiencies
- quantitating platelets
- assessing platelet function
- detecting inappropriate coagulation or fibrinolysis
- measuring levels of certain inhibitors
- monitoring anticoagulant therapy

The discussion of laboratory assays presented here will be based on the aspect of hemostasis being evaluated and in conjunction with discussions of hemostatic defects.

■ SCREENING TESTS

The **prothrombin time, activated partial thromboplastin time,** and **thrombin time** may be used as screening tests to exclude the presence of significant hemostatic defects prior to surgery or in patients with liver disease and are useful as a starting point for determination of the etiology of bleeding disorders. The prothrombin time (PT) and activated partial thromboplastin time (APTT) are also used to monitor anticoagulant therapy.

The **PT** is one of the more frequently requested laboratory coagulation assays and primarily assesses the extrinsic pathway of coagulation. It is used routinely to monitor therapy with the anticoagulant warfarin (Coumadin). Although the test name would appear to imply measurement of prothrombin, factor II is only one of five factors measured by the PT and the test is more sensitive to levels of factor VII (Ravel, 1995) than it is to prothrombin. The test is performed by adding a tissue extract of thromboplastin with calcium to the patient's sample. Both reagents and patient plasma are warmed to 37°C prior to initiating testing. Addition of these reagents to citrated plasma (citrate is the anticoagulant used for most coagulation specimens) substitutes for *in vivo* activation mechanisms. The tissue thromboplastin reagent employed for testing also contains a phospholipid that acts as a platelet substitute (citrated plasma is "platelet poor"). The PT screens for deficiencies of **factors II, V, VII, and X,** and **to a lesser degree, factor I** (severe fibrinogen deficiencies will be detected). Laboratory PT measurement differs from the actual coagulation cascade in the body (compare Figures 15–3 and 15–5). The test will not be affected by levels of factor IX and will not reflect platelet defects or coagulation defects of the intrinsic pathway prior to the prothrombin to thrombin conversion because the thromboplastin reagent used serves to activate the extrinsic pathway and to bypass the intrinsic pathway. The endpoint of the test is clot detection, generally by automated methods such as photo-optical detection.

Results of PT testing are reported in various ways depending on the testing laboratory and clinician preferences. A common reporting method provides the time (in seconds) required for detection of a clot along with the laboratory's reference range. Variations of this method include reporting the patient time along with a control time and reporting a ratio of the patient time divided by the mean of the reference range and multiplied by 100. It is important that "reference" and "control" values are not confused or used interchangeably. Reference ranges reflect a statistical determination of values from a "normal" population. Control values are derived from commercially prepared substances used to evaluate test conditions and aid in ensuring valid data. (See Chap. 1 for a more detailed discussion of reference ranges and controls.) Prothrombin time test results are sometimes reported in percent activity, but this is an outdated method and is not recommended (Lotspeich-Steininger, 1992). (Percent activity compares the patient results to a

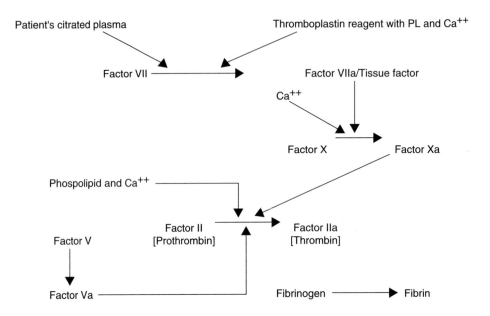

FIGURE 15–5. Prothrombin time.

standard curve prepared with increasing dilutions of plasma.) More recently some laboratories have begun to report PT results in terms of an international normalized ratio (INR) that has been proposed as a standard reporting method. This method is intended to reduce the test variations seen as a consequence of varying test methods and differences in tissue thromboplastin reagents. Disagreement as to how well INR reporting minimizes these differences continues, but a number of clinicians prefer this method of reporting. This method of reporting is appropriately used for the monitoring of anticoagulant therapy after the patient is stabilized. The method is more widely used in Europe than in the United States. Some laboratories may choose to report results in both number of seconds (along with reference range) and as an INR value. **Reference ranges** should be established by each laboratory and vary depending on methodology and the type of thromboplastin used. Ranges are generally about 11 to 13 seconds for automated methods, with slightly longer times being typical of manual clot detection.

The **APTT** is a sensitive test for factor deficiencies in the intrinsic coagulation pathway and is the test of choice for monitoring heparin therapy. It is more sensitive to defects in the common pathway than the PT and can detect deficiencies in all of the coagulation factors except factors VII and VIII (the test bypasses the extrinsic pathway). Platelet abnormalities, however, will not affect APTT results. The predecessor to the APTT was the PTT. The discovery that addition of certain "activator" substances added to the reagent resulted in rapid, consistent activation of factor XII (contact factor) and increased the test's sensitivity to heparin result-ed in the APTT in use in today's laboratories (Ravel, 1995). Like the PT, the APTT is usually performed by automated or semi-automated methods, but can be performed manually. Also like the PT, detection of fibrin clot formation by photo-optical, mechanical, or visual (manual methods) means is the endpoint of the test. Reagents for APTT testing adds a platelet phospholipid substitute with chemical or particulate substances such as kaolin (Ravel, 1995) as contact activators after the patient's citrated plasma is recalcified by the addition of calcium chloride (Fig. 15–6). Test results are reported in seconds with reference ranges varying depend-ing on the method and reagent. **Reference ranges** generally do not have a lower limit < 20 and have an upper limit of ≤ 45 seconds (Lotspeich-Steininger, 1992), with a typical range being 25 to 35 seconds (Henry, 1996).

The **thrombin time**, used less frequently than either the PT or the APTT, is a measure of the rate of formation of fibrin and assesses the fibrinogen to fibrin con-version. A commercially prepared thrombin reagent is added to the patient's plas-ma and the time required for clot formation is reported. Because the presence of fibrinogen in the patient's plasma is required for formation of a fibrin clot, fib-rinogen deficiencies will result in an abnormally high thrombin time. Elevated thrombin times may also result from the presence of fibrin degradation products or other inhibitors, including the anticoagulant heparin.

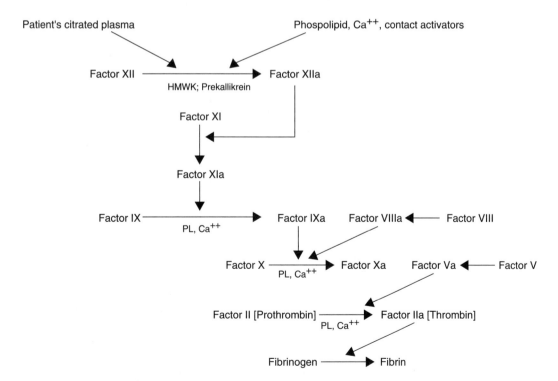

FIGURE 15–6. Activated partial thromboplastin time.

A later section of this chapter provides a discussion of the follow-up for abnormal results of the PT, APTT, and thrombin time.

■ TESTS OF PLATELET FUNCTION

The ability of platelets to effectively form an initial platelet plug in the primary hemostatic response is dependent on the presence of sufficient numbers of properly functioning platelets. Abnormalities in the number of platelets (**quantitative disorders**) or in the function of platelets (**qualitative disorders**) can lead to hemostatic defects. Discussions here will focus on qualitative defects with only a brief discussion of quantitative defects. Chapter 3 provides more detail regarding quantitative platelet abnormalities. The most common platelet abnormality is one of quantity, specifically a decreased number of platelets (thrombocytopenia). **Thrombocytopenia** may result from decreased platelet production, an increase in the destruction of circulating platelets by immune and non-immune processes, or by increased splenic sequestration. Inadequate numbers of circulating platelets increase the bleeding tendency and the risk of spontaneous bleeding.

Thrombocytosis, an abnormally increased platelet count, can be benign and transient in nature or may be pathologic. Significant thrombocytosis can increase the risk of thrombus formation or of hemorrhage (usually only with platelet counts exceeding one million [Ravel, 1995]). Platelet counts may be performed by manual or automated means as described in Chapter 3. A typical reference range for platelets is 150,000 to 400,000/μL. Significant bleeding does not usually occur with functional platelets above 50,000 or 60,000. Spontaneous bleeding is likely if platelet counts fall below 20,000. The presence of purpura is suggestive of platelet abnormality.

Qualitative platelet disorders are related to the functions of platelets in the hemostatic process (adhesion, aggregation, release). As is the case with other aspects of hemostatic responses, the platelet response to vessel injury involves a number of interrelated processes and reactions. Formation of the primary hemostatic plug begins with the exposure of platelets to subendothelial collagen or the basement membrane as a result of vessel injury causing platelets to adhere (stick to) the area of damage. The degree of platelet response to the vessel damage is partially dependent on the extent of the injury (minor injuries expose basement membrane only and elicit a lesser response than more significant injuries that also expose varying types of collagen and elicit more significant responses).

Adhesion involves an interaction between these exposed surfaces and the glycoproteins of the platelet membrane. Platelet adhesion cannot occur without the plasma protein **factor VIII:vWF** (von Willebrand factor) and a **platelet receptor called platelet membrane glycoprotein 1b**. The VIII:vWF serves to link the glycoprotein 1b platelet receptor to the exposed subendothelial tissue (Lotspeich-Steininger, 1992). A lack of either results in defective platelet adhesion as seen in von Willebrand's disease (lack of VIII:vWF) and in Bernard-Soulier syndrome (lack of platelet membrane receptor glycoprotein 1b).

Aggregation, the ability of the platelets to stick to each other, occurs in primary and secondary waves and includes changes in platelet shape with the development of pseudopods that facilitate aggregation. Aggregation begins in response to a number of **stimuli** including ADP, thromboxane A2 (TxA_2), thrombin, collagen, and epinephrine. The primary wave of aggregation follows stimulation by ADP and by surface contact (Sacher and McPherson, 1991). ADP is released from the dense granules of these activated platelets, resulting in the involvement of additional platelets in a secondary wave of irreversible aggregation. This ADP release also activates an enzyme (phospholipase) that reacts with platelet membrane phospholipids to produce arachidonic acid, a precursor to both mediators and inhibitors of aggregation. As a result of a complicated series of reactions in the prostaglandin pathway and the **cyclo-oxygenase pathway of arachidonic acid metabolism**, endoperoxidases are produced that result in **formation of thromboxane A2 (potent stimulator of aggregation and vasoconstriction)** and **prostacyclin** (PGI_2), which **inhibits platelet aggregation** (by increasing platelet levels of cyclic AMP) and causes vasodilation (Lotspeich-Steininger, 1992). A simplified schematic of the cyclo-oxygenase pathway of arachidonic acid metabolism is presented in Figure 15–7. Note that **aspirin can interfere with this process** by inhibiting the action of cyclo-oxygenase on arachidonic acid. Figure 15–8 represents the formation of the primary hemostatic (platelet) plug and subsequent fibrin stabilization.

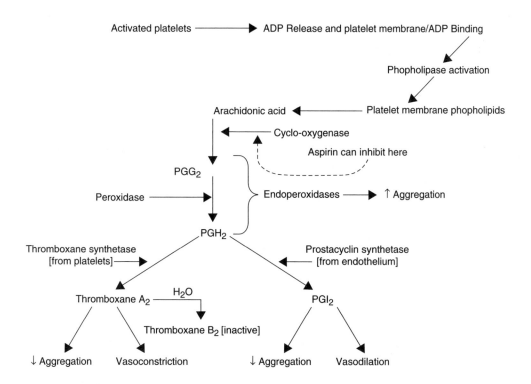

FIGURE 15-7. Cyclo-oxygenase pathway of arachidonic acid metabolism.

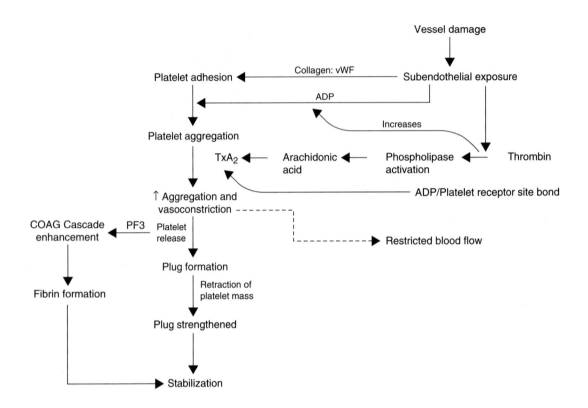

FIGURE 15–8. Primary hemostatic (platelet) plug formation.

Platelets also release a variety of substances (see earlier discussion and Table 15–1) important to the hemostatic process. When a platelet abnormality is suggested on the basis of history and/or examination but the platelet count is within acceptable ranges, a defect in platelet function should be considered. Laboratory assays of platelet function include

- bleeding time
- clot retraction
- platelet aggregation
- beta thromboglobulin
- platelet factor III
- platelet factor IV release assay
- platelet survival

The **bleeding time**, performed in a controlled and standardized manner, is probably the single best indicator of overall platelet function. Prolonged bleeding times are seen in response to both quantitative and qualitative defects such as:

- thrombocytopenia: count < 100,000 (Ravel, 1995); any etiology
- von Willebrand's disease: platelet adhesion defect
- most defects of platelet function: abnormal in most congenital defects (eg, Glanzmann's thrombasthenia) and acquired defects (eg, uremia, myelo-proliferative disorders)
- after aspirin ingestion: inhibits action of cyclo-oxygenase on arachidonic acid
- afibrinogenemia and severe hypofibrinogenemia: absent or insufficient fibrin is produced to permit formation of a stable plug
- some vascular disorders (Lotspeich-Steininger, 1992)

An incision of standardized length and depth, as well as standardized test conditions (such as pressure application), is critical to achieve reliable, reasonably reproducible results. This test evaluates the formation of a primary hemostatic plug in response to a small, clean incision in the forearm. The capillaries injured as a consequence of the incision will bleed until the damaged area is plugged by the aggregation of platelets. Pressure is maintained at a constant 40 mm Hg throughout the test. Although the same in principle, today's bleeding time differs in some important aspects from earlier versions of the procedure. In early versions of the bleeding time (Duke method and Ivy method) standardization was inadequate, particularly in terms of the depth of the incision. Modifications of the Ivy method using a template to standardize the incision (Mielke modification) improved upon the reproducibility of the test. The size of the standard incision 1 mm depth and 9 mm length) in this procedure may result in scarring. Commercially available devices (Surgicutt and Simplate) that standardize the incision and use a shorter incision (5 mm) of the same depth are now used in many laboratories. In addition to providing a means for reproducible incisions, these devices offer the added convenience of being disposable and easy to use. Devices are also available in smaller versions for use on pediatric patients. Despite significant improvements, duplication of results remains an issue with the bleeding time. Even when performed in accordance with a standardized test protocol and in a skillful manner, some variation is inherent in the procedure. Results should however, agree within at least 2 to 3 minutes (Sacher and McPherson, 1991). **Reference ranges** should be established by the laboratory in accordance with the method used and may vary somewhat in children and adults. A typical reference range is 2 to 9 minutes (Lotspeich-Steininger, 1992). Conflicting reports concerning the usefulness of the bleeding time as a predictor of surgical hemorrhage risk are found in the literature. Disagreement seems to be greater in regard to bleeding times that are elevated to a mild or moderate degree. Despite these differing reports and study results, significantly prolonged bleeding times (especially with times twice the upper limit of the reference range [Ravel, 1995]) indicate a definite increase in bleeding risk and bleeding times 1.5 times the upper limit somewhat increase the possibility of excessive bleeding during surgery. Bleeding times in excess of 15 minutes with a normal platelet count are highly suggestive of a qualitative platelet defect and should be investigated further utilizing more specific tests of platelet function (ie, von Willebrand factor, platelet aggregation tests, etc). (If the validity of initial bleeding time results is questionable, the clinician may prefer to repeat the bleeding time test prior to initiating additional procedures.)

Though infrequently utilized, the **clot retraction** test is a general measure of the ability of platelets to assist in producing a firmer clot. Clots shrink and express serum trapped within the clot. In this test, whole blood is allowed to clot in a glass tube at 37°C. After an hour clot retraction should have begun with the clot shrinking and pulling away from the sides of the tube. Full clot retraction is not achieved for about 24 hours at which time the clot will take up about half of the original blood volume. Normal clot retraction requires adequate numbers of platelets, ability of the platelets to function in the retraction process ("contractile" platelets), the presence of calcium and ATP, and a sufficient fibrinogen level. Although normal in a variety of platelet abnormalities, clot retraction is usually abnormal in thrombocytopenia, in Glanzmann's thrombasthenia, and with some fibrinogen abnormalities. The availability of more accurate, specialized tests of platelet function that rely less on subjective judgments and produce more timely results have made clot retraction an outdated test procedure.

Platelet aggregation tests evaluate the ability of platelets to stick to one another in the formation of the primary hemostatic plug. In this assay, substances known to initiate platelet aggregation *in vitro* are introduced into platelet rich plasma. As platelets begin to change shape and form aggregates in response to the aggregating agent, the plasma becomes less turbid (clearer), allowing increasing amounts of light to be transmitted through the specimen. A device called a "platelet aggregometer" is used to measure and record the changes in transmitted light. A variety of **aggregating agents** may be employed for this purpose: ADP, epinephrine, ristocetin (an antibiotic demonstrated to induce shape change and aggregation in platelets, collagen, thrombin, and arachidonic acid). Typical aggregation curves are depicted in Figure 15–9. Note that a "lag" phase occurs after the addition of collagen and is followed by a single wave of aggregation, whereas ristocetin and thrombin generally produce a biphasic (two-wave) response. Arachidonic acid responses are also usually biphasic. The aggregation curves seen with ADP and epinephrine are dependent on the concentration used (Lotspeich-Steininger, 1992). Platelet aggregation results are interpreted by comparing the results obtained with the patient's specimen to those obtained on normal control specimens (comparison with a single normal control is not generally sufficient, except with prominent abnormalities, because of the expected level of variability among individuals and the many variables involved in aggregation testing—see list). Because some degree of subjectivity is inherent in interpretation of these results, individuals charged with this responsibility must be experienced and possess a good understanding of the process of platelet aggregation, the variables affecting results, and the amount of variability expected among normal responses.

As noted previously, a number of factors may affect platelet aggregation studies. Many of these factors are related to the collection and storage of samples to be used for testing. For this reason it is imperative that specimens be collected by strict adherence to established procedures, stored only as directed, and analyzed within the acceptable time period. Other factors are concerned with specimen and reagent characteristics (eg, hematocrit of sample, concentration and pH of aggregating agent). A number of these factors are listed and described briefly as follows:

- Specimens must be collected in plastic tubes and should not come in contact with any type of glassware since glass activates platelets.
- Samples should be kept at room temperature until testing begins. Platelets will be viable longer at room temperature; refrigerated temperatures will reduce platelet responsiveness to aggregating agents.
- Testing should be completed no more than 2 hours after sample collection.
- Samples should be maintained in closed tubes to avoid carbon dioxide loss and resultant changes in pH.
- Appropriate blood to anticoagulant ratio is essential. Specimens in which the hematocrit is either significantly increased or decreased may require adjustment of anticoagulant (low hematocrit needs more anticoagulant; higher hematocrits need less [Lotspeich-Steininger, 1992]).

Assays for the measurement of specific substances released by platelets are also available and may be indicated for differential diagnosis or for confirmation of a particular diagnosis suggested by other findings. These tests include beta-thromboglobulin, platelet factor III, and platelet factor IV.

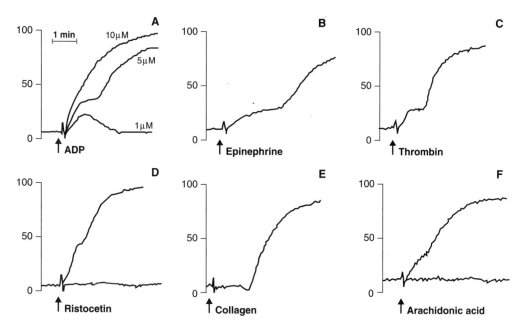

FIGURE 15–9. Platelet aggregation response curves. (From Lotspeich-Steininger C, Stiene-Martin A, Koepke J. *Clinical Hematology: Principles, Procedures, Correlations.* Philadelphia, Lippincott, 1992.)

FIBRINOGEN ASSAYS

There are a variety of methods for the measurement of fibrinogen (factor I), the precursor of fibrin. The conversion of fibrinogen to fibrin is under the influence of thrombin and is the last major step in the process of coagulation. A commonly used technique involves the addition of a high concentration of thrombin to the plasma sample and measuring the clotting time. The time required for clot detection is inversely proportional to the concentration of fibrinogen in the sample. Standards with known concentrations of fibrinogen are used to establish a standard curve from which the fibrinogen concentration in the unknown sample can be determined. Although today's techniques for this procedure are not as sensitive to the presence of heparin and FDP as some previous methods, these substances may affect results. Collection of specimens for fibrinogen testing through heparinized lines should be avoided for this reason. Testing can also be performed using certain snake venom reagents in place of the thrombin. The test principle is essentially the same, but snake venom reagents are not affected by the presence of heparin.

Immunologic assays of fibrinogen employ an antibody specific for fibrinogen and are often not readily available in most clinical settings. Both functional and dysfunctional fibrinogen are measured using this technique, because conversion of fibrinogen to fibrin is not measured, as is the case in the previously described method. For this reason, the use of these two assays together can be useful in the diagnosis of dysfibrinogenemia.

Decreased levels of fibrinogen may result either from increased conversion of fibrinogen to fibrin at a rate that does not allow adequate replacement, or from decreased liver production of fibrinogen. Increased conversion of fibrinogen to fibrin may be a result of disseminated intravascular coagulation (DIC) or the activation of fibrinolysis. (See DIC discussion in later section of this chapter.) Depleted fibrinogen levels seen in DIC are sometimes said to result from the "consumption" of fibrinogen. Fibrinogen depletion occurs, however, as fibrinogen is converted, not consumed. Liver disease can result in decreased production of fibrinogen, but significantly low levels develop only with severe damage. **Increased fibrinogen levels** may be seen in response to trauma or the onset of severe illnesses, in smokers, and as a result of genetic conditions (Ravel, 1995). Increased production of fibrinogen in trauma and severe illness is an acute reaction and the increases seen in fibrinogen are temporary. A typical **reference range** for quantitation of fibrinogen by measuring the fibrinogen to fibrin conversion subsequent to thrombin addition is 200 to 400 mg/dL.

COAGULATION FACTOR ASSAYS

There are a number of laboratory techniques available for the determination of specific coagulation factor levels. These techniques may assess the functional activity of the factor (one- and two-stage clotting methods; fluorometric and colorimetric methods) or may involve a quantitative immunoassay of the factor using electroimmunodiffusion, immunoradioometric assay (IRMA), or enzyme linked immunoassay (ELISA) techniques (Lotspeich-Steininger, 1992). One-stage clotting assays are simpler techniques that are based on modifications of the PT and APTT (depending on the factor being assayed) in which the clotting time for deficient plasma is corrected by the addition of various dilutions of plasma containing the deficient factor. A standard curve is constructed using dilutions of a known standard and the unknown factor activity is determined by converting the clotting time to percent activity from this curve. Factor assays are not as readily available as the more routine coagulation tests (eg, PT, APTT, fibrinogen) for a variety of reasons, including the length of time required for testing, the level of expertise required, and the number of frozen or commercial lyophilized reference and deficient plasma samples that must be maintained and tested. Assay of factor VIII:C (coagulant activity of factor VIII) and factor VIII:vWF (von Willebrand factor) are commonly employed in the diagnosis and differentiation of hemophilia A and von Willebrand disease. (See later discussions of hemophilias and von Willebrand's disease.) An immunologic assay is available for the measurement of another component of the factor VIII complex referred to as the factor VIII related antigen (factor VIIIR:Ag) and for the Ristocetin co-factor (the von Willebrand-Ristocetin effect on platelets). Assay of the Ristocetin co-factor assesses the functionality of vWF and may be referred to as factor VIIIR:RC or factor VIIIR:Rco.

TESTS OF THE FIBRINOLYTIC SYSTEM

Fibrinolysins (enzymes that destroy fibrinogen, fibrin, or both) may be **acquired or natural**. Natural fibrinolysins are a part of the body's normal response to intravascular clot formation and are discussed in the previous section on the fibrinolytic system. These naturally occurring fibrinolysins are also referred to as **secondary fibrinolysins** because their action is generally directed at fibrin, rather than fibrinogen, except when they are present in high concentrations. Acquired fibrinolysins are not common. They are associated with malignancy and long, extensive surgery (Ravel, 1995) and are referred to as **primary fibrinolysins** because the target of their action is fibrinogen (circulating primary fibrinolysins do not require initiation of fibrin clot formation for activation) rather than fibrin.

A variety of tests are available to detect the presence of fibrinolysins. A number of coagulation tests used primarily to assess other aspects of hemostasis can provide indirect evidence of the presence of fibrinolysins as a result of either

- decreased fibrinogen levels consequent to fibrinolysis (fibrinogen assays) or
- interference of fibrin/fibrinogen degradation products with the assay (PT, APTT, thrombin time). FDP can block the conversion of fibrinogen to fibrin by interfering with the action of thrombin.

More sensitive assays involve the detection of FDP (may refer to fibrinogen degradation products, fibrin degradation products, or both and may sometimes be called fibrin split products). Recall that in the degradation of fibrin the fibrin polymer is split into smaller fragments in a series of proteolytic steps. It is these fragments—the products of degradation—that are detected. The degradation products are not only incapable of forming clots themselves, but also may interfere with the ability of any remaining fibrinogen to participate in the clotting process. When fibrinolysis occurs, the degradation products enter the circulation and are cleared by the liver and reticuloendothelial system. It is when excessive fibrinolysis occurs, resulting in concentrations of FDP that are too high to be effectively cleared, that problems occur in hemostasis. Testing for these products is based on immunological principles (tests based on functionality cannot be employed because the products are by definition abnormal in terms of biologic activity). A commonly used FDP method utilizes latex particles that are coated with specific antibodies. Addition of this reagent will produce agglutination when added to the patient's sample if degradation products are present in sufficient quantity. Specimens producing positive results can then be diluted and tested to provide semi-quantitative test results (highest dilution producing positive results). The dilution at which agglutination last occurs can also provide information suggestive of etiology. Test results must be interpreted based on the particular method used, but general principles are as follows:

- titer of ≤ 1:10: generally considered to be normal
- titers > 1:10 but < 1:40: typical of venous thrombosis with secondary fibrinolysin response (may also produce titers above 1:40 in some cases; titers > 1:10 and < 1:40 occasionally seen in clinically normal persons [Ravel, 1995])
- titer > 1:40: suggestive of DIC; mild cases may produce lower titer

It is important to recognize that such methods do not detect all degradation products present because some FDP may be bound to fibrinogen and not detected (Henry, 1996). Assays that utilize antibodies directed at the D and E fragments (late products of degradation) are generally considered more reliable in terms of sensitivity levels than are those detecting only X and Y fragments. The protamine sulfate test, developed to detect the presence of degradation products by releasing fibrin monomers and allowing them to polymerize (Ravel, 1995), has largely been replaced by the immunologic FDP assay.

A newer FDP assay called the **D-dimer test** is abnormal in most of the same conditions as the assay previously described, but distinguishes primary and secondary fibrinolysis. In this test, an antibody specific for the cross-linked D-dimer (D-D fragment) is employed. The D-dimer can only be produced when fibrin (not fibrinogen) is broken down because cross-linkage occurs *after* fibrin formation. D-dimer testing can be performed on plasma, whereas specimens used for FDP testing are serum with a plasmin inhibitor added to avoid continued *in vitro* degradation. The ability to directly test plasma in the D-dimer assay avoids the concern that levels of FDP detected may include products of *in vitro* lysis as well. Thus the

D-dimer test is used as a specific indicator of intravascular of thrombus formation and subsequent degradation of fibrin and to verify *in vivo* fibrinolysis.

Other tests of the fibrinolytic system include the measurement of functional levels of plasminogen (the precursor of plasmin), of alpha-2-antiplasmin (an inhibitor of fibrinolysis), and of the plasminogen activator inhibitor (PAI). Because PAI is an acute phase reactant (like fibrinogen), levels may be increased following surgery. However, levels that are elevated prior to surgery correlate with an increase in the development of post-operative thrombosis (Jacobs, 1990). PAI levels may also be used in the evaluation of deep vein thrombosis and myocardial infarction (increased levels seen in patients with recurrent myocardial infarction, coronary artery disease, and deep vein thrombosis [Jacobs, 1990]). There are two separate forms of PAI; an assay specific for the PAI-1 form is under development for clinical use (Henry, 1996).

■ TESTS FOR COAGULATION INHIBITORS

A variety of substances that act to inhibit coagulation (see previous discussion of natural anticoagulants) can be measured by laboratory methods. Antithrombin III, proteins C and S, alpha-1-antitrypsin, C_1 esterase inhibitor, and the lupus anticoagulant are discussed here.

Antithrombin III (ATIII) assays include immunologic tests that measure the ATIII concentration and functional assays that provide an estimation of ATIII activity. Decreased ATIII concentrations may be seen as a result of severe liver disease and in DIC as well as in an uncommon hereditary condition. Other conditions leading to a secondary decrease in ATIII include deep vein thrombosis, extensive malignancy, nephrotic syndrome, septicemia, and major surgery (Ravel, 1995). Persons with decreased ATIII levels are generally considered to be at higher risk for the development of venous thrombosis (hereditary deficiency is associated with very high risk [Ravel, 1995]). ATIII assays are also beneficial in investigating an inadequate response to heparin therapy. When patients with decreased ATIII levels (generally 40 % or less of normal) are given standard heparin doses the expected change in the APTT may not occur, giving the appearance that the patient is "resistant" to heparin. Patients who do not respond as expected to heparin therapy should be evaluated for ATIII deficiency.

Protein C, an enzyme that is produced by the liver and is vitamin K dependent, circulates in an inactive form. When activated, it serves as an anticoagulant by inactivating the active forms of factors V and VIII, thus inhibiting both the intrinsic (factor VIIIa) and the extrinsic (factor Va) coagulation pathways. In order to be fully effective, protein C requires another liver synthesized, vitamin K dependent protein called protein S as a cofactor. A decrease in either of these proteins can result in an increased risk of vascular thrombosis. A congenital deficiency of protein C may result in recurrent thrombophlebitis and pulmonary embolism, particularly in high risk situations such as trauma, surgery, or pregnancy (Ravel, 1995). Heterozygous individuals are unlikely to develop problems before adolescence, whereas homozygous conditions produce symptoms of greater severity that are noted soon after birth. Acquired deficiencies may result from liver disease or vitamin K deficiency and may be seen in DIC and as a result of some medications (particularly Coumarin anticoagulants). Both proteins C and S are measured by similar techniques that include immunologic quantitation methods and complex methods for the evaluation of functional activity. Assays should be performed prior to the institution of Coumarin anticoagulant therapy because levels can be significantly decreased as a result. It may be desirable to first use functional activity assays when protein C or S abnormalities are suspected (Ravel, 1995), because normal quantities of the proteins may be present but lack normal functional capability. Such assays are likely to be available only in larger or more specialized laboratories.

Alpha-1-antitrypsin is an inhibitor of both the coagulation and fibrinolytic systems, but plays a more significant role in coagulation inhibition, where it acts as a powerful inhibitor of factor XIa. Hereditary deficiencies are associated with serious lung and liver disorders, but have not been linked to abnormalities of hemostasis. Assay and phenotyping of alpha-1-antitrypsin are discussed in Chapter 4.

The **C_1 esterase inhibitor** (also called C_1 *inhibitor* or C_1 *inactivator*) was first identified as a result of its role as an inhibitor in the complement system. It has subsequently been associated with inhibitory actions in the coagulation, fibrinolytic, and kinin systems as well (Lotspeich-Steininger, 1992). Its inhibitory action in the coagulation system is directed toward factors XIIa and XIa. (In the fibrinolytic system it inhibits plasmin and in the kinin system it inhibits kallikrein [Lotspeich-Steininger, 1992].) Assays for C_1 esterase inhibitor may be quantitative in nature or may assess the functional activity of the inhibitor.

The **lupus anticoagulant** inhibits the interaction of phospholipids with the coagulation factors and can lead to a prolonged APTT or PT. This immunoglobulin may also be referred to as *lupus inhibitor, phospholipid type* or as *phospholipid type anticoagulant*. Interestingly, this anticoagulant is more likely to produce thrombus formation than bleeding tendency (Sacher and McPherson, 1991). It is most often detected as part of the follow-up to an elevated APTT. Its name originated from its presence in patients with systemic lupus erythematosus (SLE), but it is more often found in persons without SLE (Jacobs, 1990, Sacher and McPherson, 1991). Assay of this anticoagulant is important in the work-up of patients with thrombosis or with elevations in the APTT and in some cases of fetal death (especially mid-term fetal death [Jacobs, 1990] and in recurrent spontaneous abortion [Sacher and McPherson, 1991]). The presence of this inhibitor is also associated with drug therapy with chlorpromazine and with some autoimmune diseases other than SLE. The lupus anticoagulant is seen in up to 50% of AIDS patients (Jacobs, 1990) and may also be present in some "normal" individuals.

■ CORRECTION STUDIES (MIXING STUDIES)

Taken together, the results of the PT and APTT can provide valuable information in regard to the nature of factor deficiencies or underlying disorders. Additional information can then be obtained by performing correction studies (also called *mixing* or *substitution studies*) and, if indicated, specific factor assays. Recall that the PT is a test of the extrinsic coagulation pathway and is sensitive to deficiencies in factors II, V, VII, and X, and to a lesser degree, factor I. The APTT is a test of the intrinsic coagulation pathway and is more sensitive to defects in the common pathway than the PT. It can detect deficiencies in all of the coagulation factors except factors VII and VIII. Table 15–4 provides a general guide to the various combinations of PT and APTT test results.

The addition of normal serum and/or fresh plasma to samples followed by repeat testing to determine whether prolonged times are corrected can provide additional information to the clinician and can be of particular importance in differentiating deficiencies of factors VIII and IX. Before undertaking such studies it is prudent to have a new specimen collected and the PT and APTT repeated, particularly in the absence of clinical indicators of abnormality. Inappropriate specimen collection may result in falsely prolonged times in both the PT and the APTT. Interpretation of **correction studies** is dependent on an understanding of the differences in plasma and serum. *In vivo,* **plasma** is the liquid part of the blood. When blood is removed from the body clotting will occur if anticoagulant substances are not promptly added to and mixed with the blood specimen. Anticoagulants used to maintain the blood in a fluid state *in vitro* act by different mechanisms including the chelation of calcium (EDTA for example) and inhibition of thrombin (heparin). Anticoagulated specimens are then centrifuged to separate cellular elements from the plasma. **Serum**, on the other hand, is the fluid that is left after blood is allowed to clot in the test tube. Clotted specimens are then centrifuged for better separation of the clot from the serum. Serum and plasma are distinctly different in terms of the coagulation proteins they contain. Fresh plasma will contain all of the coagulation proteins that are present in circulating

TABLE 15–4. Evaluation of PT and APTT Results

	Normal APTT	**Prolonged APTT**
Normal PT	No apparent abnormality	Deficiency of one or more of factors VIII, IX, XI, XII von Willebrand's disease
Prolonged PT	Isolated factor VII deficiency: result of liver disease or anticoagulant inhibition of vit. K Rare congenital factor VII deficiency	Deficiency of factor V, X or II Significant fibrinogen defects[1] Presence of inhibitors Presence of fibrinolysins DIC (high levels of FDP) Severe liver disease or combined factor deficiencies High heparin levels[1]

[1]Both usually prolonged in these cases. Factor XIII is not measured by either test—clot will dissolve in 5M urea if factor XIII is deficient.

Data from Sacher RA, McPherson RA. *Widmann's Clinical Interpretation of Laboratory Tests,* 10th ed. Philadelphia, FA Davis, 1991.

blood. Factors V and VIII are more labile than the other factors and will begin to decrease in stored plasma samples. Because the fibrinogen is converted to fibrin in the coagulation process, serum does not contain fibrinogen. Factors XIII, VIII, V, and II are also consumed or destroyed in the coagulation process and consequently are not present in serum. Factors VII, IX, X, XI, and XII are present in serum. A special type of plasma, called **absorbed plasma**, results from the addition of substances that remove the liver synthesized vitamin K dependent factors (II, VII, IX, X) from plasma. Thus absorbed plasma contains factors I, V, VIII, XI, XII and XIII. Table 15–5 summarizes the coagulation proteins found in fresh plasma, absorbed plasma, and serum.

With this knowledge and an understanding of the factors to which the PT and APTT are sensitive, tentative confirmation of a factor deficiency or the presence of an inhibitor can be made based on the correction or lack of correction of prolonged times with mixing studies. The following example is a good illustration of the application of mixing studies in follow-up to PT and APTT results.

> **Example.** A patient with a normal PT and a prolonged APTT on initial testing (confirmed by repeat analysis on a new specimen) could have a deficiency of factor VIII, IX, XI, or XII (see Table 15–4). Deficiencies of either factor VIII (hemophilia A) or factor IX (hemophilia B) could produce these results and the same clinical findings. If the APTT time is corrected following the addition of absorbed plasma, the presumptive diagnosis is a deficiency in factor VIII and can be confirmed by factor VIII assay. (Factor VIII is present in absorbed serum; factor IX is not present in absorbed plasma, but is found in serum.)

Using fresh normal plasma in mixing studies is helpful in detecting the presence of an inhibitor. Because fresh plasma contains all the circulating coagulation proteins, prolonged PT or APTT times due to factor deficiencies should be corrected by the addition of fresh plasma. If correction does not result from mixing fresh plasma (one part patient plasma and one part normal fresh plasma), the presence of an inhibitor should be suspected. (Conversely, the addition of plasma containing an inhibitor to plasma on which normal times were previously obtained will result in prolonged PT and/or APTT times [depending on inhibitor] following mixing.) Table 15–6 illustrates expected test results for the PT, APTT, and correction studies for various factor deficiencies.

TABLE 15–5. Coagulation Proteins Present in Serum and Plasma

	Coagulation Proteins Present
Fresh plasma	I, II, V, VII, VIII, IX, X, XI, XII, XIII[1]
Absorbed plasma	I, V, VIII, XI, XII, XIII[1]
Serum	VII, IX, X, XI, XII

[1]Factor XIII not measured by either PT or APTT.

TABLE 15–6. Factor Deficiency Effects on PT, APTT, and Correction Studies

Deficient Factor	PT	APTT	Correction Studies Normal Plasma	Absorbed Plasma	Normal Serum
I	↑	↑	PT/APTT corrected	PT/APTT corrected	Neither corrected
II	↑	↑	PT/APTT corrected	Neither corrected	Neither corrected
V	↑	↑	PT/APTT corrected	PT/APTT corrected	Neither corrected
VII	↑	N	PT corrected	PT *not* corrected	PT corrected
VIII	N	↑	APTT corrected	APTT corrected	APTT *not* corrected
IX	N	↑	APTT corrected	APTT *not* corrected	APTT corrected
X	↑	↑	PT/APTT corrected	APTT *not* corrected	APTT corrected
XI/XII	↑	↑	PT/APTT corrected	PT/APTT corrected	PT/APTT corrected
Inhibitor present[1]	↑	↑	PT/APTT *not* corrected	PT/APTT *not* corrected	PT/APTT *not* corrected

[1]If results suggest an inhibitor, more specific testing is indicated for identification and quantitation.

■ MONITORING ANTICOAGULANT THERAPY

The effect of anticoagulant therapy on laboratory coagulation studies is useful in achieving desired therapeutic levels. Laboratory monitoring of coumarin antico-agulants and heparin are discussed in this section. Recall that some of the coagulation proteins synthesized by the liver require vitamin K for synthesis and are thus termed *vitamin K dependent.* Coumarin anticoagulants act by inhibiting the liver cells ability to utilize vitamin K. Consequently, the factors affected by this anticoagulant are those that are vitamin K dependent—II, VII, IX, and X. Factor VII is most sensitive to the effect of the anticoagulant because it has the shortest half-life of the vitamin K dependent factors; factor II (prothrombin) is the least sensitive (Ravel, 1995). Of the various coumarin type anticoagulants, Coumadin (warfarin sodium) is the most commonly used in the United States. **Laboratory monitoring** of this anticoagulant is best achieved with the **PT**, which is sensitive to all of the vitamin K dependent factors except factor IX. The time required for blood levels of the anticoagulant to reach equilibrium is dependent on the half-life of the drug. Because the half-life varies significantly among individuals, the time required to achieve equilibrium is also highly variable. The desirable therapeutic range has generally been accepted as 2 to 2.5 times the mid-point of the reference range. However, recent recommendations (Ravel, 1995) suggest that a range 1.3 to 1.5 times this value should be used for PTs determined using rabbit brain or rab-bit brain/lung reagents (these are the reagents commonly used) and a range of 1.5

to 2.0 for when the anticoagulant is used with prosthetic valve patients. Assuming a PT reference range of 11 to 13 seconds (mid-point 12), the desired therapeutic range under the newer recommendations would be approximately 15 to 18 seconds (previously 24 to 30 seconds) and 18 to 24 seconds for prosthetic valve patients. It was previously noted that prothrombin times are sometimes reported as an INR. It is essential to note that use of the INR was developed only for use in monitoring anticoagulant therapy and only after the patient is stabilized on the therapy. Use of the INR reporting method at the initiation of therapy may produce misleading results.

Heparin acts to increase the anticoagulant effect of antithrombin III. Discovered before ATIII, heparin was initially credited with the anticoagulant effects seen following its administration. With current knowledge of ATIII, it appears that the primary anticoagulant action is the result of ATIII activity with heparin serving to significantly increase the effect when it binds to ATIII. In addition to the inhibition of thrombin, the ATIII/heparin complex also inhibits other coagulation factors to varying degrees with factors IXa and Xa being affected most. The half-life of heparin averages about 90 minutes, but a longer half-life is exhibited with increased dosage and a shorter half-life in the presence of deep vein thrombosis or pulmonary embolism (Ravel, 1995). Responses to heparin therapy are quite variable and are affected by a number of factors in addition to dosage and route of administration, including:

- antithrombin III levels
- significantly increased or decreased platelet levels: due to concentration of platelet factor 4; impact is not as significant as that of ATIII level
- presence of fibrin: fibrin can bind to thrombin preventing ATIII binding
- renal clearance: about 20 % (Ravel, 1995) of heparin in plasma is excreted by the kidneys; decreased clearance in renal failure may result in plasma levels sufficient to produce bleeding; obese patients may have decreased heparin clearance rates (Ravel, 1995)
- certain drugs: antihistamines, nicotine, phenothiazines, digitalis, tetracycline, and IV penicillin (Lotspeich-Steininger, 1992)

Heparin therapy is **monitored using the APTT**, with the **therapeutic range** generally targeted at 1.5 to 2.5 times the upper limit of the reference range. Others prefer to use a pre-therapy APTT time instead of the upper limit of the reference range. Use of this value may be preferred because a patient's pre-therapy time could be significantly lower than the upper reference range limit. For example, a therapeutic range based on a reference range upper limit of 35 would be 52.5 to 75 seconds, whereas use of the latter method for a patient with a pre-therapy time of 25 seconds would produce a range of 37.5 to 62.5 seconds. This method allows the desirable range to be "tailored" to the individual patient. Although recommendations for optimum time of specimen collection vary, the following times are generally considered appropriate:

- intermittent IV therapy: one half hour prior to next scheduled dose
- subcutaneous injection: half way between doses
- continuous IV therapy: no specified time because response is theoretically uniform (some studies have shown a circadian rhythm, with peak effect 7 PM to 7 AM; maximum 4 AM and through 7 AM to 7 PM—lowest 8 AM; other studies show no such rhythm [Ravel,1995])

Complications of heparin therapy include bleeding and thrombocytopenia. Thrombocytopenia seen as a consequence of heparin therapy is not often severe and is ordinarily reversed within a few days of the discontinuation of therapy. In some patients the thrombocytopenia may persist, with counts falling < 100,000. An even smaller percentage of patients (0.5 % [Ravel, 1995]) may develop a thrombocytopenia that is followed by the onset of arterial thrombosis (called *white clot syndrome* because of the partially white color of thrombi resulting from platelet masses [Ravel, 1995]). Heparin should be discontinued in such cases. Low molecular weight heparin is associated with a lower rate of bleeding complications and a more predictable response than is seen with high molecular weight fractions.

 TIME FOR REVIEW. After studying the preceding sections, you should be able to respond correctly to the following:

■ List the five factors detected by the prothrombin time.

■ The prothrombin time is used to monitor anticoagulant therapy with

_____.

■ The INR was developed to reduce _____ and is intended for use in monitoring _____ therapy after the patient is stabilized.

■ A test that is sensitive to factor deficiencies in the intrinsic coagulation pathway and is used to monitor heparin therapy is the _____.

■ The test that measures the rate of formation of fibrin and assesses the fibrinogen to fibrin conversion is the _____.

■ When performed in a standardized manner, this test is probably the best single indicator of overall platelet function: _____.

■ Platelet adhesion cannot occur without the plasma protein factor _____ and a platelet receptor called _____.

■ Platelet aggregation refers to the ability of platelets to _____.

■ Aggregation begins in response to a number of stimuli, including _____, _____, _____, _____, and _____.

■ Arachidonic acid metabolism results in the formation of a potent stimulator of aggregation and vasoconstriction called _____ and of an inhibitor of platelet aggregation called _____.

■ Briefly explain how aspirin interferes with platelet function.

■ List and briefly describe four tests of platelet function.

■ A number of factors influence tests of platelet aggregation. List and briefly describe five of these.

■ Indirect evidence of the presence of fibrinolysins may be provided by the results of tests usually used to assess other aspects of hemostasis. List three such tests and briefly explain how the presence of fibrinolysins produces abnormal results.

■ What is measured by the FDP test?

■ An FDP titer > 1:40 is suggestive of _____.

■ What is the primary advantage of the D-dimer test as compared to traditional FDP assays?

■ Other tests of the fibrinolytic system include the measurement of functional levels of _____, _____, and _____.

■ List and briefly describe four inhibitors of coagulation.

■ How are correction studies useful in the coagulation laboratory?

■ List the coagulation factors present in:

fresh plasma:

absorbed plasma:

serum:

■ How can correction studies be used to aid in differentiating deficiencies of factors VIII and IX?

■ When inadequate response to heparin therapy is seen, laboratory assay for this inhibitor should be performed: _____.

Check your responses by reviewing the preceding sections.

SELECTED DISORDERS

Coagulation disorders may be congenital or acquired conditions. Hemophilia A and B, von Willebrand's disease, liver disease, and disseminated intravascular coagulation (DIC) are presented in this section along with a brief summary of other inherited factor disorders. Platelet disorders are discussed in Chapter 3.

HEMOPHILIA

The term *hemophilia* is used to refer to a tendency for excessive bleeding. **Hemophilia A** (classic hemophilia) results from a congenital deficiency of factor VIII and **hemophilia B** (Christmas disease) is a consequence of an inherited deficiency of factor IX. The two conditions are virtually indistinguishable clinically and are inherited by the same patterns of genetic transmission. These conditions occur exclusively in males (with rare exceptions) as a result of X-linked inheritance. Because females have two X chromosomes (males one), those with the abnormal gene on one chromosome almost invariably have a normal gene on the other X chromosome providing sufficient factor activity to prevent clinical expression of the hemophiliac condition. If both X chromosomes have the abnormality, hemophilia may be expressed—generally in a mild form. Clinical expression of hemophilia ranges from nearly asymptomatic conditions to very severe cases. The severity of the condition is related to the percentage of factor activity (factor VIII:C for hemophilia A and factor IX for hemophilia B) present (Table 15–7).

Excessive bleeding consequent to trauma is the **major symptom** of hemophilia. Patients with severe hemophilia may bleed excessively following minimal trauma, while those with mild cases generally experience excessive bleeding only after more significant trauma. Mild cases may not be detected until excessive bleeding following a surgical procedure or tooth extraction occurs. Other symptoms include hemarthrosis (bleeding into joints; may be crippling over time), soft tissue hematomas, bleeding from the mouth, and urinary and gastrointestinal tract bleeding. Wound repair is often delayed as well. Spontaneous hemorrhaging may be seen in severe hemophiliacs in the absence of apparent trauma. Of particular concern is intracranial hemorrhage, which is relatively common in severe cases and may be fatal. Although clinical manifestations for hemophilia A and B are generally identical, hemarthrosis may not be seen as frequently in hemophilia B. This is not, however, sufficient basis for differentiation of the two conditions.

Differentiation of hemophilia A and hemophilia B is not possible based solely upon clinical symptoms and history. The two conditions were not distinguished until the early fifties. Symptoms may be identical and both follow the same pattern of inheritance. However, patients who present with symptoms suggestive of hemophilia are much more likely to suffer from factor VIII:C deficiency than from factor IX deficiency in terms of the incidence of these conditions (hemophilia A accounts for four out of five cases [Sacher and McPherson, 1991];

TABLE 15–7. Clinical Severity of Hemophilia

Clinical Severity	Factor Activity
Mild	Between 5% and 40%[1]
Moderate	Between 1 and 5%
Severe	< 1%

[1]Abnormality is usually not evident on laboratory screening until factor activity falls < 30% to 40%.

90% of cases [Ravel, 1995]). The **primary screening test** for hemophilia is the APTT, which is abnormal in response to significantly decreased activity of either factor VIII:C or factor IX. Mild or borderline cases and most carriers will not be detected by the APTT because factor activity must be significantly decreased (≤ 40% [Henry, 1996]; ≤ 30% to 35% [Ravel, 1995]; < 30% [Sacher and McPherson, 1991]) in order to produce a prolonged time. The PT, thrombin time, and, in most cases, the bleeding time are normal. Some patients (Ravel, 1995, Henry, 1996) may exhibit a prolonged bleeding time, particularly those with severe factor deficiencies. Correction studies may be used to differentiate factor VIII:C and factor IX deficiencies. Correction of the APTT with absorbed plasma and the failure of serum to correct the APTT provides a presumptive diagnosis of factor VIII:C deficiency (hemophilia A). Prolonged APTT values that result from factor IX deficiency are corrected by serum, but not by absorbed plasma (see Table 15–6). Specific factor assays are required for **definitive diagnosis** and to determine the level of factor activity. DNA probes are now available in some specialized laboratories and some specialized centers offer assays for prenatal diagnosis of hemophilia A.

Factor VIII concentrates, cryoprecipitate, and fresh frozen plasma are therapeutic sources of factor VIII. Treatment to arrest bleeding requires raising the plasma level of factor VIII to an adequate level (continuous level of at least 25% to 30% [Stein, 1993]) and is best achieved by the administration of factor VIII concentrate or cryoprecipitate. Factor VIII in these products is measured in units that are equivalent to the factor VIII activity in 1 mL of plasma. Methods for calculating dosage required to achieve desired plasma activity levels of factor VIII are

- (desired factor level – initial factor level) × plasma volume = units to administer; calculate plasma volume as 41 mL/kg body weight (hct > 35%) (formula from Stein, 1993)
- 1 unit of administered for each 2% of activity increase desired (ie, patient's factor VIII activity needs to be increased by 20%; 10 units required) "rule of thumb" (Ravel, 1995)

Because the half-life of factor VIII is about 12 hours, two doses are required in each 24-hour period. Factor VIII levels should be measured 6 hours after the dose at which time an activity of 50% to 60% is necessary to ensure that continuous levels of 25% to 30% are maintained (Stein, 1993). Surgery and dental extractions require prophylactic treatment and higher levels of factor VIII activity (50% to 60% [Stein, 1993]). Major surgical procedures should be avoided if at all possible. Patients with mild or moderate hemophilia may benefit from pharmacologic agents that act to increase the release of endogenous factor VIII (DDAVP—desmopressin acetate). This treatment avoids the use of donor products (cryoprecipitate, factor concentrates) and the associated risks of infectious disease transmission. Patients with severe hemophilia A are not sufficiently responsive to this treatment. Cryoprecipitate does not contain factor IX and thus is not a beneficial treatment for hemophilia B. Concentrates of factor IX as a single factor are not available. Concentrates of factor IX along with the other vitamin K dependent liver synthesized factors are available and can be used to raise the plasma factor IX levels. This factor concentrate contains concentrated factors II, VII, IX, and X and may be referred to as *prothrombin complex concentrate.* Fresh frozen plasma also contains factor IX.

■ VON WILLEBRAND'S DISEASE

This condition is usually inherited as an autosomal dominant trait, but autosomal recessive transmission has been described in some cases (Henry, 1996; Lotspeich-Steininger, 1992; Ravel, 1995), with rare cases of X-linked recessive transmission described (Ravel, 1995). It now appears to be the most commonly diagnosed congenital coagulation disorder. This disorder results from low levels of VIII:vWF and a resultant qualitative platelet adhesion defect. Patients with von Willebrand's disease also have a decreased level of factor VIII:C. Factor VIII nomenclature can be confusing and somewhat variable. The factor VIII complex (also referred to as VIII/vWF or factor VIII-vWF complex) includes

- VIII:C: the portion in the intrinsic coagulation pathway that serves as a co-factor in activating factor X; also referred to as pro-coagulant portion
- VIII:vWF: the portion that is important in platelet adhesion; may be referred to as simply vWF or vWF activity
- VIIIC:Ag: the part of VIII:C (procoagulant portion) to which antibodies are developed; portion measured by antibody techniques
- VIIIR:Ag: an antigen of the vWF portion of the factor VIII molecule; called factor VIII related antigen; also referred to as vWF:Ag
- VIIIR:RCo: the ristocetin cofactor involved in platelet aggregation

In most patients this coagulopathy does not produce severe clinical symptoms. Commonly seen symptoms include easy bruising, bleeding from mucous membrane and cutaneous sites, nosebleeds, and menorrhagia. Gastrointestinal bleeding and excessive bleeding following surgery or tooth extraction are also seen. The hemarthroses and soft tissue hematomas associated with hemophilia are not typical of von Willebrand's disease, but may be seen in severe cases in which the level of VIII:C is markedly decreased. The condition exists in a variety of types: type I (heterozygous, dominant inheritance with mild to moderate severity); type II, which includes subtypes (variable severity) and type III or homozygous type (a severe form inherited as a recessive trait) (Table 15–8). Laboratory findings are variable and depend, in part, upon the degree of factor VIII:C deficiency. Bleeding times are typically prolonged with a normal PT and thrombin time. The APTT may be normal or prolonged based on the activity of factor VIII:C. Factor VIII:C assays show decreased activity (to varying degrees) and VIIIR:RCo is reduced. Quantitative measurement of vWF:Ag is available by immunologic techniques (Laurell rocket method) and other methods that may be used in place of, or in conjunction with, the Laurell rocket. Measurement of the specific component activi-

TABLE 15–8. von Willebrand's Disease—Inherited Subtypes

vWF Type	Genetic Pattern[1]	Bleeding Time	PLT Count	Factor VIII	vWF:Ag	VIIIR:RCo	vWF Binding to Plts	vWF Multimer Pattern	vWF Binding to Factor VIII
1	Autosomal dominant	Often ↑	N	Often ↓	Usually ↓	Usually ↑	↓	Normal	Normal
2A	Autosomal dominant	Usually ↑	N	May be ↓	Usually ↓	↓	↓	HMW Multimers absent	Normal
2B	Autosomal dominant	Usually ↑	↓	May be ↓	Often ↓	↓	↑ (due to abnorm. vWF)	HMW Multimers may be absent	Normal
2M	Autosomal dominant	Often ↑	N	May be ↓	Usually ↓	Usually ↓	↓	Abn. structure: all HMW multimers present	Usually normal
2N	Autosomal dominant	Usually ↑	N	Markedly ↓	Usually ↓	Usually N	Usually N	Normal	Markedly ↓
3	Autosomal recessive	Markedly ↑	N	Markedly ↓	Markedly ↓	Markedly ↓	Markedly ↓	All multimers markedly ↓	Presumably normal

[1]Genetic pattern listed is most common inheritance pattern; HMW = high molecular weight.

Adapted from Henry JB. *Clinical Diagnosis and Management by Laboratory Methods,* 19th ed. Philadelphia, Saunders, 1996.

ties of the factor VIII complex is required for definitive diagnosis. Table 15–8 summarizes the various types of inherited (an acquired type of von Willebrand's results from the development of autoantibodies against vWF) von Willebrand's disease.

■ FACTOR I DISORDERS

Inherited fibrinogen disorders, which may be quantitative or qualitative in nature, are uncommon. Quantitative disorders include afibrinogenemia (a lack of fibrinogen) and hypofibrinogenemia (decreased levels of fibrinogen). **Afibrinogenemia** is inherited as an autosomal recessive trait and results in incoagulable blood. All laboratory assays dependent on the formation of fibrin (PT, APTT, fibrinogen assay, bleeding time, thrombin time, etc) will be elevated in this condition. Levels of fibrinogen in these patients are at or near 0. Fibrinogen levels in **hypofibrinogenemia** are < 100 mg/dL and generally produce prolonged times in tests that are dependent on the fibrinogen to fibrin conversion.

Structurally defective fibrinogen places the patient at risk for both bleeding and thrombus formation. The **dysfibrinogenemias** (functional defects consequent to structural disorders) can produce somewhat variable results with a number of laboratory assays, but may first be detected based on prolonged times for coagulation screening tests (especially thrombin time). In addition to abnormalities of fibrinogen structure, deficiencies in the fibrin stabilizing factor (factor XIII) may also be involved in functional fibrinogen disorders. Factor XIII deficiencies are not detected by these tests. The **reptilase time** is prolonged in the presence of structural defects in fibrinogen and may be useful because it is not elevated in response to the presence of heparin. Although the disorders are not common, there are at least 11 classifications of congenital dysfibrinogenemias, with nearly 50 conditions identified within these classifications. More specialized testing is required to determine the specific fibrinogen defect (such as release defect of fibrinogen A, B, or both; polymerization defect alone or in combination with release defects; fibrinopeptide defects of release, polymerization, or both; stabilization defects) and classify the disorder. Patients with fibrinogen disorders may exhibit easy bruising, bleeding tendencies, and poor wound healing, and, especially in the dysfibrinogenemias, may have thrombotic tendencies.

Hemostatic defects may result from a variety of inherited factor deficiencies in addition to those discussed for factors I, VIII, and IX. These are summarized in Table 15–9 along with corresponding acquired disorders.

TABLE 15–9. Congenital Factor Defects

Factor	Condition	Congenital Incidence	Acquired Defects in	Minimum Hemostatic Level[1]
I	Afibrinogenemia	Rare	Severe liver disease	
	Hypofibrinogenemia	Rare	DIC	50 to 100 mg
	Dysfibrinogenemia	Uncommon	Fibrinolysis	
II	Hypoprothrombinemia	Extremely rare	Liver disease	20% to 40%
			Vitamin K deficiency	
			Anticoagulant therapy	
V	Deficiency	1 in 1,000,000	Severe liver disease	
			DIC	10% to 25%
			Fibrinolysis	
VII	Deficiency	1 in 500,000	Liver disease	5% to 10% (Lotspeich-Steininger, 1992)
			Vitamin K deficiency	
			Anticoagulant therapy	10% to 20% (Sacher and McPherson, 1991)
VIII	Hemophilia A	1 in 10,000 males	DIC and fibrinolysis	25% to 30%
	von Willebrand's	1 in 80,000		20% to 40%
IX	Hemphilia B	~1 in 50,000 males	Liver disease	15% to 25% Lotspeich-Steininger, 1992)
			Vitamin K deficiency	
			Anticoagulant therapy	20% to 50% (Sacher and McPherson 1991)
X	Deficiency	Rare	Liver disease	
			Vitamin K deficiency	10% to 20%
			Anticoagulant therapy	
XI	Hemophilia C	Rare		10% to 25%
XII	Deficiency (Hageman trait)	Rare		0% to 5%[1]
XIII	Deficiency	Rare	Liver disease	
			DIC	1% to 3%
			Fibrinolysis	

[1]Minimum hemostatic level may differ slightly among literature sources; may not be required for adequate hemostasis.

Table compiled with data from various sources including Lotspeich-Steininger et al, 1992; Sacher and McPherson, 1991; Ravel, 1995; and Henry, 1996.

■ HEMOSTATIC DISORDERS IN LIVER DISEASE

Because of the important role of the liver in hemostasis, particularly in terms of the synthesis of coagulation factors, abnormalities should be anticipated in significant liver disease. The liver's hemostatic role is not limited to the synthesis of coagulation factors. It also plays a role in the synthesis of factors in the fibrinolytic system and in the breakdown and removal of factor complexes. Through poorly understood mechanisms, liver disease also affects the production and function of platelets. As a result, significant impairment of hepatic function can not only produce deficiencies in the coagulation proteins, but may also be complicated by excessive fibrinolysis, platelet disorders, and intravascular coagulation. The earliest and most frequently seen coagulation defect in liver disease is a deficiency in the vitamin K dependent factors (II, VII, IX, and X). Factor VII deficiency may be the first apparent defect and, when occurring alone, results in an elevation in the PT with a normal APTT. Depending on the type of liver disease, fibrinogen levels may be either increased or decreased. Normal levels of fibrinogen may be present, but dysfunctional as a result of structural abnormalities. Activity of factor VIII, vWF, and the ristocetin cofactor, which are not synthesized within the hepatocytes, may be normal or elevated. The impairment of platelet production and function consequent to liver disease is especially pronounced in alcoholics. Inability of the liver to clear activated coagulation and fibrinolytic factors results in an accumulation of these activated complexes. Hepatocellular damage sufficient to result in coagulation factor deficiencies also produces a decrease in the production of albumin and deficient levels of antithrombin III and proteins C and S. When hepatocytes are severely damaged, vitamin K administration does not produce an increase in factor synthesis.

Patients with hemostatic disorders attributable to liver damage do not commonly have spontaneous bleeding episodes in the absence of hemorrhagic lesions like esophageal varices or hemorrhagic gastritis (Sacher and McPherson, 1991). Patients may, however, experience significant post-operative bleeding or bleed excessively following liver biopsies.

■ VITAMIN K DEFICIENCY

Vitamin K is a fat soluble vitamin that promotes the hepatic synthesis of coagulation factors II, VII, IX, and X (the "vitamin K dependent" factors). Insufficient vitamin K levels lead to impaired synthesis of these factors, typically reflected by a prolonged PT. The APTT may be prolonged or normal. Vitamin K deficiency may result from inadequate dietary intake, biliary obstruction, or malabsorption. In addition, deficiency may result from the effect of antibiotic therapy on normal intestinal flora that normally synthesize vitamin K. Coumarin anticoagulant therapy acts by interfering with the synthesis of vitamin K. Vitamin K deficiency in newborns is of particular concern.

Vitamin K administration corrects coagulopathies that result from its deficiency and can also be used to help distinguish between obstructive and nonobstructive jaundice. The PT and APTT should be improved within 48 hours of vitamin K injection in cases of biliary obstruction (Sacher and McPherson, 1991). Improvement occurs because factor levels are low in this condition as a result of impaired vitamin K absorption (ie, bile salts do not reach the intestine where they aid fat absorption—vitamin K is a fat soluble substance).

■ DISSEMINATED INTRAVASCULAR COAGULATION

Disseminated intravascular coagulation (DIC) is a complex disorder that usually occurs secondary to other illnesses that may themselves be life threatening conditions even without the added complication of a bleeding disorder. It is a common cause of acquired bleeding tendency. DIC (also referred to as *consumptive coagulopathy, defibrination syndrome,* or *diffuse intravascular coagulation*) from a pathologic intravascular generation of thrombin triggered by the release of tissue thromboplastin, or other substances with similar effect, into the bloodstream. Consequently, the coagulation system is activated and fibrin or fibrin clots are deposited in small vessels throughout the body. As a result, coagulation proteins and platelets are consumed and the fibrinolytic system activated to remove the fibrin. In the absence of normal regulation, fibrinolysins encounter little hindrance in the lysis of any target coagulation proteins or platelets remaining in the circulation (ie, not used in the coagulation process). The severity of DIC is quite variable, ranging from chronic subacute cases to those of catastrophic severity. Prognosis is generally dependent on the nature of the underlying condition. Identification of the underlying disorder is crucial in order to allow the immediate institution of appropriate therapy. Initially associated with premature placental separation and amniotic fluid embolism, DIC may occur consequent to

- infectious conditions: particularly septicemia; some viral infections
- surgery: especially large scale procedures involving the brain, lungs, or genitourinary system or procedures complicated by intraoperative or postoperative shock
- obstetric conditions: amniotic fluid embolism, premature placental separation, retained fetus, septic abortion
- severe burns
- major trauma: particularly crush injuries
- leukemia and extensive solid malignancies
- tissue necrosis
- acidosis or alkalosis
- newborn respiratory distress syndrome
- vascular disorders
- liver disease: usually produces gradually developing DIC
- hemolytic transfusion reaction
- snake bites

An awareness of the conditions that predispose the development of DIC is imperative because diagnosis must be made as quickly as possible in the acute presentation of DIC (mortality rate estimated at 60% to 80% [Lotspeich-Steininger, 1992]). This disorder should be suspected in any patient who has a predisposing condition and begins to bleed or exhibits symptoms of organ damage by microemboli (hypotension, hypoxia, mental confusion, oliguria or anuria, acute respiratory failure, focal tissue infarction, etc). Bleeding may first be noted from venipuncture sites or surgical wounds. Nosebleeds, gastrointestinal tract bleeding, and widespread bruising are common. Oozing blood from tissues during surgery is a frequent warning sign (Ravel, 1995).

Specific triggers of DIC can initiate coagulation via the extrinsic pathway (thromboplastin release) or the intrinsic pathway (contact activation), or by direct activation of specific coagulation factors (II, X). Table 15–10 provides a classification of triggering mechanisms.

A number of laboratory assays may provide evidence of acute DIC as well as an indication of the nature of the underlying condition. Keeping the processes involved in DIC in mind that assists in understanding the results of laboratory assays used to confirm suspected DIC. These processes include

- activation of coagulation with the resultant generation of thrombin and fibrin formation
- consumption of coagulation factors (especially V and VIII)
- consumption of platelets
- activation of the fibrinolytic system and a subsequent increase in FDP in the circulation

TABLE 15–10. Classification of DIC Triggering Mechanisms

Extrinsic Activation	Intrinsic Activation	Direct Factor Activation
Thromboplastin release	Contact activation	Factor II or X activation
Trauma	Shock	Snake venom
Surgery	Sepsis	Pancreatitis
Sepsis	Hemangioma	Sepsis
Hemolysis	Burns	Carcinoma
Acidosis	Vasculitis	
Obstetric events	Aneurysm	
Carcinoma		
Hypoxia		
Antigen/antibody complex		

The classic laboratory picture of acute DIC includes elevations in the PT, APTT, and thrombin time in conjunction with a decreased fibrinogen concentration and platelet count. FDP tests are positive, often at a titer of > 1:40. The D-dimer test is a sensitive early indicator of DIC and may be positive as soon as 4 hours (Lotspeich-Steininger, 1992) after onset. Laboratory findings of concurrent hypofibrinogenemia and thrombocytopenia are highly suggestive of DIC. In addition, levels of ATIII are decreased. Hemoglobin and hematocrit levels are variable decreased based upon the degree of bleeding. Peripheral blood smears may show schistocytosis and evidence of leukocytosis, thrombocytopenia, and reticulocytosis. (Peripheral smear examination findings may be consistent with a microangiopathic hemolytic anemia [Ravel,1995]) Samples may show varying degrees of hemolysis, often marked, indicative of intravascular hemolysis. Laboratory findings in acute cases of classic DIC are summarized in Table 15–11. Cases of chronic DIC, as may be seen with liver disease, can be more difficult to diagnose as a result of varying degrees of platelet and coagulation factor depletion that may be only slight. Serial measurements, though variable, may be necessary to achieve definitive diagnosis in such cases.

TABLE 15–11. Laboratory Findings in Acute Presentation of Classic DIC

Laboratory Assay	Result	Comments
Fibrinogen	↓	Decreases 4 to 24 hours after onset
Platelet count	↓	Decreases 48 hours after onset
PT	↑	Degree of prolongation varies
APTT	↑	Degree of prolongation varies
Thrombin time	↑	Degree of prolongation varies
Antithrombin III	↓	
FDP	↑	Sensitive test
D-dimer	↑	May be detected 4 hours after onset; sensitive, specific test
Factor V assay	↓	Generally not performed as part of diagnostic work-up; levels of other factors also decreased
Factor VIII assay	↓	Generally not performed as part of diagnostic work-up; levels of other factors also decreased
Hemoglobin/hematocrit	Variably ↓	Dependent on degree of hemorrhage
Reticulocyte count	↑	Additional information provided, but is not primary test for DIC
WBC	↑	Additional information provided, but is not primary test for DIC
Peripheral smear	↑ Schistocytes	Additional information provided, but is not primary test for DIC

Laboratory assays also provide an indication of the underlying condition in many situations (ie, positive blood cultures with sepsis, evidence of liver damage, leukocyte abnormalities in leukemia, etc), but history may provide the best indicator in others (ie, snake bite, postoperative conditions, postpartum state, etc). As previously noted, it is imperative to determine the underlying condition because successful management of DIC must focus on treatment of the precipitating condition, as DIC will likely not be resolved until this condition is treated. This is no easy task in catastrophic conditions such as massive traumas, overwhelming sepsis, and cardiogenic shock. In addition, treatment must be implemented to maintain an adequate blood volume and to restore depleted coagulation factors and platelets. Blood components often used in the management of DIC include red blood cells to correct anemia, platelet transfusions to treat thrombocytopenia, and fresh frozen plasma and/or cryoprecipitate to replenish depleted coagulation factors. Repeat laboratory determinations should be utilized at periodic intervals to determine the levels of correction achieved. Even though some clinicians have employed heparin therapy and antifibrinolytic agents in the treatment approach to DIC, such treatment is rarely appropriate (and is at best controversial) and is only indicated in the presence of profound thrombotic events (Lotspeich-Steininger, 1992; Sacher and McPherson, 1991; Stein, 1993). Although the prognosis for patients in full blown DIC (especially when the underlying condition is critical) is not particularly bright, early recognition and immediate intervention are critical to increase the likelihood of a good outcome.

15. SELF TEST

Choose the correct response by circling the appropriate letter. The answer key may be found in the appendices.

1. **The test that screens for deficiencies of factors II, V, VII, X, and to a lesser degree factor I is the**
   A. PT
   B. aPTT
   C. thrombin time
   D. antithrombin III

2. **INR results are most useful when**
   A. used to monitor heparin therapy after the patient is stabilized
   B. used for routine prothrombin time screening tests
   C. used to monitor Coumadin therapy after the patient is stabilized
   D. used to detect deficiencies of vitamin K dependent factors

3. **The ability of platelets to change shape, develop pseudopods, and stick to other platelets is referred to as**
   A. platelet adhesion
   B. platelet release
   C. platelet aggregation
   D. platelet survival

4. **Aspirin interferes with platelet function by**
   A. activating the release of ADP
   B. direct inhibition of platelet membrane phospholipids
   C. increasing platelet aggregation
   D. inhibiting the action of cyclo-oxygenase on arachidonic acid

5. **In the primary phase of coagulation**
   A. factor X is activated
   B. blood vessels and platelets act in response to vessel injury
   C. fibrinogen is converted to fibrin

6. **Specimens may be rejected for coagulation testing if**
   A. specimen is inadequately mixed
   B. collection tube is over- or underfilled
   C. inappropriate anticoagulant is used
   D. all of the above

7. **The liver-synthesized coagulation factors that are vitamin K dependent are**
   A. I, II, VII, X
   B. II, V, VII, IX
   C. II, VII, IX, X
   D. I, V, X, XI

8. **The coagulation factor with the shortest half-life is**
   A. VII
   B. X
   C. II
   D. III

9. **The coagulation factor present in most tissues is**
   A. VII
   B. X
   C. II
   D. III

10. **This factor acts to stabilize the fibrin clot. It is not measured by either the PT or the APTT.**
    A. II
    B. VIII
    C. IV
    D. XIII

11. **This factor, though required for several hemostatic functions, is not a coagulation protein.**
    A. II
    B. VIII
    C. IV
    D. XIII

12. **Activation of the extrinsic pathway of coagulation begins with**
    A. factor III
    B. factor I
    C. factor XII
    D. factor X

13. The intrinsic pathway of coagulation is activated when vessel damage results in exposure of
    A. tissue thromboplastin
    B. plasminogen
    C. collagen
    D. arachidonic acid

14. The end result of the reactions in the fibrinolytic system is the generation of a substance important in the dissolution of fibrin clots. This substance is
    A. fibrinogen
    B. plasmin
    C. kallikrein
    D. calcium

15. This substance is an important endogenous activator of plasminogen that is released into the plasma at the site of vascular injury. It requires the presence of fibrin to function effectively.
    A. urokinase
    B. streptokinase
    C. tPA
    D. antiplasmin

16. The naturally occurring anticoagulant (coagulation system inhibitor) of primary significance is
    A. antithrombin III
    B. protein C
    C. alpha-2-antiplasmin
    D. alpha-2-antitrypsin

17. This inhibitor of fibrinolysis inactivates plasmin after consumption of alpha-2-antiplasmin and alpha-2-macroglobulin, but is also an important inhibitor of coagulation.
    A. antithrombin III
    B. protein C
    C. alpha-2-antiplasmin
    D. alpha-2-antitrypsin

18. Heparin therapy is best monitored by the
    A. PT
    B. APTT
    C. bleeding time
    D. antithrombin III

19. When a patient does not respond to standard doses of heparin, this laboratory assay may be beneficial in determining the cause of the ineffective response.
    A. PT
    B. APTT
    C. bleeding time
    D. antithrombin III

20. An FDP titer above 1:40 is
    A. considered normal by most methods
    B. typical of venous thrombosis
    C. suggestive of DIC
    D. an insignificant finding

21. This assay is a specific indicator of intravascular thrombus formation and subsequent degradation of fibrin.
    A. ATIII activity
    B. plasminogen assay
    C. D-dimer
    D. lupus anticoagulant

22. This immunoglobulin inhibits the interaction of phospholipids with the coagulation factors. Its presence may result in a prolonged PT or APTT, but is more likely to produce thrombus formation than bleeding tendency.
    A. ATIII activity
    B. plasminogen assay
    C. D-dimer
    D. lupus anticoagulant

23. When the PT is prolonged with a normal APTT, the most likely cause is
    A. factor XIII deficiency
    B. isolated deficiency of factor VII
    C. isolated deficiency of factor VIII
    D. factor IX deficiency

24. **What results would a significant deficiency of fibrinogen be expected to produce?**
    A. prolonged PT and APTT; both corrected by normal plasma, but not with absorbed plasma or normal serum
    B. normal PT and prolonged APTT corrected by absorbed plasma and normal serum, but not with normal plasma
    C. normal APTT and prolonged PT corrected by normal plasma, but not with absorbed plasma
    D. prolonged PT and APTT; both corrected by normal plasma and absorbed plasma, but not with normal serum

25. **A prolonged PT and APTT that is not corrected by normal plasma, normal serum, or absorbed plasma is suggestive of**
    A. factor VIII deficiency
    B. von Willebrand's disease
    C. presence of an inhibitor
    D. hyperfibrinogenemia

26. **A male patient presenting with symptoms consistent with hemophilia has a normal PT and a prolonged APTT. Following the results of correction studies, the physician makes a presumptive diagnosis of hemophilia A to be confirmed by specific factor assay. Choose the correction study results the physician is most likely to have received.**
    A. APTT corrected by normal and absorbed plasma, but not by normal serum
    B. APTT corrected by normal plasma and serum, but not by absorbed plasma
    C. APTT corrected by normal serum, but not by normal or absorbed plasma
    D. APTT not corrected by normal or absorbed plasma or by normal serum

27. **A prolonged bleeding time in the presence of a normal platelet count is suggestive of**
    A. thrombocytopenia
    B. platelet function disorder
    C. hypercoagulability

28. **The disorder that results from a platelet adhesion defect as a consequence of low levels of portions of the factor VIII complex is**
    A. hemophilia A
    B. hemophilia B
    C. von Willebrand's disease

29. **The laboratory findings most consistent with classic DIC are**
    A. increased fibrinogen, PT, APTT, platelet count, and FDP of 1:10
    B. increased fibrinogen and PT; decreased APTT and platelet count; FDP > 1:40 and positive D-dimer
    C. decreased fibrinogen and platelet count; prolonged PT and APTT; FDP > 1:40 and D-dimer positive
    D. decreased fibrinogen, platelet count, and PT; prolonged APTT; FDP > 1:40 and D-dimer negative

16. TRANSFUSION SERVICE TESTING

The transfusion services department of the clinical laboratory may be better known as the "blood bank" in many institutions. **Immunohematology** is the term applied to the study of blood-related antigens and antibodies in transfusion service testing, and specialized blood bank technologists are called **immunohematologists**. Although recent advances have led to the automation of some techniques within this department, immunohematology testing remains one of the areas of the clinical laboratory in which the laboratory scientist is more likely to encounter situations requiring well developed investigatory skills and clinical judgment. Testing within this department is often routine, but in a variety of situations becomes quite complex. More so than technologists in any other area of the laboratory, the technologist performing blood bank testing must recognize that errors carry the potential of serious, often life threatening, consequences.

This chapter focuses on the transfusion service testing that occurs after donor blood has been collected, screened, and prepared for transfusion. Donor selection, testing of donated blood, and the preparation of blood components is discussed only briefly. Practitioners should consult their institutional policies and procedures or other authoritative sources for the appropriate administration of blood and/or blood products as this subject is merely addressed in general terms in this text. Because an understanding of blood bank procedures requires a general knowledge of basic immunology principles, a brief overview of basic immunology and immunohematologic concepts is provided. Chapter 18 provides additional detail regarding immunology concepts.

BASIC CONCEPTS

The field of immunohematology, though sometimes complex, is interesting and varied. A variety of subject areas are integrated in the study and practice of immunohematology. As the name implies, aspects of both immunology and hematology must be applied. In addition, fundamental genetic principles are utilized in the study of blood groups and blood group characteristics. Other areas of the clinical laboratory may also be involved in some aspects of transfusion service testing, particularly in the investigation of possible transfusion reactions.

Immunohematology not only deals with the transfusion of blood and blood components, but is also involved in the determinations required for donor organ matching, sensitization issues related to organ transplantation, and in the resolution of parentage issues. Principles of immunohematology are also useful in a variety of forensic applications. An overview of basic immunology and immunohematology concepts, along with the definition of a number of frequently used terms, is provided in this section.

The term **immunity** is applied to the body's ability to resist, or protect itself against, a variety of agents. Simply stated, the immune system is capable of distinguishing between "self" and "non-self" and mounts an attack against non-self (foreign substances) in defense of self. Immunity may be natural (innate) or acquired and can be passive or active. **Natural** or innate immunity refers to the non-specific, essentially permanent defenses with which we are born. **Acquired immunity** is specific and is developed in response to exposure to particular "foreign" substances. Acquired immunity has "memory" and responses intensify with subsequent exposure to the same substance. **Active immunity** results from the development of immune mechanisms (eg, antibodies) in response to having had a disease or having been vaccinated with attenuated organisms or products produced by the organism to which an immune response is directed. **Passive immunity**, on the other hand, is produced when prepared sera containing antibodies is injected directly to provide protection. Immune responses may be cellular or humoral (involving antibodies and other substances).

The primary immunogic components involved in blood bank testing and reactions are antibodies and antigens. **Antibodies** are proteins (immunoglobulins; abbreviated Ig) produced in response to antigenic stimulation and may be specific (reacting only with a particular type of antigen) or non-specific (reacting with a variety of similar antigens). **Antigens** are any substance that can provoke antibody formation; they may also be referred to as *immunogens*. **Haptens** are substances that are too small to be immunogenic alone, but may react when attached to a carrier protein. The **immunogenicity** (or antigenicity) of an antigen refers to its potency in eliciting an immune response. Immunogenicity is influenced by a number of factors, including various biologic and chemical properties of the antigen, its molecular size, and its configuration. Highly immunogenic antigens are more likely to produce a response than those of low immunogenicity.

Although there are exceptions, antigens of primary interest in the blood bank are virtually always found on red blood cells. Over 300 antigenic configurations on the membrane of erythrocytes have been discovered and classified. These antigens are usually proteins or glycolipids. These red cell antigens are important in transfusion service testing because they can elicit antibody formation when red cell products are transfused to a recipient. Once such antibodies are present in the patient's serum, future transfusion of red cells containing the same antigen can produce a significant, and frequently quite perilous, immune response.

Antibodies formed in response to antigenic stimulation are then capable of reacting with that antigen. Antibodies produced in response to and capable of reacting with a foreign antigen are called **alloantibodies**. **Autoantibodies** are directed at and react with an individual's own (self) antigens. An **immunoglob-**

ulin molecule typically consists of four polypeptide chains and are held together by disulfide bonds: two identical **heavy chains** and two identical **light chains**. Heavy and light designations are made based on relative differences in mass. Light chains are of two types designated kappa (κ) and lambda (λ), but the light chains of a given immunoglobulin will either both be κ or both λ. There are five different types of heavy chains (both heavy chains in a given Ig are of the same type) also designated by Greek letters: α, δ, ε, γ, and μ. Immunoglobulins are divided into regions of fairly stable amino acid composition (C regions) and regions which are highly variable (V regions). The variable region of the immunoglobulin contains the sites for antigen binding called **Fab fragments** (fragment antigen binding). The Ig molecule is Y shaped with a hinge region in the middle that provides a degree of freedom for the short arms containing binding sites (Figure 16–1). Immunoglobulins vary in size and structure and are classified according to these and other properties into five general classes: IgG, IgA, IgM, IgD, and IgE. The two antibody classes of primary importance in the blood bank are IgG and IgM. **IgG antibodies** are monomers (composed of one Ig molecule) with a half-life of about 3 weeks. They are much smaller (molecular weight 160,000) than the **IgM antibodies**, which are pentamers (composed of five Ig molecules; molecular weight 900,000) with a half-life of about 5 days.

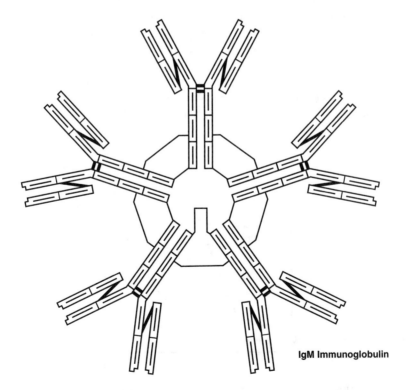

IgM Immunoglobulin

FIGURE 16–1. An IgG monomer is made up of one Ig molecule; an IgM pentamer is 5 Ig molecules connected by short peptide chains called *J chains.*

Antibody responses are classified as primary or secondary. The **primary response** involves the formation of antibodies upon initial exposure to an antigen. Production begins slowly in what is called a **lag phase** and then rapidly increases in the **log phase**. The log phase is followed by a **plateau phase** of relatively stable production and a final **decline phase** in which the antibody level decreases. Subsequent exposure to the same (or a very similar) antigen results in a **secondary**, or **anamnestic, response**. Secondary responses have a shorter lag phase and a longer plateau. Antibody levels reach much higher titers in a secondary response and stay higher much longer (longer decline phase). Figure 16–2 illustrates the differences in primary and secondary, or anamnestic, responses.

When antibodies bind to antigens, an **antigen-antibody complex** is formed. **Complement** may be activated via the classical pathway by antigen-antibody complexes. Complement is a group of proteins, primarily synthesized in the liver, that form a "cascade" in which an activated complement component serves to catalyze activation of another component and amplify the response. The complement system can be activated **through two separate pathways, classical and alternative**, either of which can initiate the **final common pathway**. Antibodies are capable of binding to or "fixing" complement only after reacting with an antigen. This reaction causes a change in the antibody that reveals a site capable of binding with the first complement component **C1** (specifically the **C1q** molecule). Activation of complement produces three primary consequences: clearance of complexes, release of mediator substances, and direct lysis of cells. Refer to Chapter 18 for a more detailed explanation of complement.

The detection of antigen-antibody reactions is of primary importance in transfusion service testing. These reactions are detected by examination for the presence of **agglutination** of red cells (hemagglutination), which results when antibodies attach to red cell antigens and then form a "lattice" of cross-linked cells.

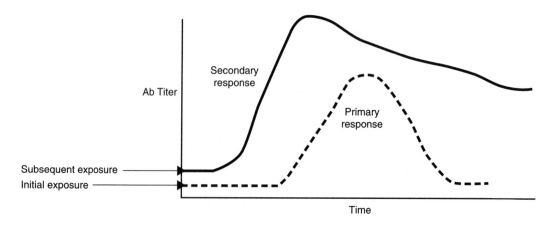

FIGURE 16–2. Primary and secondary immune responses.

The strength of the reaction is determined based on the degree of agglutination observed. Antigen-antibody reactions may also be detected by the presence of **hemolysis** in response to specific test procedures. Hemolysis may occur as a result of complement activation. Because the detection of hemolysis in response to antigen-antibody complex formation is essential in the blood bank, *it is imperative that samples collected for use in transfusion service testing be free of hemolysis.* The presence of hemolysis as a result of traumatic venipuncture may prevent the detection of reactions critical to the appropriate interpretation of testing results.

A variety of tests are performed in transfusion services, but are generally based on the common principles of the detection of specific antibodies and antigens. Test procedures also involve determinations of compatibility and quantifying the concentration of antibodies present. Some routine blood bank procedures are listed in Table 16–1.

THE ABO BLOOD GROUP SYSTEM

The ABO blood group system is of paramount importance in transfusion medicine and is perhaps the blood group system with which the majority of persons are most familiar. Karl Landsteiner discovered this system in 1900 by mixing the serum and cells of his colleagues and noting the reactions observed. He found that the serum of some persons would agglutinate the red cells of others. These studies led him to the discovery of the A, B, and O blood groups. The fourth blood group of the ABO system, AB, was later discovered by some of Landsteiner's students. This blood group system is unique in that antibodies directed against the antigens *not* present on an individual's erythrocytes are almost always found as naturally occurring antibodies in the serum. This principle is called *Landsteiner's law* and will be better understood as the discussion of the ABO system progresses.

The ABO system is more complex than it may initially appear to be. The major antigens of this system are the A and B antigens; the major antibodies are anti-A and anti-B. The genes that determine the presence or absence of these antigens are found on chromosome 9. These so-called A and B genes do not, however, directly produce antigens. Instead they are responsible for the production of a transferase enzyme that attaches a sugar molecule to the carbohydrate chain of a basic precursor substance. The linkage of this sugar molecule is required to give the anti-

TABLE 16–1. Routine Blood Bank Procedures

Procedure	Basis of Test
ABO group determination	Forward typing: red cell antigen detection
	Reverse typing: antibody detection
RH typing	Red cell antigen detection
Antibody screen	Detection of unexpected antibodies
Antibody identification	Determination of antibody specificity
	using known red cell antigens
Compatibility testing	Detection of antigen-antibody complex formation
	between donor component and recipient

gen its specificity. The gene responsible for the O blood group does not cause production of the transferase enzyme and thus results in no antigen expression (such genes are called *amorphs*). Another antigen, **H**, is required for either the A or B antigen to be produced. The H gene codes for another specific transferase that is responsible for attaching a sugar (L-fucose) to the second carbon of the galactose molecule at the end of the precursor chain. Fucose must be attached to the precursor first in order for A and B activity to be expressed. The H gene is independent from the ABO locus, and is believed to be located on chromosome 19 (Henry, 1996). Another locus on chromosome 19, the **SE** locus, is also involved in the expression of the A and B antigens because the SE gene regulates the function of the H gene. The SE gene determines what is referred to as *secretor status*. Persons with a dominant SE gene are called **secretors**, which means that soluble H, A, and B substances are found in their saliva and in other secretory fluids; 80 % of the population are secretors. Inheritance of two recessive (se/se) genes results in nonsecretor status.

Expression of the **A antigen** results from the attachment of **N-acetyl-galactosamine** to the number three carbon of galactose. The attachment of **galactose** in the same location results in expression of the **B antigen**. Recall that fucose must first be attached to the number 2 carbon of the terminal galactose in the precursor chain or the sugars responsible for specificity of the A and B antigens cannot be added. ABO antigens are present on the surface of red cells as well as in tissue and endothelial cells. As alluded to previously, they may also be found in soluble form in body secretions in the majority of the population (secretors).

◼ PATTERNS OF INHERITANCE

Inheritance of ABO antigens follows simple Mendelian principles. A and B behave like dominant genes and O behaves like a recessive gene. Before proceeding with a discussion of ABO blood group inheritance, it is important to recall the distinction between phenotype and genotype. **Genotype** refers to the genes actually present on the chromosome, whereas **phenotype** refers to the expressed characteristic. In the case of the ABO system, the phenotype is what is determined by routine testing. The ABO genes are alleles (allelic genes occupy the same locus on a chromosome and determine the heredity of a specific characteristic) so they are interchangeable at their locus and each of the paired chromosomes may have any one of the three genes. In other words, an individual may have an A gene on one of the paired chromosomes and an O gene on the other. This individual's genotype would be AO, but the phenotype (what is expressed and detected by routine testing) would be A—the person has blood group A. Note that the genotype AA would result in the same phenotype—blood group A. A person with both an A gene and a B gene would have the AB blood group phenotype (A and B are co-dominant) and an AB genotype. An individual with blood group O phenotype must have the genotype OO because the O phenotype is not expressed in the presence of either A or B. Note that detection of either the AB phenotype or the O phenotype tells us what the corresponding genotype must be: AB and OO, respectively. The A phenotype and the B phenotype each have two possible genotypes: AA or AO and BB or BO, respectively. Table 16–2 summarizes the inheritance of ABO blood groups in terms of the possible genotypes of offspring and Table 16–3 provides the same information in terms of phenotypes.

The H antigen is also inherited in simple mendelian fashion, with each parent contributing either an H gene or an h gene. Offspring may then be HH, Hh, or hh. Either HH or Hh inheritance will produce the H antigen. The H antigen is extremely common, with over 99% of the population having this antigen on their red cells. Only those individuals with the hh genotype do not produce the H antigen. A very rare occurrence, this genotype results in what is called the **Bombay phenotype** or O_h blood group. Individuals with this phenotype are always type O because a lack of the H antigen prevents the attachment of fucose required for subsequent attachment of the sugars responsible for expression of the A or B antigen. However, these persons differ from other type O persons who do have H antigen and fucose attachment to the precursor substance. The Bombay phenotype is very rarely encountered, but may be detected by testing for the presence of the H antigen. Antisera specific for the H antigen is derived from a seed extract of *Ulex europaeus* and is commercially available for use in testing. Because the use of this reagent is rarely indicated, it is not generally stocked in most laboratories.

■ ABO BLOOD GROUP DETERMINATION

ABO blood group determination is accomplished in the laboratory using known reagent antisera and red cells of known antigenic composition. Because individuals are expected to possess antibodies directed toward the A or B antigen absent from their own red cells, both red cells and serum are used to establish and confirm ABO groups. Specific antisera are used to detect red cell antigens

TABLE 16–2. ABO Blood Group Inheritance (Possible Genotypes of Offspring)

Parent #2	Parent #1				
Genotype	AA	AO	BB	BO	OO
AA	AA	AA; AO	AB	AB; AO	
AO	AA; AO	AO; OO	AB; BO	AB; AO; BO; OO	AO; OO
BB	AB	AB; BO	BB	BB; BO	BO
BO	AB; AO	AB; OO	BB; BO	BB; BO; OO	BO; OO
OO	AO	AO; OO	BO	BO; OO	OO

TABLE 16–3. ABO Blood Group Inheritance (Possible Phenotypes of Offspring)

Parent #2	Parent #1				
Genotype	AA	AO	BB	BO	OO
AA	A	A or O	AB	AB or A	A
AO	A or O	A or O	AB or B	AB or A or B or O	A or O
BB	AB	AB or B	B	B	B
BO	AB or A	AB or O	B	B or O	B or O
OO	A	A or O	B	B or O	O

in what is called **forward typing** (also called *direct typing*). Forward typing involves the addition of reagent antisera of known specificity to a suspension of the patient's red cells. It is important that red cells and antisera be present in appropriate ratios to ensure optimal reactions. Anti-A, anti-B, and anti-A,B are used in forward typing procedures. Anti-A,B (as opposed to use of only the separate anti-A and anti-B) may be useful in the detection of weaker antigens such as A subgroups (see later discussion), because anti-A,B reacts more strongly with either group A or B cells than anti-A or anti-B alone. The monoclonal reagents available today produce stronger reactions than do naturally occurring antibodies. Agglutination will occur when anti-A reagent is added to patient cells containing the A antigen and when anti-B reagent is added to cells containing the B antigen. Both A cells and B cells will react with the anti-A,B reagent. Red cells from individuals with blood group O will not agglutinate with anti-A, anti-B, or anti-A,B because they contain neither the A nor the B antigen.

Reagent red cells are used in **reverse typing** (*indirect testing*) to detect the presence of antibodies as a confirmatory typing procedure. Individuals of blood group A lack the B antigen and thus are expected to have the B antibody (anti-B) in their serum. Likewise, those of group B lack the A antigen and should have anti-A in their serum. Because group O individuals lack both the A and B antigens, both anti-A and anti-B should be present in their serum. Reverse typing is performed by testing the patient's serum against known A and B cells. The reagent red cells will agglutinate when added to the patient's serum if the corresponding antibody is present. Thus the reagent B cells should react with the anti-B in the serum of a group A individual; reagent A cells should agglutinate when added to the serum of a group B individual containing anti-A. Serum from a group O individual should agglutinate both A and B reagent red cells. Persons with group AB are not expected to have either anti-A or anti-B in their serum and therefore none of the reagent red cells should agglutinate. Using both A_1 and A_2 cells is useful in detecting A subgroups. Table 16–4 provides the expected reactions for the ABO blood groups in forward and reverse typing. Table 16–5 shows the phenotype frequencies of the four common ABO blood groups, which differ among racial groups.

■ DISCREPANCIES IN ABO TYPING

Although the results of forward and reverse typing generally produce consistent findings, discrepancies are seen in some situations. When **ABO typing discrepancies** (ie, forward typing indicates one group and reverse typing indicates a different group) occur, they must be resolved in order for an accurate determination of the patient's ABO group to be made. **Further testing with additional antisera and/or known red cells** may be employed to resolve these discrepancies. It is prudent to first **recollect the specimen** and **repeat all testing** to rule out incorrectly identified cells or serum and the possibility of technical errors. **Appropriate reagent reactivity should also be assured** through quality control procedures. In many cases, the **patient's medical history** and/or clinical findings may provide clues as to the cause of the discrepant results. Situations may

TABLE 16–4. Expected Reactions in ABO Forward and Reverse Typing

Patient's Blood Group	Patient Cells with:			Patient Serum with:		
	Anti-A	Anti-B	Anti-A,B	A_1 cells	B cells	A_2 cells
O	0	0	0	+	+	+
A	+	0	+	0	+	0
B	0	+	+	+	0	+
A,B	+	+	+	0	0	0
A_2[2]	$+^w$	0	+	$+$[1]	+	0

0 = negative; no agglutination; + = positive; agglutination; reaction strength is not depicted in this table (ie, 4+, 3+, 2+, 1+).

[1]Occurrence of anti-A_1 is variable.
[2]Testing with anti-A_1 lectin required for confirmation; see A subgroup discussion.

occur in which immediate transfusion is required without sufficient time to resolve the typing discrepancy and definitively establish the patient's ABO group. In such cases, emergency transfusion of group O packed red cells (no A or B antigens) and/or group AB fresh frozen plasma (no A or B antibodies) may be warranted. It is important to ensure that an adequate pre-transfusion specimen has been obtained to allow investigation of the discrepancy between the forward and reverse typing results. Possible causes of discrepancies between forward and reverse ABO typing are described below.

Inaccurate Reverse Type

WEAK OR ABSENT ANTIBODIES. The absence of an expected antibody (or antibodies) should be reported because it may be indicative of a serum protein abnormality or of an unusual blood group.

- Anti-A and anti-B are not detectable until 3 to 6 months of age and may react only weakly at this time. These antibodies do not reach maximum strength until about 5 years of age (Ravel, 1995). Hence, reverse typing is not appropriate in the newborn (use forward typing results; antibodies found in cord blood or neonatal serum should be considered to be of maternal origin) and may be misleading in infancy.

TABLE 16–5. ABO Phenotype Frequencies

ABO Phenotype	Frequency (%) in US Population				Approx. Overall Frequency
	White	Black	Native American	Asian	
O	45	49	79	40	45
A	40	27	16	28	41
B	11	20	4	27	10
AB	4	4	<1	5	4

Adapted from Sacher RA, McPherson RA. *Widmann's Clinical Interpretation of Laboratory Tests,* 10th ed. Philadelphia, FA Davis, 1991, with overall frequency from Whitlock SA. *Immunohematology: Delmar's Clinical Laboratory Manual Series.* Albany, NY, Delmar Publishers, 1997

- Aged patients may have weakly reacting antibodies.
- Immunosuppressed patients or immunodeficient patients may have weak or undetectable antibodies.

PRESENCE OF UNEXPECTED ANTIBODIES

- Cold reacting autoantibodies such as anti-I or anti-IH. If this is suspected as the cause of discrepant results a cold panel (see antibody identification discussion later in this chapter) should be performed using an auto control and O cells for confirmation.
- Alloantibodies that are reactive at room temperature such as those in the MN and P systems. Antibody should be confirmed and identified.
- Passively acquired anti-A and/or anti-B.
- Subgroup of A with anti-A1 in serum.

PRESENCE OF ROULEAUX FORMATION. *Rouleaux* refers to a group of red cells that are stacked together in a formation that resembles a stack of coins. Rouleaux formation may be seen in patients with conditions that result in protein abnormalities, particularly the presence of monoclonal gamma globulins. Plasma expanders may cause the same phenomenon. Significant rouleaux may be mistaken for agglutination and can be particularly troublesome for the less experienced technologist. True agglutination and rouleaux can be distinguished by saline dispersion (rouleaux can be dispersed with saline, true agglutination cannot).

Inaccurate Forward Type

RED BLOOD CELL ANTIGEN ABNORMALITIES

- Weak antigens such as those seen in A or B subgroups
- Suppressed antigens as occasionally seen in leukemia.
- Cells heavily coated with warm autoantibody. Elution and identification of the antibody are required.
- Acquired abnormalities that may be seen occasionally with carcinoma and some bacterial infections; an acquired B antigen is associated with some cases of colon and gastric malignancies and with intestinal obstruction.

BONE MARROW TRANSPLANTS. "Mixed field" agglutination with reagent antisera may be noted as the transplanted marrow begins to produce red cells.

TRANSFUSION OF NON-SPECIFIC ABO GROUP CELLS. Mixed field agglutination may also be noted when red cells outside the patient's ABO group have been transfused.

◼ ABO SUBGROUPS

Although **subgroups** of both A and B occur, B subgroups are rare and are encountered much less frequently than A subgroups. Subgroup classifications are made based on serologic test results reflecting the antigenic variations.

Subgroup antigens are the same chemically, but vary quantitatively in terms of antigen sites available for antibody binding. The major subgroups of the A phenotype are A_1 and A_2. Most individuals of the A phenotype are A_1 (about 80%). The A_2 subgroup (found in about 20% of the population) becomes important in terms of transfusion medicine when an antibody directed toward the A_1 antigen is developed. An anti-A_1 lectin reagent prepared from *Dolichos biflorus* is used to distinguish A subgroups. Agglutination with this reagent is seen with A_1 cells (and to a lesser degree with the cells of an intermediate A subgroup, A_{int}), but not with cells of the A_2 subgroup or other A subgroups. A similar reagent giving the same results is prepared from the serum of group O or group B individuals after absorption with A_2 cells. The presence of the anti-A_1 antibody in the serum of individuals of the A_2 subgroup or other subgroups of A is detected by using A_1 reagent red cells. This antibody will agglutinate A_1 red cells, but will not agglutinate A_2 reagent red cells. The occurrence of the A_1 antibody in A subgroups is variable, but the rare subgroup A_x usually has detectable anti-A_1. Table 16–6 summarizes the serologic differences of the ABO subgroups that may be used for identification and classification along with the differences in serum transferase levels and the number of antigen binding sites found on the erythrocyte membrane. The typical strength of agglutination reactions is depicted in the table and may sometimes provide the initial clue to the presence of a subgroup. Routine subgroup classification is not necessary, and is of greater academic interest than of clinical importance. However, *subgroup classification becomes important clinically in cases involving:*

- Forward and reverse type discrepancies
- The presence of anti- A_1

Likewise, the transfusion of subgroup-specific red blood cells is not a routine consideration in the transfusion services department. In fact, donor units are not routinely classified as A_1, A_2, etc, but rather simply as group A. If anti-A_1 is detected in the serum of an A subgroup individual, donor units may be screened with anti-A_1 lectin to identify A_2 cells for transfusion if desired. Many consider the presence of anti-A_1 to be of no clinical significance, but there are some reports of anti-A_1 resulting in the increased destruction of transfused A_1 cells (Mollison, 1989).

Of the subgroups listed in Table 16–6, A_2 is the most commonly encountered, occurring in about 20% of those expressing an A phenotype. However, fewer than 10% of those individuals of this subgroup are found to have an antibody to A_1. The other A subgroups are not commonly encountered and the B_3 subgroup occurs only rarely. A comparison of the test results for ABO subgroups to the expected reactions given in Table 16–4 demonstrates how ABO subgroups may result in inconsistent forward and reverse ABO typing results. Consider the following examples for purposes of illustration. Note that the problematic results may occur in either forward typing or reverse typing. Consequently, *in the absence of supporting data,* one should not assume the reverse type to be in error and the forward type reflective of the "true" ABO type.

TABLE 16–6. Serologic Differentiation and Characteristics of ABO Subgroups

ABO Phenotype	Patient Red Cells with Anti					Patient Serum with Reagent Red Cells			Other Characteristics	
	A	A_1	B	A,B	H^1	A_1	B	O	Level of Transferase in Serum	Antigen Sites Per RBC $\times 10^3$
A_1	++++	++++	0	++++	0/+	0	++++	0	Normal	810 to 1170
A_{int}	++++	++	0	++++	++	0	++++	0		
A_2	++++ or +++	0	0	++++	+++	$0/+^2$	++++	0	Decreased	240 to 290
A_3	$++^{mf}$	0	0	$++^{mf}$	+++	$0/+^2$	++++	0	Low	30
A_x	$0/\pm$	0	0	++	++++	$+^3$	++++	0	Very low	4
A_m	0^4	0	0	0	++++	0	++++	0	Low (A_1 or A_2 enzyme may be present)	0.2 to 1.9
B	0	0	++++	++++	++	++++	0	0	Normal	750
B_3	0	0	$++^{mf}$	$++^{mf}$	+++	++++	0	0	Low	
O	0	0	0	0	++++	++++	++++	0	Normal	1700
O_h	0	0	0	0	0	++++	++++	++++	Normal	

[1]Testing not routinely performed.
[2]Anti-A_1 may or may not be present.
[3]Anti-A_1, usually, but not always, present.
[4]A antigen specifically demonstrated only after adsorption/elution procedures.
mfMixed field.

Adapted from Henry JB. *Clinical Diagnosis and Management by Laboratory Methods,* 19th ed. Philadelphia, Saunders, 1996

Example 1. An A₂ individual with antibody to A₁.

- Forward typing results are consistent with *group A.*
- Reverse typing results are consistent with *group O.*

RESOLUTION: Patient's red cells will not agglutinate with anti-A1 lectin. Patient's serum will not agglutinate reagent A2 cells. Reverse type was misleading.

Example 2. An individual with B₃ subgroup.

- Forward typing results are consistent with *group O.*
- Reverse typing results are consistent with *group B.*

RESOLUTION: Recollect specimen and repeat testing—this subgroup is not commonly encountered! If repeat testing confirms the initial testing results, check for mixed field agglutination in forward testing. The presence of mixed field agglutination may be indicative of circumstances other than a subgroup that may be ruled out by reviewing the patient's history: Is the patient a bone marrow transplant recipient? Has the patient been recently transfused? With which ABO type? If mixed field agglutination is present with anti-B and anti-A,B and cannot be otherwise explained, the B₃ subgroup is suspected. Additional testing is required for confirmation. It may be necessary to refer the sample to a specialty reference laboratory because appropriate resources are not likely to be available in the transfusion services department of most clinical laboratories. If the patient is a secretor, B substance can be detected along with H substance in the saliva (no B substance would be detected if the patient were truly type O or if the individual is a nonsecretor). The level of transferase in the serum is low in the B_3 subgroup, but normal in group O. Should transfusion be urgently required prior to resolution of the ABO discrepancy, type O packed red cells may be used. *Forward type was misleading.*

As noted previously, it is important to resolve any discrepancies encountered in ABO typing results in order for an accurate determination of the patient's ABO group to be made. Fortunately, discrepant results are encountered on a relatively infrequent basis. Nonetheless, it is essential that the blood bank technologist be cognizant of the potential causes of discrepant typing results, alert to their occurrence, and knowledgeable of the appropriate follow-up necessary for resolution.

■ ABO ANTIBODIES

The ABO antibodies found in serum as described in Landsteiner's law are typically referred to as "naturally occurring." Despite this commonly accepted terminology, detectable levels of these antibodies are not present at birth and appear to be developed in response to exposure to natural antigenic substances that are widely distributed in the environment. The same sugar linkages required for expression of the A and B antigens are present in the cell walls of bacteria providing one source of environmental exposure. Plant pollens (Henry, 1996) may also serve as the stimulus for production of these "natural" antibodies. ABO antibodies are usually detectable in serum by the sixth month of life (3 to 6 months).

The **naturally occurring antibodies** of the ABO system (anti-A, anti-B, and anti-A,B) are **primarily IgM** antibodies with an optimal reactivity at 4°C. On the other hand, immune forms of these antibodies developed in response to immune stimulus (eg, ABO incompatible pregnancy, infusion of ABO incompatible red cells) are **primarily IgG** immunoglobulins. These forms react equally well at 37°C and 4°C and usually are present in higher titers than their naturally occurring counterparts. **Anti-A$_1$** is considered to be a naturally occurring antibody when found in the serum of A subgroups. As previously noted, it is generally considered to be of little clinical significance. **Anti-H** is generally encountered as a harmless cold autoantibody. Nearly all red cells contain the H antigen, but the quantities of the antigen vary among the different ABO types (Figure 16–3). In fact, methods for the identification of the anti-H cold autoagglutinin involve comparisons of reaction strength with red cells of the various ABO groups. Group O individuals have the greatest amount of H antigen activity and group AB individuals have the least (with the exception of the Bombay phenotype, in which there is no H activity). The anti-H cold reactive autoantibody is most frequently found in individuals of blood groups A$_1$ and A$_1$B, the blood groups with the least amount of H antigen activity. The anti-H found in individuals with the rare Bombay phenotype is much more problematic. In this instance, anti-H is a powerful antibody that strongly agglutinates or hemolyzes red blood cells. Because all red cells from individuals other than those with this rare phenotype contain at least some H

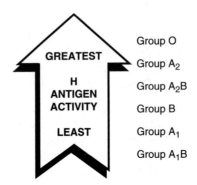

FIGURE 16–3. Relative activity of H antigen.

antigen, serum from those with the Bombay phenotype will agglutinate virtually all red cells, making compatibility determinations extremely troublesome. To further complicate this situation, the anti-H that is found in the Bombay phenotype is reactive throughout a broad temperature range.

 TIME FOR REVIEW. After studying the preceding sections, you should be able to respond correctly to the following:

■ Define the following terms:

active immunity:

passive immunity:

antibody:

antigen:

hapten:

immunogenicity:

alloantibody:

autoantibody:

■ The portion of the immunoglobulin that is capable of antigen binding is located in the _____ (variable/constant) region and is called the _____.

■ Antigen-antibody complexes may activate complement through the _____ pathway.

■ Antigen-antibody reactions may be detected in the blood bank by the presence of _____ or _____.

■ The ABO blood group system is unique in that an individual's serum contains antibodies directed against _____.

■ Expression of the A antigen results from the attachment of _____ to the number 3 carbon of galactose.

■ Expression of the B antigen results from the attachment of
_____.

■ In order for either the A or B antigen to be expressed, another antigen called
_____ is required to attach fucose to the galactose molecule.

■ In forward ABO typing, the patient's _____ are tested with reagent _____ in order to detect the presence
of specific _____ (antigens or antibodies).

■ In reverse ABO typing, the patient's _____ is tested for the presence of specific _____ (antigens or antibodies).

■ Distinguish between the terms *genotype* and *phenotype*.

■ List all the possible genotypes and corresponding phenotypes that are possible
for the offspring of the pairs of parents listed.

Parents with genotypes AA and AB:

Parents with genotypes BO and AO:

Parents with phenotype A and phenotype B:

Parents with phenotype AB and phenotype O:

■ List and briefly explain three possible causes for discrepancies in forward and reverse ABO typing.

■ Explain how A_1 and A_2 phenotypes can be distinguished by serologic testing.

■ Anti-H is most significant in this rare phenotype: _____.

■ The ABO group containing the most H antigen activity is group _____.

■ Naturally occurring anti-A and anti-B are usually of this immunoglobulin class Ig____ .

Check your responses by reviewing the preceding sections.

THE RH SYSTEM

The Rh system is second only to the ABO system in terms of clinical importance. It is likely the most complex red cell antigen system encountered, and nomenclature for this system can be equally complex. The system includes over 50 antigens with a number of phenotypic variants. The intricacies of the Rh system cannot be presented in an in-depth fashion in this text. Basic concepts and routine clinical application are provided in this section.

The designation of this system as "Rh" comes from the first experiments involving the antigens of this system by Landsteiner and Wiener in 1940. These animal experiments involved the use of red blood cells from the rhesus monkey to immunize guinea pigs and rabbits. They found that the antiserum produced as a result of this immunization would cause 85% of human red blood cells to agglutinate. The antigen responsible for antibody production was called the *Rh factor*. The antibody produced in response to this antigen was later found to have the same specificity as an antibody reported earlier by Levine and Stetson in their study of hemolytic disease of the newborn.

RH NOMENCLATURE

Three different **nomenclatures** have been used to describe this system: the Fisher-Race; the Wiener; and the Rosenfield. Both the Fisher-Race and the

Wiener systems are based on different theories of inheritance. The Rosenfield system is independent of the genetic inheritance of the antigens. The **Wiener** system is based on the theory of eight common alleles found at the same locus. The alleles are called *agglutinogens* and individuals inherit two—one from each parent. Each agglutinogen is, in turn, composed of up to three different antigenic factors or determinants. **Fisher and Race** later proposed a theory of inheritance based on three closely linked loci with the alleles Cc, Ee, and Dd. The three genes are inherited as a single unit. It was later determined that no actual "d" allele exists, but this designation is often used to indicate the lack of the D antigen. The nomenclature systems used with each of these theories, along with the Rosenfield system, are summarized in Table 16–7. Table 16–8 further illustrates the Fisher-Race and Wiener systems. **Rosenfield** uses numerical designations to name the antigens of the Rh system (eg, Rh1, Rh2, Rh3) and, as previously noted, does not infer any genetic theory of inheritance. The Fisher-Race and Wiener systems are both currently used, but the Fisher-Race method is generally considered simpler, easier to remember, and more practical for most routine situations. Although most experts believe the Wiener theory is probably the most accurate representation of this system (Ravel, 1995), its unwieldy terminology reduces the use of this system in many situations. It is important to understand both systems of nomenclature because both are used in blood banking and in the literature. Recent evidence from studies involving the analysis of gene products and using DNA cloning and nucleotide sequencing points to inheritance that differs from both the Wiener and Fisher-Race theories (Henry, 1996). These studies suggest two closely linked genes—one for the D antigen and another for the CE antigens—that may have developed from one common "ancestor" gene.

RH ANTIGENS

The Rh antigens are lipoproteins located on the surface of erythrocytes. Unlike the ABO antigens, which protrude from the outer layer of the red cell membrane and can be found on tissue cells and in soluble form in body fluids, the Rh antigens are found only on red cells, where they are an integral part of the cell membrane. Also unlike the ABO system, antibodies to antigens not located on the red cell are not naturally occurring in the Rh system. Instead, they are produced in response to the introduction of cells that do contain the antigen.

TABLE 16–7. Fisher-Race, Wiener, and Rosenfield Antigens

Fisher-Race	Wiener	Rosenfield
D	Rh$_o$	Rh1
C	rh'	Rh2
E	rh"	Rh3
c	hr'	Rh4
e	hr"	Rh5

TABLE 16–8. Fisher-Race and Wiener Nomenclatures

Fisher-Race		Wiener		Frequency In United States			
Genes	Antigens	Gene	Factors	White	Black	Native American	Asian
DCe	D, C, e	R¹	Rh$_o$, rh', hr"	0.42	0.17	0.44	0.70
DcE	D, c, E	R²	Rh$_o$, hr', rh"	0.14	0.11	0.34	0.21
Dce	D, c, e	R⁰	Rh$_o$, hr', hr"	0.04	0.44	0.02	0.03
DCE	D, C, E	R^Z	Rh$_o$, rh', rh"	Very rare	Very rare	0.06	0.01
dce	c, e	r	hr', hr"	0.37	0.26	0.11	0.03
dCe	C, e	r'	rh', hr"	0.02	0.02	0.02	0.02
dcE	c, E	r"	hr', rh"	0.01	Very rare	0.01	Very rare
dCE	C, E	r^y	rh', rh"	Very rare	Very rare	Very rare	Very rare

Frequencies from Whitlock, 1997

The **primary antigen** in the system is **D (Rh$_o$)**. Inheritance of this antigen from either parent or from both parents results in an individual who is **Rh positive**. When this antigen is not inherited from either parent, the individual is **Rh negative** regardless of what other Rh antigens may be present. In other words, the designations Rh positive and Rh negative are made solely based on the presence or absence of the D antigen. The D antigen is **highly immunogenic** and readily provokes antibody production when introduced to an individual lacking the antigen (ic, transfusion or pregnancy). This high immunogenicity (antigenicity) resulted in D being the first Rh antigen to be identified. Until the development of prophylactic Rh$_o$ immune globulin (RhoGam), exposure of Rh negative (D negative) pregnant women to Rh positive (D positive) red cells of their unborn child frequently resulted in severe cases of hemolytic disease of the newborn (HDN; see later section).

Common Rh phenotypes have antigen sites on each erythrocyte in the range of 10,000 to 33,000 and react well at room temperature with modern antisera to give clear-cut, strong positive reactions. Other individuals possess the D antigen, but their red cells react weakly or not at all at room temperature. These reactions may be enhanced by 37°C incubation or, in some cases, cannot be detected without the use of the anti-human globulin (AHG; see later discussion) technique. This **weak D, or D (Rh$_o$) variant** as it is sometimes called, can be produced in at least three different situations. (This weakly-reacting D was previously referred to as **D^u**, but this terminology is no longer commonly used.) A weak D may occur in several circumstances:

- a reduced number of D antigen sites on the erythrocyte; quantitative difference
- a variation in the D protein produced by the gene; qualitative difference
- a missing piece of the antigen (D antigen referred to as a "mosaic"—structure includes several different parts; one or more of these parts may not be present)

Individuals with a weak D antigen or D variant are treated as Rh positive in some circumstances and as Rh negative in other instances. When blood from such individuals is **transfused** to a recipient it is **treated as Rh positive** because a D negative recipient could produce antibodies to the weakened or variant D antigen. If an individual with a weakly-reacting D antigen is to receive blood they are **treated as an Rh negative recipient** and given D negative blood. This precaution is taken because individuals with a weak D as a result of an absence of part of the mosaic may produce antibodies when exposed to the missing piece on donor red cells. Consequently, it is important to perform the additional test procedures necessary to detect a weak D antigen on donor blood. However, it is not necessary to distinguish between D negative and weak D individuals as recipients because D negative blood will be administered in either case. For this reason, many institutions perform only routine D testing as a part of their standard pre-transfusion testing.

Although there are numerous other Rh antigens, only the most common will be discussed here. The four most common Rh antigens, after the D antigen, are those resulting from the **Cc and Ee** alleles. The other antigens are not as clinically significant and are either quite rare or require rare antibodies to be detected. Because one gene is inherited from each parent, a variety of antigen combinations are possible including the following partial list provided as an example:

CCEE
CCee
CCEe
CCEe
ccEE
ccEe
CcEe
Ccee

Variants of these antigens have also been described, but are not frequently encountered. These variant forms are often associated with a particular racial group. For example, the C^W antigen, which is either a variant of C or a low incidence antigen produced on a variant Cc protein, is found primarily in the white population. Approximately 2% (Henry, 1996) of the white population, usually of the DCe phenotype, have the C^W antigen. On the other hand, a variant of the e antigen that is rarely encountered in the white population is seen in about one fourth of the black population. Some evidence (ie, number of e variants; development of e-like antibodies by individuals positive for the e antigen) now exists to suggest that the e antigen may also be mosaic in structure.

Rh phenotype is determined by testing for the presence of the D, C, E, c, and e antigens using antisera specific for each antigen. From the phenotyping results, the **most probable genotype** can be determined based on the incidence of each antigen (as opposed to testing parents and other family members to determine genotype). Not performed as a component of routine testing, such determinations do become important in some circumstances such as locating compatible blood in the presence of an unexpected antibody or parentage determinations. Tables similar to that shown in Table 16–9 can be used to determine the most probable genotype for a given set of Rh phenotyping results.

The designation **Rh$_{null}$** is used to denote rare individuals who have no Rh antigens present on their red cells. This rare phenotype seems to have two genetic mechanisms for inheritance. Because individuals of the Rh$_{null}$ phenotype also have depressed levels of some other red cell antigens (S, s, and U) and lack the high frequency antigen Fy^a, and Rh related proteins (Henry, 1996), the Rh proteins may be required for appropriate expression of some membrane glycolipids. Still other blood group antigens (M, N, Kidd, and others) are enhanced in the Rh$_{null}$ phenotype. Though very rarely encountered in the transfusion services department, Rh$_{null}$ individuals who have been immunized by virtue of pregnancy or prior transfusion may present extremely complex transfusion problems. Because their red cells contain none of the 50 plus known Rh antigens, prior immunization may lead to the development of antibodies directed at any or all of the missing antigens to which they have been exposed. The presence of a number of such antibodies would make it virtually impossible to locate compatible blood for transfusion. The presence of an antibody designated as anti-Rh29 (Henry, 1996) presents particular difficulty, as it will react with all red cells except those from an individual of the Rh$_{null}$ phenotype.

Another blood group system, **LW**, was previously thought to be a part of the Rh system. It is now known to be a separate system that is closely associated with the

TABLE 16–9. Determination of Most Probable Rh Genotype

Rh Phenotype Results					
Patient Red Cells with Anti-					
D	C	E	c	e	**Possible Genotypes in Order of Frequency[1]**
+	+	0	+	+	Dce/dce or DCe/Dce or dCe/Dce
+	+	0	0	+	DCe/DCe or DCe/dCe
+	+	+	+	+	DcE/Dce or DCe/dce or DCE/dce or DCE/Dce or dCE/Dce
+	0	+	+	0	DcE/DcE or DcE/dcE
+	0	0	+	+	Dce/dce or Dce/Dce
0	0	0	+	+	dce/dce
0	+	0	+	+	dCe/dce
0	0	+	+	+	dcE/dce
0	+	+	+	+	dCe/dcE or dCE/dce
0	+	0	0	+	dCe/dCe
0	0	+	+	0	dcE/dcE
+	+	+	0	+	DCE/DCe or DCE/dCe
+	+	+	+	0	DCE/DcE or DCE/dcE
+	+	+	0	0	DCE/DCE or DCE/dCE
0	+	+	0	+	dCE/dCe
0	+	+	+	0	dCE/dcE
0	+	+	0	0	dCE/dCE

+ indicates positive reaction; 0 indicates negative reaction.

[1]Overall frequency; most probable genotype may vary somewhat based on race or ethnicity. Possible genotypes in o rder of frequency from Henry, 1996

Rh system as a result of a relationship that is not entirely clear. It is now believed that the antibody originally described by early workers was anti-LW (named for Landsteiner and Wiener) instead of anti-D. Although many characteristics of this system remain to be definitively described, varying amounts of the antigen may produce the various LW phenotypes. Those of the Rh_{null} phenotype lack the LW antigen and may be the only individuals who are truly LW negative.

■ RH ANTIBODIES

Antibodies may be formed following exposure to any Rh antigen not found on an individual's own red cells. Of the common Rh antigens, D is most likely to provoke antibody production because of its high antigenicity. However, not every D negative person exposed to the D antigen as a result of transfusion or pregnancy will produce anti-D. Exposure by transfusion is more likely to result in antibody production than pregnancy (frequency varies among sources, but about 20% in pregnancy and between 50 and 70% in transfusion), as a result of the much larger number of red cells. Despite the higher likelihood of antibody development in response to transfusion, anti-D resulting from transfusion exposure is less likely to be encountered in practice because donor and recipient Rh types are matched except in rare emergency circumstances requiring immediate transfusion when D-negative blood is not immediately available. The resultant antibodies are **principally IgG**. Although some IgM forms may be seen early in the response, they quickly disappear. IgG anti-D can remain for a lifetime. The presence of Rh antibodies is frequently not detected until the 37°C phase of testing. Some may not be detected until the AHG test phase. Rh antibodies are generally not associated with the ability to activate complement. These antibodies coat the surface of the red cells that contain the antigen against which they were formed. Coated cells are destroyed (hemolyzed) and cleared from the circulation by the reticuloendothelial system. Avoiding subsequent exposure to the offending antigen is of extreme importance. Because IgG antibodies may remain in the circulation throughout a lifetime, a second exposure produces a swift and potent anamnestic response. It is this response that results in **hemolytic transfusion reactions** and **hemolytic disease of the newborn**. Such reactions can be produced by antibodies to any of the Rh antigens, but are more commonly seen with D. Hemolytic transfusion reactions and HDN are discussed in later sections of this chapter.

■ RH TYPING

Anti-D reagent serum is used for routine Rh determinations. A positive reaction is indicated by agglutination of the patient's red cells by the anti-D reagent. Red cells that produce a positive reaction are called Rh positive. Those that produce a negative reaction on direct testing must be tested further before they can be called Rh negative because a weak D antigen may not be detected with direct testing only. (Testing for weak D is not required for recipients, because they will be given Rh negative blood regardless.) Procedures may vary slightly among institutions and with different reagents; a typical test procedure is depicted in Figure 16–4.

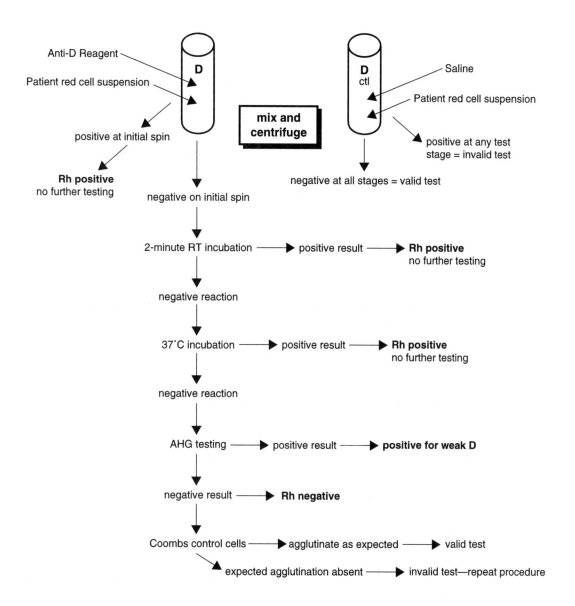

FIGURE 16–4. Determination of Rh type.

A 3% to 5% suspension of the patient's red cells is prepared and tested with anti-D reagent. Another test tube should contain the patient's cell suspension with saline (instead of the anti-D reagent) to be used as a test control. Agglutination in the control tube at any stage of testing (excluding following the addition of Coombs control cells) renders the test invalid. The cause of the positive control must be determined and resolved before accurate Rh determination can be made. Patients are designated as Rh positive if the anti-D reagent agglutinates their red cells at any of the following stages of testing:

- at initial spin: patient cells and anti-D are mixed in the appropriate ratio and centrifuged
- following room temperature incubation: If agglutination is not observed at initial spin, test tubes are allowed to stand at room temperature (if specified by the reagent manufacturer), centrifuged, and examined again for agglutination.
- following 37°C incubation: If agglutination is not observed after RT incubation, test tubes are incubated at 37°C for a specified time (usually 22 to 30 minutes), centrifuged, and examined again for agglutination.

Red cells that do not show agglutination following 37°C incubation are tested with AHG. Agglutination appearing only in this phase of testing indicates the presence of a weak D antigen. Red cells that still show no agglutination are considered Rh negative. An additional control procedure is required following this stage to ensure the validity of test results. Cells that are coated with IgG antibody are added to both the control and patient test tubes and centrifuged. Agglutination must be present following addition of these antibody-coated cells in order for results to be considered valid and reported (see AHG testing section for a better understanding of this control procedure).

Testing for other Rh antigens (eg, C, c, E, e) is not routinely performed in pretransfusion testing and has no bearing on the designation of Rh positive or Rh negative. However, donor blood is tested for these antigens if the recipient demonstrates the corresponding antibody, and maternal and fetal cells are tested if HDN is associated with maternal antibody to one of these antigens.

OTHER BLOOD GROUP SYSTEMS

The hundreds of known red cell antigens have been classified into 22 blood group systems. The antigens and antibodies of many of these systems are not frequently encountered in routine transfusion medicine. Red cell antigens vary in terms of their clinical significance as well. Only those blood group systems that are more commonly dealt with in the clinical setting are discussed in this text. Some of the antigens in these systems are found on the red cells of most of the population and are thus referred to as **high frequency antigens**. Those antigens that are only rarely found are termed **low frequency antigens**. When an antibody is developed to a high frequency antigen, finding compatible red cells for transfusion is more difficult because the erythrocytes of most donors will carry that antigen. Antibodies to low frequency antigens do not as often present difficulty in the location of compatible blood, but can be difficult to identify as the corresponding antigen may not be present on the reagent red cells used to screen for the presence of unexpected antibodies. A more complete discussion is provided in the section of this chapter on antibody identification.

The clinical significance of the antibodies in these other blood group systems is related to a number of factors, including:

- the immunogenicity of the antigen
- type of antibody formed
- ability of the antibody to cause HDN or hemolytic transfusion reaction (HTR)

Other characteristics that are important to blood bank technologists include the test phase in which the antibody is most likely to be detected and the probability of finding compatible blood when an antibody is present. Table 16–10 summarizes important information for the most commonly encountered antibodies. The blood group systems discussed here are presented based upon the type of antibody produced. The antibodies are typically classified as "warm" or "cold" depending on the temperature of optimum reactivity. Those that react best or only at 37°C or in the AHG phase are called **warm reacting** and those that react best at room temperature or at 4°C are called **cold reacting**. This is a somewhat "loose" classification, because antibodies do not always react optimally at the same temperature. It is nonetheless a convenient classification for discussion purposes.

■ BLOOD GROUP SYSTEMS WITH COLD REACTIVE ANTIBODIES

Antibodies that react best at room temperature or lower, the cold reactive antibodies, are usually of the IgM class. These antibodies are less often clinically significant because they are more likely to react at temperatures lower than normal body temperature. It is important to note that the only blood bank rule to which there is no exception is the rule that there is an exception to every rule. Although an antibody directed at a particular antigen may virtually always be seen as an IgM antibody reacting at lower temperatures, warm reactive IgG forms may also be seen. Antibodies of the Lewis, MNS, P, and I blood group systems are cold reactive IgM antibodies.

Lewis Blood Group System
The **Lewis system antigens** are Lewis a (Le^a) and Lewis b (Le^b). These antigens are not initially found on the red cell even though they are produced from the same precursor chain as the ABO substances. Rather than being directly synthesized on the red cell membrane, the Lewis antigens are produced in secretions and then carried in the plasma by lipoproteins that are absorbed onto the erythrocyte surface. This process of erythrocyte absorption is reversible. Because these antigens are not well developed at birth, cord blood types are negative for both antigens even though one or both may have been inherited. The LE and le alleles are found on chromosome 19. Possible **Lewis phenotypes** are **Le (a+ b–); Le (a– b+); and Le (a– b–)**. A fourth phenotype, Le (a+ b+) is sometimes seen in infants or young children who later become Le (a– b+). The mechanisms by which these phenotypes are determined are quite complex and cannot be fully dealt with here. Nonetheless, the following points, in conjunction with Figure 16–5, provide a general basis for understanding Lewis phenotype development:

TABLE 16–10. Characteristics of Common Alloantibodies

Antibody	Ig Class	Most Common Phase of Reactivity			Clinical Significance		Approx. % Compatible Donors	
		sal/RT	37°C/Alb	AHG	HTR	HDN	White	Black
D	IgG	Few	✓	✓	Yes	Yes	15	8
C	IgG		✓	✓	Yes	Yes	30	68
E	IgG	Few	✓	✓	Yes	Yes	70	98
c	IgG		✓	✓	Yes	Yes	20	1
e	IgG		✓	✓	Yes	Yes	2	2
Cw	IgG/IgM	Some	✓	✓	Yes	Yes	98	100
K	IgG	Rare		✓	Yes	Yes	91	97
k	IgG			✓	Yes	Yes	0.2	0.1
Kpa	IgG	Rare		✓	Yes	Yes	98	99.9
Kpb	IgG			✓	Yes	Yes	<0.1	0.1
Jsa	IgG			✓	Yes	Yes	>99.9	81
Jsb	IgG			✓	Yes	Yes	<0.1	1
Fya	IgG			✓	Yes	Yes	34	90
Fyb	IgG			✓	Yes	Yes	17	77
Jka	IgG			✓	Yes	Yes	23	9
Jkb	IgG			✓	Yes	Yes	28	5
M	IgM	✓			Few	Yes	22	30
N	IgM	✓			Rare	Rare	28	26
S	IgG/IgM		Some	✓	Yes	Yes	45	69
s	IgG			✓	Yes	Yes	11	3
U	IgG			✓	Yes	Yes	0	1
Lua	IgM	✓			?	Yes	92	96
Lub	IgG			✓	Yes	Mild	<0.1	<0.1
P1	IgM	✓	Some		Rare	No	21	6
P	IgM	✓	Some	Some	Probable	Yes	<0.1	0.1
PP1Pk	IgG/IgM	✓	Some	Some	Probable	Yes	<0.1	0.1
Lea	IgM	✓	Some		Yes	No	78	77
Leb	IgM	✓			Yes	No	28	45
I	IgM	✓	Few		Rare	No	<0.1	<0.1
i	IgM	✓	Few		?	No	<0.1	<0.1

Adapted from Henry JB. *Clinical Diagnosis and Management by Laboratory Methods,* 19th ed. Philadelphia, Saunders, 1996

- Persons who are **homozygous for the le allele** (le/le) develop neither the Lea nor the Leb antigen and are of the **Le(a– b–) phenotype**.
- The LE gene codes for a specific enzyme that adds fucose to a sugar on the precursor chain, resulting in **formation of the Lea antigen**.
- **Leb antigen production** depends on gene interactions (LE, SE, H) similar to those of the ABO system: SE inheritance allows production of type I H substance; addition of fucose (by the enzyme coded for by inheritance of the LE gene) to a specific location on type I H substance results in formation of the Leb antigen.
- Only secretors can form Leb antigen (H substance is precursor).
- LE and H produced enzymes compete to add fucose to the precursor chain and form Lea and Leb respectively; Leb is more readily absorbed by red

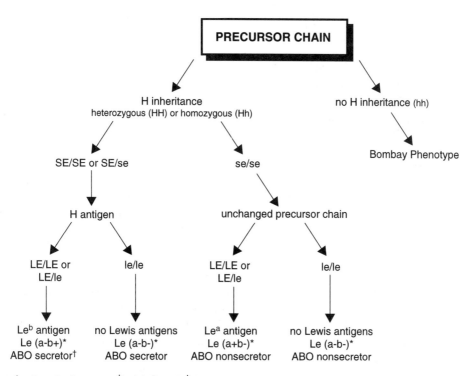

FIGURE 16-5. Production of Lewis blood group antigens.

cells producing an **erythrocyte Lewis phenotype of Le (a– b+) in secretors** even though **secretor saliva contains both Le^a and Le^b**.

The **antibodies of the Lewis system** are most frequently seen in individuals of the Le (a– b–) phenotype. Lewis antibodies can be present naturally with exposure to the corresponding antigen or may be formed in response to antigen exposure. They are most often IgM antibodies that react best at or below room temperature. They also react relatively well at 37°C (especially the Le^a antibody). Because they easily activate complement, the Lewis antibodies may be detected in the AHG phase when a polyspecific reagent (polyspecific AHG detects complement; see later section on AHG testing) is used. Lewis antibodies reacting in this phase of testing or showing in vitro hemolysis should be considered clinically significant and blood lacking the corresponding antigen selected for transfusion. Hemolytic transfusion reactions as a consequence of anti-Le^a have been reported, although none have been reported due to anti-Le^b. These antibodies do not cause HDN for two reasons:

- Antibodies are usually IgM and thus do not cross the placenta.
- Lewis antigens are not well developed by birth and therefore do not stimulate maternal antibody production.

The MNSs Blood Group System

The **MNSs blood group system** antigens of primary importance are M, N, S, s, and U. M and N are alleles and S and s are alleles. Therefore, an M or an N is inherited from each parent and an S or an s is inherited from each parent. Resultant MN genotypes could be either MM, NN, or MN and S genotypes could be either SS, Ss, or ss. U is a high frequency antigen found on nearly all red cells. Red cells lacking the U antigen have been found in < 1% of the black population and are apparently the consequence of a missing, or markedly reduced, protein on which the U antigen would be found in the red cell membrane. These individuals also lack both the S and s antigens, which would be found on the same protein. This phenotype (negative for S, s, and U) and a similar phenotype (S and s negative and U positive) that is found rarely in the black population are believed to result from a rare allele at the S locus. This allele is referred to as S^u. Antigens of the MNSs blood group system are frequently used in paternity determinations.

Antibodies to the M and N antigens are usually cold reactive IgM antibodies. They may be naturally occurring or developed in response to exposure to the antigen. Anti-M is seen more commonly than anti-N (rare) and although both are generally not clinically significant, there are rare reports of HTR associated with these antibodies. The M and N antibodies demonstrate what is referred to as **dosage effect**. Dosage effect refers to instances in which an antibody reacts more strongly with cells containing stronger antigen. In this case, an anti-M antibody produces a stronger reaction (2+, for example) with red cells that are homozygous for M (MM) than with cells that are MN (1+, for example). In some circumstances, knowledge of which antibodies exhibit the dosage effect and the antigen make-up of reagent cells used for antibody screening can be of assistance in the antibody identification process.

Antibodies to the Ss antigens are usually immune stimulated IgG antibodies that react at 37°C and may only be detected in the AHG phase of testing. Discussed in this section because they are a part of the MNS system, these antibodies are not classified as cold reactive antibodies. These antibodies may produce either HTR or HDN, so antigen negative blood must be administered in the presence of the antibody. The anti-U antibody is not commonly encountered because most red cells contain this "universal" antigen. This antibody is also usually immune stimulated and of the IgG class. It too, has been implicated in both HTR and HDN.

The P Blood Group System

Inheritance of the three **antigens of the P system** appears to be controlled by two separate genetic systems via a complex biochemical process that is not described here. Because the terminology used to refer to the antigens and to the phenotypes of this system is similar, care must be exercised to distinguish between the two. The antigens are P, P_1, and P^k, while the phenotypes resulting from dif-

TABLE 16–11. Lewis Phenotype Frequencies

	Frequency (% US Adults)	
Phenotype	*White*	*Black*
Le(a- b+)	72	55
Le(a+ b-)	22	23
Le(a- b-)	6	22

Frequencies from Whitlock, 1997

ferent antigen combinations are P_1, P_2, P_1^k, P_2^k, and p. The most common phenotype (94% of the black population and 79% of the white population) is P_1 in which the P_1 and P antigens are produced. The P_2 phenotype in which only the P antigen is produced is the second most common phenotype (21% of the white population and 6% of the black population). The other phenotypes (P_1^k—no P antigens; P_2^k—P_1 and P^k antigens; p—P^k antigen) are all very rare in both the black and white populations (Henry, 1996). The antigens of this system are found not only on red cells, but also on platelets, leukocytes, and tissue cells. The degree of expression of the P_1 antigen varies among individuals.

The antibody of the P system most commonly encountered is **anti-P_1** that is produced by persons of the P_2 phenotype. This antibody is usually a weak, cold reactive IgM antibody that occurs without immune stimulation. The antibody may also be detected in the AHG phase of testing with polyspecific reagent because it has the ability to bind complement. If anti-P_1 is reactive with pre-warming techniques or produces *in vitro* hemolysis, P_1 antigen negative units should be used for transfusion. This antibody has been reported to cause HTR. It has not, however, been implicated in HDN and would not be expected to cause this condition because the antibody is usually IgM (does not cross placenta) and the P_1 antigen is not well developed at birth.

I and i Antigens/Antibodies

Cold reactive antibodies specific for the **I and i antigens** may also be encountered in transfusion services. These antigens do not technically constitute a blood group system, and are present in varying amounts on virtually all red cells. In general terms, the erythrocytes of newborns contain the most i antigen and adult erythrocytes contain the most I antigen. At birth, the red cells are essentially negative for the I antigen on serologic testing (tests as I negative and i positive). The strength of the i antigen begins to gradually decrease and the expression of the I antigen becomes increasingly stronger. Eventually, at about 18 months of age, the red cells test as I positive and i negative. This transformation does not occur in very rare individuals.

Anti-I occurs as either an auto- or alloantibody, but the alloantibody is not common. Auto anti-I is a relatively common, cold reactive IgM antibody that is usually present in low titer. Although its presence is not often significant, it may be seen in individuals with an acquired autoimmune hemolytic anemia. A high titer

TABLE 16–12. MNSs Antigen and Phenotype Frequencies

Antigen	Frequency[1] (% U.S. Adults) White	Frequency[1] (% U.S. Adults) Black	Phenotype			Frequency[2] (% U.S. Adults) White	Frequency[2] (% U.S. Adults) Black
M	78	70	M+	N–		28	26
N	72	74	M+	N+		50	44
S	55	31	M–	N+		22	30
s	89	97	S+	s–	U+	11	3
			S+	s+	U+	44	28
			S–	s+	U+	45	69
			S+	s–	U–	0	<1
			S–	s–	U+	0	Rare

[1]Antigen frequencies from Whitlock SA. *Immunohematology: Delmar's Clinical Laboratory Manual Series.* Albany, NY, Delmar Publishers, 1997.
[2]Phenotype frequencies from Henry JB. *Clinical Diagnosis and Management by Laboratory Methods,* 19th ed. Philadelphia, Saunders, 1996.

of anti-I is associated with *Mycoplasma pneumoniae* infections (sometimes referred to as "atypical pneumonia"). **Anti-i** occurs less frequently and has been seen only as an autoantibody. It is seen most frequently in individuals who have, or have recently had, infectious mononucleosis. It has also been reported in alcoholic cirrhosis (Henry, 1996).

■ BLOOD GROUP SYSTEMS WITH WARM REACTIVE ANTIBODIES

Warm reactive antibodies are generally of greater clinical significance because they react at body temperature. Antibodies in this classification are usually of the IgG class and thus are capable of crossing the placenta and producing HDN. These antibodies are also more likely to cause HTR. They are reactive at 37°C and usually react in the AHG phase of testing.

The Kell Blood Group System

The **Kell blood group system** was first identified as a result of investigation of a case of HDN. This system is now known to be a complex system of over 20 antigens. The inheritance of Kell antigens is controlled by three closely linked loci on chromosome 7. The Kk alleles are found at one locus; the Kp^a and Kp^b alleles at another; and the Js^a and Js^b alleles at the third. Although a mechanism of biosynthesis of these antigens has been hypothesized, it has not been proven and is not yet clearly understood. The **primary antigens** of the Kell system are **K** and **k**. With inheritance of one allele from each parent, possible phenotypes are KK, Kk, and kk. The k antigen is a high frequency antigen found on the erythrocytes of 99% of the white population and more than 99% of the black population. For this reason, the KK phenotype is quite rare. The phenotype seen in greatest frequency is K negative, k positive. The Js^a and Js^b alleles most commonly produce the phenotype Js (a– b+) and the most common phenotype resulting from the Kp^a and

Kp^b alleles is Kp (a– b +). There are **two very rare Kell phenotypes** called the **K$_o$** (Kell null) phenotype and the **McLeod** phenotype. As implied by its name, no Kell antigens are expressed in the K$_o$ phenotype. The McLeod phenotype is characterized by a weakened expression of the Kell antigens and abnormal red cell morphology consequent to an abnormality in a protein associated with the expression of Kell antigens (Henry, 1996).

The anti-k antibody is not often produced by immune stimulation because most red cells have the corresponding antigen. **Anti-K**, on the other hand, is one of the more frequently encountered alloantibodies in the blood bank. Because only about 9 % of the white population and 2 % of the black population are positive for the K antigen, finding K negative blood for transfusion to an individual with anti-K is generally not difficult. Excluding the ABO system antigens (ie, A and B), the K antigen is second only to D in immunogenicity. The Kell antibodies are usually IgG antibodies reacting at 37°C and many are detectable only in the AHG phase of testing. All of the antibodies of the Kell system are capable of causing both hemolytic transfusion reactions and HDN.

The Kidd Blood Group System

The **Kidd blood group system** contains only two known antigens, Jk^a and Jk^b, which are coded for by allelic genes. The chromosome containing the Kidd locus has not been conclusively determined. The most common Kidd phenotype in the white population (49 %) is Jk (a + b +) and the most common in the black population (57 %) is Jk (a + b–). The least common phenotype for both the white and black populations (23 % and 9 % respectively) is Jk (a– b +). A fourth phenotype, Jk (a– b–) or Kidd null, is very rarely seen outside the Polynesian population, in whom its frequency approaches 1 % (Henry, 1996).

Antibodies of the Kidd system are notorious for the difficulty encountered in their detection and identification and are (not so affectionately) dubbed the "treacherous Kidds" by some blood bankers. The antibodies of this system are immune stimulated antibodies of the IgG class detectable only in the AHG phase of testing. These antibodies have several characteristics that contribute to the difficulties encountered in their detection and identification:

- usually present in low titer
- weak avidity (*avidity* refers to total binding strength of all antigen binding sites together)
- disappear rapidly after immunization, but produce a potent anamnestic response on subsequent exposure
- demonstrate dosage effect

Despite the difficulty that may be encountered in detecting these antibodies, their detection and identification is important because Kidd antibodies cause both HTR and HDN. Kidd antibodies are sometimes detected only as a result of an anamnestic response produced by a secondary exposure to the corresponding Kidd antigen. In other words, these antibodies are sometimes not detected until HTR occurs. Kidd antibodies are very effective in activating complement and thus can produce significant *in vivo* hemolysis. Blood banks often use only polyspecific reagents in the AHG phase of testing because this reagent detects complement, due to the chance that a complement dependent Kidd antibody may be missed when using monospecific IgG AHG reagent. Kidd antibodies are responsible for more than three fourths of severe, delayed HTRs (Henry, 1996). Careful evaluation of all test results is imperative when a Kidd antibody is suspected.

The Duffy Blood Group System

The Duffy blood group system consists of a number of antigens, the most common of which are the Fy^a and Fy^b alleles. Inheritance of these antigens is controlled by a locus on chromosome 1. Duffy antigenic phenotypes differ considerably between the black and white populations, as illustrated in Table 16–13. Interestingly, the Fy (a– b–) phenotype is associated with resistance to infection with the malarial parasite *Plasmodium vivax.* (As an interesting aside, a different red cell antigen may offer protection from the deadly consequences of severe infection with another malarial organism, *Plasmodium falciparum,* as reported in the February 1998, issue of *Laboratory Medicine.* This antigen, Sl^a or KN4, is from the Knops system and appears to play a role in the progression of the disease caused by *P. falciparum* infection and prevent death.) Both anti-Fy^a and anti-Fy^a are immune-stimulated IgG antibodies detected only in the AHG phase of testing, but anti-Fy^b is the more commonly encountered of the two. Both are capable of producing HTR and HDN.

The Lutheran Blood Group System

The Lutheran blood group system consists of eight antigens from four pairs of alleles. The primary antigens of this system are the Lu^a and Lu^b alleles to which the other three pairs of alleles are closely linked. The genes that code for the Lutheran antigens are found on chromosome 19. The most common Lutheran phenotype in both the black and white populations is Lu (a– b +) and the Lu (a– b–) phenotype is very rarely seen in either. **Antibodies** to Lu^a and Lu^b are not commonly encountered and are rarely associated with HTR and HDN. Anti-Lu^a is particularly uncommon because Lu^a is a high frequency antigen. These antibodies are an example of the inadequacy of a simplistic classification of antibody systems as cold or warm reactive. Anti-Lu^a is usually predominantly a cold reactive IgM antibody and anti-Lu^b is predominantly warm reactive IgG antibody. Both antibodies may

TABLE 16–13. Duffy Phenotype Frequencies

	Frequency (% US Adults)	
Phenotype	*White*	*Black*
Fy (a+ b+)	49	1
Fy (a+ b-)	17	9
Fy (a- b+)	34	22
Fy (a- b-)	Very rare	68

be seen as a mixture of the IgG, IgM, and IgA antibody classes. Lutheran antibodies are associated with a **characteristic mixed field agglutination** pattern in which a small red cell agglutinates are seen against a background of cells that are not agglutinated.

 TIME FOR REVIEW. After studying the preceding sections, you should be able to respond correctly to the following:

■ The primary antigen in the Rh system is _____.

■ List three situations in which a weak D antigen may be produced.

■ The four most common Rh antigens, after the D antigen, are ____, ____, ____, and ____ .

■ Designation of Rh positive or negative depends solely on the presence/absence of the ____ antigen.

■ Individuals with a weak D antigen may be treated as Rh positive or Rh negative depending on the circumstances. Indicate whether these individuals are treated as positive or negative in the cases listed below:

   Transfusion recipient:

   Blood donor:

■ Complete the chart below to compare the three nomenclature systems for Rh antigens.

FisherRace	Wiener	Rosenfield
D		
	rh'	
		Rh3
c		
	hr"	

■ Refer to Table 16–9 to provide the most probable genotype for the sets of testing results provided.

Rh Phenotype Results					
Patient Red Cells with Anti-					
D	C	E	c	e	Most Probable Genotype
+	+	0	+	+	
+	0	0	+	+	
+	+	+	+	+	
0	+	+	+	0	

■ Individuals who have no Rh antigens on their red cells are called _____.

■ Of the five common Rh antigens, _____ is most likely to provoke antibody production.

■ Rh antibodies are primarily of the Ig____ class.

■ A second exposure to the D antigen results in a swift, potent secondary response called an _____ response.

■ HTR and HDN _____ (do/do not) result from antibodies to all of the common Rh antigens.

■ Provide the appropriate Rh type for red cells that are agglutinated by reagent anti-D:

at initial spin:

after a 2-minute RT incubation:

after 37°C incubation:

after AHG phase only:

do not agglutinate at any test phase:

■ A positive result in the control tube means the test is _____.

■ A negative result after the addition of _____ cells means the test is invalid.

■ List three factors that affect the clinical significance of an antibody.

■ Antibodies that react best at or below room temperature are called _____ reactive.

■ Refer to Table 16–10 to respond to the following regarding alloantibodies:

usual Ig class of:

E

e

D

M

N

S

s

P_1

Le^a

Le^b

K

Jk^a

Jk^b

Lu^a

Lu^b

Fy^a

■ The Le^b antigen can only be produced in _____ (secretors/non-secretors).

■ List two reasons why Lewis antibodies do not cause HDN.

■ Antibodies to the M and N antigens demonstrate dosage effect. What does this mean?

■ Antibodies to the Ss antigens are usually _____ stimulated Ig ____ antibodies.

■ The most common antibody of the P blood group system is anti- _____.

■ Which antigen, I or i, is stronger on normal adult red cells?

■ A high titer anti-I autoantibody is associated with _____ infection.

■ Anti-i occurs only as an _____ antibody and is seen most frequently in individuals who have, or have recently had, _____.

■ The Kell phenotype seen in greatest frequency is: K ____/k ____.

■ Excluding the A and B antigens, the _____ antigen is second only to D in immunogenicity.

■ Antibodies of the _____ system are notorious for difficulties encountered in their detection and identification.

■ List three characteristics of the antibodies referred to in the previous question that contribute to the difficulty in detecting and identifying them.

■ The antigen phenotypes of this blood group system differ markedly between the black and white populations and the phenotype most commonly seen in the black population is associated with resistance to infection by the malarial organism *Plasmodium vivax*. What is this blood group system?

■ _____ antibodies are associated with a characteristic mixed field aggutination pattern.

Check your responses by reviewing the preceding sections.

OVERVIEW OF PRE-TRANSFUSION TESTING

Pre-transfusion testing is the term applied to the testing employed to ensure the highest degree of safety that can reasonably be achieved in the transfusion of blood or blood products. The testing required depends on the product to be transfused, with the most thorough testing required for transfusion of red cell products. Pre-transfusion testing is aimed at the prevention of adverse effects of transfusion, including the transmission of infectious disease and immune responses.

■ DONOR SELECTION

Transfusion service departments in a hospital clinical laboratory do not generally collect and process donor blood. This function is usually left to larger regional blood collection facilities such as the American Red Cross. A variety of regulatory agencies oversee donor selection and testing as well as the administration of blood and blood products. These agencies include the FDA (Food and Drug Administration), HCFA (Health Care Financing Administration), the State Health Department, and OSHA. In addition, standards are established by the JCAHO, CAP, and the AABB (American Association of Blood Banks) that must be met in order to be accredited by these organizations. The AABB establishes standards for testing that are generally accepted by the other accrediting organizations.

As previously noted, donor selection and testing will not be dealt with in detail in this text. However, an overview is presented in order to provide a general understanding of donor requirements and the processing of donor blood. Prior to acceptance as a blood donor, individuals are screened on the basis of medical history and an abbreviated physical examination. Donors respond to questions developed to determine whether they are at high risk for certain infectious diseases, particularly HIV. In addition, mechanisms are provided to allow the donor to confidentially exclude himself/herself as a donor even after blood has been collected. This may be accomplished by placing a designated bar code on the registration form or on the blood bag itself. Such procedures are useful for situations in which a prospective donor may have been less than truthful in response to the donor questionnaire, but realizes that he/she has engaged in risky behaviors that increase the risk of infectious diseases. Prospective donors concerned with the embarrassment of being deferred based on responses to questions can then exclude themselves at any point, even after the unit of blood has been collected.

Although the history provided by the prospective donor is an important part of donor selection, donor centers do not, of course, rely solely on the honesty of prospective donors. A variety of test procedures are performed to rule out the presence of, or exposure to, a variety of conditions, as discussed below. Donors must meet criteria established for physical examination related to

- age: minimum age of 18 or, with parental permission, 17 when state law allows; previous upper age limits are no longer in place
- weight: minimum of 110 lbs required for full donation; donors of lower weight may be approved if the amount of blood withdrawn is adjusted; unexplained weight loss of more than 10 lbs, regardless of body weight, excludes a potential donor
- temperature: potential donors with a temperature above 99.5°F are deferred because of the possibility of an underlying infectious process
- pulse and blood pressure: pulse rate in the range of 50 to 100 and regular; systolic pressure no higher than 180 and diastolic no higher than 100; blood bank physician is given some discretion in regard to pulse and blood pressure requirements
- hemoglobin: screening method of testing is used to ensure hemoglobin level of at least 12.5 g/dL

Donors may be deferred permanently or temporarily. Causes for such deferrals are summarized in Table 16–14. The information in this table is provided only for general information and is not a comprehensive listing of all situations in which a donor may be deferred.

DONOR TESTING

Prospective donors who are not excluded in the initial screening process are accepted for blood donation. All donated units of whole blood are tested according to established protocols prior to the preparation of components (eg, packed red cells, fresh frozen plasma, platelets) for transfusion. Donors with unacceptable test results are notified and are either deferred or retested for confirmation. Donors with confirmed positive test results for HIV or hepatitis are permanently excluded and blood collected from such donors is discarded. Table 16–15 summarizes the testing performed on donor blood.

GENERAL RECIPIENT TESTING

Recipient blood samples are tested to determine **ABO group** and **Rh type**. As previously noted, it is not necessary to test for the presence of a weak D antigen on recipient blood samples because the recipient will be treated as Rh negative in the presence of weak D. Although not required, some laboratories may choose to complete testing for weak D. An **antibody screen** is performed on the recipient to detect the presence of any "unexpected" antibodies that have the potential to

TABLE 16–14. Donor Deferral

Permanent Deferral	*Temporary Deferral*
HIV positive	Childbirth within 6 weeks
Hemophiliac	Blood donation within last 2 months
Past or present IV drug use	Current antibiotic treatment
Symptoms of AIDS	Active disease (cold, flu, other infections)
Any person who has engaged in sex for money or drugs since 1997 and men who have had sex with other men since 1977	Malaria risk: recent travel to endemic area; immigrant from endemic area (3-year deferral); previous malaria diagnosis (deferred for 3 years
Positive tests for hepatitis B surface antigen, hepatitis B core antigen or hepatitis C antibody	after asymptomatic)
History of viral hepatitis	Recent vaccination (2 weeks to 1 month depending on type of vaccination)
Serious bleeding tendencies	Incarcerated for ≥ 72 hours (1-year deferral)
Chronic cardiopulmonary disease and chronic disease of the liver or kidneys	Tattoo within last 12 months
Most malignant solid tumors	Transfused with blood component within last 12 months
Hematologic malignancies	Close contact with viral hepatitis (1-year deferral)
Chemotherapy	High-risk sex within last 12 months
Previous donation in which recipient developed hepatitis or became HIV positive; no other donors involved	Rape victim (1-year deferral)
Positive test for human T-cell lymphotropic virus	Administration of hepatitis B immune globulin or rabies treatment following animal bite (1-year deferral)
Treatment of psoriasis with the drug etretinate	Certain medications, including Accutane (1 month)
	Does not meet physical exam criteria

TABLE 16–15. Summary of Testing on Donor Blood

Test	Comments
ABO group	Required to facilitate administration of type specific blood; retested for confirmation prior to transfusion
Rh type	Required to facilitate administration of Rh compatible blood; retested for confirmation prior to transfusion; weak D positive blood considered Rh positive
Antibody screen	To detect the presence of any unexpected antibody; if detected, red cells can be transfused but plasma cannot and is either discarded or used for reagent preparation
Hepatitis B surface antigen (Hb$_s$Ag)	Confirmed positive test results in permanent donor deferral; blood is discarded
Hepatitis C core antibody	Confirmed positive test results in permanent donor deferral; blood is discarded
Antibody to hepatitis C virus	Confirmed positive test results in permanent donor deferral; blood is discarded
Syphilis test	Confirmed positive test results in permanent donor deferral; blood is discarded
HIV antibody tests	Confirmed positive test results in permanent donor deferral; blood is discarded
HIV antigen test	Confirmed positive test results in permanent donor deferral; blood is discarded
Antibody to HTLV	Confirmed positive test results in permanent donor deferral; blood is discarded
ALT	Previously required testing; nonspecific test that is no longer required, but may be performed

result in hemolytic transfusion reactions. If clinically significant antibodies are detected, **antibody identification** techniques are employed to determine the specificity of the antibody. Donor red blood cells can then be tested to locate erythrocytes that are negative for the antigen toward which the antibody is directed. Compatibility testing (crossmatch) is performed prior to transfusion of red cell products. **Compatibility testing** includes testing the donor red cells with the patient's serum (major crossmatch) in various test phases to detect reactions that may occur *in vivo* and result in serious transfusion complications. ABO and Rh typing have been discussed in previous sections. A discussion of the additional test procedures involved in pre-transfusion recipient testing follows.

A **check of previous blood bank records** on recipients is another important component of pre-transfusion procedures. Strict record retention regulations are applied to the blood bank and workers are required to compare current test results to those previously obtained if the patient has been tested at their facility in the past. Although ABO and Rh type do not change (except in bone marrow transplant recipients who receive marrow of differing ABO type), the comparison of current test results to those obtained previously is an important measure aimed at detecting typing errors, incorrectly identified specimens, or misidentified patients. In the event that a discrepancy exists between the ABO and Rh type obtained on the current specimen and that included in previous patient records, the discrepancy should be resolved before proceeding with testing. A new sample should be collected from the patient, ensuring proper patient and sample identification and ABO and Rh testing repeated. Results of any previous antibody detection procedures and compatibility testing must also be reviewed. This review may alert the technologist to previous compatibility problems and their resolution. It is also important that the blood bank be aware of any potentially immunizing event (ie, pregnancy, transfusion) in the patient's history, particularly those occurring subsequent to any previous testing.

ANTIBODY DETECTION AND IDENTIFICATION

Excluding the antibodies of the ABO system occurring as described in Landsteiner's law, the presence of antibodies in the serum or coating the red cells of a recipient is an unexpected finding in the blood bank. Hence, the reference to the detection of "unexpected" antibodies. While it is of paramount importance to detect antibodies with the potential to cause HTR, other antibodies amount to little more than a bothersome presence that may interfere with other procedures.

ANTIBODY DETECTION

The **antibody screen** is used to detect the presence of unexpected antibodies in the serum. It is standard practice to screen the serum of recipients for such antibodies. The antibody screen is also routinely used in other situations, including:

- screening for the presence of unexpected antibodies in donated blood
- screening during pregnancy to detect maternal antibodies capable of producing HDN
- as a part of the investigation of a hemolytic transfusion reaction (see later discussion)

If the antibody screen is positive, the specificity of the antibody must be determined using **antibody identification** techniques (**antibody panel**). In some situations it is also necessary to determine the titer of the antibody by determining the highest dilution at which the antibody remains capable of agglutinating red cells. Another test, the **direct antiglobulin test, or DAT**, is used to detect antibodies coating the red cells. These antibodies can be removed from the red cells by elution and then identified using the antibody panel. The need to perform DAT testing may first be apparent as the result of a positive reaction in the **auto control** of the antibody screen.

The **antibody screen** is performed using reagent red cells of known antigenic make-up. These cells are always group O cells to avoid agglutination as a result of naturally occurring anti-A and anti-B. AABB standards dictate that these reagent cells cannot be pooled—that is, they must come from an individual donor. At least two, and sometimes three, screening cells are used and should be selected to ensure that all of the red cell antigens corresponding to the most frequently encountered antibodies are present in one of the cell populations. Red cells used for antibody detection are generally obtained from commercial sources. The manufacturer tests the cells for a variety of antigens and provides the blood bank with an **antigram** for each lot number of reagent. The antigram (Fig. 16–6) is a listing of the antigens present on the reagent red cells. Cells that are homozygous for antigens corresponding to antibodies that exhibit the dosage effect are preferred to detect more weakly reacting antibodies. A particular antigram can only be used to interpret results obtained from the reagent and lot number specified on the antigram. Use with any other reagent, including reagents made by the same manufacturer but of a different lot number, **will** produce erroneous findings.

Because different antibodies have varying reaction characteristics, antibody screening and identification procedures vary in terms of incubation time and temperature and enhancement media depending on the type of antibody to be detected or identified. Most laboratories do not include room temperature incubation in their antibody screening protocol because antibodies reacting only at this temperature are not considered clinically significant. The aim of the antibody screen is to detect clinically significant antibodies, which are generally reactive at 37°C or in the AHG test phase. A typical antibody screen protocol involves adding the reagent screen cells (which are a 3% to 5% red cell suspension) to the patient's serum in the ratio specified by the manufacturer to provide the appropriate serum:cell ratio for optimal reactivity. This is generally one volume of reagent cells to two volumes of patient serum (ie, 1 drop cells in 2 drops serum; 2 drops cells in 4 drops serum). An auto-control tube containing the patient's serum with and a 3% to 5% suspension of the patient's cells added in the same ratio used for the reagent cells and patient serum is included in some testing protocols. After thorough mixing, the tubes may be centrifuged and examined for agglutination or immediately placed in a 37°C heat block for incubation. (Some laboratories omit the initial spin reading for the same reasons discussed above for omission of a room temperature incubation phase.) Some laboratories use an enhancement medium (eg, albumin, low ionic strength saline [LISS]) for the 37°C incubation period. Incubation time is dependent on whether or not an enhancement medium

XYZ Screen Cells   **Lot #: 1234567**   **Expiration Date: 04/19/9X**

Shaded areas indicate antibodies that are generally of the IgM class

CELL	Rh System							MNSs System				P	Lewis		Lutheran		Kell System					Duffy		Kidd	
	D	C	E	c	e	Cw	V	M	N	S	s	P1	Lea	Leb	Lua	Lub	K	k	Kpa	Jsa	Jsb	Fya	Fyb	Jka	Jkb
I	+	+	0	0	+	0	0	+	0	+	+	+	+	0	0	0	+	0	+	0	0	0	+	+	+
II	+	0	+	+	+	0	0	0	+	0	+	+	0	+	0	+	+	+	+	0	0	+	+	0	+

Sample antigram for illustration purposes only; cannot be used to evaluate the results of antibody screening.

FIGURE 16–6. Sample antigram for antibody screening.

is used and the specific type of medium used, but generally is in the range of 15 to 30 minutes. Following incubation, the tubes are centrifuged and examined for agglutination of the red cells (hemolysis is also an indication of a positive reaction). The cells are then washed four times with saline, tested with AHG, and examined again for agglutination or hemolysis.

Although the antibody screen itself does not provide definitive identification of antibodies that are detected, it can provide a significant amount of useful information if results are carefully examined. The possibilities of the antibody (or antibodies) present may be narrowed based on whether one or both of the reagent screen cells were agglutinated by the patient's serum by examination of the antigram. The phase of testing in which a positive reaction was noted, whether the reaction was demonstrated by agglutination or hemolysis, the strength of reactions seen in various phases, and other factors can also provide a hint of the antibody's identity. Some examples are provided following the sample antigram. Note that a negative antibody screen does not ensure the absence of antibodies, only that antibodies were not detected to the antigens on the reagent red cells. No antibody screen can include all red cell antigens. Antibodies may be present even with a negative antibody screen in at least two situations:

- the antibody is directed at an antigen not found on either of the screen cells
- a weakly reactive antibody is not detected even though its corresponding antigen is present (eg, Kidd antibodies, other antibodies showing dosage effect and reagent red cell is heterozygous for the corresponding antigen)

A positive antibody screen (positive reaction with one or both screen cells) requires further testing to identify the antibody (or antibodies) present. A positive auto-control also requires additional testing. Figure 16–7 depicts the flow of testing for detection and identification of unexpected antibodies. Table 16–6 presents examples of antibody screening results.

ANTIBODY IDENTIFICATION

An antibody panel is performed in the same manner as an antibody screen, but consists of a greater number of reagent red cells (group O) for which the antigens are known. Although the number of panel cells used varies, most panels include at least eight reagent red cells. In selecting an antibody panel, it is important to have a number of cells sufficient to identify most antibodies but not so many as to make testing impractical. Results are recorded for the various test phases and identification made by using a systematic method of evaluation that includes elimination and examination of patterns of reactivity. Elimination is accomplished by noting the first reagent red cell for which no reaction was seen in any phase of testing. Antibodies to the antigens found on that cell are eliminated. The next cell for which there were no reactions in any

TABLE 16–16. Examples of Antibody Screening Results

Cell	Results			Comments
	Initial Spin	*37°C*	*AHG*	
I	0	2+	3+	The antibody detected reacts with an antigen that is found on both screen cells (D, e, s, P_1, Lu^b, k, Js^b, Fy^b, Jk^b). Though none can be ruled out without further testing, it is unlikely that anti-k is present (rare Ab) and anti-P_1 usually reacts at lower temperatures. Anti-Lu^b is also not frequently encountered. Duffy antibodies are usually only detected with AHG; Kidd antibodies generally produce weak reactions. Antibodies of the Rh system typically react well at 37°C and with AHG. These results are suggestive of anti-D or anti-e. No determination can be made without an antibody identification panel.
II	0	2+	3+	
I	0	0	0	This antibody reacts with an antigen on cell II that is *not* on cell I (E, c, N, Le^b, K, Fy^a). None of the six can be ruled out without further testing, but anti-N is rare and usually reacts best at lower temperatures. Neither anti-N nor anti-Le^b is expected to react at 37°C or with AHG. Anti- E or anti-c could produce these results, but usually react more strongly than indicated here at 37°C. These results are most suggestive of an anti-K or anti-Fy^a; anti-K is the more likely choice as it is more commonly encountered. No determination can be made without an antibody identification panel.
II	0	+/-	2+	
I	2+	1+ w/hemolysis	+/- w/hemolysis	This antibody reacts with an antigen on cell I that is not on cell II (C, M, S, S, Le^a, Jk^a). It reacts best at lower temperature, which is not consistent with anti-C, anti-S, or anti-Jk^a. Anti-M is not often reactive at 37°C or with AHG. Anti- Le^a reacts best at or below room temperature, but also reacts fairly well at 37°C and may be detected with polyspecific AHG. Hemolysis after 37°C incubation is associated with Lewis (Le) and Kidd (Jk) antibodies (as well as some other antibodies directed at antigens other than the six under consideration here). These results are most consistent with the expected reaction pattern of anti-Le^a. No determination can be made without an antibody identification panel.
II	0	0	0	

Examples based on the presence of a single antibody; the presence of multiple antibodies increases the difficulty of interpreting results. Interpretive comments based on sample antigram in Figure 16-6.

phase of testing is treated in the same manner and this process continued until the antibodies corresponding to the antigens on all reagent red cells with no reactions are eliminated. Systematic elimination may not narrow the antibody choices sufficiently. Knowledge of characteristic reactivities of the commonly encountered antibodies may provide additional guidance. Patterns of reactivity can be an important component of interpretation of panel results as well.

In some cases, further testing will be required for a definitive identification. This is often the case when multiple antibodies are present and/or with antibodies that exhibit the dosage effect. Additional testing may include the use of an **enzyme panel**. Proteolytic enzymes such as ficin or papain are often used for this purpose. Such enzymes enhance the reactivity of some antigen-antibody complexes and inhibit others by destroying the antigens. Enzyme panels must be used in conjunction with routine panels and must not be used alone. Use of an enzyme panel without an untreated panel may result in a failure to detect clin-

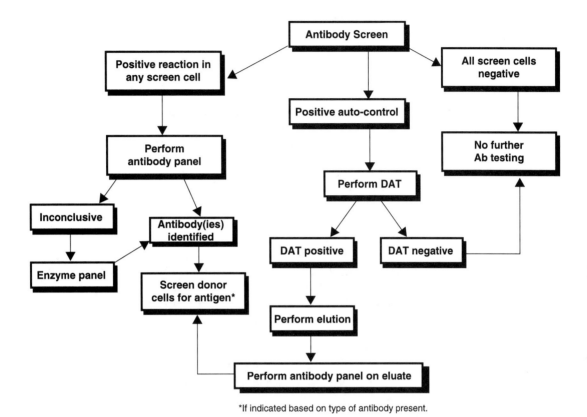

*If indicated based on type of antibody present.

FIGURE 16–7. Antibody detection and identification.

ically significant antibodies. Enzyme panels may be performed using commercial enzyme treated panels. These panels consist of red cells that have been pretreated with an enzyme and the excess enzyme removed. This is usually the most practical method, although direct addition of enzyme to the serum/cell mixture may produce stronger effects. Variation of reaction temperatures may also be helpful in the identification process when multiple antibodies are present, particularly if the antibodies involved have different optimum temperatures of reactivity. For example, incubation of the panel cells at 4°C (refrigerator temperature) will enhance the reaction of antibodies with optimal reactivity in this range, but reduce the reactivity of an antibody optimally reactive at 37°C. This approach may be of benefit when an IgM antibody of relatively broad thermal range is present in conjunction with other antibodies. Other specialized techniques, such as absorption techniques and the use of rare reagent red cells, are available to aid in particularly challenging cases. When antibodies reacting at 37°C or with AHG cannot be identified, specimens can be referred to immunohematologists at a regional reference lab for more extensive testing. These specialists are often available by telephone to provide guidance and suggestions in difficult cases. When a clinically significant antibody is identified, donor red cells must be tested for the corresponding antigen prior to transfusion. Donor cells that do not contain the antigen against which the antibody is directed should be chosen for transfusion. Donor units are tested with specific reagent antisera for this purpose. When the antibody detected corresponds to a low frequency antigen, random testing of units usually identifies cells that are suitable for transfusion fairly quickly. However, antibodies to higher frequency antigens may require the testing of an inordinate number of units. Knowledge of antigen and phenotypic frequencies may be helpful in narrowing the prospective units. A **positive DAT** indicates that the red cells are coated with antibody. The antibody is removed from the red cells through a process called *elution* and the eluate containing the antibody is tested in the same manner as described for serum. Commercial reagents for antibody elution are available that allow antibodies to be eluted with relative ease when the manufacturer's instructions are followed exactly.

It is important to note that no method for the detection and identification of antibodies is foolproof. Blood bank procedures should be developed to ensure that clinically significant antibodies are likely to be detected. However, antibodies can elude detection by even the most experienced and conscientious blood bank technologist following all appropriate procedures. As referred to previously, the antibodies of the Kidd blood group system are particularly troublesome. In many cases, the presence of a Kidd antibody is not detected until an antibody screen is performed subsequent to a transfusion that resulted in a delayed hemolytic transfusion reaction (see Adverse Effects of Transfusion, later in this chapter). Blood bank workers responsible for compatibility testing and choosing appropriate units for transfusion probably fear nothing more than a call for investigation of a possible transfusion reaction. Even when no errors in identification, testing, or judgment were made, it is difficult for these individuals to avoid feeling responsible in the face of serious clinical consequences resulting from the transfusion of blood they deemed compatible.

Figures 16-8, 16-9, and 16-10 are sample antibody panel identification sheets.

The crossmatch is usually performed at the same time as antibody screening procedures, unless it is performed subsequent to a "type and screen" procedure (also called "type and hold"; discussed in a later section). The crossmatch, or compatibility testing, involves procedures designed to

- serve as a final check of ABO compatibility
- provide an opportunity to detect clinically significant antibodies directed at antigens not found on screen cells or antibodies otherwise not detected by screening
- provide reasonable assurance of serologic compatibility between the donor cells and the recipient's serum

The AABB establishes acceptable procedures for compatibility testing. Methods used must include those that will demonstrate ABO incompatibility and detect clinically significant unexpected antibodies, if either is present, and must also

CELL #/PHENOTYPE		Rh							MNSs					P	Lewis		Lutheran		Kell				Duffy		Kidd		Patient Results			
		D	C	E	c	e	f	Cʷ	M	N	S	s		P₁	Leᵃ	Leᵇ	Luᵃ	Luᵇ	K	Kpᵃ	Jsᵃ		Fyᵃ	Fyᵇ	Jkᵃ	Jkᵇ	#	IS	37°	AHG	CC
1	rr	0	0	0	+	+	+	0	+	0	+	+	+	+	+	0	0	+	0	0	0	+	+	+	+	0	1	0	0	0	2+
2	rr	0	0	0	+	+	+	0	+	0	+	+	+	+	0	+	0	+	+	0	0	+	+	+	+	+	2	0	0	2+	
3	r'r	0	+	0	+	+	+	0	+	+	0	0	+	+	0	+	+	+	+	0	0	+	0	+	0	+	3	0	0	0	2+
4	r"r	0	0	+	+	+	+	0	0	0	0	+	+	0	0	+	0	+	+	+	0	0	0	0	0	+	4	0	0	0	2+
5	rr	0	0	0	+	+	+	0	0	+	0	+	+	+	0	+	0	+	+	0	0	0	+	0	+	+	5	0	0	0	2+
6	R₀r	+	0	0	+	+	+	0	0	+	0	+	+	0	0	+	0	+	+	+	0	+	0	+	0	+	6	0	0	0	2+
7	R₁R₁	+	+	0	0	+	0	0	0	0	+	0	+	0	0	+	0	+	+	0	+	0	+	+	0	+	7	0	+/-	2+	
8	R₁R₁	+	+	0	0	+	0	0	+	0	+	0	+	0	0	+	0	+	+	0	0	0	+	0	+	0	8	0	+/-	2+	
9	R₁R₁ʷ	+	+	0	0	+	0	+	+	0	0	+	+	+	0	0	0	+	+	0	0	+	0	+	0	+	9	0	0	0	2+
10	R₂R₂	+	0	+	+	0	0	0	0	+	0	0	+	+	+	0	0	+	+	0	+	+	0	+	+	0	10	0	0	0	2+
11	rr	0	0	0	+	+	+	0	0	0	0	0	+	+	+	+	+	+	+	+	0	+	0	+	+	0	11	0	0	0	2+
																											auto	0	0	0	2+
																											SCI	0	0	0	2+
																											SCII	0	+/-	2+	
																											cord				
																											A₁ cells				
																											B cells				

Patient Name: Edith Anglin   Physician: Charles William, M.D.

Hospital Number: 22334455   Room #: 233

ABO: A   Rh: Neg   DAT: Neg

This is an example of a simple, straightforward antibody identification panel with a single antibody present. The systematic elimination process has been started by eliminating antibodies to all of the antigens present on cell 1, since there were no reactions at any test phase with this cell. The eliminated antigens have been marked through. Figure 16.9 on the following page continues this process.

Specimen Collected: 02/09/9X   14.00

Specimen Tested: 02/09/9X   16.00

Technologist: Alex Timms, MT, SBB (ASCP)

INTERPRETATION: _____

CC = COOMBS CONTROL

SC = SCREEN CELL

XYZ Screen Cells   Lot #: 1234567   Expiration Date: 04/19/9X

shaded areas indicate antibodies that are generally of the IgM class

		Rh System						MNSs System					P	Lewis		Lutheran		Kell System				Duffy			Kidd			PT. RESULTS		
CELL		D	C	E	c	e	Cʷ	M	N	S	s	V	P₁	Leᵃ	Leᵇ	Luᵃ	Luᵇ	K	k	Kpᵃ	Jsᵃ	Fyᵃ	Fyᵇ	Jsᵇ	Jkᵃ	Jkᵇ	IS	37°	AHG	CC
1		+	+	0	0	+	0	+	0	+	0	0	+	0	+	0	+	0	+	0	0	+	0	+	+	+	0	0	0	2+
II		+	0	+	+	0	0	0	+	0	+	0	+	0	+	0	+	+	+	0	0	+	+	0	0	+	0	0	+/-	2+

FIGURE 16–8. Sample antibody identification sheet.

CELL #/Rh PHENOTYPE		Rh						MNSs				P	Lewis		Lutheran		Kell						Duffy		Kidd		Patient Results				
		D	C	E	c	e	Cw	M	N	S	s	P1	Lea	Leb	Lua	Lub	K	k	Kpa	Kpb	Jsa	Jsb	Fya	Fyb	Jka	Jkb	#	IS	37°	AHG	CC
1	rr	0	0	0	+	+	0	+	0	+	+	+	+	0	0	+	0	+	0	+	0	+	+	+	+	0	1	0	0	0	2+
2	rr	0	0	0	+	+	0	+	0	+	+	+	0	+	0	+	+	+	0	+	0	+	+	0	+	+	2	0	0	2+	
3	r'r	0	+	0	+	+	0	0	+	+	0	+	0	+	0	+	0	+	0	+	0	+	0	0	0	+	3	0	0	0	2+
4	r"r	0	0	+	+	+	0	+	0	0	+	0	0	+	+	+	0	+	0	+	0	+	0	0	0	+	4	0	0	0	2+
5	rr	0	0	0	+	+	0	+	0	+	0	0	0	+	0	+	0	+	0	+	0	+	+	+	+	+	5	0	0	0	2+
6	R0r	+	0	0	+	+	0	+	0	0	+	+	+	0	0	+	0	+	0	+	0	+	0	+	+	+	6	0	0	0	2+
7	R1R1	+	+	0	0	+	0	0	+	+	0	0	0	+	0	+	+	+	0	+	0	+	0	+	0	+	7	0	+/-	2+	
8	R1R1	+	+	0	0	+	0	+	0	0	+	+	+	0	0	+	+	+	0	+	0	+	0	+	+	+	8	0	+/-	2+	
9	R1R1w	+	+	0	0	+	+	+	+	+	+	0	0	+	0	+	0	+	0	+	0	+	+	0	+	0	9	0	0	0	2+
10	R2R2	+	0	+	+	0	0	+	0	0	0	+	+	0	0	+	0	+	0	+	0	+	0	+	0	+	10	0	0	0	2+
11	rr	0	0	0	+	+	0	0	+	0	0	+	0	+	+	+	0	+	+	0	+	0	+	+	0	+	11	0	0	0	2+
																											auto	0	0	0	2+
																											SCI	0		0	2+
																											SCII	0	+/-	2+	
																											cord				
																											A1 cells				
																											B cells				

CC = COOMBS CONTROL

SC = SCREEN CELL

Patient Name: Edith Anglin   Physician: Charles William, M.D.

Hospital Number: 22334455   Room #: 233

ABO: A   Rh: Neg   DAT: Neg

Specimen Collected: 02/09/9X   14:00

Specimen Tested: 02/09/9X   16:00

Technologist: Alex Timus, MT, SBB (ASCP)

INTERPRETATION: Anti-K

The elimination process started in Figure 16.8 is continued for each cell in which there were no reactions at any phase of testing—cells 3, 4, 5, 6, 9, 10, and 11. When this process is completed, only the K antigen remains. The pattern of reactivity for the patient results matches that of anti-K and the K antigen is present on each cell with which there was a reaction. The identification panel is interpreted as anti-K. Since anti-K is usually an IgG antibody, detected in AHG, capable of reacting at body temperature, and associated with HTR, donor cells must be screened and K-negative blood provided for transfusion.

XYZ Screen Cells   Lot #: 1234567   Expiration Date: 04/19/9X

shaded areas indicate antibodies that are generally of the IgM class

	Rh System							MNSs System				P	Lewis		Lutheran		Kell System						Duffy		Kidd		PT. RESULTS			
CELL	D	C	E	c	e	Cw	V	M	N	S	s	P1	Lea	Leb	Lua	Lub	K	k	Kpa	Kpb	Jsa	Jsb	Fya	Fyb	Jka	Jkb	IS	37°	AHG	CC
I	+	+	0	0	+	0	0	0	+	+	+	+	+	0	0	+	0	+	0	+	0	+	0	+	+	+	0	0	0	2+
II	+	0	+	+	0	0	0	0	0	0	+	+	0	+	0	+	+	+	0	+	0	+	+	+	0	+	0	+/-	2+	2+

FIGURE 16-9. Sample antibody identification sheet.

522

FIGURE 16–10. Sample antibody identification sheet.

Patient Name: Michael Edwards   Physician: Valerie Cole, M.D.

Hospital Number: 00112244   Room #: 422

ABO: O   Rh: Pos   DAT: Neg

Specimen Collected: 02/09/9X   14:00

Specimen Tested: 02/09/9X   16:00

Technologist: Cami Brooks, MT, SBB (ASCP)

INTERPRETATION: Anti-E and Anti-Fyᵃ

CC = COOMBS CONTROL

SC = SCREEN CELL

Systematic elimination on these routine panel results rules out the antibodies to all of the antigens listed except E, C^w, Js^a, & Fy^a. [eg, no reaction at any phase with cells 5, 6, 7. For cell 5 this eliminates antibodies to c, e, M, S, Lu^b, k, Jk^a, & Jk^b. Elimination is continued for cells 6 & 7.] The **enzyme panel results show an enhancement of the reaction in cells 4 & 10 and significant depression of the reaction in cells 1, 2, 3, 8, & 9.** These results suggest the presence of 2 antibodies—one that is enhanced by enzyme treatment; one reading more weakly. Note that cells 4 & 10 both contain the E antigen and **enzyme enhancement of antibody activity is demonstrated in the Rh system.** Cells 1, 2, 3, 8, & 9 all contain the Fy^a antigen. **Enzyme treatment inhibits the Fy^a antigen** by destroying antigen sites on the red cell. Although antibodies to C^w & Js^a have technically not been ruled out, they are unlikely to be present. In addition, in order to identify antibodies with an acceptable degree of confidence, at least 2 cells should contain the corresponding antigen.

Main Panel — Rh Phenotype

CELL #	Rh PHENOTYPE
1	rr
2	rr
3	rr
4	r'r
5	rr
6	R₀r
7	R₁R₁
8	R₁R₁
9	R₁R₁ʷ
10	R₂R₂
11	rr

Initial Panel Results

#	IS	37°	AHG	CC
1	0	0	2+	
2	0	0	2+	
3	0	0	2+	
4	0	2+	2+	
5	0	0	0	2+
6	0	0	0	2+
7	0	0	0	2+
8	0	0	2+	
9	0	0	2+	
10	0	2+	2+	
11	0	0	0	2+

Enzyme Panel Results

#	IS	37°	AHG	CC
1	0	0	+/-	
2	0	0	+/-	
3	0	0	+/-	
4	0	4+	4+	
5	0	0	0	2+
6	0	0	0	2+
7	0	0	0	2+
8	0	0	+/-	
9	0	0	+/-	
10	0	4+	4+	
11	0	0	0	2+

Controls (enzyme):

	IS	37°	AHG
auto	0	0	0
SCI	0	0	2+
SCII	0	2+	2+
cord			
A₁ cells			
B cells			

XYZ Screen Cells   Lot #: 1234567   Expiration Date: 04/19/9X

shaded areas indicate antibodies that are generally of the IgM class

CELL	D	C	E	c	e	Cᵂ	V	M	N	S	s	P₁	Leᵃ	Leᵇ	Luᵃ	Luᵇ	K	k	Kpᵃ	Jsᵃ	Jsᵇ	Fyᵃ	Fyᵇ	Jkᵃ	Jkᵇ	IS	37°	AHG	CC
I	+	+	0	0	+	0	0	+	0	+	+	+	0	+	0	+	0	+	0	0	+	0	+	+	+	0	0	0	2+
II	+	0	+	+	+	0	0	+	+	0	+	+	+	0	0	+	+	+	0	0	+	+	+	0	+	0	0	2+	3+

(Rh System | MNSs System | P | Lewis | Lutheran | Kell System | Duffy | Kidd | PT. RESULTS)

523

include an antiglobulin test. Historically, the crossmatch was divided into "major" and "minor" testing. A **minor crossmatch** consisted of testing the patient's cells with donor serum. This form of testing is no longer used because all donor blood is now screened for the presence of antibodies. The **major crossmatch** tests serum from the intended recipient with the donor's red cells in order to determine compatibility and to ensure that when transfused, the donor red cells will have acceptable survival and will not cause clinically significant destruction of the recipient's red cells. Although the major crossmatch is the best test available to determine compatibility and to predict satisfactory transfusion outcomes, it cannot guarantee that the patient has no antibodies to donor antigens, that the transfused red cells will survive normally, or that the recipient will have no adverse effects related to the transfusion.

Compatibility testing is performed using the different test phases described for antibody screens and antibody identification: initial spin, 37° incubation, and AHG. (Some institutions use only the initial spin—or immediate spin—crossmatch when no clinically significant antibodies have been detected in an antibody screen and the recipient has no previous history of unexpected antibodies.) Agglutination seen upon initial spin is generally indicative of an ABO incompatibility; thus ABO testing should be repeated on both the intended recipient and on the donor cells before further testing or problem solving is undertaken. The appropriate identification of the original sample and the serum removed from the collection tube must be verified. If the original ABO testing results are confirmed by repeat testing, a new sample should be collected and tested.

Other causes of *in vitro* incompatibility in the crossmatch may result from a variety of causes including:

- the presence of an autoantibody
- the presence of an alloantibody—if the antibody screen is negative, the antibody present in the patient's serum may be to an antigen not present on the reagent screening cells
- contamination of reagents
- contamination of saline used in washing procedure
- rouleaux which may give the appearance of incompatibility, but can be distinguished from true agglutination by saline dispersal

No matter the underlying cause, incompatibility problems should be resolved prior to the issue of blood (Figs. 16–11 and 16–12). In some cases the need for transfusion is extremely urgent and the risks associated with delaying transfusion may outweigh those associated with the infusion of blood that has not been demonstrated to be compatible. Such circumstances preclude identification of the problem and location of compatible blood prior to administration of red cells. Most institutions require the requesting physician to sign a statement of release indicating that he/she is aware of the risks of transfusion of incompatible red blood cells, but must proceed with transfusion as a life saving measure. In the event that transfusion must proceed, the least incompatible units should be selected for transfusion and the investigation of the problem continued.

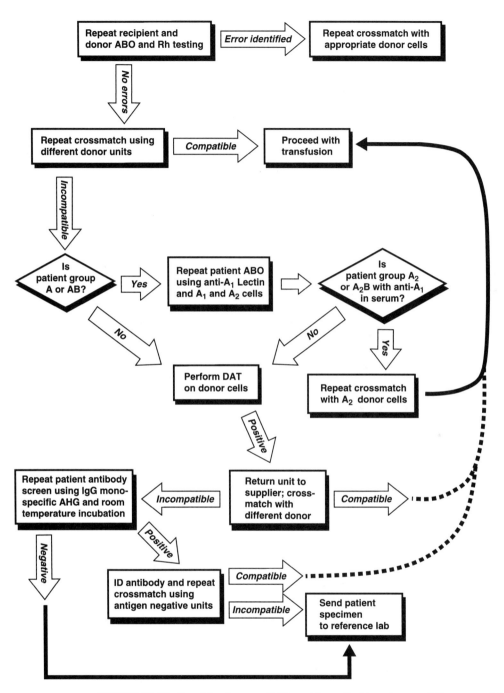

FIGURE 16–11. Resolving incompatibility problems. Problem: Incompatible crossmatch; negative antibody screen; negative autocontrol.

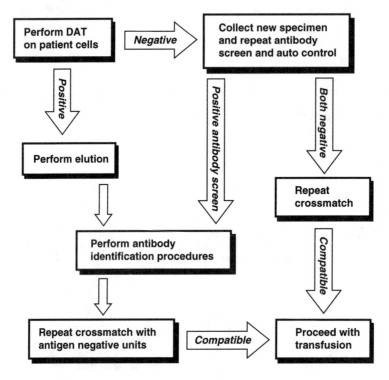

If problem is not resolved, refer patient specimen to a reference laboratory for additional investigation and/or specialized testing.

FIGURE 16–12. Resolving incompatibility problems. Problem: Incompatible crossmatch; negative antibody screen; positive autocontrol.

An incompatible crossmatch with a negative antibody screen and a negative auto-control may be seen when

- donor sample is contaminated
- ABO incompatibility due to clerical or technical errors
- anti-A_1 is present in the serum of a group A_2 or A_2B patient
- the donor has positive DAT
- strong I antigens on donor cells react with weak cold autoagglutinin in patient serum
- the patient has an antibody to a low incidence antigen found on donor cells, but not on reagent cells used for antibody screen
- the recipient has an antibody reacting with homozygous donor cells but not heterozygous screen cells

The **selection of donor units for transfusion** is based on the ABO and Rh type of the intended recipient. Ideally, ABO and Rh specific units should be chosen (ie, an A negative recipient should receive A negative red cells; an AB positive individual should receive AB positive red cells). However, emergency situations often present less than ideal circumstances that may require the transfusion of blood with little or no pretransfusion testing. Regardless of the circumstances, it is vital that a pre-transfusion sample be obtained from the recipient, so that testing can be performed as soon as possible. It is almost always possible to at least determine the ABO group of the recipient and to test for the presence of a D antigen that reacts upon initial spin, so that ABO group specific cells can be administered. In situations in which blood must be transfused before even the ABO group is determined, O cells are transfused. The most important consideration in selecting red cells for transfusion is to choose red cells lacking antigens to which the recipient has antibodies. Antibodies present in donor plasma are less important because packed red cells contain very little donor plasma. Further, the dilutional effect seen when donor plasma is administered lessens the likelihood of significant recipient red cell destruction. Transfusion of red cells that are not type specific may also be required when the administration of a large number of units is required in massive hemorrhage and a sufficient number of type specific donor units are not immediately available.

Some institutions require the physician to sign a form documenting the medical necessity for releasing blood for transfusion without compatibility testing and/or for releasing donor cells that are not type specific. As previously stated, it is important to obtain a blood sample from the recipient prior to the transfusion of donor cells because the completion of required testing is still necessary. This sample would also be important to the investigation of any adverse effects experienced by the recipient.

When type specific red cells cannot be administered, donor cells with the least likelihood of introducing antigens to which the recipient has antibodies or that could produce immunization must be selected. Table 16–17 provides the ABO groups that may be transfused to recipients.

Because the goal is to choose donor cells that do not contain antigens to which the recipient has antibodies, group AB recipients can be transfused with any ABO group as they have neither anti-A nor anti-B. Group O recipients, on the other hand, have both anti-A and anti-B and thus can only be transfused with group O

TABLE 16–17. Selection of Donor Red Cells

Recipient ABO	Donor ABO
A	A; O
B	B; O
AB	AB; A; B; O
O	O
Unknown	O

red cells. **The concept of group O as a "universal donor" ONLY applies to packed red cells and IS NOT applicable to whole blood transfusion.** Transfusion of group O whole blood would introduce both anti-A and anti-B into the recipient's circulation.

Even though anti-D is not naturally occurring and thus no immediate harm results from administering D positive cells to D negative individuals, this practice is avoided for important reasons. First, because the D antigen is highly immunogenic, most D negative recipients will develop anti-D in response to exposure to the antigen. Subsequent transfusion of D positive cells to a recipient with anti-D would result in hemolytic transfusion reaction. However, unless the subsequent transfusion was also required under emergency circumstances precluding completion of pretransfusion testing, the presence of the anti-D would be detected and D negative cells transfused. It is especially critical to avoid transfusion of D positive cells to D negative females who have not passed the age of childbearing to avoid HDN in D positive children they may later bear. Consequently, the decision to transfuse D positive red cells to a D negative recipient is simpler, in relative terms, if the intended recipient is male or is a female beyond childbearing age. When death is imminent without transfusion and D positive red cells are the only available product for transfusion, D positive cells are administered regardless of the patient's sex and age. In all other cases, D positive cells should not be administered to a D negative recipient.

■ TYPE AND SCREEN

Type and screen procedures are used for situations in which the need for transfusion of red cells may arise, but is not usually necessary. A type and screen consists of a determination of the patient's ABO and Rh type and an antibody screen. If the antibody screen is positive, antibody identification procedures are completed. Donor units may be screened for the corresponding antigen. Units are not selected for transfusion and tested with the patient's serum because the likelihood of transfusion is small. However, should transfusion become necessary, the blood bank has already completed much of the required pre-transfusion testing and can immediately begin compatibility testing. Many institutions identify those procedures for which type and screens should be ordered on a document called a maximum surgical blood order schedule (MSBOS), which also lists the number of units generally appropriate for procedures warranting crossmatch. A sample MSBOS is included in the appendices.

OTHER TEST PROCEDURES

This section provides a brief explanation of some of the other procedures used in transfusion service testing. These procedures may be indicated as part of the resolution of problems encountered in routine testing or in the identification of antibodies.

■ ANTIGLOBULIN TESTING

Antibodies may attach to antigen sites on the red cell surface without resulting in agglutination. Such red cells are said to be "coated" with antibody. Red cells may also be coated with complement. Anti-human globulin (AHG) is a reagent used to detect the presence of antibody or complement coated red cells. AHG is available in polyspecific form or as a monospecific reagent. **Polyspecific AHG** reacts with the different immunoglobulin classes and with the C3d fraction of complement and is generally used initially. **Monospecific** reagents are developed to detect the presence of a particular class of immunoglobulin (eg, specific for IgG) or of complement. Red cells may become coated *in vivo* or *in vitro. In vitro* coating is useful to aid in the identification of antibodies or serologic incompatibility between donor and recipient. AHG testing is the final stage of compatibility testing and antibody procedures, as discussed previously. Testing for the *in vitro* coating of red cells is called an **indirect antiglobulin test** because the AHG is added following incubation of red cells with serum that may contain antibodies. The antibodies are given the opportunity to attach to the red cell in the incubation phase for detection in the AHG phase of testing. Testing for *in vivo* coating of red cells is called the **direct antiglobulin test**, or **DAT**. The DAT involves no incubation period. Red cells are tested directly after washing with saline to remove all serum from the sample. A positive DAT is never a normal finding and should always be investigated. A positive DAT indicates that red cells are being coated *in vivo* and may be seen in a number of circumstances, including:

- hemolytic disease of the newborn
- autoimmune hemolytic anemia
- red cell sensitization in some disease states
- red cell sensitization with some drugs
- hemolytic transfusion reactions

All positive DATs should be investigated using monospecific reagents to determine the nature of the substance coating the red cells. A drug-induced positive DAT will likely require testing by a specialized laboratory for confirmation.

Testing with AHG requires strict adherence to established protocols to ensure valid results. Inadequate washing is one of the major causes of false negative antiglobulin tests (direct or indirect). Incomplete washing allows antibodies that may be present in the serum (but not attached to the red cells) to remain in the sample. These antibodies can neutralize the AHG reagent and result in a negative test result despite the presence of antibody-coated red cells. Fortunately, antibody-coated control cells (called *Coombs control cells*) are used to check the reactivity of the AHG reagent in each test tube yielding a negative reaction following completion of patient testing. If agglutination is not observed following the addition of Coombs control cells, the test is invalid and must be repeated. Delays between steps in the test procedure can also result in false negative reactions. If the washing process is delayed or the AHG is not added immediately following the last wash, globulins bound to the red cell may be eluted and neutralize the AHG reagent. These situations would also be detected by a failure of the Coombs control cells to agglutinate. Causes of false positive and false negative reactions in AHG testing are summarized in Table 16–18.

ELUTION

When red cells are coated with an antibody, the antibody must be removed from the red cell surface to be identified. This is accomplished by a procedure called **elution**. A variety of methods may be employed for elution depending, in part, on the nature of the antibody coating the cells. Some methods employ **chemicals** and others rely on **temperature changes** (eg, heat elution, freeze-thaw elution). All methods consist of a variety of steps used to detach the antibody from the red cells and all begin with a series of washes. The decanted saline from the last wash is saved to test along with the **eluate** (the liquid harvested from the elution procedure). Both the eluate and the last wash are tested in the same manner as serum for antibody identification. The last wash serves as a control to ensure that any antibody detected in the eluate is a result of the elution procedure rather than serum contamination resulting from inadequate washing. Red cells that have been subjected to the elution procedure must be discarded and are not to be used for further testing because red cells and antigen sites are usually destroyed in the process of removing antibodies from the red cell surface.

ADSORPTION

Adsorption refers to the removal of antibodies from serum using specially treated red cells. The type of red cells used to provide antigens for the removal of antibodies depends on the purpose for which the adsorption is undertaken. Specific test conditions such as the time and temperature of incubation depend on the type of antibody and its thermal range of reactivity. An appropriate serum to cell ratio is important to successful adsorption, with a low antibody (serum) to antigen (red cell) ratio usually producing the most effective antibody adsorption. The primary

TABLE 16–18. Causes of False Positive and False Negative Reactions in AHG Testing

False Negative Reactions	False Positive Reactions
Inadequate washing	Contaminated reagent
Contaminated AHG reagent	Sample collected in serum separator tube
Failure to add AHG	Rouleaux
Delay in washing	Overcentrifugation
Delay in adding AHG after last wash	Incorrect strength of red cell suspension
Loss of reactivity in expired AHG reagent	Inaccurate interpretation of results
Inappropriate incubation time or temperature	
Incorrect strength of red cell suspension	
Inappropriate centrifugation	
Inaccurate interpretation of results	

use of the adsorption procedure is to remove particular antibodies in order to facil-itate the detection and/or identification of other antibodies (ie, multiple antibod-ies, alloantibodies masked by autoantibody). Adsorption is also used in conjunc-tion with elution (called adsorption-elution procedures) in the classification of some rare ABO subgroups. Table 16–19 summarizes the uses of adsorption.

ANTIBODY TITERS

Antibody titration is used to determine the amount of antibody present and is accomplished using serial twofold dilutions of the serum being tested. The diluted serum is tested with the antigen corresponding to the antibody and examined for agglutination at each level of dilution. The highest dilution in which agglutination is detected macroscopically indicates the titer, which is expressed as the reciprocal of the dilution. For example, dilutions of 1:2; 1:4; 1:8; 1:16; 1:32; and 1:64 may be tested. If macroscopic agglutination is observed in all dilutions except the 1:64 dilu-tion, the titer is reported as 32. Antibody titers are most often used in

- assessing the risk of HDN when maternal IgG antibodies are present: increasing titers indicate that the corresponding antigen is present on

TABLE 16–19. Applications of Antibody Adsorption Procedures

Purpose	Explanation
Autoantibody removal	The presence of autoantibodies (whether warm or cold reacting) can mask the presence of underlying alloantibodies that may be clinically significant. These antibodies can generally be adsorbed onto the patient's red cells that have been enzyme treated. The serum can then be tested for the presence of alloantibodies and any detected antibody identified.
Single alloantibody removal	When multiple antibodies are detected in a patient's serum, identification of the individual antibodies can be difficult at best. Positive reactions may be seen with all panel cells, making elimination impossible. Enzyme panels may facilitate identification, but may be inadequate in some cases depending on the antibodies present. Individual antibody removal can be accomplished by using cells with the antigen for the antibody suspected. This technique is especially helpful when an antibody to a high frequency antigen is suspected.
Rare ABO subgroup classification	Some of the less frequently encountered ABO subgroups may have antigens so weakly expressed that red cells will not be agglutinated by the corresponding antisera. Adsorption can be combined with elution to facilitate the identification of these subgroups. If anti-A or anti-B can be absorbed on to the red cell surface and then eluted and identified with the appropriate reagent cells, the presence of the corresponding antigen on the red cells is indirectly proven.

fetal cells and stimulating the production of additional antibody; a titer that does not increase with periodic testing, or decreases, is suggestive of fetal cells that do not contain the corresponding antigen and a lower risk of HDN

- classifying high titer, low avidity (HTLA) antibodies: these antibodies produce very weak reactions (low avidity) in testing, but when titration is performed react (though weakly) at dilutions of 1:64 or higher. On the other hand, other antibodies producing very weak test reactions will not react in serum dilutions at all or react only in the initial 1:2 dilution.

■ WARM AUTOANTIBODIES

Autoimmune hemolytic anemia (AIHA) may result from the presence of antibodies directed toward antigens on the individual's own red cells. Most cases of AIHA are caused by warm reactive autoantibodies. The development of these antibodies may be idiopathic or secondary to another disease process, particularly another autoimmune process. A positive DAT is seen in these cases as a result of the antibody coating of red cells. These autoantibodies present significant challenge in the blood bank because they usually have a broad specificity and react with nearly all red cells. For this reason, transfusion is generally avoided as long as possible in patients with AIHA caused by warm autoantibodies. If transfusion becomes necessary, transfusion of the least incompatible units is used if the specificity of the autoantibody cannot be determined. *It is essential to rule out the presence of alloantibodies prior to transfusion.*

■ COLD AUTOANTIBODIES

Cold autoantibodies are usually benign, significant only in terms of their interference with other blood bank procedures. They may be clinically significant in some circumstances (eg, when patient body temperature is lowered, as in some cardiac surgeries) depending on their thermal range of reactivity. Commonly encountered cold reactive autoantibodies include anti-I, anti-i, anti-H, and anti-IH. Table 16–20 shows how these autoantibodies can be differentiated.

BLOOD COMPONENTS

A variety of blood products can be prepared from one unit of donated whole blood and used for a variety of therapeutic purposes. Whether or not pre-transfusion testing is required for blood products is dependent on the type of product to be administered. Red cell products require the most extensive testing. Components also vary in terms of storage requirements and shelf life. These characteristics of blood components are summarized for the most common products in Table 16–21. This table also lists the indications for therapeutic use of these components and their contents. Blood components are not addressed beyond this summary in this text.

TABLE 16–20. Differentiation of Cold Autoantibodies

Test Cells	Reaction with Patient Serum[1]			
Adult O cells	3+	0	3+ - 4+	4+
Cord O cells	0 or +/-	3+	3+ - 4+	1+
A₁ cells	3+	0	+/-	+/-
A₂ cells	3+	0	2+	2+
Antibody interpretation	Anti-I	Anti-i	Anti-H	Anti-IH

[1]Reaction strengths shown are relative; although strengths may vary, interpretation is made based on the strength of a given reaction relative to the other reactions (ie, anti-H reaction with A₁ cells may be 1+ instead of +/-, but will be less than reaction of anti-H with A₂ cells).

TABLE 16–21. Summary of Common Blood Components

Component	Content and Volume	Storage and Shelf Life	Indications and Effect
Packed red cells	70% to 80% RBC's with some plasma, WBC's, plts; ~ 250 mL volume	1° to 6°C; 21, 35, or 42 days depending on anticoagulant or additive solution	To increase red cell mass one unit raises HCT ~ 3%
Washed red cells	> 80% RBC's suspended in saline; ~ 250 mL volume	1° to 6°C; 24 hours after wash (open system)	To increase red cell mass in patients with history of febrile reactions due to leukocyte antibodies 1 unit raises HCT ~ 3%
Leukocytes	WBC's > 1.0 × 10¹⁰ granulocytes, some plts and plasma, RBC (about 10% HCT) single donor volume ~ 250 mL	24 hours room temperature	Severe granulocytopenia (<500/mm³) with sepsis (unresponsive to antibiotics)
Platelets	1 unit concentrate: ≥ 5.5 × 10¹⁰ plts 1 single donor apheresis unit: ≥ 3.0 × 10¹⁰ plts; can be HLA matched; both contain WBCs and plasma (~50 mL concentrate; ~ 250 mL apheresis)	5 days (1 day if open system) at room temperature with constant, gentle agitation	Bleeding due to thrombocytopenia or some platelet disorders; also used as prophylactic therapy; may be indicated in massive red cell transfusions—6 to 8 units plt conc per 10 units RBCs; each unit plt conc raises plt by 5000 to 8000; 6 to 10 units usually given—raises 30,000 to 80,000
Fresh frozen plasma	Plasma, coagulation factors and complement; contains 0.7 to 1.0 units of factors II, V, VII, VIII, IX, X, XI, XII, XIII and 500 mg fibrinogen in total volume of 200 to 250 mL	Frozen: 1 year at −18°C Thawed: 6 hours	Bleeding due to deficiency of multiple coagulation factors such as in liver disease or DIC; with massive transfusion of RBCs (2 units FFP/10 units RBCs); should not be used for volume expansion only
Cryoprecipitate	Factor VIII:c (80 units), von willebrand factor, fibrinogen (200 mg), factor xiii, other plasma proteins volume 10 to 25 ml	Frozen: 1 year at −18°C Thawed: 6 hours Entered or pooled: 4 hours	von Willebrand's disease, factor XIII deficiency, hypofribinogenemia; also will increase factor VIII level in hemophilia A, but factor VIII concentrate preferred
Factor VIII concentrate	Amount of factor VIII indicated on vial; provided lyophilized and reconstituted to 25 mL	2 years at 2° to 8°C	Hemophilia A
Albumin	5%: 5 g/ 100 mL 25%: 25 g/ 100 mL small amt of alpha and beta globulins	3 years room temperature 5 years at 2° to 8°C	Plasma volume expansion or hypoproteinemia

See donor testing requirements discussed previously; required rechecks on donor for some products—especially ABO/Rh confirmation. Information summarized from AABB Technical Manual, 11th ed, 1993 and AABB standard's, 17th ed, 1996.

ADVERSE EFFECTS OF TRANSFUSION

The majority of transfusions are completed without incident and with no subsequent complications. Nonetheless, the possibility of adverse effects is always present. The term **transfusion reaction** is used to refer to a number of these adverse effects or unfavorable events. Although the most feared and most serious reaction to transfusion is an **acute hemolytic transfusion reaction**, in which the donor red cells are lysed upon entry into the circulation by recipient antibodies, a variety of other reactions may be encountered. Adverse effects of transfusion may be categorized as **immune or antibody mediated reactions** involving the action of immunoglobulins, or as **nonimmune** (not associated with immune antibodies). These effects may be further classified as **acute** (effects seen immediately) or as **delayed** (time lapse before effects are evident). This system for the classification of adverse effects of transfusion is presented in Table 16–22. Other means of classification are also used.

■ FEBRILE NON-HEMOLYTIC TRANSFUSION REACTION

The most commonly encountered transfusion reaction is a febrile non-hemolytic transfusion reaction (FNHTR). A reaction of this type is defined as a rise in temperature of 1° or more during or immediately following transfusion that is not explained by any other cause. It occurs as a result of an immune attack against donor white cells and is characterized by fever, headache, shaking chills, and general malaise. Although this type of transfusion reaction is usually mild and limited, similar symptoms are seen in more serious reactions (acute immune hemolytic and as a result of bacterial contamination). Consequently, transfusion must be immediately halted and the blood bank notified to begin investigation of the suspected transfusion reaction (even if the patient has a known history of leukoag-

TABLE 16–22. Classification of Adverse Effects of Transfusion

Acute	Delayed
Immune	
Hemolytic (incompatible RBCs)	Hemolytic (anamnestic antibody response to RBC antigen)
Nonhemolytic	Alloimmunization (exposure to donor antigens not present on
Febrile (antibody to donor WBC's)	recipient cells)
Uticarial (antibody to plasma proteins)	Post-transfusion purpura (development of platelet antibodies
Anaphylactoid (antibody to IgA)	Graft vs Host disease (engraftment and mulitiplication of
	immunocompetent donor lymphs in immunodeficient recipient)
Nonimmune	
Hemolytic (bacterial contamination)	Infectious disease (hepatitis, AIDS, cytomegalovirus)
Volume overload	Iron overload
Metabolic (electrolyte and/or metabolic	
changes such as hyperkalemia,	
hypocalcemia, hypernatremia)	

glutinins). Even though it is not practical to perform compatibility testing for white cell or HLA antigens, FNHTR can be prevented in red cell transfusion by using filters designed to reduce the number of white cells introduced to the recipient or by transfusion of washed or deglycerolized red cell products. These methods are indicated for any patient with a history of FNHTRs. Removal of white cells from platelets is more difficult, but the newest platelet filters restrict the passage of white cells. Patients may also be pre-medicated with an antipyretic agent. FNHTRs occur in about 1% to 3% of all red cell transfusions and in about 30% of platelet transfusions (Henry, 1996), but are seen more frequently in patients who have been previously transfused or as a result of sensitization by fetal white cell antigens in pregnancy. The greater the number of transfusions and/or pregnancies, the greater the risk of FNHTR.

■ UTICARIA

The second most commonly encountered adverse reaction to transfusion, **uticaria**, results from allergy (IgE antibodies) to plasma proteins in the donor unit. Characterized by hives, itching, and local erythema, this type of reaction is treated (or prevented when history of this response to transfusion is known) with antihistamines to block the action of the histamine producing IgE antibodies. Slowing the transfusion rate may also be indicated, and with more severe allergic reactions that may include bronchospasm, ending the transfusion may be indicated (Sacher and McPherson, 1991). If a more severe immunologic reaction is suspected, the transfusion should be immediately stopped.

■ DELAYED HEMOLYTIC TRANSFUSION REACTIONS

A **delayed hemolytic transfusion reaction** (DHTR) occurs as a result of the introduction of red cell antigens to which the recipient has immune antibodies that were not detectable in the recipient's serum during pre-transfusion testing. Antibodies of the Kidd system are most often implicated in this anamnestic type of reaction, but antibodies of the Duffy and Rh systems are also associated with DHTRs. These reactions are often suspected when sustained improvement in hemoglobin level and hematocrit cannot be achieved in the absence of active bleeding. Symptoms of DHTRs may occur up to 14 days after transfusion and include fever, falling hemoglobin level, mild jaundice in some cases, positive DAT, increased bilirubin, and sometimes, reversible renal failure. In some cases, the drop in hemoglobin level and hematocrit may be the only manifestation. Although not as severe as acute hemolytic transfusion reactions, these reactions can be serious. An occurrence of a DHTR must become a part of the patient's transfusion history and the information, including the antibody implicated, should be provided to the patient to keep in his/her possession should the need for transfusion arise in the future. With this information available, blood bank staff involved in providing blood for any future transfusion can ensure that antigen negative blood is used even if the antibody has decreased to an undetectable level.

■ ACUTE HEMOLYTIC TRANSFUSION REACTIONS

Despite uncommon occurrence, **acute hemolytic transfusion reactions** are the most feared effect of transfusion therapy. These reactions are the **most serious, life threatening consequences of transfusion** and are **almost always attributable to major ABO incompatibility** resulting from a **clerical error or to errors in identification** of either the recipient or the recipient blood sample. Certainly errors in ABO typing are a possible cause of these reactions as well, but are not usually involved. When red cells containing the A or B antigen are introduced into the circulation of an individual with the corresponding antibody, immediate intravascular hemolysis occurs as a result of rapid complement activation. Virtually all ABO incompatibilities can be avoided, with the rare exception of the presence of very weak or atypical antibodies. With such grave consequences possible, it is imperative that each institution has established protocols for the identification of the patient from whom pretransfusion samples are collected, the sample itself, the donor unit to be transfused, and the recipient of the transfusion. Mechanisms for the detection of clerical and identification errors should be an important part of the protocol. Such mechanisms include scanning barcoded identification bracelets and checks of identifying information by at least two individuals before release of blood from the blood bank and again before initiation of transfusion. Major ABO incompatibility may result from carelessness or errors that result in the following situations:

- pre-transfusion sample collected from wrong patient
- administration of donor product to the wrong patient
- clerical error in identifying information for donor or recipient
- ABO typing error or other testing errors

ABO incompatibilities should be detected on initial spin in compatibility testing with the rare exception previously noted for atypical or very weak antibodies (which would often be suspected as a result of discrepant ABO forward and reverse typing results).

The **symptoms** of an acute hemolytic transfusion reaction are noted almost immediately and include shaking chills, fever, drop in blood pressure, nausea, chest pain, flushing, dyspnea, back pain, pain at the infusion site, shock, generalized bleeding, and oliguria or anuria. Patients who are anesthetized are at the greatest risk for a fatal outcome because they cannot recognize the onset of symptoms. Diffuse bleeding at the surgical site and a drop in blood pressure signal the possibility of an acute hemolytic transfusion reaction in these patients. **DIC and renal failure** may occur as a result of this type of reaction. Treatment must begin promptly and is aimed at maintaining blood pressure and renal blood flow and correcting coagulation abnormalities. Transfusion must be stopped immediately upon suspicion of reaction and the IV line kept open with saline. Investigation, as outlined in Figure 16–13, must begin quickly.

LABORATORY INVESTIGATION OF SUSPECTED TRANSFUSION REACTIONS

When symptoms consistent with a significant adverse reaction to a transfused product are noted, immediate action is called for. As is evident from the previous descriptions of some of the reactions that may be encountered, the presenting symptoms may initially be the same for less serious reactions and for life threatening ones. Thus the transfusion should be halted upon the first indication of a reaction and the IV line kept open with saline infusion in case immediate treatment for hypotension is required. The patient must be closely monitored and the attending physician notified so that appropriate intervention can be initiated. All identifying information, for both patient and donor product, should be rechecked. The blood bank must be promptly notified of the suspected reaction and, if possible, a urine specimen obtained. Laboratory investigation should be started quickly. Initial findings determine how the remainder of the investigation should proceed and investigation protocols may vary somewhat among institutions. The initial goal of the investigation is to determine whether or not the reaction is due to acute intravascular hemolysis by immune mechanisms resulting from an ABO incompatibility. If this is determined to be the case, the investigational focus turns to the cause of the transfusion of incompatible blood. Testing may continue to determine the extent of the complications associated with acute intravascular hemolysis. When results of the investigation do not indicate an acute hemolytic transfusion reaction, other reaction types are evaluated. Figure 16–13 depicts a general investigation protocol for suspected transfusion reactions and Figure 16–14 illustrates the relative response times for plasma and urine hemoglobin and for serum haptoglobin and bilirubin levels in intravascular hemolysis.

HEMOLYTIC DISEASE OF THE NEWBORN

Hemolytic disease of the newborn (HDN), also called *erythroblastosis fetalis,* involves the destruction of antibody coated (sensitized) infant red blood cells, resulting in a hemolytic anemia and jaundice. In this condition, the mother is exposed to fetal red cells as a result of fetal-maternal or transplacental hemorrhage (TPH). When these fetal cells contain an antigen not present on maternal red cells, immune IgG maternal antibodies may be produced. IgG antibodies are capable of crossing the placenta and entering the fetal circulation, where they attach to the corresponding antigen on the fetal red cells. The antibody coated red cells are removed from the fetal circulation by the reticuloendothelial system and destroyed (*extravascular hemolysis*). This increased red cell destruction results in increased bilirubin and other bile pigments, which is cleared (after diffusion across the placenta) from the maternal circulation by the maternal liver. Some bile pigments may remain in the amniotic fluid. If the fetal bone marrow is not capable of adequately replacing the destroyed red cells, a progressive fetal anemia will evolve. The severity of HDN depends on the level of fetal red cell destruction, and ranges from a mild condition with slight jaundice seen in the newborn to *in utero* fetal death near the time of delivery (hydrops fetalis). The primary clinical indications

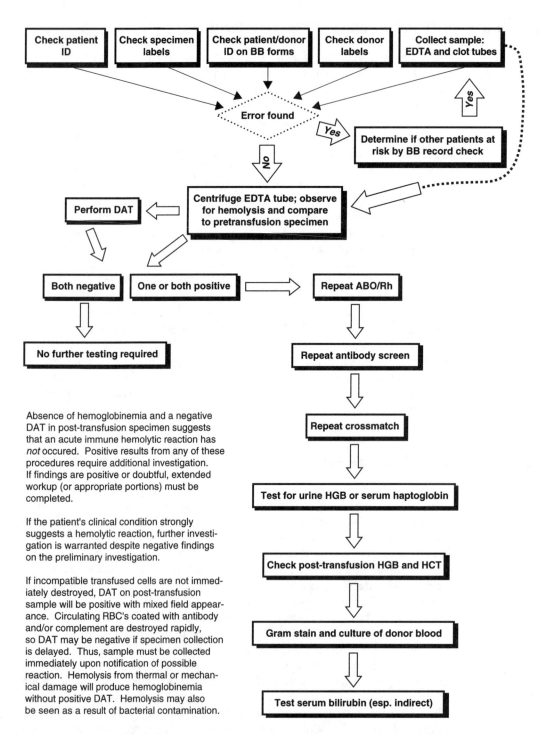

Absence of hemoglobinemia and a negative DAT in post-transfusion specimen suggests that an acute immune hemolytic reaction has *not* occured. Positive results from any of these procedures require additional investigation. If findings are positive or doubtful, extended workup (or appropriate portions) must be completed.

If the patient's clinical condition strongly suggests a hemolytic reaction, further investigation is warranted despite negative findings on the preliminary investigation.

If incompatible transfused cells are not immediately destroyed, DAT on post-transfusion sample will be positive with mixed field appearance. Circulating RBC's coated with antibody and/or complement are destroyed rapidly, so DAT may be negative if specimen collection is delayed. Thus, sample must be collected immediately upon notification of possible reaction. Hemolysis from thermal or mechanical damage will produce hemoglobinemia without positive DAT. Hemolysis may also be seen as a result of bacterial contamination.

FIGURE 16–13. Laboratory investigation of suspected transfusion reaction.

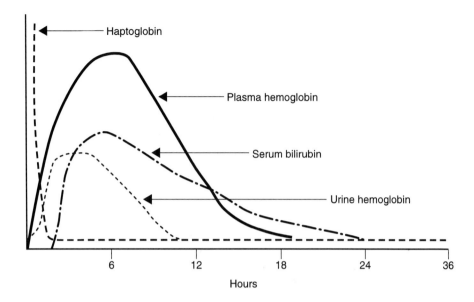

FIGURE 16-14. Relative response time for change in intravascular hemolysis. (Adapted from Henry JB. *Clinical Diagnosis and Management by Laboratory Methods,* 19th ed. Philadelphia, Saunders, 1996.)

of Rh_o-HDN are anemia and jaundice that develops rapidly. High reticulocyte counts are characteristically found as the bone marrow attempts to replace the red cells that have been destroyed.

Although some amount of transplacental hemorrhage is normally anticipated during pregnancy and is particularly evident at about 28 weeks gestation, the volume of fetal-maternal hemorrhage is greater at birth and may be increased in response to amniocentesis and manual repositioning of the baby from breech. Spontaneous or induced abortion may also increase transplacental hemorrhage.

■ RH HEMOLYTIC DISEASE OF THE NEWBORN

Any maternal IgG antibody can cause HDN if the fetal cells contain the corresponding antigen, but severe HDN is more commonly associated with Rh antibodies. Maternal anti-D is first produced in response to an immunizing event such as pregnancy or transfusion. Because D positive red cells are rarely administered to women who are (or will subsequently be) capable of childbearing, immunization usually occurs as a result of pregnancy and/or childbirth. Although the first D positive child born to a D negative mother is not often affected (unless the mother has been exposed to D positive red cells prior to the pregnancy), subsequent exposure to the D antigen results in a potent response. In addition to the characteristic findings noted previously (anemia, jaundice, elevated indirect bilirubin, reticulocytosis), a positive DAT provides evidence of HDN, as it signifies the *in vivo* coating of red cells by antibody.

Significant HDN resulting from a D positive fetus carried by a D negative woman is rare today because of testing in the prenatal period and the administration of Rh immune globulin. Prior to the development of Rh immune globulin (RhoGam), nearly half of all deaths in the perinatal period were attributable to $Rh_0(D)$-HDN (Sacher and McPherson, 1991). Once maternal antibodies have been developed, the process cannot be reversed. Consequently, the goal is to prevent initial sensitization and the subsequent development of HDN. Every pregnant woman should routinely be tested for Rh type and have an antibody screen performed early in pregnancy. If the antibody screen is still negative at 28 weeks gestation, a prophylactic dose of Rh immune globulin is recommended (American College of Obstetricians and Gynecologists [ACOG]). It has been demonstrated that mothers who have not been sensitized can almost always be protected from fetal sensitization by the administration of high-titer anti-D in gamma globulin. This exogenous antibody prevents sensitization by destroying fetal cells as they enter the maternal circulation and before maternal antibody production is stimulated. It, in effect, "tricks" the maternal immune system into seeing a protective mechanism in place to attack the foreign antigen presented by the fetal red cells. Spontaneous or induced abortion, ectopic pregnancy, and amniocentesis should also be treated with immune Rh-Ig administration. The ACOG recommended dose is 300 µg at 28 weeks (a 50 µg dose is often used when abortion occurs before 12 weeks gestation). Additional Rh-Ig is administered within 72 hours of delivery. In most cases, the standard 300 µg dose is sufficient protection, as it neutralizes about 30 mL of fetal whole blood. However, in some cases the transplacental hemorrhage is greater than this amount and additional units are indicated.

Laboratory procedures are available to approximate the amount of hemorrhage and the Rh-Ig dosage required. A screening test is often performed first, with a quantitative test performed when indicated. The **qualitative fetal screen** is available in commercial kits and involves incubation of red cells from a maternal sample with anti-D. After incubation the cells are washed and Rh positive indicator cells are added to the sample. The indicator cells will bind to any anti-D bound to fetal cells in the maternal circulation in a manner that produces a rosette appearance when the cells are observed microscopically. Positive fetal screens are followed by a **quantitative test** called the **Kleihauer-Betke acid elution stain**. This test employs an acid buffer to liberate the hemoglobin of adult red cells. Fetal hemoglobin is resistant to this acid buffer. A stain of a maternal blood smear treated with the acid buffer will reveal maternal cells that are very pale (termed "ghost" cells) and more darkly stained fetal cells on microscopic examination. The percentage of fetal cells is determined and used to calculate the volume of fetal-maternal hemorrhage and the Rh-Ig dosage required to neutralize the fetal red cells (1 unit or 300 µg for each 15 mL red cells or 30 mL whole blood). Rh-Ig may be detectable for up to 3 to 6 months in the maternal circulation. D negative women carrying a D positive child who are not treated with Rh-Ig have about a 10% incidence of sensitization. Those treated post-partum with Rh-Ig have an incidence of 1% to 2% and those treated both ante-partum and post-partum have an incidence of only 0.1% to 0.2% (Ravel, 1995).

When the initial or 28-week **maternal antibody screen is positive for anti-D** (or other antibodies implicated in HDN), continued monitoring is required. Anti-D (or other Rh antibodies) should be titered with subsequent titers performed every 2 weeks (Sacher and McPherson, 1991; 2 to 3 weeks [Henry, 1996]). A low titer (< 1:16) that does not increase is indicative of lower fetal risk. Titers of ≥ 1:16 or a rising titer indicate higher risk and the need for evaluation of bile pigments in amniotic fluid. The amount of bilirubin present in the amniotic fluid related to gestational age provides a value that can be classified as low risk, moderate risk, or severe risk. A severe risk classification indicates that fetal death is imminent. As indicated by these results and other testing to determine fetal lung maturity, the clinician must make a determination as to the appropriate management strategy, such as intrauterine transfusion or premature delivery.

Bilirubin levels may become dangerously elevated in the HDN infant following birth. The excess bilirubin that had been released into the maternal circulation, where it was bound with albumin, conjugated in the liver, and then excreted, now accumulates in the neonatal circulation. The infant's immature liver cannot effectively manage the increasing levels and there is a limited amount of serum albumin available for binding. The excess bilirubin is deposited in the cells of the nervous system and, because of the immature blood-brain barrier, may be deposited throughout the brain tissue. Permanent brain damage or death may result. In the most severe cases of HDN the newborn may require exchange transfusion, but most can be effectively treated without this intervention. Bilirubin levels are used as the major standard for monitoring the effectiveness of other treatment, such as phototherapy, and for deciding if and when exchange transfusion is warranted. Although sources may vary somewhat in recommendations, phototherapy is usually instituted at bilirubin levels of ≥15 mg/dL, with exchange transfusion considered when levels reach 20 mg/dL ([Sacher and McPherson, 1991]; 18 mg/dL [Henry, 1996]). **Blood used for exchange transfusion** should be

- ABO compatible: maternal serum used for crossmatch; if mother and baby are not same ABO type, group O cells should be transfused; if maternal serum cannot be obtained, infant serum with eluate from the coated RBCs can be used
- < 7 days old: to provide maximum 2,3-DPG levels and lower potassium levels
- cytomegalovirus (CMV) negative: if mother is CMV positive, CMV negative transfusion is not required
- warmed close to body temperature
- irradiated if infant weighs < 1200 g or may be immunocompromised

ABO HEMOLYTIC DISEASE OF THE NEWBORN

Hemolytic disease of the newborn resulting from maternal-fetal ABO incompatibility is generally a relatively mild condition. The mother and infant are often of different ABO groups, but most antibodies of the ABO system are IgM antibodies that cannot cross the placenta. However, some of the antibody present may be of the IgG form, particularly in group O individuals. Therefore ABO-HDN is more likely to be seen when the maternal blood group is group O and the fetal red cells are group A, B, or AB. Prior immunization as a result of pregnancy or transfusion is not required for the development of ABO-HDN. This condition is almost always mild and rarely calls for intensive treatment.

■ HDN WITH OTHER ANTIBODIES

Any maternal IgG antibody can cause HDN if the fetal cells carry the corresponding red cell antigen. Antibodies to the other Rh antigens, as well as antibodies to antigens of the Kell, Duffy, and Kidd systems, are capable of producing HDN. Like that resulting from anti-D, HDN in these cases ranges from mild to severe. Anti-c, anti-K, and anti-E are the most frequent cause of HDN excluding ABO and D cases. Detection of these IgG antibodies in maternal antibody screens performed during pregnancy also require continued monitoring. Unlike anti-D, the titer of these antibodies in maternal serum has not been adequately correlated with fetal outcome (Ravel, 1995). Amniotic fluid examination is used to evaluate fetal risk in the presence of these antibodies. The need for intrauterine transfusion or premature delivery of the infant is very unlikely with HDN mediated by these antibodies.

 TIME FOR REVIEW. After studying the preceding sections, you should be able to respond correctly to the following:

■ List four causes for temporary donor deferral.

■ List four causes for permanent donor deferral.

■ List the procedures commonly included in pre-transfusion recipient testing for the administration of red cell products.

the antigram provided:

XYZ Screen Cells   **Lot #: 123456**   **Expiration Date: 04/19/9X**

shaded areas indicate antibodies that are generally of the IgM class

CELL	Cell	Rh System					MNSs System				P	Lewis		Lutheran		Kell		Duffy		Kidd		PT. RESULTS			
		D	C	E	c	e	M	N	S	s	P_l	Le^a	Le^b	Lu^a	Lu^b	K	k	Fy^a	Fy^b	Jk^a	Jk^b	IS	37°	AHG	CC
I	I	+	+	0	0	+	+	0	+	+	+	+	0	0	+	0	+	0	+	+	+	0	0	0	2+
II	II	+	0	+	+	+	0	+	0	+	+	0	+	0	+	+	+	+	+	0	+	0	+/-	2+	

■ List three instances in which a positive DAT would be expected.

■ List three purposes served by compatibility testing.

■ Define the following terms and provide an example of when each might be indicated:

elution:

adsorption:

■ List three causes of false negative and of false positive results in AHG testing.

■ Which class of antibodies is capable of crossing the placenta and thus causing HDN?

■ Briefly describe the procedures used to approximate the volume of transplacental hemorrhage.

■ The most commonly encountered transfusion reaction is _____.

■ Briefly describe the processes involved in development of delayed hemolytic transfusion reactions.

■ List three errors that may result in an acute hemolytic transfusion reaction consequent to ABO incompatibility.

■ Why should transfusion be halted when symptoms of adverse reactions are noted?

■ Outline the laboratory testing used in the investigation of a suspected transfusion reaction.

■ Review the tables and figures presented in this chapter.

Check your responses by reviewing the preceding sections.

16. SELF TEST

 Choose the best response for each item. The answer key may be found in the appendices.

1. **Antibodies formed in response to and capable of reacting with a foreign antigen are referred to as**
    A. autoantibodies
    B. alloantibodies
    C. haptens

2. **IgG antibodies are composed of _____ Ig molecules.**
    A. 5
    B. 3
    C. 1

3. **Subsequent exposure to an antigen results in a response with a shorter lag phase and a longer plateau than that of the initial exposure. This type of response is called the**
    A. decline phase
    B. log phase
    C. primary response
    D. anamnestic response

4. **ABO forward typing consists of**
    A. patient cells with specific reagent antisera
    B. patient serum with specific reagent cells
    C. patient cells tested with reagent cells
    D. patient serum tested with reagent antisera

5. **The antibody/antibodies expected to be found in the serum of a group A individual is/are**
    A. anti-A
    B. anti-B
    C. anti-A,B
    D. no antibodies expected

6. The antibody/antibodies expected to be found in the serum of a group O individual is/are
   A. anti-A
   B. anti-B
   C. anti-A,B
   D. no antibodies expected

7. The antibody/antibodies expected to be found in the serum of a group AB individual is/are
   A. anti-A
   B. anti-B
   C. anti-A,B
   D. no antibodies expected

8. Which of the following phenotypes could be seen in the offspring of a parent with the A phenotype and a parent with the B phenotype?
   A. A and B only
   B. A, B, and AB only
   C. A, B, AB, and O

9. The Bombay phenotype refers to a rare condition in which an individual, always group O, is
   A. homozygous (HH) for the H antigen
   B. heterozygous (Hh) for the H antigen
   C. homozygous hh and does not produce the H antigen

10. Immunodeficient patients may have a discrepancy in their ABO type. The discrepant results would be seen in the
    A. forward testing only
    B. reverse testing only
    C. results of both forward and reverse testing would be invalid

11. What results would individuals of the A_2 subgroup with anti-A_1 in their serum produce?
    A. negative reaction with A_1 cells in reverse testing and negative results with anti-A_1 lectin in forward testing
    B. positive reaction with A_1 cells in reverse testing and positive results with anti-A_1 lectin in forward testing
    C. negative reaction with A_1 cells in reverse testing and positive results with anti-A_1 lectin in forward testing
    D. positive reaction with A_1 cells in reverse testing and negative results with anti-A_1 lectin in forward testing

12. The ABO group containing the most H antigen activity is group
   A. A
   B. B
   C. AB
   D. O

13. The five most common Rh antigens are
   A. r, D, d, C, c
   B. D, d, C, c, E
   C. D, C, c, E, e

14. The most immunogenic of the Rh antigens is
   A. D
   B. C
   C. c

15. Rh antibodies are primarily of the _____ class.
   A. IgM
   B. IgG
   C. IgA

16. Individuals with a weak D antigen are treated as
   A. Rh positive in all situations
   B. Rh negative in all situations
   C. Rh negative as a donor, but Rh positive as a recipient
   D. Rh positive as a donor, but Rh negative as a recipient

17. Rare individuals who have no Rh antigens on their red cells are designated as
   A. Rh_o
   B. R^o
   C. Rh"
   D. Rh_{null}

18. The Le^b antigen is produced by
   A. non-secretors only
   B. secretors only
   C. both secretors and non-secretors

19. Choose the group of antigens for which all the corresponding antibodies would be expected to cause HTR and HDN.
   A. M, N, D, K, I, i, P_1
   B. P, Le^a, Le^b, M, N
   C. K, D, c, E, Jk^a, Jk^b, Fy^a, Fy^b
   D. K, M, N, Le^a, Le^b, P_1

20. Antibodies of this blood group system are notorious for being difficult to detect because of their low titer, weak avidity, rapid disappearance, and demonstration of dosage effect.
    A. Kidd
    B. Duffy
    C. Kell
    D. Rh

21. The test used to detect antibody-coated red cells is the
    A. antibody screen
    B. antibody panel
    C. adsorption
    D. direct antiglobulin test

22. The procedure used to remove antibody from the surface of red cells is called
    A. adsorption
    B. elution
    C. AHG testing
    D. antigram

23. Assuming type specific blood is not available, which of the following transfusions should *not* take place?
    A. group O transfused to group A
    B. group B transfused to group O
    C. group A transfused to group AB

24. Rouleaux may be confused with
    A. a negative test reaction in AHG testing
    B. a positive test reaction in AHG testing by resembling agglutination
    C. a positive test reaction in AHG testing by resembling hemolysis

25. The process of removing antibodies from serum using specially treated red cells is called
    A. adsorption
    B. elution
    C. washing

26. The concept of O as the universal donor applies to
    A. packed red cells
    B. fresh frozen plasma
    C. whole blood
    D. all of the above

27. **Anti-H would react most strongly with**
    A. A_1 cells
    B. B cells
    C. O cells
    D. A_2B cells

28. **Hemophilia A is best treated with which of the following blood components or derivatives?**
    A. factor VIII concentrate
    B. fresh frozen plasma
    C. cryoprecipitate
    D. albumin

29. **Which of the following transfusion reactions is an acute, immune reaction?**
    A. post-transfusion purpura
    B. volume overload
    C. non-hemolytic febrile
    D. infectious disease

30. **Acute hemolytic transfusion reactions are almost always attributable to**
    A. ABO incompatibility
    B. cold reactive autoantibodies
    C. WBC antibodies
    D. allergic response to plasma proteins

31. **The type of HDN that is usually mild and is more frequently seen when the maternal blood group is O is**
    A. Rh
    B. ABO
    C. Kell
    D. Duffy

32. **Which of the following results on maternal serum is most indicative of a high-risk situation?**
    A. maternal anti-M detected on initial screen and again at 28 weeks gestation
    B. Rh positive mother with anti-I detected on initial antibody screen
    C. anti-D of 1:8 titer on initial screening; subsequent titers of 1:16, then 1:32
    D. all sets of results indicate the possibility of severe HDN

17. BASIC MICROBIOLOGY

Microbiology, the study of living organisms that cannot be seen with the naked eye, was introduced by the French chemist Louis Pasteur. Such organisms were actually first described nearly 200 years earlier (1675) by Leeuwenhoek as he studied the tiny creatures he called "animalcules." He observed these organisms in saliva, water, and intestinal contents of normal individuals using a single lens capable of 200X magnification. He drew and described what we now know to be bacilli, cocci, and spirochetes. It was to be many years and many researchers later before the "germ theory" of disease was generally accepted in 1876.

Microbiology today is a complex and still growing field encompassing the study of bacteriology, mycobacteriology, parasitology, virology, and mycology. Depending on the size and scope of testing of the laboratory, these areas of study may be included in one department or each area may be a separate department. Virology and mycobacteriology testing may be limited or not performed at all in smaller institutions. Infectious diseases are still common and new infectious agents continue to be identified. Further, microbes have been linked to a number of conditions (some forms of cancer, peptic ulcers, and others) in which they were previously unsuspected. To illustrate the continued growth of the field, a few of the infectious agents identified since 1975 are listed in Table 17–1.

Comprehensive treatment of this subject area is beyond the scope of this text. This chapter presents a review of basic concepts and then focuses on the application of these principles in the identification and treatment of some of the more common conditions resulting from infectious agents.

BASIC CONCEPTS

Most of the microorganisms found in nature are not **pathogenic**, or disease producing, for humans and are not able to invade the body. The body contains a number of organisms considered to be **normal flora**. These organisms are found in various sites, including the skin, the upper respiratory tract, the intestines, and the vagina. The type of organisms considered to be normal flora is dependent on the site. That is, organisms that are ordinarily harmless at one site may be pathogenic in another. These organisms may also produce disease under circumstances

TABLE 17–1. Examples of Infectious Agents Identified Since 1975

Infectious Agent	Resultant Disease
Borrelia burgdorferi	Lyme disease
Clostridium difficile	Pseudomembranous colitis
Helicobacter pylori	Gastritis
Hepatitis C virus	Hepatitis
Hepatitis E virus	Hepatitis
Hepatitis G virus	Hepatitis
Human immunodeficiency virus	AIDS
Legionella pneumophila	Legionnaires' disease
Human herpes virus 8	Kaposi's sarcoma
Parvovirus B19	Fifth disease

Adapted from Greenwood, 1997

that result in impairment of the body's defense mechanisms. In such cases, organisms that are usually innocuous become **opportunistic pathogens**.

Microorganisms are relatively simple in structure and are usually unicellular. These cells may be of the more primitive **prokaryotic** type or of the more advanced **eukaryotic** type. Bacteria and related organisms are prokaryotic and fungi and protozoa are eukaryotic. Viruses, on the other hand, are not true cells and rely on the host cell and its biochemical processes. In most cases viruses are visible only with the use of an electron microscope.

Even before the discovery of microscopic organisms, it was recognized that certain illnesses were rarely contracted a second time. Individuals who had recovered from illnesses like smallpox seemed to be somehow protected from acquiring the disease when exposed to it again. This recognition eventually led to the development of methods to provide "artificial" immunity. Refinement of initial methods led to the development of **live attenuated** (reduced virulence) **vaccines** that are effectively used against a number of diseases, including measles and poliomyelitis. Other vaccines, such as those for typhoid fever and whooping cough, are not live vaccines and use organisms that have been killed instead. Protection from diphtheria and tetanus, diseases in which bacterial toxins produce serious effects, is provided by **antitoxins** or **toxoids** that neutralize the specific toxin produced. Toxoids are prepared by methods that make the bacterial toxin non-poisonous.

The knowledge that an antibody produced in response to a particular microbial antigen has a high specificity for that antigen led to development of serologic methods of identification of these organisms. **Specific antiserum** can be used to detect the presence of the corresponding microbial antigen. These techniques have been further refined with the development of monoclonal antibodies from single antibody producing cells. **Monoclonal antibodies** have absolute specificity for their target antigen.

Specimens collected for microbiologic studies must be collected according to established protocols in order for organisms to be recovered and identified. These organisms are quite particular about their living conditions and do not remain viable under adverse circumstances. Some of these conditions include:

- *Oxygen requirements:* Some organisms thrive in the presence of oxygen. They may derive energy solely from oxygen dependent metabolic pathways (**obligate aerobes**) or require energy for growth, but at a lower concentration (**microaerophilic aerobes**). Other organisms have oxygen independent metabolic pathways and are inhibited or killed by oxygen at atmospheric levels (**obligate anaerobe**). Another group of organisms is a bit more adaptive and can generate energy via oxygen dependent or oxygen independent pathways though their preference is for the oxygen-dependent pathway. These organisms are **facultative anaerobes**. **Aerotolerant anaerobes** derive energy only from oxygen independent pathways, but are not killed by atmospheric oxygen levels.
- *Nutrient requirements:* Different organisms require varying nutrient mediums to remain viable and to grow.
- *Temperature:* Organisms must be maintained at appropriate temperature levels to thrive.

Other considerations for the appropriate collection of specimens may depend on the site from which the specimen will be obtained. The microbiology department should provide a complete specimen collection protocol to all individuals charged with the responsibility of obtaining specimens. This protocol should be followed exactly with any questions referred to the microbiology department prior to undertaking specimen collection. As with other areas of laboratory analysis, the results obtained are dependent on the specimen used for testing. Improperly collected specimens jeopardize the validity of test results. In some instances (eg, wrong container used), it will be immediately apparent to the microbiology staff that an unsuitable specimen has been submitted and the specimen will be rejected with a request for recollection. In other cases (eg, storage conditions prior to delivery of specimen), an unsuitable specimen may not be readily apparent. In such cases, testing may yield a report indicating the absence of clinically significant organisms when such organisms are in fact present. General considerations for proper specimen collection are provided below. Specific collection instructions must be obtained from the testing laboratory.

- Collect specimens prior to initiating antibiotic therapy; if the patient is already on antibiotic therapy, the microbiology department must be notified in order to facilitate testing decisions.
- Use sterile collection containers (stool specimens are an exception).
- Use only the type of container indicated for the type of specimen being collected.
- Ensure that the collection container is tightly closed or appropriately sealed to prevent leakage and avoid contamination of the specimen and of other surfaces with the specimen contents; improperly or inadequately sealed containers will likely be rejected.
- Collect a sufficient quantity of material to allow complete testing.
- Ensure that the specimen is completely and accurately labeled.

- Deliver the specimen to the laboratory promptly with the time of collection appropriately documented; if immediate delivery is impossible ensure appropriate storage conditions are maintained during the delay; delayed delivery and/or improper storage can result in death of the organisms found in the specimen; CSF specimens require immediate delivery.
- Ensure all required information (such as the specimen source, time of collection, any antibiotic therapy, special instructions from requesting physician) is made known to the testing staff.

BACTERIOLOGY

Bacteriology is perhaps the area of microbiology that is most familiar and most frequently encountered. A large portion of our knowledge of bacteria comes from studying their growth. When these organisms are in an environment with suitable nutrients and proper physical and chemical conditions, the cell will grow and divide, providing sufficient material for examination and testing. Growth of the organism in the laboratory is important for detection and identification purposes and for susceptibility studies that determine the effect of various antibiotics on the organism. Growth is visualized in the laboratory by the appearance of colonies on solid growth media and by turbidity in liquid broth media. A bacterial colony can be seen after about 20 to 30 cell divisions (Greenwood, 1997) of a single bacterium or clump of bacteria. Many organisms produce colonies that are characteristic in appearance and thus of importance in the identification process. The time required for adequate growth of organisms contributes heavily to the amount of time required to receive definitive results from the bacteriology laboratory. However, in relative terms the rate of growth and reproduction is astronomic, with the number of organisms doubling in several minutes or several hours depending on the particular type of organism. Automated methods have significantly shortened the time required to detect bacterial growth in many instances. Examination of the growth of organisms in broth media provides a visualization of the growth curve, as depicted in Figure 17–1. The specific characteristics of the growth curve are organism dependent and in many cases can be beneficial in identification procedures. However, general characteristics are widely applicable. When first placed in a broth medium, the number of organisms remains fairly constant, a period called the **lag phase**. Following this phase an increase in cell numbers becomes detectable and the rate of reproduction increases rapidly until a maximum rate is achieved (**exponential phase**; sometimes referred to as *log phase*). Because growth at this rate cannot be continued indefinitely within a closed system with a finite amount of available nutrients, growth ultimately slows, with the bacterial cell number reaching a maximum and stabilizing (**stationary phase**). The final phase of the growth curve is the **decline phase**, in which cell death occurs as a result of nutrient depletion and accumulation of metabolic waste products.

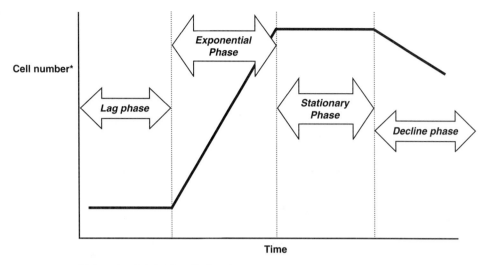

*Cell number plotted on logarithmic scale.

FIGURE 17–1. Representative growth phase.

■ NORMAL FLORA

As previously noted, the body contains a number of organisms considered to be normal flora. A general knowledge of the type of organisms expected to be found in a given site is important for at least two reasons: first, to recognize their presence as non-pathogenic and second, to avoid contamination of specimens with indigenous flora (ie, by disinfecting the surrounding area, such as skin for blood culture venipuncture, genital area for urine collection, etc.). Table 17–2 lists some of the more frequently isolated organisms constituting normal flora for various sites. This listing is not comprehensive; a number of other sites contain organisms considered to be normal flora.

TABLE 17–2. Frequently Isolated Normal Flora for Selected Sites

Site	Organisms	Frequency
Skin	*Staphylococcus epidermidis*	Almost always present
	Corynebacterium species	Almost always present
	Propionibacterium acnes	Almost always present
	Malassezia furfur	Almost always present
	Staphylococcus aureus	Frequently present
	Candida species	Occasionally present
	Veridans streptococci	Occasionally present
Mouth and oropharynx	*Veridans streptococci*	Almost always present
	Fusobacterium species	Almost always present
	Veillonella species	Almost always present
	Staphylococcus epidermidis	Usually present
	Treponema species	Usually present

(Cont.)

TABLE 17–2. *(Cont.)*

Site	Organisms	Frequency
Mouth and oropharynx *(cont.)*	*Streptococcus pneumoniae*	Frequently present
	Lactobacillus species	Frequently present
	Neisseria species	Frequently present
	Bacteriodes species	Frequently present
	Porphyromonas species	Frequently present
	Prevotella species	Frequently present
	Candida species	Frequently present
	Staphylococcus aureus	Occasionally present
	Enterococcus species	Occasionally present
	Actinomyces species	Occasionally present
	Peptostreptococcus species	Occasionally present
	Hemophilus influenzae	Occasionally present
	Hemophilus species	Occasionally present
Small intestine	*Lactobacillus* species	Usually present
	Bacteroidaceae	Usually present
	Enterococcus species	Frequently present
	Clostridium species	Frequently present
	Enterobacteriaceae	Frequently present
	Mycobacterium species	Frequently present
Large intestine	Enterobacteriaceae	Almost always present
	Bacteroidaceae	Almost always present
	Clostridium species	Almost always present
	Lactobacillus species	Frequently present
	Veridans streptococci	Usually present
	Enterococcus species	Usually present
	Staphylococcus aureus	Occasionally present
	Staphylococcus epidermidis	Occasionally present
	Group B streptococcus	Occasionally present
	Actinomyces species	Occasionally present
	Pseudomonas species	Occasionally present
	Treponema species	Occasionally present
	Mycobacterium species	Occasionally present
	Candida species	Occasionally present
Vagina	*Lactobacilllus* species	Almost always present
	Candida species	Frequently present
	Clostridium species	Frequently present
	Staphylococcus epidermidis	Occasionally present
	Group B streptococcus	Occasionally present
	Veridans streptococci	Occasionally present
	Enterococcus species	Occasionally present
	Bacteroidaceae	Occasionally present
	Actinomyces species	Occasionally present
	Bifidobacterium species	Occasionally present
	Propionibacterium acnes	Occasionally present
	Peptostreptococcus species	Occasionally present
	Acinetobacter species	Occasionally present
	Enterobacteriaceae	Occasionally present
	Gardnerella vaginalis	Occasionally present
	Mycoplasma species	Infrequently present
	Ureaplasma urealyticum	Infrequently present

Adapted from Henry JB. *Clinical Diagnosis and Management by Laboratory Methods,* 19th ed. Philadelphia, Saunders, 1996

▩ NOMENCLATURE

Standardized, consistent nomenclature is important to avoid confusion and ambiguity in the literature and in the reporting of bacteriologic results. The International Committee of Systematic Bacteriology, which publishes an approved list of names, regulates bacterial nomenclature. In reviewing the names of bacteria, such as the listing in Table 17–2, one would not list brevity and ease of pronunciation as characteristics. Bacteria are referred to by **genus** and **species**, with the capitalized genus name appearing first followed by the species, which is not capitalized. When written, the terms are usually italicized. For example, in the name *Staphylococcus aureus,* staphylococcus is the genus and aureus is the species.

▩ METHODS OF IDENTIFICATION

Methods employed for the detection and identification of bacteria may be classified as direct methods or indirect methods. **Direct methods** include:

- *Microscopic examination:* morphology and staining characteristics allow preliminary classification to be made; Gram stains, acid fast bacillus (AFB) staining, direct examination, and fluorescent microscopy are some of the methods used
- *Culture characteristics:* appearance of colonies on solid media (size, shape, translucency, color); range of conditions that support growth (temperature, oxygen requirements, type of media)
- *Biochemical reactions:* metabolic differences, such as whether the organism is gas producing, whether it possesses certain enzyme activities (eg, catalase, oxidase) and whether particular end products are produced (indole, hydrogen sulfide)

Indirect methods include:

- *Antibody reactions:* use of antibodies against a particular antigen in serologic testing; highly specific monoclonal antibodies are now used in many tests; tests that are based on the reaction of specific antibodies include latex agglutination, counter-immunoelectrophoresis, hemagglutination, and enzyme linked immmunoassay-sorbent (ELISA)
- *DNA probes:* uses separated strands of cloned fragments of DNA that recognize complementary sequences in the microorganism
- *Immunofluorescence:* utilizes antibodies "labeled" with a fluorescent dye

A variety of **typing techniques** are employed to differentiate similar strains of a particular type of bacteria that may differ only in terms of minor characteristics. Different bacteria can be typed using a number of methods, including:

- serotyping: using antibodies against particular surface structures of bacteria
- phage typing: susceptibility to lysis by certain bacteriophages or viruses that infect and parasitize bacteria
- bacteriocin typing: susceptibility to naturally occurring antibacterial substances
- protein typing: using electrophoretic techniques
- gene probe typing: using cloned fragments of DNA that recognize complementary sequences within the microorganism
- polymerase chain reaction: allows specific sequences of DNA to be amplified by making multiple copies of a defined region of the genome; can be used to mediate DNA "fingerprinting," a technique that uses the variable regions of DNA

■ PRELIMINARY IDENTIFICATION

Certain methods of distinction are employed in the laboratory as a means of classifying bacteria and narrowing the possibilities for the organism detected. Experienced bacteriologists have a solid knowledge of the characteristics of a wide range of bacteria, of the normal flora indigenous to a particular site, and of the pathogens most commonly isolated from a particular type of specimen. Initial preliminary classifications are necessary to determine how the evaluation process will proceed and which test methods should be employed. Figure 17–2 and Table 17–3 provide an overview of a system for preliminary identification.

■ THE GRAM STAIN

Although the preparation of a Gram stained smear is a relatively simple procedure, incorrect performance can yield misleading results. It is important that the smear itself be prepared in a manner that minimizes distortion of organisms that may be present and that the smear is of a thickness allowing appropriate staining reactions. The procedural steps involved in the preparation of a Gram stain are outlined below.

1. *Preparation of the smear:* the smear should be thin and taken from a representative site; a clean (in some instances, sterile) microscope slide should be used; the slide must be appropriately labeled
2. *Air drying:* the smear should be allowed to completely air dry
3. *Fixation:* smears are "fixed" with gentle heat or with methanol; excessive heat fixation will distort bacterial cells and white cell morphology
4. *Staining:* times may vary, but should be the same in relative terms (ie, same length of time for crystal violet and Gram's iodine); adhere to times established in institutional procedures:

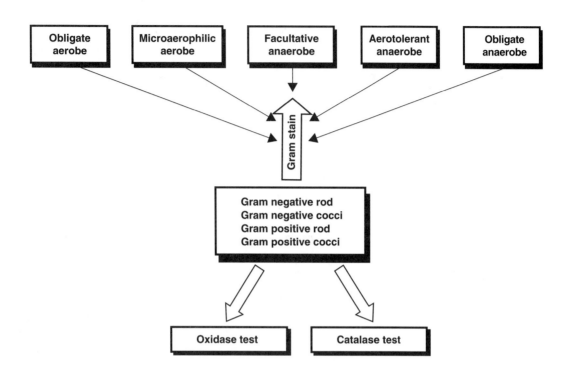

FIGURE 17-2. Preliminary identification system. Based on the results of preliminary procedures, the classifications in Table 17-3 can be established, with each including one or more, often several, organisms fitting that description.

— flood the slide with crystal violet and allow it to stand for 10 seconds
— flood the slide with Gram's iodine for 10 seconds; rinse it with tap water
— decolorize with ethanol, acetone, or ethanol/acetone mixture: *critical step;* care must be taken to avoid over- or underdecolorizing; ethanol decolorizes more slowly than acetone; the required time is usually 1 to 5 seconds; thick smears may be difficult to appropriately decolorize; rinse the slide with tap water
— counterstain with safranin for 10 seconds; rinse and allow the slide to air dry or gently blot dry with bibulous paper

Additional biochemical testing, some of which is now semi-automated, provides further narrowing of the possible organisms present.

TABLE 17–3. Preliminary Classification

Obligate Aerobe	Microaerophilic Aerobe	Facultative Anaerobe	Aerotolerant Anaerobe	Obligate Anaerobe
Gm neg rod, oxidase pos	Gm neg rod, oxidase and catalase pos	Gm neg rod, oxidase pos	Gm pos rod, catalase neg	Gm neg rod, catalase pos
Gm neg rod, oxidase neg		Gm neg rod, oxidase neg	Gm pos cocci, catalase pos	Gm neg rod, catalase neg
Gm neg cocci, oxidase pos		Gm pos rod, catalase pos		Gm pos rod, catalase pos
Gm pos rod, catalase pos		Gm pos rod, catalase neg		Gm pos rod, catalase neg
Gm pos rod, catalase neg		Gm pos cocci, catalase pos		Gm pos cocci, catalase pos
Gm pos cocci, catalase pos				Gm pos cocci, catalase neg
				Gm neg cocci, catalase pos
				Gm neg cocci, catalase neg

Staining characteristics are important in the identification of bacteria. The organisms are differentially stained based on the structural characteristics of the bacterial cell wall. They are classified as gram positive or gram negative based on whether they resist decolorization. **Gram positive** bacteria resist decolorization and remain stained the dark purple color resulting from crystal violet and Gram's iodine. **Gram negative** organisms are decolorized and then take up the safranin stain to produce a lighter pink color. Improper decolorization can make it very difficult to distinguish the two groups of organisms. The greater permeability of the cell walls of gram negative organisms is believed to render these cells more susceptible to decolorization and counterstaining. Control slides should be used to ensure appropriate technique.

Morphologic characteristics are also used to classify bacteria. **Bacilli** are cylindrical, rod-shaped cells (often referred to as *rods* rather than *bacilli*) and **cocci** are spherical, or nearly spherical, in shape. **Vibrios** and **spirilla** are rod-shaped cells that are curved or twisted in contrast to the relatively straight bacilli. The organisms within these shape categories are subdivided further based on additional morphologic characteristics:

- *cocci:* cocci are relatively uniform in size; main subdivisions are based on prevailing manner of cell grouping (ie, chains, clusters, pairs) and Gram staining characteristics (most cocci are gram positive); very few species are motile

- *bacilli:* main subdivisions based on Gram staining characteristics and presence or absence of endospores (size, shape, and position of spores may be distinguishing); some have flagella that give motility; shape variations among the bacilli include slightly curved, ovoid and club shapes and smaller pleomorphic shapes; some grow in chains or filaments; Vibrios are short, comma shaped rods; spirilla are gram negative spiral filaments and are usually motile with polar flagella

■ GRAM POSITIVE COCCI

The name **staphylococcus** is derived from the Greek words for "bunch of grapes" and "berry or grain," indicative of the characteristic cell groupings of irregular clusters resembling a bunch of grapes. They may also be seen as single cells or pairs of cells. The bacteria of this genus are **gram positive**, **catalase positive**, **facultative anaerobes** that grow well under either aerobic or anaerobic conditions and on a variety of nutrient media. Of the approximately 30 species of the staphylococcus genus, *Staphylococcus aureus* is the *major pathogen.* This species is characterized by an enzyme called **coagulase** that has the capability to clot blood by converting fibrinogen in citrated human plasma to fibrin. Coagulase testing is used to differentiate *Staph aureus* from other species of this genus, as none of the other species are coagulase positive. Individual *Staph aureus* colonies are seen on blood agar after incubation at 37°C as circular, opaque colonies of about 2 to 3 mm diameter (Greenwood, 1997). The surface of the colonies is characteristically smooth and shiny with yellow or cream pigmentation frequently seen. *Staph aureus* can be selectively isolated using media containing sodium chloride with mannitol (mannitol salt agar). If necessary, *Staph aureus* can be confirmed by detection of another enzyme, thermonuclease (a heat-stable anti-DNA enzyme), produced by the organism.

Staph aureus is frequently present as normal flora in the nose and on the skin. It typically causes infection when resistance is lowered by damage to the skin or mucus membranes. The **most common site of infection** with *Staph aureus* is the **skin**. Although most infections with this organism are confined to minor lesions or pustules, it occasionally produces widespread impetigo in children. *Staph aureus* is also associated with serious infection of wound sites. It is associated with purulent inflammation, notably the production of abscesses. In a few cases, generally in otherwise debilitated individuals, serious pneumonia, meningitis, and septicemia are caused by this organism. *Staph aureus* causes about one fourth (Ravel, 1995) of infectious endocarditis cases and produces one type of food poisoning. In cases of food poisoning that result from *Staph aureus,* the symptoms seen result from ingestion of bacterial toxins rather than enteric infection with living organisms. *Staph aureus* has been linked to toxic shock syndrome as well.

Importantly, *Staph aureus* is associated with infections acquired during hospitalization. Of particular concern are those that produce an enzyme called **beta-lactamase**. This enzyme renders the organism resistant to antibiotics that contain a beta-lactam ring (penicillins and cephalosporins). Beta-lactamase splits this ring, rendering the antibiotic ineffective. The term *methicillin resistant Staph aureus*

(**MRSA**) is applied to these beta-lactamase producing organisms. Tests are available to show bacterial beta-lactamase production. Organisms yielding a positive beta-lactamase test should be considered resistant to penicillin, ampicillin, and first and second generation cephalosporins until susceptibility testing is completed. Other organisms, including *Staph epidermidis* and *Hemophilus influenzae* type B, may also produce beta-lactamase.

Staph aureus can be typed based on the endotoxin (A, B, C, D, and E toxins) produced by the organism. These toxins may be produced singly or in combination. It is the ingestion of these toxins that produces the nausea, vomiting, and diarrhea of staphylococcal food poisoning within a few hours of ingestion.

Most of the **coagulase negative staphylococcal organisms** isolated are *Staph epidermidis*. **Staph epidermidis** is almost always found as normal skin flora and is a frequent contaminant in cultures from the skin area and in cultures collected by skin puncture (eg, blood cultures) without the area being adequately disinfected. Although usually considered to be a skin contaminant when isolated from most cultures, *Staph epidermidis* is capable of producing disease. It may be associated with infections related to indwelling catheters, prosthetic joint devices, bacteremia in immunosuppressed patients, endocarditis (especially in persons with an artificial heart valve), and infections following eye surgery (Greenwood, 1997). *Staph epidermidis* is often resistant to many antibiotics. Another coagulase negative staphylococcal organism, *Staph saprophyticus,* is sometimes isolated in urinary tract infections in young women. Some laboratories may not speciate coagulase negative staphylococcal organisms, reporting them simply as "coagulase negative *Staphylococcus.*"

Streptococci are **gram positive** cocci that typically **occur in chains** of varying lengths or in pairs. These organisms are generally facultative anaerobes, but some strains are microaerophilic or anaerobic. Streptococci are catalase negative. Streptococcal organisms are part of the normal flora in various sites, most notably the upper respiratory tract. Some streptococcal species, *Streptococcus pyogenes* (group A strep) in particular, can cause a variety of diseases that range in severity from mild to life threatening. The classification of streptococcal organisms is traditionally based on the type of hemolysis the organism produces on blood agar. Those that produce a **clear zone** of hemolysis are called β-hemolytic (beta hemolytic); those that produce a **narrow green colored zone** are called α-hemolytic (alpha hemolytic); and those that **do not produce a zone** of hemolysis should be called **non-hemolytic** (these organisms have been referred to as γ-hemolytic, but *non-hemolytic* is the preferred term). The majority of the streptococcal species producing disease in humans are β-hemolytic. The hemolytic streptococci can be classified serologically (using antisera directed at polysaccharide antigens contained in the cell wall and specific for each group) into Lancefield groups designated by the letters A–H and K–V. Further subdivision of the organisms is possible based on their surface protein antigens (M, T, and R–M are of most importance clinically). Such typing is of importance in epidemiology studies of outbreaks of infection, but is not in routine clinical use. Table 17–4 lists the medically important streptococci.

TABLE 17–4. Medically Important Streptococci

Species	Lancefield Group	Type of Hemolysis
Streptococcus pyogenes	A	β
Streptococcus agalactiae	B	β
Streptococcus equisimilis	C	β
Streptococcus zooepidemicus	C	β
Streptococcus bovis	D	α or none
Streptococcus equinis	D	α or none
Streptococcus faecalis	D	α or none; classified as Enterococcus along with with *Strep durans* and *Strep faecium*; see Table 17-5
Streptococcus milleri [1]	A, C, G, or F	α, β, or none
Streptococcus pneumoniae	None	α
Streptococcus sanguis	None	α
Streptococcus mitior [2]	None	α
Streptococcus mutans	None	None

[1]Includes strains designated as *Strep intermedius, Strep constellatus,* and *Strep anginosus.*

[2]Includes strains *Strep mitis* and *Strep oralis.*

Adapted from Greenwood D, Slack R, Peutherer J. *Medical Microbiology: A Guide to Microbial Infections—Pathogenesis, Immunity, Laboratory Diagnosis and Control,* 15th ed. New York, Churchill Livingstone, 1997

Group A β-hemolytic streptococci (Strep pyogenes) produce about 20 different enzymes and toxins that cannot currently be definitively linked individually (or in combination) with particular syndromes or infections. Some of these substances are

- streptolysin O: lyses red cells; also cytotoxic to neutrophils, platelets, and cardiac tissue; inactivated by oxygen; responsible for subsurface hemolysis on blood agar
- streptolysin S: not inactivated by oxygen; responsible for surface hemolysis on aerobic blood agar plates; has leukocidal action
- streptokinase: enzyme that promotes fibrinolysis; may enhance the spread of the organism; used therapeutically as a fibrinolysin
- hyaluronidase: may be associated with the spread of the organism through connective tissue
- DNAases: enzymes that hydrolyze nucleic acids and nucleoproteins; pathogenic role unknown
- erythrogenic toxins: three distinct toxins; induce lymphocytes to produce and release cytokines that result in fever, tissue damage, and shock

The **most common infection caused by group A strep** is an **acute sore throat**. Although beta hemolytic group A strep may be isolated from some clinically normal children, it is difficult to reliably distinguish the carrier state from true pathogens. Because prompt treatment is believed to reduce the risk of developing rheumatic fever and acute glomerulonephritis, the presence of these organisms in throat or nasopharyngeal cultures of children is considered a pathogenic finding regardless. The virulence of *Strep pyogenes* is related to the M protein surface antigen.

Other infections resulting from group A strep that are relatively frequent are **wound infections** and **localized cellulitis**. Less commonly encountered infections include **bacteremia**, **impetigo**, **scarlet fever**, and the rapidly progressing infection called **necrotizing fascitis** that causes significant tissue destruction necessitating surgical removal of damaged tissue. **Rheumatic fever** and **acute glomerulonephritis** may occur subsequent to infection with some strains of group A beta strep.

Commercial kits are available for the rapid detection of group A strep. Although these tests are highly specific, the sensitivity of the tests is relatively low. For this reason, it is important for all *negative tests to be followed by culture* for confirmation. A culture report of beta hemolytic strep is not clinically useful without grouping of the organism. **Bacitracin sensitivity testing** is used to presumptively identify group A beta hemolytic strep, as these organisms are generally much more sensitive to bacitracin than other groups. Bacitracin sensitivity is considered to provide **presumptive identification** because some non-group A organisms may also demonstrate sensitivity. Specific tests for accurate, definitive grouping are available commercially. Features of some additional streptococci are summarized in Table 17–5.

Viridians streptococci lack lancefield antigens and produce alpha hemolysis on sheep blood agar. These organisms are the most common cause of infectious endocarditis and may also cause urinary tract infections, pneumonia, and wound infections.

Streptococcus pneumoniae (also called *pneumococcus* and sometimes *Diplococcus pneumoniae*) are **gram positive diplococci** (small, paired cocci) frequently seen as normal flora in the throat. This organism is a common cause of **bacterial pneumonia**, which results in bacteremia in about 20 % (Ravel, 1995) of cases. Middle ear infections in children and meningitis in older children and adults (especially if debilitated) may result from *Strept pneumoniae* as well.

■ ENTEROBACTERIACEAE

Enterobacteriaceae are a large family of **gram negative rods** found primarily in the intestinal tract. Many of these organisms cause disease in other locations or if an overgrowth of certain types is present. Contaminated food or water introduces other organisms in this group. **Salmonella** and **Shigella** are **always pathogens** that are introduced from the environment. Organisms in this family are either **facultative anaerobes or aerobes** and are **oxidase and catalase positive**. Table 17–6 summarizes the laboratory differentiation of members of the

TABLE 17–5. Features of Selected Non-Group A Streptococci

Lancefield Group	Species	Most Frequently Associated Infection	Comments
B	*Streptococcus agalactiae*	Neonatal septicemia Neonatal meningitis Post-partum endometritis Post-partum bacteremia	Found in genital tract of 20–30% of women of childbearing age; mother may be screened during pregnancy or just prior to delivery (controversy as to when and whether all women should be screened in pregnancy); this organism also causes mastitis in cows
C	*Streptococcus anginosus* (and others)	Pharyngitis Meningitis	Usually an animal pathogen; only occasionally causes human infection
D	*Streptococcus faecalis* *Streptococcus bovis* *Streptococcus equinis* (and others)	Endocarditis Urinary tract infection Biliary tract infection Mixed wound infections Intra-abdominal infections	Majority of serious group D infections caused by enterococci—certain group D species normally in intestinal tract with particular lab characteristics; may be placed in separate *Enterococcus* genus to include species of *faecalis, faecium, durans,* and others; group D strep would include species *bovis* and *equinus*
F	*Streptococcus milleri* (*anginosus*)	Dental abscesses Bacteremia	Infections uncommon

Information from Greenwood, 1997; Henry, 1996; Ravel, 1995

Enterobacteriaceae family. Brief discussions of some of these organisms follow Table 17–5.

Much of the morbidity and mortality associated with Enterobacteriaceae results from endotoxins within their cell walls. Symptoms, including fever, chills, and hypotension, are effects of these endotoxins. In addition, they may produce an increase in granulocytes, decreased platelets, activation of both complement pathways, and disseminated intravascular coagulopathy (DIC). When blood levels of substances producing vasoconstriction and proteolytic enzymes reach significant levels, diminished cardiac output and endotoxic shock results.

Laboratory isolation of Enterobacteriaceae is accomplished using differential (varying organisms produce different characteristics with media) and selective (selective for growth of certain organisms only; does not support growth of other organisms) media. This is of particular importance in stool cultures because of the presence of so many organisms.

Salmonella organisms are a major cause of food borne illnesses throughout the world. They characteristically possess two sets of antigens that can be demonstrated serologically in the laboratory.

- O antigens: also called *somatic antigens;* heat stable polysaccharides in the cell wall; different antigens designated by number; some also produce a surface polysaccharide, notably the *Salmonella typhi* Vi antigen
- H antigens: flagellar antigens; made up of structural proteins from flagella; two "phases"—phase 1 and phase 2—of antigens: phase 1 designated by lower case letters and phase 2 designated by number/letter combinations

TABLE 17–6. Laboratory Differentiation of Enterobacteriaceae

Test	Salmonella typhi	Other Salmonella serotypes	Shigella	Escherichia Coli	Citrobacter	Klebsiella	Enterobacter*	Proteus	Providencia
Motility	+	+	–	+	+	–	+	+	+
Gas from glucose	–	+	–	+	+	+	+	v	v
Acid from lactose	–	–	–	+	+	+	+	–	–
Urease	–	–	–	–	–	v	–	+	–
Citrate utilization	–	+	–	–	+	+	+	v	+
H$_2$S production	+	+	–	–	v	–	–	v	–
Indole	–	–	v	+	v	v	v	v	+
PPA Test	–	–	–	–	–	–	–	+	+
Gluconate oxidation	–	–	–	–	–	+	+	–	–

+ = positive; – = negative; v = variable; * includes *Serratia;* PPA = phenylpyruvic acid.

From Greenwood D, Slack R, Peutherer J. *Medical Microbiology: A Guide to Microbial Infections—Pathogenesis, Immunity, Laboratory Diagnosis and Control,* 15th ed. New York, Churchill Livingstone, 1997

Thus the more than 2000 serotypes of *Salmonella* can be described in terms of antigenic structure using a three part formula beginning with the numbers describing the O antigen, followed by the lower case letter(s) of the phase 1 H antigen and the number or letter designation of the phase 2 H antigen. Although not routinely important, these designations allow each different serotype to be referred to consistently and can be of assistance in epidemiological studies. Three examples are provided for illustration purposes:

Salmonella typhi	9, 12, (Vi) : d : –
Salmonella typhimurium	1, 4, 5, 12 : i : 1, 2
Salmonella enteritidis	1, 9, 12 : g, m : 1, 7

Illnesses produced by *Salmonella* species are summarized in Table 17–7.

The **Shigella** genus is divided into four species based on serologic and biochemical testing: *Shigella dysenteriae, Shigella flexneri, Shigella boydii,* and *Shigella sonnei. Shigella* organisms produce bacillary dysentery characterized by frequent bloody, mucopurulent stools. (A similar dysentery caused by amoeba is termed *amoebic dysentery.*) *Shigella* organisms usually remain localized to the colon, whereas *Salmonella* may enter the bloodstream early in infection. Stool culture is the main diagnostic test.

Escherichia coli, another member of the Enterobacteriaceae family, is a gram negative coliform (used to refer to any Enterobacteriaceae by some and by others

TABLE 17–7. Infections Produced by *Salmonella*

Infection	Species	Comments
Typhoid fever	*Salmonella typhi*	Transmitted through fecal contamination of food and water; blood culture usually positive in first 2 weeks (Ravel, 1995), stool culture later; antibody tests also available; incubation period variable, but usually about two weeks; symptoms include high fever, GI symptoms, splenomegaly, necrosis and "typhoid ulcers" of lymphoid tissues
Paratyphoid fever (enteric fever)	*Salmonella typhimurium*[1] *Salmonella enteritidis (paratyphi)*[1]	Clinically similar to typhoid fever, but milder
Salmonella gastroenteritis	*Salmonella typhimurium*[1] (most common)	Most frequent *Salmonella* infection; short incubation time; abdominal pain, nausea, diarrhea, leukocytosis, positive stool culture
Bacteremia	Various[1]	Seen occasionally; more common in patients with systemic lupus erythematosus, AIDS, leukemia, or lymphoma; rare cases of pneumonia, meningitis, and endocarditis may also be seen

[1]Infection with species other than *Salmonella typhi,* which is spread by fecal contamination, results from contaminated poultry and other animals and from inadequately cooked eggs.

to describe only lactose fermenting Enterobacteriaceae) bacteria present in the intestinal tract (especially the large intestine). Its presence is used as an indication of fecal contamination in water. *E coli* has a number of different strains and is **serotyped based** on the distribution of **O, H, and K antigens** (Greenwood, 1997). It is the **most common cause of urinary tract infections** and the most common cause of gram negative septicemia (usually subsequent to a urinary tract infection). This organism also causes meningitis and septicemia in neonates. **E coli** is a frequent cause of diarrhea in infants and is associated with "traveler's" diarrhea. Because the organism is normally found in the colon, it was thought that only certain strains were capable of producing diarrhea. However, a number of exceptions have since been noted. One specific strain, **E coli 0157:H7**, that causes a particularly severe diarrhea with bloody stools is found primarily in cattle. Some outbreaks of infection with this strain have been seen as a result of improperly handled or inadequately cooked beef.

Klebsiella organisms are gram negative rods that are usually somewhat shorter and thicker than those of the other Enterobacteriaceae. Members of the genus are differentiated on the basis of biochemical testing. *Klebsiella* organisms (particularly *Klebsiella pneumoniae*) are a relatively common cause of urinary tract infections (including those acquired in the hospital). A resistant, necrotizing pneumonia characteristically found in alcoholics and debilitated patients (Friedlander's pneumonia) is caused by *Klebsiella pneumoniae*. Klebsiella is usually resistant to ampicillin, amoxicillin, and most other penicillins, but is usually sensitive to cephalosporins. Organisms of the **Enterobacter** genus are closely related to *Klebsiella* organisms, but are usually motile, whereas *Klebsiella* is nonmotile. *Enterobacter aerogenes* and *Enterobacter cloacae* are the species of primary clinical importance. They are primarily seen in urinary tract infections.

The genus **Proteus** consists of two species: *Proteus mirabilis* and *Proteus vulgaris*. The *Providencia* genus is closely related to the *Proteus* genus and some organisms previously classified as *Proteus* are now considered to be of the *Providencia* genus. **A characteristic feature of Proteus** organisms is their **ability to "swarm"** (growth that starts at the edge of the colony and then spreads over the surface of the media, rather than being confined to a discrete colony of growth) on solid culture media. *Proteus* is a fairly prevalent cause of urinary tract infections. Although septicemia may occur, it is usually only seen in patients with serious underlying conditions. It is also seen in infected surgical wounds and bedsores in hospitals.

Other members of the Enterobacteriaceae family are less commonly seen as pathogens, but are associated with a number of infections, especially in the presence of diminished host resistance. **Citrobacter** and **Serratia** are two examples of these organisms. *Serratia,* perhaps the most serious of this group, usually causes urinary tract infections, particularly following cytoscopy or urinary tract surgery and in association with indwelling catheters. Many *Serratia* urinary tract infections are asymptomatic and thus may go untreated for some time. Bacteremia results in about 10% (Ravel, 1995) of cases.

■ OTHER GRAM NEGATIVE BACILLI

Of the *Pseudomonas* genus, *Pseudomonas aeruginosa* is the species most commonly associated with human disease. *Pseudomonas* organisms are **gram negative bacilli** that grow on a variety of media and are **usually motile**, having one or two polar flagella. The organism is characterized by the production of a **grape-like odor** when grown on culture media in the laboratory. The primary importance of *P aeruginosa* lies in its capacity to act as an **opportunistic pathogen** in immunocompromised patients, particularly individuals with cystic fibrosis or chronic granulomatous disease (Greenwood, 1997). The organism is well suited to the role as an opportunistic pathogen by virtue of its adaptability and resistance to a number of antibiotics and disinfectants. It is the cause of about 10 % of nosocomial infections (Ravel, 1995) and can infect virtually any external site. Community acquired infections are generally less severe than those that are acquired in a hospital setting. **Infections associated with *Pseudomonas*** include urinary tract infection, pneumonia, infection of burn sites, septicemia, and infections obtained from whirlpool tubs.

Most species of the *Hemophilus* genus are found normally in the nasopharynx. They are quite **small, pleomorphic gram negative bacilli** sometimes referred to as *coccobacilli.* These organisms require blood or certain blood constituents in order to grow on culture media (the name *hemophilus* is derived from Greek meaning "blood loving"). The major pathogen in this genus, ***Hemophilus influenzae,*** is the most common etiology of meningitis in children between the ages of 2 months and 5 years. A vaccination for *H influenzae* type B is now available and significantly reduces the occurrence of HIB mediated meningitis. It also reduces the pharyngeal carriage of the organism (Greenwood, 1997). Most of these cases result from type B *H influenzae* (HIB), a capsulated form of the organism. *H influenzae* is also associated with a variety of other infections, including pneumonia, acute epiglottitis (croup), sinusitis, childhood otitis media, bronchitis, and septic arthritis. Other species of clinical importance include *Hemophilus parainfluenzae, Hemophilus aphrophilus,* and *Hemophilus paraphrophilus,* which may be seen in some cases of endocarditis, dental infections, and abscesses in the lung or brain.

Campylobacter and *Helicobacter* are both spiral bacteria with flagella that are especially suited to colonization and penetration of mucus membranes. ***Helicobacter pylori*** was not discovered until 1983 even though it colonizes about one half of the population. Its discovery was facilitated by the development of fiberoptic endoscopy and the ability to biopsy gastric mucosa. Several additional *Helicobacter* species, not all associated with humans, has since been identified. Although most *H pylori* infections are symptomless and the endoscopic appearance of the stomach is normal, some infected persons develop **peptic ulcers**. The identification of this organism as the causative agent of idiopathic peptic ulceration and as a significant risk factor for gastric malignancy was a significant discovery. Infections are responsive to a number of antibiotics. The most successful treatment regimens combine two or more antibiotics with bismuth subsalicylate (Pepto-Bismol) or combine an antibiotic with an acid pump inhibitor. The first regimen eliminates infection in the majority of patients (>90% according to Greenwood [1997]; 87% reported by Stein [1993]) and involves 2 weeks of therapy composed of daily doses of 5 to 8 Pepto-Bismol tablets, 250 mg of tetracycline four times daily, and 250 mg of metronidazole three times daily (Stein, 1993).

Even though the organism produces no reaction in most standard biochemical tests, it produces a very powerful **urease** enzyme that can be detected in biopsy tissue. A small portion of infected tissue can be placed in a urea solution containing an indicator to detect pH changes as ammonia is formed by the action of the urease produced by the organism. Positive results may be detected in a few minutes or up to 2 hours later. Light infections may not be detected by this method. *H pylori* can be detected by other methods, including:

- gram stains of tissue and special histologic staining procedures
- culture (rarely utilized except in epidemiologic studies or if sensitivity tests are required): serologic methods to detect antibodies to the organism or its products (significant number of false positive results in some circumstances)
- DNA probes with polymerase chain reaction (PCR) amplification (not routinely available at present)

The ***Campylobacter*** genus was first identified in the early 1900s as a cause of spontaneous abortion in sheep and was originally classified as a vibrio with the first species called *Vibrio fetus* (Greenwood, 1997). That organism, now called *Campylobacter fetus,* is a major cause of abortion in both sheep and cattle but rarely infects humans. It is, however, associated with bacteremia in individuals with immuneodeficiencies (Greenwood, 1997; Ravel, 1995) and is seen in rare cases of septic abortions (Greenwood, 1997). More frequently seen in human infections are the species ***Campylobacter jejuni*** and ***Campylobacter coli.*** These species are small, spiral Gram negative rods with a single flagellum at one or both ends that confers the organisms with rapid motility. They grow best at 42°C in microaerophilic conditions. Although inactive in a number of biochemical tests, they are strongly oxidase positive. The enteritis produced by *Campylobacter* is one of the most common causes of diarrhea in most developed countries. Animals, particularly poultry, are the main source of infection. Features of some additional gram negative bacilli are summarized in Table 17–8.

■ GRAM NEGATIVE DIPLOCOCCI

The two pathogenic ***Neisseria*** species, *Neisseria meningitidis* and *Neisseria gonorrhoeae,* have similar morphologic and culture characteristics but cause very different diseases. They appear on Gram stain as **gram negative diplococci** that are slightly oval with a flat or bean-shaped side. Occurring in **pairs**, the flat (or bean-

TABLE 17–8. Summary of Additional Gram Negative Bacilli

Genus	Summary Information
Bordatella	Most important species is *Bordatella pertussis,* etiologic agent of pertussis (whooping cough); highly contagious; detected by culture, serologic testing, or direct antigen testing on nasopharyngeal swabs
Brucella	Gram negative coccobacilllus with three primary species; organisms cause rare febrile disease called *brucellosis;* infection with one species transmitted from cattle, another species from goats, and the third from swine; detected by culture with special media (blood culture is positive in nearly half of cases) or, most frequently, by serologic testing
Yersinia	Three important species are *Yersinia pestis* (cause of septicemic, pneumonic, and bubonic plagues), *Yersinia enterocolitica* (most common of the three; causes acute enteritis), and *Yersinia pseudotuberculosis* (found in animals; rarely seen in humans, but can produce enteritis with symptoms similar to appendicitis diagnosed by stool culture in enteritis or by lymph node culture in mesenteric adenitis)
Francisella	Medically important species is *Francisella tularensis,* which causes tularemia; very small, gram negative coccobacillus that requires special media to grow; major reservoir is wild animals, especially wild rabbits
Legionella	Natural habitat is water; several species, but most infections caused by *Legionella pneumophila* (rapidly progressing pneumonia called *Legionnaire's disease*); preferred diagnostic method is immunofluorescent staining using monoclonal antisera
Vibrio	Small, curved, gram negative rods; most important species is *Vibrio cholerae* (produces cholera by an enterotoxin) and is divided into many serotypes; infection occurs from drinking contaminated water or eating shellfish from contaminated water; diagnosis traditionally by stool culture; recently developed tests use monoclonal antibody

Information in summary compiled from Greenwood, 1997; Henry, 1996; Ravel, 1995

shaped) sides face each other. The organisms (especially *N gonorrhoeae*) may be seen within polymorphonuclear cells and referred to as **intracellular**, gram negative diplococci. ***Branhamella catarrhalis,*** normally found in the upper respiratory tract, closely resembles the *Neisseria* species. *Neisseria* requires specific conditions to grow well on culture, but grow well on chocolate and Thayer-Martin media when incubated at 35° to 37°C in a moist environment with 5% to 10% carbon dioxide. The two species can be differentiated based on sugar fermentation reactions. The meningococcus usually ferments both glucose and maltose; gonococcus ferments glucose only. Neither species ferments lactose nor sucrose.

Neisseria meningitidis infection may result in a variety of diseases, but **meningitis** and **septicemia** are the most commonly encountered. It is believed that the organism passes through the mucosa of the nasopharyngeal area to enter the bloodstream (positive blood cultures are frequently seen early in infection). Meningitis due to this organism occurs only in individuals who lack a bactericidal antibody to the strain of the infecting organism. Incidence is highest in young children, who rarely have this antibody. Upon acquiring the organism, an individual may either become ill or develop immunity by antibody production. Factors determining the virulence and communicability of meningococcus are not fully understood. When meningococcal meningitis is suspected, specimens for both **blood cultures and CSF culture** should be obtained. In addition to culture, a cell count and differential may be performed on the CSF. **Immediate examination of a Gram stain on CSF** is important to initiate antibiotic therapy. Meningococci are divided into three primary serogroups—A, B, and C—with group A being the group generally associated with epidemic meningitis. A purpuric rash may accompany meningococcal meningitis and septicemia due to meningococcus infection. Both septicemia and meningitis may be present together in some patients. These infections have a **significant mortality rate** and require immediate treatment.

Neisseria gonorrhoeae is never found as normal flora and is an exclusively human pathogen spread almost without exception by sexual contact. The organism has a **short incubation** period and infected males often present clinically a few days after exposure with an acute urethritis. Most seek treatment fairly quickly in response to **dysuria** and a purulent penile **discharge**. Although males are rarely asymptomatic, infected females may first seek treatment in response to their partner's symptoms. Dysuria and vaginal discharge are only seen in about half of infected females. **Asymptomatic carriage** of the organism can result in significant complications if the gonococci ascend (during menstruation, after instrumentation, termination of pregnancy, etc) to the fallopian tubes, producing acute salpingitis, pelvic inflammatory disease, and possible sterility. The eyes of babies born to infected women are susceptible to infection that rapidly leads to blindness if untreated. Disseminated infection may occur resulting in painful joints, fever, and occasional septic skin lesions. *Neisseria gonorrhoeae* infection is usually diagnosed and treated with relative ease. The presence of intracellular, gram negative diplococci on gram stain is indicative of *N gonorrhoeae* and therapy is usually initiated based on this finding with culture results pending. Most strains of the organism are **highly susceptible to penicillin**, although resistant strains have arisen. Single dose therapy is adequate for most cases (excluding disseminated infections) and offers the advantage of complete compliance.

■ OTHER BACTERIA TRANSMITTED BY SEXUAL CONTACT

Nongonococcal urethritis in men is most commonly caused by ***Chlamydia trachomatis*** (Ravel, 1995). (There are four species of *Chlamydia;* infections also occur in the eye and in the respiratory tract.) In women, the organism may produce cervicitis and urethritis. Many women and some men are asymptomatic. The organisms are **small gram negative bacteria that stain poorly** on Gram stain and may be better demonstrated with other staining techniques. They are **obligate intracellular parasites** (ie, like viruses, they depend on the host cell for energy production). Infections are usually localized in males, but untreated infections in females can result in ascending infection causing endometritis, salpingitis, and pelvic inflammatory disease. Tubal damage and infertility or ectopic pregnancy may result. Infants born to infected mothers may develop pneumonitis as a result of infection with the organism (Greenwood, 1997). The effect of untreated infection on male fertility is not yet known. **Specimens for culture** must be collected exactly according to established protocol and **delivered immediately** to the laboratory using **special transport media** in order to maintain viability of the organism. Inappropriately transported or stored specimens will not produce valid results.

Gardnerella vaginalis is a small gram negative (usually stains gram negative) bacillus or coccobacillus that may cause **vaginitis**. However, isolation of the organism is not diagnostic of vaginitis because it is seen as **normal flora** in up to half of the female population. Vaginal discharge is usually the only symptom of infection in women and males exhibit no symptoms.

Table 17–9 presents some of the bacterial pathogens isolated with relative frequency in selected conditions.

■ ANAEROBES

A wide variety of anaerobic bacteria exist as **normal flora** in the **mouth** and oropharynx, in the **gastrointestinal tract**, and in the **female genital tract** (Table 17–10). These organisms can result in infection as opportunistic pathogens. Infection with anaerobes can also result from animal or human bite wounds with the infecting organism coming from the mouth. Anaerobes **typically produce a foul**, **repulsive odor** and a large amount of pus. They should be suspected in deep abscesses, when no organisms are isolated aerobically from pus, and when infection is associated with necrotic tissue. Additional indications of anaerobic (non-clostridial) infection are listed in Table 17–11 and selected anaerobes are summarized in Table 17–12. **Specimens** collected for anaerobic culture should be collected in anaerobic transport media and delivered promptly to the laboratory. These organisms are **typically slow growing** and may require several days for detection.

■ SPIROCHETES AND RICKETTSIA

The spirochetes includes the genera *Treponema* and *Borrelia,* with various species included in each genus. These organisms are **thin spiral or helical rods** that are actively **motile with flagella** at each pole and around the cell body. Infections with treponemal and borrelial organisms typically result in conditions with distinct clinical stages that may be separated by periods of remission. The infecting organism may be difficult to detect in later stages, but is usually detectable in early lesions. Infections spread from the initial site to the bloodstream and other organs, where untreated conditions may progress to fatality. Spirochetes include both pathogenic organisms and those that are found normally in the mouth, intestines, and genital tract.

TABLE 17–9. Common Bacterial Pathogens for Selected Conditions

Condition	Frequently Encountered Pathogens
Acute bronchitis	*Streptococcus pneumoniae* *Hemophilus influenzae*
Sore throat	*Streptococcus pyogenes* (group A, β-hemolytic)
Sinusitus/otitis media	*Streptococcus pneumoniae* *Hemophilus influenzae*
Urinary tract infection	*Escherichia coli* *Proteus* *Klebsiella*
Gastrointestinal infection	*Salmonella* *Campylobacter* *Shigella* *Escherichia coli*
Endocarditis	Streptococci (esp. viridians) Enterococci *Staphylococcus epidermidus* *Staphylococcus aureus*
Septicemia	*Escherichia coli* *Staphylococcus epidermidus* *Staphylococcus aureus* *Streptococcus pneumoniae*
Genital tract infections	*Neisseria gonorrhoeae* *Chlamydia trachomatis* *Gardnerella vaginalis*
Meningitis	*Neisseria meningitidis* *Hemophilus influenzae* (type B) *Streptococcus pneumoniae* Group B *Streptococcus* *Escherichia coli* (esp. neonates)
Skin infection	*Staphylococcus aureus* *Streptococcus pyogenes* (group A, β-hemolytic)

TABLE 17–10. Anaerobic Bacteria Found as Normal Flora

Organism	Skin	Mouth	Gastrointestinal Tract	Genitourinary Tract
GRAM POSITIVE BACILLI				
Actinomyces	–	+	+	+
Bifidobacterium	–	+	+	+
Clostridium	–	–	+	+
Eubacterium	–	+	+	+
Lactobacillus	–	+	+	+
Propionibacterium	+	+	+	+
GRAM POSITIVE COCCI				
Coprococcus	–	–	+	–
Gaffkya	–	–	+	+
Gemmiger	–	–	+	–
Peptococcus	+	–	+	+
Peptostreptococcus	+	+	+	+
Ruminococcus	–	–	+	–
Sarcina	–	–	+	–
Streptococcus	+	+	+	+
GRAM NEGATIVE BACILLI				
Anaerobiospirillum	–	+	+	?
Anaerorhabdus	–	–	+	?
Bacteroides	–	+	+	+
Bilophila	–	–	+	+
Butyrivibrio	–	–	+	–
Centipeda	–	+	+	?
Desulfomonas	–	–	+	–
Fusobacterium	–	+	+	+
Leptotrichia	–	+	+	–
Mitsuokella	–	+	+	?
Porphyromonas	–	+	+	+
Prevotella	–	+	+	+
Selenomonas	–	+	+	–
Succinimonas	–	–	+	–
Succinivibrio	–	–	+	–
Wolinella	–	+	+	–
GRAM NEGATIVE COCCI				
Acidaminococcus	–	–	+	+
Megasphaera	–	–	+	–
Veillonella	–	+	+	+
SPIROCHETES				
Treponema	–	+	+	+
Other spiral forms	–	+	+	+

From Greenwood D, Slack R, Peutherer J. *Medical Microbiology: A Guide to Microbial Infections— Pathogenesis, Immunity, Laboratory Diagnosis and Control,* 15th ed. New York, Churchill Livingstone, 1997

TABLE 17–11. Clinical Indications of Nonclostridial Anaerobic Infection

Foul smelling pus, discharge, or lesion
Large amount of pus/abscess formation
Failure to isolate organisms from pus
Infection associated with necrotic tissue
Gas formation in tissues
Failure to respond to conventional antibiotic therapy
Infected human or animal bite wound
Gram negative bacteremia
Septic thrombophlebitis

Adapted from Greenwood, 1997

TABLE 17–12. Summary of Selected Anaerobic Bacteria

Organism	Summary
Clostridium	Gram positive spore-producing bacilli
C difficile	C difficile is most frequently proven cause for antibiotic associated diarrhea; usually occurs after antibiotic therapy and causes varying degrees of diarrhea; may progress to inflammation of colon mucosa with the most severe form (pseudomembranous colitis) destroying portions of the mucosa; intestinal perforation and sepsis may occur; detected by culture on special media or by testing for the endotoxin produced
C perfringens	C perfringens is common cause of gas gangrene, characterized by rapidly spreading edema, myositis, and tissue necrosis; usually results from contamination of wound with soil containing animal or human fecal material; organisms produce a wide range of potent toxins; other organisms may also be present; immediate, intensive treatment (surgical and antibiotic) required; also seen in septic abortion, peritoneal infections, and food poisoning
C tetani	Different strains of C tetani produce neurotoxins that vary in toxigenicity, some are extremely toxic; neurotoxins affect motor impulses; pain and stiffness usually first symptoms followed by spasms; primarily derived from soil contaminated with animal feces, but spores are present in a wide variety of locations
C botulinus	C botulinus produces severe food poisoning (botulism) due to ingestion of food contaminated with neurotoxin produced by the organism; not common, but may be associated with insufficient heating in the canning process; special cultures or tests for toxin usually only performed in reference laboratories; stool usually tested—vomitus and gastric contents may be tested—and suspected food should also be tested; toxin is heat labile, so specimens must be refrigerated
Bacteroides	Most frequent organisms in anaerobic infections; several species; infection usually results in abscess or gangrene; Bacteroides fragilis is most commonly isolated (accounts for about one fourth of all anaerobes isolated from clinical specimens); Bacteroides organisms seen in intra-abdominal and soft tissue infections, sometimes with focal lesions of GI tract, appendicitis, septic abortion, pelvic abscess in females, and aspiration pneumonia
Gram positive anaerobic cocci	Frequently seen in association with Bacteroides infections, but may produce disease themselves; part of normal flora in mouth, GI tract, genitourinary tract and skin—may cause infections of these sites in some situations; may be isolated from various clinical sites including decubitus, foot ulcers, blood cultures, human or animal bites, abdominal infections, pleural infections, dental abscesses and root canals, and other sites

Table developed based on information from Greenwood, 1997; Henry, 1996; Ravel, 1995

Some of the treponemal pathogens are:

- *Treponema pallidum:* causes syphilis; usually acquired by sexual contact
- *Treponema pertenue:* causes yaws, a disease endemic to rural populations in tropical climates
- *Treponema carateum:* causes pinta, a disfiguring disease confined to the skin; now seen only in certain regions of Mexico, Central America, and Colombia (Greenwood, 1997)

Only **T pallidum** is discussed here. **T pallidum** is primarily transmitted by sexual contact and enters tissues by penetration of intact mucosa or through skin abrasions. The organism rapidly enters the lymphatic system and travels throughout the body via the bloodstream. It may affect various organs. After an incubation period, a lesion (chancre) typical of **primary syphilis** is formed at the site of initial infection. Such lesions may be inconspicuous and remain unnoticed, especially in females. Untreated, syphilis is a progressive disease with stages identified as primary, secondary, latent, and tertiary:

- *Primary:* begins after incubation period of approximately 3 to 6 weeks (incubation may be < 2 weeks or up to 13 weeks [Ravel, 1995]); manifested by formation of shallow painless lesions that usually heal during the 4- to 8-week period of this stage
- *Secondary:* most patients develop rash (especially on the palms of hands and soles of feet) and generalized lymphadenopathy; secondary, widespread, highly contagious lesions appear, especially on trunk and extremities; in the latter part of this stage (which lasts about 12 weeks) visible lesions disappear
- *Latent:* lasts an average of 3 to 5 years; many patients in this stage have active disease relapse during the first year; by end of this stage, about half of untreated patients either do not develop further evidence of disease or have "spontaneous cure"; about one fourth remain in the latent phase; remaining fourth enter tertiary stage; individuals usually not considered infectious in late latent stage, but infection can still be transmitted during pregnancy and blood transfusion
- *Tertiary:* may not develop for decades after initial infection; slowly progressive and destructive effects may be seen in any organ—neurologic, cardiovascular, and ocular syphilis are common; rarely possible to isolate organism in this stage; tertiary syphilis may be fatal

Laboratory diagnosis of syphilis may be accomplished by a variety of methods depending on the clinical circumstances. Some of these methods are summarized in Table 17–13.

Borrelia species are associated with **relapsing fever** and **Lyme disease**. Infections with a number of species in this genus are acquired as a result of tick bites. Lyme disease is named for the city in Connecticut in which the investigation of a cluster of cases of suspected juvenile rheumatoid arthritis led to its dis-

TABLE 17–13. Methods for Laboratory Diagnosis of Syphilis

Test	Explanation	Comments
Microscopic examination	Organism can be directly observed in preparations from syphilitic lesions using a special microscopy technique called *dark-field microscopy* (requires special condenser)	Was only diagnostic method prior to development of immunologic methods; may be beneficial in early primary stage before antibodies are developed; requires specimen collected according to specific protocol and skill/experience for proper interpretation
Non-specific immunologic tests	*T pallidum* infection produces both non-specific and specific antibodies; cardiolipin and reagin tests (VDRL and RPR) detect the non-specific antibodies; RPR is newer, easier to use; VDRL preferred for CSF samples; both give similar results and can be quantitated (titer reported)	Used as screening tests; should be confirmed with more specific test; may not be positive in tertiary syphilis; positive results also seen as a result of other infections (viral, other treponemal organisms, non-treponemal bacteria) or hypersensitivity reactions (usually return to negative in few weeks), some systemic or chronic illnesses including rheumatoid arthritis; false positives higher in older individuals
Specific immunologic tests	Fluorescent treponemal antibody (FTA) and a modification, the FTA-ABS (FTA with absorption); specific antibody test using fluorescent dye viewed with UV microscope	Generally available only in reference labs; not suitable for screening; relatively good sensitivity after early primary stage; only occasional false positives, esp when absorption used

covery in 1975. The causative organism is *Borellia burgdorferi.* Studies suggest that the disease was endemic to the United States more than 10 years earlier and the same clinical manifestations have been known in Europe since the early 1900s (Greenwood, 1997). Natural hosts of *B burgdorferi* are wild and domesticated animals, including rodents and deer. Transmission of the organism to humans occurs as a result of bites from ticks that have become infected by feeding on an infected animal. The most easily recognized manifestation of Lyme disease is a characteristic expanding rash (erythema chronicum migrans, or ECM) seen at the site of the tick bite. Lyme disease can be a progressive, multisystem illness and is divided into three stages. The first stage is characterized by ECM and secondary lesions. Other symptoms may include fever, fatigue, headache, malaise, neck stiffness, sore throat, and generalized lymphadenopathy. Stage two of the illness includes a fading of skin lesions with development of musculoskeletal symptoms or intermittent arthritis and cardiac or neurologic abnormalities. This stage may occur weeks to months after stage one. Stage three may occur months or years later and patients who develop this stage have chronic dermatologic, neurologic, or rheumatologic problems. Chronic cardiac manifestations may also be seen. Laboratory confirmation of suspected Lyme disease typically involves serologic testing for the presence of antibodies to the organism. IgM antibodies typically develop within 3 to 6 weeks (Greenwood, 1997) of infection. After 4 weeks of disease onset, IgG antibody tests are more reliable (Henry, 1996). Initial testing may be performed using enzyme immunoassay or immunofluorescence techniques with Western blot techniques used as follow-up testing for positive or equivocal results (Henry, 1996). Negative screening specimens may warrant testing of a convalescent specimen 2 to 4 weeks after the initial negative specimen. False positive results may be seen as a result of cross-reactivity with antibodies to other spirochetes and other bacteria or in patients with connective tissue diseases or other conditions resulting in the formation of immune complexes. False negative results may be seen when detectable levels of antibodies are slow in developing or in immunosuppressed patients. Although a definitive diagnosis can be made by culturing *B burgdorferi* from appropriate biopsy material (Greenwood, 1997), the organism can be difficult to detect and the procedure involves lengthy, specialized techniques that are not readily available in most clinical environments.

■ ANTIBIOTIC SUSCEPTIBILITY

The positive aspects of widespread antibiotic availability have been accompanied by the development of a number of resistant strains of organisms. Although the sensitivity pattern of many bacteria are usually predictable, laboratory sensitivity studies are often performed on all clinically significant isolates because of the widespread occurrence of bacterial resistance, particularly that of organisms for which sensitivity to β-lactam antibiotics was previously assumed. Appropriate antibiotic therapy is important to reduce the occurrence of such resistance. However, the large number of infections seen in some practices makes it impractical to fully investigate each case and wait for susceptibility studies to be completed prior to the initiation of antibiotic therapy. In other cases, when infection is severe and/or rapidly progressive immediate intervention is warranted. Still, antibiotics should be used only when necessary and avoided in conditions of viral etiology that are responsive to symptomatic treatment. When practical, antibiotic choices should be made on the basis of culture and sensitivity reports and if antibiotic therapy is started while sensitivity results are pending, the report should be evaluated when available. The sensitivity report is especially helpful in such situations if the organism is not susceptible to the antibiotic being administered or to determine if an equally effective, less expensive alternative is available. Sensitivity reports may also be useful for dosage modification of the antibiotic in use. As noted earlier, culture specimens are best collected prior to the initiation of antibiotic therapy and the laboratory should be notified when culture specimens are collected from patients currently on antibiotic therapy. Sensitivity reports are generally available 24 hours after an organism is isolated. With the number of antibiotic agents available continually increasing, microbiologists must determine which antibiotics will be used for testing. Most test representative samples of the various groups of agents. Institutions may have established policies that limit antibiotic choices to some extent or define "preferred" agents. Reports typically indicate whether an organism is sensitive, resistant, or moderately sensitive (intermediate) to each agent tested. Although *in vitro* sensitivity or resistance is generally indicative of the expected *in vivo* response, individual responses may vary.

Antibiotic agents act by differing **mechanisms to inhibit or destroy the infecting organism**, ideally without harming the host (selective toxicity). Antibiotic sites of action include:

- bacterial cell wall: most bacteria have a rigid cell wall; because human cells do not, the cell wall is the primary target for selective toxicity agents; agents with beta lactam rings bind to proteins involved in cell wall construction; penicillins, cephalosporins, and other compounds are in this group
- protein synthesis: bacterial ribosomes sufficiently differ from those of humans to allow selective inhibition of bacterial protein synthesis; tetracylines, aminoglycosides, chloramphenicol, and other agents are in this group
- DNA synthesis: bacterial DNA synthesis may be inhibited directly (quinolones, nitrofurans, and nitromidazoles) or indirectly (by interfering with folic acid metabolism—sulfonamides and diaminopyrimidines)
- RNA synthesis: bacterial RNA synthesis is inhibited by rifamycins

Other factors considered in the selection of an antibiotic (or other antimicrobial agent) include:

- any known allergies
- site of infection
- host renal and/or hepatic function
- host immune mechanisms
- route and frequency of administration
- absorption and excretion attributes
- cost

Laboratory **methods for antibiotic susceptibility testing** are generally based on inhibitory activity rather than on lethal activity. Commonly employed methods are

- disk diffusion: paper disks containing a specified amount of antibiotic agents are placed on a freshly inoculated agar surface; the antibiotic diffuses into the agar; the zone of growth inhibition around the disk is measured; the zone is inversely related to MIC (minimum inhibitory concentration)—that is, the larger zone; the lower MIC
- serial dilution: series of tubes containing various dilutions (and thus antibiotic concentration) are inoculated with the organism; the lowest concentration inhibiting visible growth is the MIC

Therapeutic monitoring of serum antibiotic levels may be indicated for some agents, particularly those with a narrow therapeutic range or those with significant toxic effects. Monitoring is particularly important in patients with impairment of renal function or other underlying conditions that may alter the pharmacokinetics of the antibiotic agent. Collection of specimens at the appropriate time is essential to accurate monitoring. Some antibiotics are best monitored by peak levels (level of highest serum concentration) and others by trough levels (lowest serum concentration). Both peak and trough levels are often most beneficial. The ideal time of collection for peak levels varies according to the **half-life of the antibiotic**, but in general terms specimens for peak levels are collected:

- 30 (60 minutes for vancomycin) minutes after IV infusion completed, or
- 60 minutes after IM injection, or
- 1 to 2 hours after oral dose

Trough levels are generally collected just prior to administration of the next scheduled dose.

Tables 17–14 and 17–15 provide additional information regarding antibiotic therapy.

■ MYCOPLASMAS

The Mycoplasmataceae family is composed of several genera, including the *Mycoplasma* genus and the *Ureaplasma* genus. Organisms belonging to this family are the smallest prokaryotic cells capable of growing in cell free media. They are **pleomorphic** appearing in spherical, coccoid, coccobacillary, ring, and dumbbell forms. Two organisms from this family are presented here. First, *Ureaplasma urealyticum* (formerly known as *T mycoplasma*) is found in the cervix or vagina of up to 80 % (Ravel, 1995) of healthy females and has been isolated from the urethra of both sexes. Evidence suggests that it may be capable of producing placental and fetal infection in pregnant women colonized by the organism.

Mycoplasma pneumoniae (formerly called *pleuropneumonia-like organisms,* or PPLO) causes a lower respiratory tract infection often referred to as *primary atypical pneumonia.* Many cases appear as upper respiratory infections of varying severity. White cell counts are normal with most *M pneumoniae* infections. Cultures can be performed using either sputum or nasopharyngeal swabs. Special transport media is required for swabs because the organisms are very sensitive to drying and special media (generally available only in reference laboratories) is required for growth. Elevated cold agglutinins (antibodies that will agglutinate group O red cells at low temperatures), though non-specific, are elevated in more than half of patients. Even though elevations may be produced by other conditions, in the presence of an acute respiratory syndrome a cold agglutinin titer of more than 1:32 is generally associated with mycoplasmal pneumonia. Serologic complement fixation tests for the detection of antibodies (antibody usually appears in second week after infection) are also used for diagnosis, but are being replaced by less time consuming immunofluorescent techniques.

TABLE 17–14. Organisms with Generally Predictable Susceptibility

Organism	Usually Susceptible to[1]
Streptococci	Penicillin Erythromycin Vancomycin
Enterococci	Ampicillin Vancomycin
Staphylococci	Gentamicin Vancomycin Clindamycin Flucloxacillin
Anaerobic cocci	Penicillin Erythromycin Metronidazole
Hemophilus influenzae	Erythromycin Tetracycline Cefotaxime
Escherichia coli	Gentamicin Ciprofloxamine Cefotaxime
Proteus mirabilis	Gentamicin Ciprofloxacine Cefotaxime
Pseudomonas aeruginosa	Gentamicin Ciprofloxacine Ceftazidime Azlocillin Imipenem
Bacteriodes fragilis	Metronidazole Cefoxitin
Chlamydia	Tetracyclines Rifampicin Macrolides

[1]List is not all inclusive.

Adapted from Greenwood D, Slack R, Peutherer J. *Medical Microbiology: A Guide to Microbial Infections—Pathogenesis, Immunity, Laboratory Diagnosis and Control*, 15th ed. New York, Churchill Livingstone, 1997

TABLE 17–15. Differential Toxicity of Selected Aminoglycosides

Antibiotic	Nephrotoxicity	Ototoxicity
Gentamicin	++	++
Amikacin	+	++
Neomycin	++	+++
Streptocmycin	±	+++
Tobramycin	++	++
Kanamycin	++	++

Relative toxicities from Greenwood, 1997

TIME FOR REVIEW. After studying the preceding sections, you should be able to respond correctly to the following:

■ Define the following terms:

pathogenic:

normal flora:

opportunistic pathogen:

obligate aerobe:

microaerophilic aerobe:

facultative anaerobe:

obligate anaerobe:

■ List three conditions important to microbial growth.

■ List and briefly explain seven general principles for the collection of specimens for culture.

■ List and briefly describe the four stages of bacterial growth.

■ In the term *Escherichia coli,* _____ indicates the genus and _____ indicates the species.

■ List three *direct* methods used in bacterial identification.

■ Methods of typing different bacterial strains include _____, which uses antibodies against particular surface structures; _____ based on susceptibility to lysis by certain bacteriophages; _____ using susceptibility to a naturally occurring antibacterial substance; and _____ using electrophoresis techniques.

■ A critical step in the Gram stain, which if performed incorrectly can result in confusion of gram positive and gram negative organisms, is _____ .

■ Preliminary identification of bacteria can be accomplished based on oxygen requirements, Gram stain results, and the _____ and _____ tests.

■ Staphylococci are gram _____ cocci typically appearing in irregular clusters. They are catalase _____ (positive/negative).

■ The major staphylococcal pathogen is *Staphylococcus* _____.

■ A major laboratory distinction between *Staph aureus* and *Staph epidermidis* is their reaction in the _____ test.

■ The most common site of infection with *Staph aureus* is the _____.

■ *Staph aureus* organisms that produce an enzyme called _____ are called methicillin resistant staph aureus (MRSA).

■ Streptococci that produce a clear zone of hemolysis are called _____ hemolytic.

■ Streptococcus pyogenes is a _____-hemolytic, group _____ strep that most commonly causes an acute sore throat.

■ List three enzymes or toxins produced by group A beta-hemolytic strep.

■ _____ sensitivity testing is used for presumptive identification of group A beta-hemolytic strep.

■ Group _____ strep are most frequently associated with neonatal septicemia and meningitis and with post-partum septicemia and endometritis.

■ *Strep* _____ is a common cause of bacterial pneumonia and may also be seen in middle ear infections and meningitis.

■ _____ and _____ of the Enterobacteriaceae family are always pathogens introduced from the environment.

■ Enterobacteriaceae are gram _____ bacilli that are oxidase and catalase _____ (positive/negative).

■ _____ is a major cause of food poisoning and possesses two types of antigens called _____ antigens and _____ antigens.

■ List three infections caused by *Salmonella* species.

■ The organism that produces bacillary dysentery is _____.

■ The most common cause of urinary tract infection and gram negative septicemia is _____.

■ The specific strain of the above organism associated with a particularly severe diarrhea with bloody stools seen as a result of improperly cooked beef is _____.

■ A characteristic feature of _____ organisms is their ability to swarm on solid culture media.

■ _____ is a gram negative rod that typically produces a grape-like odor and is an important opportunistic pathogen in immunocompromised patients. The organism is associated with urinary tract infection, infected burn sites, infections obtained from whirlpools.

■ This genus consists of small, pleomorphic gram negative bacilli (coccobacilli) that require blood or certain blood constituents for growth _____.

■ _____ (include genus, species, and type) is the most common etiology of meningitis in children between the ages of 2 months and 5 years.

■ _____ , a spiral gram negative bacillus, was discovered in 1983 and is associated with the development of peptic ulcers.

■ _____ *jejuni* is the most common cause of diarrhea in most developed countries.

■ The highly contagious etiologic agent of whooping cough is _____.

■ The two primary species of *Neisseria* are _____ and _____. List the infection(s) caused by each species.

■ These two *Neisseria* species are very similar morphologically and are gram _____ diplo_____.

■ The normal inhabitant of the upper respiratory tract that closely resembles *Neisseria* is _____.

■ The organisms most commonly seen as the cause of nongonococcal urethritis in men is _____.

■ Anaerobes typically produce a large amount of pus and a _____.

■ The anaerobe _____ is the most common proven cause of antibiotic associated diarrhea.

■ _____ is a common cause of gas gangrene.

■ _____ causes tetanus.

■ _____ produces a severe food poisoning called botulism.

■ The anaerobe most commonly isolated from clinical specimens is _____.

■ The spirochetes include the genera _____ and _____.

■ The causative agent of syphilis is _____.

■ List and briefly describe the four stages of syphilis.

■ List and briefly describe four methods for laboratory diagnosis of syphilis.

■ The organism identified in Lyme disease is _____, which may be contracted as a result of _____ bite.

■ List four mechanisms of antibiotic action with at least one example of each.

■ List and briefly describe two laboratory methods for antibiotic susceptibility testing.

■ Therapeutic antibiotic monitoring is especially important for antibiotics with a narrow _____ and in hosts with impaired _____ function.

■ The appropriate time to collect specimens for antibiotic monitoring is dependent on the _____ _____ of the antibiotic being tested.

Check your responses by reviewing the preceding sections.

MYCOBACTERIOLOGY

The *Mycobacterium* genus consists of numerous species. The **Mycobacteria** (fungus-bacteria) are **acid-fast bacilli** with **thick, waxy cell walls**. The "acid-fast" designation refers to their characteristic ability to retain a carbol fuchsin or other arylmethane dye and resist subsequent decolorization with an acidic agent such as acid alcohol. This ability is related to the structure of the organism's cell wall. Although tuberculosis in humans may result from infection with one of four closely related species of *Mycobacteria,* the most common cause by far is **Mycobacterium tuberculosis** (*Mycobacterium bovis,* a bovine tubercle bacillus, causes some cases; *Mycobacterium microti* very rarely, if ever; and *Mycobacterium africani* mainly in equatorial Africa [Greenwood, 1997]).

These slow growing organisms require special, enriched media (Lowenstein-Jensen media is most commonly used) for growth and require weeks for colonies to become evident. Once culture growth is evident, biochemical and growth tests are performed to identify the organism. **Conventional culture and biochemical testing** may require up to 6 weeks for completion. Instrumentation has been developed that reduces identification time to < 1 week. **Acid-fast smears** of sputum are used for rapid presumptive diagnosis of **pulmonary tuberculosis**. Appropriate specimen collection is essential and most laboratories screen submitted specimens, rejecting those that are inadequate for testing. **DNA probes and DNA probes with PCR** amplification are now available for the specific identification of *M tuberculosis*. These methods, generally available only at reference laboratories, allow direct detection of the organism in clinical specimens. **Renal tuberculosis** is not usually clinically evident for many years and most patients do not have systemic symptoms such as fever. Pyuria with negative urine culture and microscopic hematuria are frequent findings in renal tuberculosis; gross hematuria may be seen in some patients. Some patients may have a positive urine culture with another pathogen in addition to the *M tuberculosis* organism. Because routine urine culture methods cannot detect the *M tuberculosis* organism, the laboratory must be informed of a suspicion of renal tuberculosis or a specific AFB culture requested.

The organism ***Mycobacterium leprae*** is the causative agent of **leprosy**, a disease resulting in deformity and disfigurement. Worldwide, about 600,000 new cases are still reported each year (Greenwood, 1997). Clinical diagnosis is confirmed by histologic examination of skin biopsies and by detection of the organism in nasal discharge, scrapings of nasal mucosa, or tissue fluid and cells taken from superficial incisions in the skin.

Other mycobacterial organisms normally exist in soil and water (**environmental mycobacteria**) and are implicated in opportunistic infections. These organisms are classified into four groups (called *Runyon groups* for the botanist who developed the classification system) based on pigment production and rate of growth. Table 17–16 summarizes features of some of these species.

TABLE 17–16. Selected Environmental Mycobacteria Causing Human Disease

Species	Runyon Group	Associated Diseases
M. marinum	I	Swimming pool granuloma
M. kansasii	I	Pulmonary disease
M. scrofulaceum	II	Lymphadenopathy
		Lymphadenopathy
M. avium complex	III	Pulmonary disease
		Disseminated disease
		(AIDS related & non-AIDS related)
M. terrae	III	Post-trauma abscesses
M. malmoense	III	Pulmonary
M. fortuitum	IV	Post-trauma abscesses
M. chelonae	IV	Non-AIDS related disseminated disease
		Post-trauma abscesses

Table compiled based on information from Greenwood, 1997 and Henry, 1996

VIROLOGY

Viruses are capable of growth only within living cells and are generally composed of a single strand of either DNA or RNA in a protein shell called a *capsid*. The capsid is sometimes enclosed in a lipoprotein envelope, the constituents of which are largely obtained from the host cell. They are the **most frequent cause of infectious disease in humans**—diseases that range from the common cold and childhood diseases to AIDS. Many of the commonly encountered viral infections (eg, influenza, respiratory syncytial virus [RSV] and others) display seasonal differences. A variety of laboratory methods (Table 17–17) are now available for the diagnosis of viral diseases. Some of these methods have made it possible for some level of virology testing to be available in most clinical laboratories. Other methods, those that are particularly expensive or complex or those that are infrequently requested, are generally available only in reference laboratories.

TABLE 17–17. Laboratory Methods for Detection of Viral Disease

Method	Comments
Tissue culture	Uses living cell preparations of various types; labor intensive and highly specialized; requires several days for growth and identification of organism
Antigen or nucleic acid detection	Direct detection of viral antigen or nucleic acids; variety of procedures including latex agglutination, fluorescent techniques, (ELISA), and DNA probes
Antibody detection	Serologic tests for detection of antibodies produced in response to viral infections; available for most viruses; techniques include latex agglutination, fluorescent techniques, ELISA, hemagglutination, and complement fixation
Special stains	Histologic staining procedures for detection of herpes simplex or varicella-zoster infections; scrapings from skin vesicles are used

As with other laboratory samples, it is essential for **specimens for viral culture** to be collected, transported, and stored in accordance with established procedures to maintain viability of the organism. Improperly maintained specimens are unlikely to contain viable organisms and thus are unsuitable for testing. These specimens should be rejected for testing or clearly indicated as improperly collected specimens on laboratory reports to avoid reporting invalid results. Special transport media is commercially available and should be kept on hand for the collection of these specimens. Questions or uncertainties regarding the optimal methods for collection, transport, and storage should be directed to the testing laboratory prior to obtaining samples for testing. **Specimens for culture or for detection of viral antigens** should be collected during the acute stage of the illness. Antibody development generally occurs about 1 to 2 weeks after the onset of illness. Antibody detection without demonstration of rising titer does not differentiate current or recent infections from past infections. Therefore, **specimens for diagnosis of infection by antibody detection** should be collected in both the early stages (**acute** specimen) and in latter stages (**convalescent** specimen) for comparison of antibody titer. In some cases (eg, rubella) antibody titers are used to demonstrate immunity in the patient rather than for the detection of disease.

A comprehensive listing and discussion of viral syndromes and their causative agents is beyond the scope of this text. Table 17–18 lists the primary types of viruses that cause human disease and some examples of the viruses in each group. Selected syndromes and viral agents are discussed briefly in this section.

■ RESPIRATORY INFECTIONS OF VIRAL ETIOLOGY

Viruses are responsible for most respiratory infections. Viral infections of the upper respiratory tract are not frequently of sufficient severity to require laboratory testing. Such infections commonly include the common cold caused by a vari-

TABLE 17–18. Primary Viruses Causing Human Disease

Virus	Examples
RNA Viruses	
Orthomyxoviruses	Influenza viruses A, B, and C
Paramyxoviruses	Parainfluenza viruses; mumps; measles; respiratory syncytial virus (RSV)
Rhabdoviruses	Rabies virus
Filoviruses	Ebola virus and Marburg virus
Togaviruses	Rubella virus
Flaviviruses	Yellow fever virus; Dengue virus; Japanese encephalitis virus
Caliviruses	Hepatitis E virus
Picornaviruses	Poliovirus; Coxsackie A and B; echovirus; enterovirus; hepatitis A virus; rhinovirus (common cold)
Retroviruses	Human immunodeficiency virus (HIV); human T lymphocyte virus (HTLV) types I and II
Reoviruses	Rotaviruses
DNA Viruses	
Poxviruses	Variola; vaccinia
Herpesviruses	Herpes simplex viruses I and II; varicella-zoster virus; cytomegalovirus; Epstein-Barr virus
Adenoviruses	Many serotypes
Polyomaviruses	Papillomaviruses (warts)
Hepadnaviruses	Hepatitis B virus
Parvovirus	B19 virus

Adapted from Greenwood D, Slack R, Peutherer J. *Medical Microbiology: A Guide to Microbial Infections— Pathogenesis, Immunity, Laboratory Diagnosis and Control,* 15th ed. New York, Churchill Livingstone, 1997

ety of serotypes of the **rhinovirus** and viral pharyngitis. Viral infections of the lower respiratory tract more frequently result in the submission of specimens for laboratory testing. In the adult, influenza viruses are the most important pathogen; in children, RSV, the parainfluenza virus, and adenovirus are important pathogens in addition to influenza. Features of viral syndromes of the lower respiratory tract are summarized in Table 17–19.

■ HERPES SIMPLEX VIRUS INFECTIONS

There are two serotypes (1 and 2) of herpes simplex virus (HSV) that cause infections in humans and most adult sera contain detectable levels of antibody to one or both types. However, antibody detection is not useful in predicting immunity because individuals with antibody may still be susceptible to infection with another strain of the virus. The virus persists in a latent or dormant form in the basal root ganglia of peripheral nerves and may be reactivated. Primary infection may be asymptomatic or lesions called *vesicles* may be produced. Primary infection or reinfection is ordinarily acquired from close contact with an infected individual. Although HSV 1 and HSV 2 are distinctly different viruses, they are closely related and share some of the same antigens. **HSV 1** is associated with **non-genital infections** that include:

- mouth lesions (canker sores)
- blisters on the border of the lips (cold sores) *(cont.)*

TABLE 17–19. Viral Infections of the Lower Respiratory Tract

Viral Syndrome	Causative Agents	Comments
Influenza	Influenza A virus Influenza B virus	Acute febrile respiratory tract infection with short incubation period and systemic symptoms including chills, headache, myalgia and anorexia; type A more common and usually more serious than B; annual winter outbreaks; antibodies produced in previous infections often provide no protection because of viral antigen mutation and recombination of nucleic acid segments; best diagnosed in first 2 to 3 days of illness by culture, but may not be positive for 2 to 7 days
Bronchiolitis	Respiratory syncytial virus (RSV) Parainfluenza 3 Influenza A virus Influenza B virus Adenovirus Measles	RSV important cause of serious lower respiratory tract infection in young children and infants; may also cause severe disease in elderly and immunocompromised; transmitted by oronasal aerosol and close contact; immunity resulting from prior infection incomplete and short lived; rapid diagnosis important to prevent spread; barrier precautions (ie, masks, gowns, etc.) and isolation minimize hospital spread; organism unlikely to remain viable if transport delayed; detection of RSV by direct fluorescent staining or ELISA provide rapid results and are as sensitive, or more sensitive than cultures
Croup	Parainfluenza 1, 2, and 3 RSV Influenza A virus Influenza B virus Adenovirus Measles	Laryngotracheobronchitis; most commonly caused by parainfluenza virus; "barking" cough and obstructed breathing pattern are characteristic; direct fluorescent staining and ELISA provide rapid results, but are less sensitive than culture and should be followed by culture if negative
Pneumonia	RSV Influenza A virus Influenza B virus Parainfluenza 3 Adenovirus Measles Cytomegalovirus Varicella-zoster virus	Infections may progress to severe pneumonia; pneumonia and influenza together have significant morbidity and mortality (9% of deaths in flu season [Henry, 1996]); primary influenza pneumonia may occur during outbreak and may be fatal after very short illness (sometimes 1 day or less) especially in the young adult and in elderly (Greenwood, 1997)

Table compiled based on information from Greenwood, 1997; Henry, 1996; Ravel, 1995

- corneal ulcers (keratitis)
- focal lesions on fingers
- encephalitis (usually temporal lobe; severe condition)

HSV 2 produces **genital lesions** and is a sexually transmitted disease. The incubation period for a primary symptomatic infection averages about 1 week, but may be significantly shorter or longer. Systemic symptoms, including fever, malaise, and myalgia, are experienced by about half of patients. Some patients may have a mild, self-limiting aseptic meningitis (Ravel, 1995). In addition to genital ulceration, lesions may occur elsewhere on the body, particularly (but not limited to) the groin area. Urethral involvement is seen in about half of patients. Most patients with HSV genital lesions have **recurrent infections**, which differ notably from primary infection. Few patients exhibit systemic symptoms with recurrent infection and extragenital lesions are not commonly seen. The **infection may be acquired by neonates** during the delivery process, but may not be evident for days or weeks following exposure. Initial symptoms may be consistent with sepsis or meningitis. Most delivery infected infants are born of mothers who were not symptomatic at the time.

Laboratory methods for the detection of HSV include:

- culture: special transport media required; specimens from vesicular lesions are better than material from ulcerative lesions; material from crusted lesions provides the least suitable specimen for detection of the organism; lesions from primary infection are more likely to produce positive culture than lesions in reinfection or recurrence
- antigen detection: more rapid results than culture; most methods can distinguish types 1 and 2, but some cross-reactivity may occur; sensitivity varies considerably among different tests, but is usually greater with mucocutaneous lesions than with genital lesions (Ravel, 1995); DNA probe methods have high sensitivity and specificity
- direct staining methods: includes the Tzanck smear for detection of multinucleated epithelial cells
- antibody detection: acute and convalescent specimens should be obtained 2 weeks apart; four-fold increase in titer indicates recent onset of infection, but is unlikely to be seen in recurrent infection; diagnostic titer increase most often seen in primary HSV 2 infections

■ VARICELLA-ZOSTER VIRUS

Varicella-Zoster is a member of the herpesvirus family and is spread by **direct contact** with lesions or via **droplet inhalation**. Infection with this virus (the varicella virus and the zoster virus have been confirmed as identical [Greenwood, 1997]) is seen in two forms:

- varicella: chicken pox; primary infection; seen predominantly in children; generalized vesicular skin eruption; virus enters through upper respiratory tract or conjunctiva and multiplies in lymph nodes before entering the bloodstream; incubation period averages 2 weeks; individuals are infectious 2 days before (thus the rapid spread among children) and up to 5 days after onset while new vesicles are appearing (Greenwood, 1997);

ranges from a mild condition with few scattered lesions to a severe febrile condition with widespread vesicles; a more serious condition with greater likelihood of complications in adults and older children, and particularly in immunocompromised individuals (complications may involve variety of organs and include thrombocytopenia, myocarditis, arthritis, pneumonitis, CNS complications, and glomerulonephritis); secondary bacterial infection of lesions is the most common complication in young children

* zoster: shingles; reactivated infection; localized unilateral eruption; pathogenesis is not well described and stimulus of reactivation is not known; frequency of occurrence increases with age; more frequent in patients who are immunocompromised and those with malignancy; neuralgia is the most common symptom; a rash is usually present; it generally involves single dermatome; disseminated infection is indicated by lesions at distant sites or involvement of organs such as lung or brain; complications include postherpetic neuralgia (intractable pain persisting more than 1 month after rash; more common in older patients; may be a disabling condition lasting a year or more), ocular involvement, and encephalitis

■ HEPATITIS VIRUS

A comprehensive discussion of hepatitis viruses is beyond the scope of this text. Important general information is presented in summary fashion in Tables 17–20 and 17–21. See Chapter 4 for liver function tests in hepatitis.

TABLE 17–20. Hepatitis Virus Infections

Condition	Type of Virus	Incubation Period	Mortality (Acute)	Chronic Form	Laboratory Testing
Hepatitis A	Enterovirus 72 (Picornavirus)	28 days (14-45 days)	<1%	No	HAV antigen in stool; HAV-IgM Ab = current or recent infection; HAV-IgG Ab = old or convalescent infection
Hepatitis B	Hepadnavirus	2-3 months (29-180 days)	~ 1.4%	5% to 10% in adults (more in infants and children)	See Table 14.20
Hepatitis C	Flavivirus	6-8 weeks (2 wks to 1 year)	1-2%	>60%	HCV-IgG Ab = current, convalescent, or old infection
Hepatitis D	Delta virus (requires assistance from hepadnavirus)	3-13 weeks	up to 30%	10%-15%	HDV Ab (total) for screening HDV Ab-IgM = higher in acute infection
Hepatitis E	Calicivirus	6 weeks (14-63 days)	1%-2% (much higher in pregnant women)	No	No test methods specific for hepatitis E are commercially available yet

Table developed based on information from Greenwood, 1997; Henry, 1996; Ravel, 1995

TABLE 17–21. Hepatitis B Tests

Test	Abbreviation	Comments
Hepatitis B surface antigen	HB$_s$Ag	Immunoassay or nuclei acid probe methods; presence indicates current, active infection; persistence over 6 months indicates chronic/carrier state; usually detectable 2-6 weeks after exposure (sooner by nucleic acid probes); jaundice may be present before antigen detected in some patients
Hepatitis B surface antibody	HB$_s$Ab	Appears about 2-6 weeks after surface antigen disappears; peaks 2-8 weeks after appearance; usually persists for life in lower titer; about 10% of patients do not develop detectable levels of antibody; shows previous infection and immunity
Hepatitis B core antibody—IgM	HB$_c$Ab-IgM	Appears about 2 weeks after disappearance of HB$_s$Ag and becomes undetectable about 3-6 months after appearance
Hepatitis B core antibody—Total	HB$_c$Ab-Tot.	Appears 3-4 weeks after disappearance of HB$_s$Ag and remains elevated for life at gradually lower titer

Compiled from Greenwood, 1997; Henry, 1996; Ravel, 1995

■ CYTOMEGALOVIRUS

Cytomegalovirus (CMV) is a member of the herpesvirus group and is the most common intrauterine infection. Most affected infants are asymptomatic at birth. The organism's name (meaning "large cell") comes from the swelling seen in infected cells in culture and tissues. Infection is acquired through contact with

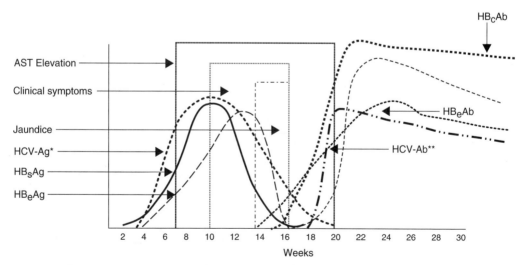

FIGURE 17–3. Development of hepatitis antigens and antibodies, AST elevation and clinical symptoms. * = HCV-Ag by RNA Probe; **HCV-IgG Ab. Diagram is approximation for illustration purposes only; antibodies depicted reflect total antibodies (ie, IgG and IgM) unless otherwise noted; diagram developed based on information from Henry, 1996; Ravel, 1995; Sacher, 1991; and Figures 17–3 through 17–7 in Ravel, 1996.

cervical secretions, semen, saliva, breast milk, blood, and urine. Infection more commonly occurs during the fetal and early childhood periods or in late adolescence and early adulthood. Most infected individuals are totally asymptomatic or have only mild symptoms. However, serious or even life threatening infection may be seen in the neonate or in immunocompromised hosts. Diagnosis may be made by culture or by serologic testing for the presence of antibodies. Culture methods are best for immunocompromised patients who may not produce detectable antibody levels. Serologic testing is used to determine the CMV status of blood for transfusion or organs for transplantation.

■ EPSTEIN-BARR VIRUS

Epstein-Barr virus (EBV) is also a herpesvirus and is the causative agent of **infectious mononucleosis** (IM). It has also been associated with Burkitt's lymphoma, nasopharyngeal carcinoma, and chronic fatigue syndrome. Although its role is not entirely clear, EBV is linked to the development of some malignancies in immunocompromised patients, especially those with AIDS, and may play some role in Hodgkin's disease. Like other members of the herpesvirus family, EBV becomes latent after primary infection and its presence is not necessarily indicative of current infection. The virus is difficult to culture from infected persons, so preferred testing is based on the detection of antibodies. These methods include techniques for the detection of **heterophile antibodies** and for **specific antibodies**. Most rapid slide tests for mononucleosis involve the detection of heterophile antibodies and thus, although highly suggestive of IM, are not specific for mononucleosis. More specific serologic tests for EBV are summarized in Table 17–22. Interpretation of EBV testing results is summarized in Table 17–23.

TABLE 17–22. Laboratory Tests for EBV Antibodies

Antibody	Summary
EBV-VCA, IgM	Antibody to viral capsid antigen; detectable about the same time as symptoms develop and peak about 1 week later; remain detectable for 2-3 months and occasionally up to 1 year
EBV-VCA, IgG	Appear about 3 days after onset of symptoms and peak during second week; detectable levels, though lower, persist for life
EBV-EA-D	Antibody to early antigen-diffuse (antigen spread throughout cytoplasm); appears during first week, peaks in 2-3 weeks, and disappears during convalescent stage; most patients with IM produce detectable levels; typically elevated in EBV-associated nasopharyngeal carcinoma
EBV-EA-R	Restricted antigen found in only one area of the cytoplasm; found in some IM patients (esp children < 2 years old) and is usually elevated in patients with EBV-related Burkitt's lymphoma
EBV-NA, IgG	Antibody to nuclear antigen; appear about 3 weeks after onset, peak at about 8 months and persist for life
EBV-NA, IgM	Detectable about the same time as symptoms develop and peak about 1 week later; remain detectable for 2-3 months and occasionally up to 1 year

Information from Henry, 1996; Jacobs, 1990; Ravel, 1995

TABLE 17–23. Interpretation of EBV Antibody Results

	VCA-IgM	VCA-IgG	EBNA-IgG	EA-D	Heterophile
Presumptive primary infection					+ (with symptoms)
Primary infection	+		0		+ or 0
Reactivated infection	0	+	+	+	0
Previous infection (old)	0	+	+	0	0
Never infected	0	0			

+ = positive; 0 = negative

Information from Henry, 1996; Ravel, 1995

■ RUBELLA VIRUS

Although infections can occur in adulthood, **rubella infections (German measles)** is a common infection of childhood. It assumes particular importance during pregnancy, because **congenital infection** may occur. Although cultures are available, serologic testing provides more rapid results and allows quantitation of antibody levels to assess immune status. A variety of methods are available, with latex agglutination, enzyme immunoassay, and passive hemagglutination techniques most commonly used (Sacher and McPherson, 1991). **Titers at or above 1:8 are evidence of immunity** to rubella. Immunity may be active (as a result of the disease itself) or passive (resulting from immunization).

■ HUMAN IMMUNODEFICIENCY VIRUS

The human immunodeficiency virus (HIV) is an RNA retrovirus and the causative agent of acquired immune deficiency syndrome (AIDS). Two different HIV viruses have been detected: HIV-1 and HIV-2 (recently found in West Africa and also appears to be associated with AIDS). The HIV-1 antigen is detectable serologically shortly after the virus is acquired, but antibodies may not be detected (seroconversion) for several weeks to years later. Active viral reproduction and infection continue even in the presence of antibodies directed against the antigen (similar to that seen in herpesvirus group). **Opportunistic infections** (particularly with *Pneumocystis carnii, Candida albicans, Cryptococcus neoformans, Mycobacterium avium,* and protozoans *Toxoplasma* and *Crytosporidium;* the malignancy, Kaposi's sarcoma, is also commonly seen) are the hallmark of AIDS. The disease is not covered in detail in this section, but diagnostic tests are summarized in Table 17–24. Performing absolute or relative measurements of the **CD4 lymphocytes** (the cells selectively infected by HIV) are used to **assess immune status**. Quantitative measurement of viral load is available using polymerase chain reacion (PCR) techniques.

TABLE 17–24. Tests for Diagnosis of HIV-1 Infection

Test	Summary
Antigen detection	Direct antigen detection by methods including fluorescent techniques, ELISA, and nucleic acid probes with PCR amplification; sensitivity varies, but nucleic acid probes are generally more sensitive; antigen can be detected earlier than antibodies; development of antigen detection tests is recent and tests are generally only available in reference laboratories; positive antigen tests are evidence of infection with the HIV virus, not of the development of the associated disease of AIDS
Antibody detection	Seroconversion (production of detectable antibodies) generally occurs 6-10 weeks after exposure, but may not occur for years; IgM antibodies are detectable first and are no longer detectable after about 2-4 months; IgG antibodies appear about 1-2 weeks after IgM antibodies and persist for life (may disappear shortly before death resulting from overwhelming infection); enzyme immunoassay techniques used
Confirmatory	Western blot (an immunochromatographic technique) is "gold standard" confirmatory test; immunofluorescence techniques are also available and ELISA and latex agglutination tests that utilize genetically engineered HIV proteins have been recently developed
Culture	May detect organisms prior to serologic detection of antigen, but is quite difficult and takes several days; more often positive in early stages than in later; detects only one half or fewer of infected neonates in the first month of life

MYCOLOGY

Fungi are non-photosynthetic organisms with rigid cell walls, including molds, mushrooms (higher fungi), lichens, and yeasts. Many forms are pathogenic to animals and human. The detection and identification of these organisms takes place in the mycology department of the laboratory. Mold **fungi** grow in branching filaments called **hyphae** that form a mesh-like appearance called **mycelium**. Reproduction occurs by formation of various kinds of spores from the mycelium. **Yeasts** are oval or spherical cells that may reproduce by budding or by spore formation. They do not form true mycelium, but yeast-like fungi from pseudomycelium and dimorphic fungi produce vegetative (feeding) mycelium in cultures but are yeast-like in infected lesions. *Actinomycetes* and *Nocardiae* are *bacteria* that produce diseases that resemble fungal infections. **Laboratory tests** for the diagnosis of fungal infections are summarized in Table 17–25 and selected organisms are discussed briefly in this section. In addition to the laboratory methods discussed, **skin tests** are available for some of these organisms. Skin tests can produce positive results in subsequent serologic testing.

TABLE 17–25. Laboratory Methods for Fungal Infection

Method	Description

Direct observation:
  Wet prep
  KOH prep
  India ink prep
  Stained smears
  Tissue biopsy
	Organisms may be observed microscopically using various techniques, including the wet preparation—wet prep or wet mount (exudate or fresh swab specimen in saline); KOH prep (exudate, scrapings, fresh swab specimen in 10% potassium hydroxide); India Ink prep (preparation used to visualize cryptococcus organisms); other stains including Gram stain, Wright's or Giemsa for histoplasmosis, and Papanicolaou stain; tissue biopsy specimens may be stained with periodic acid-Schiff or methenamine silver stains to demonstrate organisms

Culture	Permits isolation and identification of specific organism; requires special culture media and several days to grow; properly obtained specimens are necessary to ensure adequate yield and viable organisms upon laboratory receipt
Serologic tests	Tests for presence of antibodies; especially useful when appropriate specimens for other tests are difficult to obtain or when results of other tests are negative with clinical indications of fungal infection; acute and convalescent specimens are often required and should be collected one to two weeks apart; methods include latex agglutination, enzyme immunoassay, complement fixation, and immunodiffusion

◼ HISTOPLASMOSIS

Histoplasmosis, caused by ***Histoplasma capsulatum,*** is the most commonly encountered systemic fungal infection and is most frequently in the Mississippi and Ohio Valley areas. Certain birds, especially chickens and starlings (Ravel, 1995), transmit the disease to humans, placing farmers in a particular risk group. Just over half of infected individuals in endemic areas are asymptomatic, with others developing pulmonary disease ranging from mild to severe or serious disseminated infections. The disease begins with a primary pulmonary lesion that may resemble the early lesions of tuberculosis. Histoplasmosis infection is most commonly demonstrated by the use of serologic tests for the demonstration of antibodies. **Complement fixation** is the most commonly used method. **Antibody titers of ≥ 1:32** are strongly suggestive of infection (Ravel, 1995), as is a **fourfold rise in titer** between acute and convalescent specimens. Titers < 1:32 provide presumptive evidence of infection.

◼ BLASTOMYCOSIS

Blastomyces dermatitidis, a dimorphic fungus, produces a chronic infection of the lungs with granulomatous lesions resembling the early lesions of tuberculosis. Infection may spread to other tissues, especially the skin. Infection results from the inhalation of spores and is seen more commonly in the midwestern United States and eastern Canada (Greenwood, 1997). The illness progresses slowly and, untreated, has a poor prognosis. **Skin tests are unreliable**

for blastomycosis, producing positive results in only about half (Ravel, 1995) of cases and exhibiting cross-reactivity with histoplasmosis and coccidioidomycosis (Greenwood, 1997). Many serologic tests are similarly unreliable. **Serologic tests** must be chosen and interpreted carefully with knowledge of the **specificity** and **sensitivity** of the particular method, because some methods have low sensitivity (detecting less than half of cases) and show cross-reactivity with histoplasmosis. **Newer immunodiffusion and ELISA methods** are best used for diagnosis as they have more adequate sensitivity and specificity levels.

■ CRYPTOCOCCOSIS

Pigeon feces is the primary source of infection with *Coccidioides immitis,* a fungus most frequently infecting the CNS and the lungs. Persons with diminished immune mechanisms are particularly susceptible. Pulmonary infections are more common and may be subclinical in many cases. CNS infections is typically slowly progressive and may be severe. The thick capsule that is characteristic of the organism can be visualized microscopically using **India Ink** or nigrosin preparations. Serologic tests for the demonstration of both antigen and antibody are available. Diagnosis may also be made by culture or by staining of tissue biopsy.

■ CANDIDIASIS

Infections with *Candida* species may either be superficial or disseminated. *Candida albicans* is the most frequently encountered pathogenic species and causes infection as an opportunitistic pathogen. Localized infections of the skin, oral cavity (thrush), and vagina are not uncommon and are easily diagnosed. Presumptive diagnosis is often made based on results of KOH and/or wet preps. The organism grows readily on a variety of media. Disseminated candidiasis is often more difficult to diagnose as organisms may not be easily isolated from the blood. Infections with this organism are associated with antibiotic therapy, diabetes, and conditions resulting in suppression of the immune system. In addition to culture techniques, serological tests using immunodiffusion and latex agglutination are available.

PARASITOLOGY

Infection with parasitic agents is diagnosed either by direct visualization of the organism or by using serologic tests for the detection of antibodies produced in response to the agent. As emphasized for various other laboratory areas, it is imperative that specimens be collected and maintained according to established procedures. Some parasites are more hardy and easily detected, but others will not likely be detected in unsuitable specimens. A detailed presentation of parasitology procedures and the diseases resulting from parasitic pathogens cannot be addressed in this text. However, some of the principal pathogens are presented briefly in Tables 17–26, 17–27, and 17–28.

TABLE 17–26. Selected Protozoan Pathogens

Pathogen	Disease	Laboratory Detection
Plasmodium faciparum Plasmodium vivax Plasmodium ovale Plasmodium malariae	Malaria	Microscopic exam of stained blood smear (quickest method and, with experienced observer, most reliable) Indirect immunofluorescence DNA probes
Toxoplasma gondii (found in intestinal tract of cats)	Toxoplasmosis	Indirect immunofluorescence Enzyme immunoassay
Entamoeba histolytica	Amoebic dysentery	Microscopic exam for detection of active amoebae or of cysts; serologic tests occasionally helpful
Giardia lamblia	Fat malabsorption and diarrhea	Microscopic examination for detection of trophozoite form or of cyst
Trichomonas vaginalis (transmitted sexually)	Vaginitis	Microscopic exam for detection of organism with typical appearance and characteristic motility (has four anterior flagella and one prominent lateral flagellum)

TABLE 17–27. Selected Intestinal Helminths

Species	Common Name	Laboratory Detection
Ascaris lumbricoides Ancylostoma duodenale Necator americanus Trichurius trichuria	Roundworm Hookworm Hookworm Whipworm	Microscopic examination of stool specimen subsequent to special methods of concentration for observation of ova; adult Ascaris worms sometimes recovered from stool or vomitus
Strongyloides stercoralis		Examination as above for larvae; serologic tests
Enterobius vermicularis	Pinworm	Microscopic examination of perianal swab specimen for ova or of Scotch tape prep for ova or adult worms; adult worms occasionally seen on stool

TABLE 17–28. Other Parasites

Parasite	Comments
Trichinella spiralis	Tissue nematode seen worldwide; may be detected in muscle biopsies or with serologic tests
Fasciola hepatica	Trematode seen worldwide; detected by stool concentration methods or serologic testing(sheep liver fluke)
Taena saginata and Taena solium	Beef (saginata) and pork (solium) tapeworms; detected by presence of mature segments on stool
Diphyllobothrium latum	Fish tapeworm; detected by presence of ova in stool

17. SELF TEST

Choose the best response for each item. The answer key may be found in the appendices.

1. **Microorganisms that require oxygen for growth and derive energy solely from oxygen dependent metabolic pathways are called**
   A. obligate aerobes
   B. obligate anaerobes
   C. aerotolerant

2. **The phase of bacterial growth in which the rate of reproduction increases rapidly until a maximum rate is achieved is called**
   A. lag phase
   B. exponential or log phase
   C. stationary phase
   D. decline phase

3. **This organism is the major pathogen of a group of gram positive cocci that typically appear in clusters. It is catalase positive and coagulase positive and is associated with skin infections, wound infections, and food poisoning.**
   A. *Staphylococcus epidermidis*
   B. *Streptococcus pyogenes*
   C. *Staphylococcus aureus*
   D. *Streptococcus group B*

4. **Organisms that produce the enzyme beta lactamase are**
   A. incapable of producing human disease
   B. highly susceptible to all antibiotics
   C. resistant to penicillins and cephalosporins

5. **These organisms are gram positive cocci that typically occur in chains. They produce a clear zone of hemolysis on blood agar and are sensitive to bacitracin.**
   A. *Staphylococcus aureus*
   B. Group B, β-hemolytic *Streptococcus (S agalactiae)*
   C. Group A, β-hemolytic *Streptococcus (S pyogenes)*
   D. Group D, α-hemolytic *Streptococcus (S bovis)*

6. The streptococcal organism most frequently associated with neonatal septicemia and meningitis and with post-partum endometritis and septicemia is
    A. group C, α-hemolytic *Streptococcus (S anginosus)*
    B. group B, β-hemolytic *Streptococcus (S agalactiae)*
    C. group A, β-hemolytic *Streptococcus (S pyogenes)*
    D. group D, α-hemolytic *Streptococcus (S bovis)*

7. These two members of the Enterobacteriaceae family are always pathogens.
    A. *E coli* and *Proteus*
    B. *E coli* and *Salmonella*
    C. *Proteus* and *Shigella*
    D. *Salmonella* and *Shigella*

8. This organism is the most common cause of urinary tract infection and of gram negative septicemia.
    A. *Proteus mirabilis*
    B. *Pseudomonas aeruginosa*
    C. *Escherichia coli*
    D. *Shigella boydii*

9. This organism is an important opportunistic pathogen associated with infections from whirlpool baths, infection of burn sites, urinary tract infection, and about 10% of nosocomial infections.
    A. *Proteus mirabilis*
    B. *Pseudomonas aeruginosa*
    C. *Escherichia coli*
    D. *Shigella boydii*

10. Discovered in the early 1980s, this organism is associated with the development of peptic ulcers.
    A. *Campylobacter jejuni*
    B. *Pseudomonas aeruginosa*
    C. *Escherichia coli*
    D. *Helicobacter pylori*

11. Gram negative diplococci are observed on a gram stain:
    A. the organism is known to be either *Neisseria meningitidis* or *Neisseria gonorrhoeae*
    B. the organism is known to be *Neisseria gonorrhoeae*
    C. the organism may be *Neisseria meningitidis*, *Neisseria gonorrhoeae*, or *Branhamella catarrhalis*
    D. the organism is known to be pathogenic

12. **This organism is the most common cause of nongonococcal urethritis in men and, if untreated in the female, can lead to infertility.**
    A. *Gardnerella vaginalis*
    B. *Chlamydia trachomatis*
    C. *Neisseria gonorrhoeae*

13. **The organisms seen most frequently in anaerobic infections are**
    A. *Bacteroides*
    B. *Clostridium tetani*
    C. *Anaerobic streptococci*

14. **The causative agent of syphilis is**
    A. *Neisseria gonorrhoeae*
    B. *Chlamydia trachomatis*
    C. *Gonorrhoeae syphiliticus*
    D. *Tremponema pallidum*

15. **Penicillin and cephalosporin antibiotics act on bacteria to**
    A. inhibit DNA synthesis
    B. interfere with cell wall construction
    C. inhibit ribosomal protein synthesis
    D. interfere with RNA synthesis

16. **The organism associated with a lower respiratory tract infection sometimes referred to as atypical pneumonia is**
    A. *Hemophilus influenzae*
    B. *Streptococcus pneumoniae*
    C. *Pneumococcus pneumoniae*
    D. *Mycoplasma pneumoniae*

17. **Acid-fast bacilli that have thick, waxy cell walls belong to this *genus*.**
    A. *Tuberculosis*
    B. *Mycoplasma*
    C. *Mycobacterium*

18. **The causative agent of the common cold is a/an**
    A. retrovirus
    B. othomyxovirus
    C. togavirus
    D. rhinovirus

19. This organism is an important cause of lower respiratory tract infections in young children and infants and can be detected by fluorescent staining or ELISA in addition to culture techniques.
    A. RSV
    B. CMV
    C. EBV

20. _____ produces a sexually transmitted disease characterized by genital lesions and periods of latency and recurrence.
    A. HBV-2
    B. HSV-1
    C. HSV-2
    D. HCV

21. Detection of HB$_s$Ab in serum is
    A. evidence of prior hepatitis B infection and immunity
    B. diagnostic for current hepatitis B infection
    C. indicative of a chronic state if detectable for more than 6 months
    D. meaningless unless the corresponding antigen can also be demonstrated

22. The causative agent of infectious mononucleosis and the organism also associated with Burkitt's lymphoma and chronic fatigue syndrome is
    A. CMV
    B. EBV
    C. RSV
    D. HBV

23. The test results shown in the boxes below are most indicative of:

VCA-IgM	VCA-IgG	EBNA-IgG	EA-D	Heterophile
0	+	+	+	0

    A. primary EBV infection
    B. reactivated EBV infection
    C. previous (old) EBV infection
    D. individual never infected with EBV

24. In terms of HIV infection, the term seroconversion refers to
    A. the time that the HIV-1 antigen is detectable
    B. production of antibody to HIV-1
    C. primary exposure to HIV-1

25. A systemic fungal infection seen more commonly in the Mississippi and Ohio Valley areas that begins with a pulmonary lesion similar to that seen in tuberculosis and transmitted primarily by birds is
    A. histoplasmosis
    B. blastomycosis
    C. cryptococcosis
    D. candidiasis

26. Pigeon feces is the primary source of _____, a fungal infection that most frequently affects the lungs and CNS.
    A. histoplasmosis
    B. blastomycosis
    C. cryptococcosis
    D. candidiasis

27. This infection is seen in the oral cavity, vagina, or as a skin condition as the result of an opportunistic fungal pathogen.
    A. histoplasmosis
    B. blastomycosis
    C. cryptococcosis
    D. candidiasis

28. This parasite is the causative agent of amoebic dysentery.
    A. *Trichomonas vaginalis*
    B. *Giardia lamblia*
    C. *Entamoeba histolytica*
    D. *Trichenella spiralis*

29. This parasite is transmitted sexually and is identified on microscopic examination by its characteristic appearance and motility.
    A. *Trichomonas vaginalis*
    B. *Giardia lamblia*
    C. *Entamoeba histolytica*
    D. *Trichenella spiralis*

30. This parasitic organism produces malaria.
    A. *Toxoplasma gondii*
    B. *Enterobius vermicularis*
    C. *Plasmodium vivax*

18. TESTS FOR DISORDERS OF IMMUNE FUNCTION

The body has a number of mechanisms that provide protection from disease. These distinct, but interrelated mechanisms mount defensive responses to a variety of challenges. Disorders of immune function are manifested in a variety of clinical conditions, including autoimmune disorders, immunodeficiencies, and hypersensitivity reactions. Immunology is both an exciting, interesting field and a dreaded study of complex, intricately overlapping reactions. The latter view is well expressed by a physician quoted in Peakman and Vergani (1997) who termed immunology as "an invention of the devil, who is making it up as he goes along."

An in depth treatment of the subject of immunology is not undertaken in this text. Instead an overview of the immune system is provided, followed by a brief discussion of the laboratory evaluation of selected disorders of autoimmunity and immunodeficiency.

BASIC CONCEPTS OF IMMUNOLOGY

The immune system must be able to distinguish between **self** and **non-self** in order to respond appropriately to the daily challenges presented by viruses, bacteria, fungi, parasites, and toxins. When non-self, or foreign, antigens are recognized the immune system must mount an appropriate defense, including processes aimed at destruction of the offending substance. The average individual has a better grasp of basic immunologic concepts than he or she might think because observations made in our daily experiences familiarize us with some of these basic concepts. For instance, we may note that

- newborns are more susceptible to infections
- after contracting certain childhood illnesses, we are unlikely to develop the same illness on subsequent exposure
- resistance to some diseases can be provided by vaccination
- immunity to one illness does not protect us from another illness (ie, having chicken pox does not provide resistance to measles)
- within the same environment, some of us become ill while others do not
- open wounds are much more likely to become infected than intact skin

These common observations illustrate a number of immunologic principles as listed below.

- We are born with some immunity (**natural, or innate, immunity**), but additional protection is acquired later (**acquired immunity**).
- Protection from some illnesses is afforded by actively having the disease (**active immunity**).
- Protection from some diseases can be artificially provided without actually contracting the disease itself (**passive immunity**).
- Acquired immunity has **memory** and is **specific** in response.
- **Immunocompetence**, or the level of immune response mounted, varies among individuals.
- **Physical barriers**, such as the skin, provide protection from infection.

The immune system can be discussed in terms of **physical and chemical barriers** and **three major types of immunity** that work together closely to protect the body from "foreign invaders." Physical and chemical barriers are summarized in Table 18–1. The three major types of immune responses are

- humoral immunity (antibody production)
- complement
- cellular immunity

Humoral immunity refers to the production of **antibodies (immunoglobulins)** in response to exposure to a foreign **antigen**. An *antigen* is defined as any substance capable of inducing antibody production. The antibodies produced are specific for the antigen stimulating their production. Immunoglobulins are specific **glycoproteins** that are **produced by stimulated B-lymphocytes** following antigen activation. Antibody responses may be either **primary** (upon **first exposure** to a particular antigen) or **secondary** (**subsequent exposure** to same or very similar antigen produces secondary, or anamnestic, response that is more rapid than the initial response).

Immunoglobulins are complex molecules that occur in different types and perform varying functions. A simplified description of immunoglobulins to provide basic understanding can be based on visualization of the **basic immunoglobulin**

TABLE 18–1. Physical and Chemical Barriers to Infection

Barrier	Action
Skin and mucosa	Provides physical barrier against invasion by microorganisms
Cilia	Aids in removal of foreign matter and debris
Saliva	Cleanses oral cavity
Tears	Cleanse conjunctiva and aid in removal of foreign matter
Gastric acid	Kills many microorganisms unable to withstand acid pH

molecule as a Y shaped structure. The two short arms of the Y are identical each having the ability to bind antigen. The base or trunk of the Y contains special sites that are capable of interacting with the complement proteins or with specific cellular receptors on cells like granulocytes and mast cells. There is a **hinge region** where the two short arms and the trunk meet that allows some flexibility in the molecule, which is particularly important to the short arms in antigen binding. The entire molecule is made up of four polypeptide chains held together by disulfide bonds: **two heavy chains** and **two light chains**, designated as such on the basis of relative mass differences. There are two kinds of light chains and five major heavy chains, each designated by Greek letters. Each immunoglobulin molecule has either two kappa (κ) chains or two lambda (λ) chains and heavy chains that are both either α, δ, ε, γ, , or μ. Each of the polypeptide chains has a segment in which the amino acid sequence is relatively constant among the different antibodies (**constant, or C region**) and an area that varies extensively from one antibody to another (**variable, or V region**). The variable region includes the antigen binding sites found on the **Fab fragments** (fragment, antigen binding). The **Fc fragment** (crystallizable fragment) contains the sites for interaction with complement and cellular receptors. The basic immunoglobulin molecule is depicted in Figure 18–1.

The different **classes of immunoglobulins** are named based on their heavy chain: IgA, IgD, IgE, IgG, and IgM. IgG and IgA are further divided into subclasses. Primary humoral responses principally involve **IgM**, a pentamer consisting of five basic immunoglobulin molecules. **IgG**, the **most abundant immunoglobulin,** is a monomer consisting of one basic immunoglobulin molecule and is the antibody produced in **secondary immune responses**. Antibodies have a variety of roles in addition to targeting infective organisms. They also neutralize toxins, aid in removal of foreign antigens from the circulation, and activate other substances involved in the immune response. Clinical uses of antibodies include the administration of pooled immunoglobulins for passive protection and in the laboratory identification of various conditions and organisms.

After binding with an antigen, the antibody undergoes a change in conformation that exposes a site that can bind with the first component of the complement cascade. Antibodies can only bind to complement ("fix" complement) after they have reacted with their corresponding antigen. The varying antibodies are not equally capable of fixing complement. **Complement** refers to a large number of heat labile proteins (primarily synthesized in the liver) that assist antibody destruction of organisms. In a fashion similar to that seen in the coagulation cascade, complement forms cascades with each activated component serving as a catalyst for activation of subsequent components. Also analogous to the coagulation cascade, the complement cascade can be activated by one of **two different pathways (classical and alternative)** that come together in a **final common pathway** and includes a number of regulatory substances. **Antigen-antibody complexes** activate the **classical complement pathway** as do aggregated immunoglobulins, and certain stimuli such as DNA and C-reactive protein. The alternate complement pathway has a continuous slow reaction that can be activated by certain insoluble polysaccharides and the surface of some non-self cells

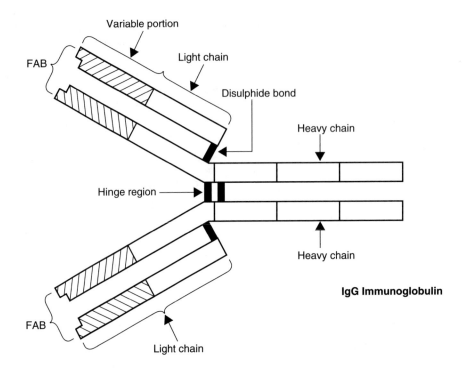

FIGURE 18–1. Basic immunoglobulin structure. IgG is a monomer. IgM is a pentamer consisting of five of these basic immunoglobulin molecules.

(such as bacteria) in the presence of the complement component C3b. The final common complement pathway is initiated by a C5 convertase produced by either the classical or alternate pathway. The final product of complement activation is a **membrane attack complex** that attacks the membrane of the offending cell and results in **lysis and death of the cell**. (Figure 18–2 provides a simplified schematic of the complement cascade.) The complement cascade is controlled in at least two ways:

- complement components are labile proteins
- presence of various circulating and membrane bound regulatory proteins including complement receptors found on the surface of cells of the immune system

There are many elements of the cellular immune system, several of which are present and functional at birth (innate immunity). Cellular elements are also involved in functions of aquired immunity. Some of the processes involved in cellular immunity are described below in terms of particular cell types.

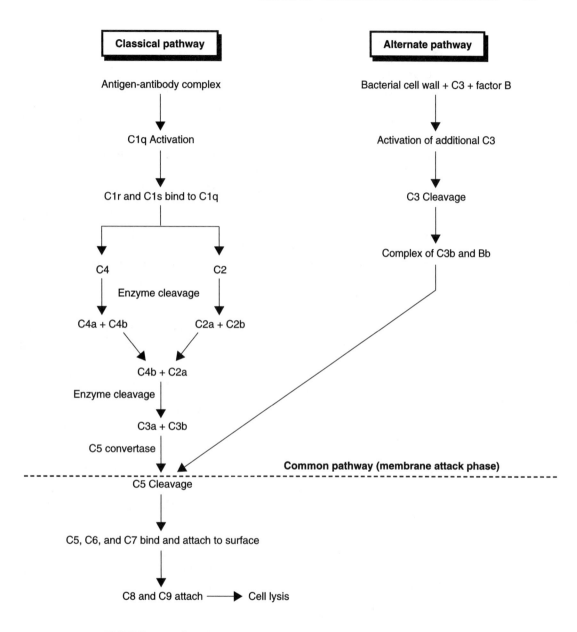

FIGURE 18–2. Complement cascade.

Granulocytes (neutrophils, eosinophils, and basophils—see Chapter 3 for detailed descriptions of these cells) are capable of migrating to tissues and mast cells are tissue residents. These four cell types contain cytoplasmic granules to which some of their immune functions are related. **Neutrophils** are an important component of the cellular immune system involved in the killing and removal of bacteria and fungi. Following activation, they are attracted by special chemicals, move toward them in a process called *chemotaxis,* and engulf microorganisms by phagocytosis. The primary role of **eosinophils** is in the control of parasitic infections. They also have low affinity IgE receptor sites and are involved in allergic responses. **Basophils and mast cells** both possess histamine containing granules and high affinity IgE receptor sites. They appear to have similar roles in blood (basophils) and in tissue (mast cells). The effect produced by the release of granules from basophils and mast cells depends on the stimulus and site and ranges from a mild localized reaction to anaphylactic shock.

Mononuclear phagocytes (MNPs) include monocytes and macrophages. They are an important component of immunity and not only serve as sophisticated phagocytes, but also play a role in

- the processing and presentation of antigens to T-cells: other cells are also involved in antigen presentation, including B-lymphocytes and dendritic cells
- release of cytokines: cytokines are small, soluble peptides involved in immune communication and influencing cellular function; specialized functions when fixed in tissue includes ingestion and killing of intracellular parasites and chronic immune responses
- cytotoxicity

B-lymphocytes begin as immature cells in the bone marrow and develop into the B-cells found in the lymph nodes and spleen that have not yet encountered antigens (may be referred to as "virgin" B-cells). **Mature B-cells** have **antigen specificity** expressed in surface immunoglobulin molecules. A complex set of interactions that take place between B-cells and T-cells are important in immune responses and illustrate the interrelatedness of the cellular and humoral immune systems. These interactions are not addressed in this text beyond the summary of the primary results of these interactions listed below:

- B-cell activation
- B-cell differentiation
    antibody producing plasma cells
    memory B-cells that retain memory of antigen encounters
- T-cell activation

T-lymphocytes influence most aspects of immune function through cytokine secretion and direct cell-to-cell interactions with B-cells. T-cells are divided into three subsets based on function:

- T-helper cells: stimulate B-cells to produce antibodies to processed antigens; stimulate B-cells to further divide
- T-suppressor cells: regulatory cells that limit antibody production
- T-killer cells (cytotoxic T-cells): cytotoxic cells with the ability to lyse target cells

T-cells have large glycoprotein **receptor sites** (T-cell receptor; **TCR**) that interact with a short amino acid segment (called a *peptide antigen*) derived from intact antigens by proteolysis. Like antibodies, these receptors have regions that are highly variable between different molecules and interact with antigens. The function of the TCR is to recognize and bind a specific antigen. These sites are not capable of reacting with intact antigens and can only react with peptide antigens when they are "held" and presented by other glycoproteins. This function is served by major histocompatibility complex (MHC) molecules, a collection of genes on chromosome 6 and known in humans as **human leukocyte antigens** (HLA) (Peakman and Vergani, 1997). T-cells will only kill target cells that present both a specific antigen and the appropriate HLA molecule. The HLA genes are polymorphic. Although this polymorphism provides broader protection against potential pathogens, it also presents significant obstacles to organ transplantation. In addition to the TCR, T-cells have specific antigenic markers on their surface called *cellular determinants* (CD) that are identified by number. More than 50 cellular determinants have been described, but those of primary importance to this discussion are

- CD3: required for T-cell function
- CD4: on approximately two thirds of T-cells; provides adhesion for interacting cells and signal for T-cell activation; T-helper cells have CD4 marker and thus are also referred to as CD4 cells or T4-lymphocytes; it is the cellular receptor for HIV
- CD8: similar to CD4; has some cell adhesion and stabilizing properties; T-suppressor cells have CD8 marker and the designation CD8 cells or T8-lymphocytes

The functions of the T-lymphocytes include:

- inducing the activation of B-cells and maturation to plasma cells or memory cells
- signaling for an increase in B-cells
- recruiting and activating MNPs
    specialized T-cells that are cytotoxic to viruses
- secretion of cytokines that promote growth and differentiation of
    other T-cells
    macrophages
    eosinophils

AUTOIMMUNE DISEASES

Autoimmune diseases result when an immune response is mounted against healthy self components (ie, immune system does not appropriately distinguish between self and non-self). Autoimmune diseases are probably the result of both genetic and environmental factors. The autoimmune reactions in these diseases may be directed against **specific target organs or tissues** (**organ-specific** autoimmune diseases) or against **structures that are common to a variety of tissues** and found throughout the body (**systemic** autoimmune diseases; non-organ specific autoimmune diseases). An occasional disease shows overlap between the two categories. A number of mechanisms of autoimmunity have been identified and are summarized in Table 18–2.

Because the same immune responses that occur in response to pathogens can occur in autoimmune disease, significant **damage** can result from these attacks on self. Damage may be caused by the effects of cytotoxic T-cells, by the effect of cytokine recruitment of MNPs and increased HLA expression, and by B-cell production of autoantibodies that activate complement. Results include:

- organ dysfunction: seen in Graves' disease, where the autoantibody binding to thyrotropin receptor stimulates production of thyroid hormone
- cell death: seen in diabetes mellitus type 1 (insulin producing beta cells) and in Hashimoto's thyroiditis

Diagnosis of autoimmune diseases, particularly systemic conditions, can be complicated because of the number of conditions producing similar results in laboratory testing. Diagnosis is accomplished by evaluation of clinical symptoms in conjunction with general screening tests (tests that indicate the possible presence of autoimmune reactions, but are not specific for a particular disorder or may be seen in non-autoimmune conditions) and more specific or confirmatory laboratory assays.

TABLE 18–2. Mechanisms of Autoimmunity

Mechanism	Description	Examples
Defective regulation	Reduction in number of suppressor cells; defective suppressor cell function	Autoimmune diseases of thyroid, islet cells, and liver
Molecular imitation (mimicry)	Pathogen and autoantigen have cross-reactive epitopes; anti-pathogen immune response leads to anti-self response	Coxsackie (pathogen) and glutamic acid decarboxylase (autoantigen) in type 1 diabetes
Hidden self antigens	Tolerance to obscure antigens ("immunologic ignorance") is broken upon release or presentation of these antigens	Sympathetic ophthalmia; Dressler syndrome (post-myocardial infarction complications)
Cytokines	Cytokines provide additional signals to activate resting autoreactive cells	Autoimmune thyroid disease following interleukin-2 therapy

Adapted from Peakman M, Vergani D. *Basic and Clinical Immunology.* New York, Churchill Livingstone, 1997

Treatment for autoimmune diseases may involve replacement therapy for specific conditions (eg, insulin in type 1 diabetes; thyroxine in Hashimoto's thyroiditis) or a blanket suppression of the immune system with corticosteroids and management of symptoms and complications. Recent clinical trials with drugs that are more selective in their inhibition of immune responses (eg, cyclosporin A) may provide another alternative (Peakman and Vergani, 1997). These methods of treatment carry significant risks, including various side effects and reduced protection from other diseases, and are generally initiated only after carefully weighing the risks and benefits of therapy. Research efforts continue for the development of more specific therapy that can block or prevent the particular autoimmune response without compromising protective immunity.

■ SYSTEMIC AUTOIMMUNE DISEASES

These diseases are referred to as **rheumatic diseases** (a reference to the pain encountered in these diseases; from the Greek for flowing pain), **connective tissue diseases**, or **collagen diseases** (references to the components typically affected in the disease process). Many of these diseases present clinically with joint and/or muscle symptoms, but other manifestations dominate the clinical picture in others such as systemic lupus erythematosus and ankylosing spondylitis. Although much progress related to the mechanisms involved in systemic autoimmune disease has been made in the last decade, classification of these conditions remains difficult as the etiology for most of them has not yet been firmly established. Specific autoantibodies that can be detected by various laboratory methods have been identified for many of these conditions and provide diagnostic specificity not previously available. Laboratory methods for the detection of autoantibodies to nuclear antigens or intracellular antigens include:

- immunofluorescent microscopy (IFM)
- enzyme linked immunoassay (ELISA)
- immunodiffusion (ID)
- counterimmunoelectrophoresis (CIE)

Table 18–3 lists a classification of systemic rheumatic diseases and related disorders. Selected disorders are discussed in the following sections.

Systemic lupus erythematosus (**SLE**; often called simply *lupus*) is a disease that can affect **essentially every organ system**, some more commonly than others. It has a poorer prognosis than many of the other rheumatic diseases, with **renal failure** being the major cause of morbidity and mortality. The course of SLE includes periods of spontaneous remission and exacerbation. **Clinical manifestations** vary in severity and may involve

- skin: "butterfly rash" on cheeks and bridge of the nose is characteristic, but not seen in all patients; rash in sun exposed areas may accompany

exacerbations; patchy (occasionally extensive) alopecia seen with relative frequency
- joints: joint pain and arthritis are seen in majority of patients
- kidneys: most patients have Ig deposits in glomeruli; clinically significant glomerulonephritis in half of patients
- neurologic features: can affect any CNS area; manifestations range from psychosis to seizures; mild cognitive dysfunction, depression, and anxiety common (Peakman and Vergani, 1997)
- thrombotic disease
- vasculitis
- impaired hematopoiesis
- pleural and/or pericardial inflammation

Table 18–4 lists the criteria for SLE diagnosis developed by the American Rheumatism Association (ARA). The presence of four criteria at any time during the course of the disease is required for diagnosis. Because there are a number of persons who have variously classified lupus-like illnesses in the presence of fewer than four of the ARA criteria, an additional system has been recommended (the Schur system) using the same ARA criteria. Using this system, patients would be classified based on the presence of varying numbers of diagnostic criteria:

- classic SLE: presence of many ARA criteria
- definite SLE: four or more criteria
- probable SLE: three criteria
- possible SLE: two criteria

Some patients in the last two categories may be subsequently diagnosed with classic or definite SLE with the presentation of additional criteria, while others will be diagnosed with other rheumatic diseases having a better prognosis than SLE.

TABLE 18–3. Classification of Systemic Rheumatic Diseases

Systemic lupus erythematosus (SLE)
Discoid lupus erythematosus (DLE)
Lupus-like syndrome
Drug-induced lupus erythematosus
Sjögren syndrome
Scleroderma and CREST syndrome
(calcinosis cutis, Raynaud's phenomenon, esophogeal dysmotility, sclerodactyly, telangiectasia)
Rheumatoid arthritis
Dermatomyositis and polymyositis
Overlap syndromes:
Mixed connective tissue diseases (MCTD)
Other disorders
Connective disease syndromes that have been poorly defined as to clinical category

Henry JB. *Clinical Diagnosis and Management by Laboratory Methods,* 19th ed. Philadelphia, Saunders, 1996

TABLE 18–4. Criteria for SLE Diagnosis

Criteria	Comments
Malar rash	Characteristic "butterfly rash"
Discoid rash	Erythematous raised patches
Photosensitivity	
Oral ulcers	Oral or nasopharyngeal ulcers
Arthritis	Involving two or more peripheral joints
Serositis	Documented pleuritis or pericarditis
Renal disorder	3+ proteinuria (or > 0.5g/24 hours) or cellular casts
Neurologic disorder	Without other identifiable cause
Hematologic disorder	Anemia or leukopenia/lymphopenia or thrombocytopenia
Immunologic disorder	Any one of:
	anti-double stranded DNA
	anti-Sm
	positive LE cell preparation (test rarely, if ever, used because better tests are available) false positive syphilis serology for 6 months
Antinuclear antibody	Elevated ANA titer by immunofluorescence or equivalent method in the absence of drugs known to produce elevated ANA titer

Criteria set by the American Rheumatism Association; diagnosis requires that four criteria be present at any time during the course of the disease.

Antinuclear antibodies with a homogeneous or speckled pattern (Table 18–5) are seen in virtually all patients, but are also seen in a variety of other autoimmune diseases (ie, high sensitivity, low specificity). Anti-dsDNA is seen in about 70 % of patients and anti-Sm in 30 % of patients (Peakman and Vergani, 1997). A variety of other autoantibodies may be detected in SLE, including anti-phospholipid antibodies associated with thrombotic episodes and recurrent abortions and antibodies against various blood cells (lymphocytes, platelets, erythrocytes). Development of SLE has been associated with specific HLA alleles. Many of the complications and organ associated features of SLE are produced as a result of deposited immune complexes.

Rheumatoid arthritis (RA) is a systemic, chronic inflammatory disease that characteristically affects peripheral joints in a symmetric manner. RA commonly results in cartilage destruction, bone erosion, and significant joint deformity. Vasculitis and subcutaneous nodules (called *rheumatoid nodules*) are seen in some patients. Nodules may also be seen in the pleura and myocardium. Sjögren syndrome frequently occurs in conjunction with RA. There is a clear genetic component in RA with predisposition conferred by certain HLA genes. Patients typically present with joint pain aggravated by movement with evident joint

TABLE 18–5. Antinuclear Antibody Patterns in Systemic Rheumatic Disease

Pattern	Associated with
Homogeneous	SLE; various other rheumatic diseases
Speckled	SLE; Sjögren's syndrome; mixed connective tissue disease; polymyositis; dermatomyositis; CREST syndrome; scleroderma (systemic sclerosis)
Peripheral	SLE; scleroderma
Nucleolar	SLE

swelling and warmth. Morning stiffness lasting for more than 1 hour is a characteristic finding. The erythrocyte sedimentation rate (ESR) and C-reactive protein (CRP) are elevated and serve as reliable indicators of the severity of disease for purposes of monitoring. The disease is associated with a variety of autoantibodies, including rheumatoid factor. **Rheumatoid factor** (RF) is an antibody directed against the Fc fragment of the IgG antibody molecule and may be detected prior to the development of clinical symptoms. RF is not, however, specific for RA and may be positive in a variety of other conditions and chronic infections. Other autoantibodies associated with RA include antikeratin antibody (AKA; good specificity, but not very sensitive); antiperinuclear factor (APF; good sensitivity, but less specific than AKA); antibody to RA associated nuclear antigen (RANA); and anti-RA33 (Henry, 1996). Table 18–6 lists the criteria for diagnosis of RA.

Sjögren syndrome (SS) is a chronic, progressive inflammatory autoimmune disease with genetic predisposition indicated by specific HLA genes. Recent evidence seems to indicate an association with retroviruses (Peakman and Vergani, 1997). SS may be seen as a primary condition in which it occurs alone or as a secondary condition seen with other systemic autoimmune diseases (particularly RA and SLE). The lacrimal, salivary, and other exocrine glands are affected and are infiltrated with lymphocyte aggregates. Clinical features include dry eyes with a "gritty" feeling and dry mouth with a high incidence of caries. Dry food dysphagia and vaginal dryness may also be seen. Extraglandular manifestations include fatigue, joint pain, muscle pain or soreness, lymphadenopathy, and cutaneous vasculitis. A speckled or homogeneous pattern of ANA and elevated RF are seen in most patients (two thirds and 90%, respectively [Peakman and Vergani, 1997]). More specific autoantibodies found in Sjögren syndrome include those directed toward the extractable nuclear antigens: anti-SS-A/Ro and anti-SS-B/La. These autoantibodies are also seen in a small percentage of SLE patients, but are rarely seen in any other condition. A polyclonal hypergammaglobulinemia is frequently seen. The disease tends to culminate in a monoclonal hypergammaglobulinemia and is associated with a significant increase in the incidence of lymphoma.

TABLE 18–6. Diagnosis of Rheumatoid Arthritis

Criteria	Comments
Morning stiffness	In and around joints, lasting 1 hour or more; must be present for at least 6 weeks
Arthritis (≥ 3 joint areas)	With soft tissue swelling or joint effusions; observed by physician; present at least 6 weeks
Arthritis of hand joints	Observed by physician; present for at least 6 weeks
Symmetric arthritis	Same joint on both sides of body; observed by physician; present for at least 6 weeks
Rheumatoid nodules	Subcutaneous nodules observed by physician
Serum rheumatoid factor	Elevated; any method
Radiographic changes	Hand/wrist; must include erosions or unequivocal bony decalcification

Four of the seven criteria must be met for diagnosis of RA.

■ ORGAN-SPECIFIC AUTOIMMUNE DISEASES

The autoimmune reaction in these diseases is directed against specific target organs or tissues. The ensuing tissue damage is cell specific and results in organ failure or dysfunction that produces the clinical syndrome. Many conditions involving a variety of organs or tissues have been associated with autoimmune processes including those affecting the

- skin
- endocrine glands
- liver
- pancreas
- muscles
- gastrointestinal tract
- kidneys
- central nervous system

In many cases the pathogenic role of autoantibodies in these conditions is either unproven or has not been fully elucidated; however, research continues in regard to these autoantibodies and the nature of their target antigens. Discussion of individual organ-specific autoimmune diseases is not presented in this text, however, examples of such diseases are listed in Table 18–7.

TABLE 18–7. Organ-Specific Autoimmune Diseases

Disease	Target Organ	Associated Autoantibodies
Hashimoto's thyroiditis	Thyroid gland	Thyroglobulin
Graves' disease	Thyroid gland	Microsomal thyroid peroxidase
Addison's disease	Adrenal gland	Adrenalcorticol
Insulin dependent diabetes mellitus	Pancreas	Islet cells
Insulin resistant diabetes mellitus	Pancreas	Insulin receptors
Primary biliary cirrhosis	Liver	Mitochondrial
Autoimmune hepatitis	Liver	Smooth muscle; ANA; microsomal
Polymyositis	Muscle	Nuclear antigens, including DNA
Atrophic gastritis	GI tract	Gastric parietal cell
Pernicious anemia	GI tract	Intrinsic factor; gastric parietal cell; salivary duct glands
Crohn's disease	GI tract	Reticulum; epithelial cells
Multiple sclerosis	CNS	Myelin, myelin associated glycoprotein
Guillain–Barre syndrome	CNS	Peripheral nerve myelin components
Amyotrophic lateral sclerosis	CNS	Ganglioside (GM1)
Myasthenia gravis	CNS	Acetylcholine receptor
Lambert–Eaton syndrome	CNS	Pre-synaptic structures
Goodpasture syndrome	Kidney	Glomerular basement membrane
Pemphigus	Skin	Intracellular substance (desmoglein 1) of epidermis or mucosa
Vitiligo	Skin	Melanocytes, tyrosinase (enzyme in melanin synthesis)

Table compiled based on information from Henry JB. *Clinical Diagnosis and Management by Laboratory Methods,* 19th ed. Philadelphia, Saunders, 1996 and from Peakman M, Vergani D. *Basic and Clinical Immunology.* New York, Churchill Livingstone, 1997

IMMUNODEFICIENCY

Immunodeficiencies may be **primary** (genetic abnormality) or, more commonly, **secondary** to another condition or substance. The nature of the resulting condition is dependent on the nature of the deficiency and the part of the immune system that is affected. The clinical picture is important in determining which laboratory assays should be performed because it is not feasible to comprehensively evaluate all components of the immune system. Clinical manifestations usually conform to a particular pattern that not only aids in test selection, but is suggestive of a particular diagnosis. Thus a comprehensive history and physical examination are indispensable diagnostic tools in immunodeficiency disorders. Immunodeficiency typically leads to an increased susceptibility to infection, frequently with opportunistic pathogens. Immunodeficiencies are classified on the basis of the decreased or deficient component. Classification may, however, be difficult in some cases because of the various interactions of immune system components. Immunodeficiency categories of classification are:

- T-lymphocyte deficiency
- B-lymphocyte deficiency
- combined T-lymphocyte and B-lymphocyte deficiency
- neutrophil defects
- complement component deficiency

Tables 18–8 and 18–9 provide information useful in narrowing the possibilities of the immune defect in cases of apparent immunodeficiency. Repeated infection with opportunistic or unusual pathogens may provide the first clinical indication of an immune disorder. Table 18–8 provides some typical patterns of infectious organisms encountered in the various types of immunodeficiency. Table 18–9 correlates various clinical symptoms with the type of immunodeficiency usually producing the symptom. Selected immunodeficiencies are summarized in Table 18–10.

Deficiencies in one or more of the complement components may also be encountered. Laboratory assay of CH50 provides a screen of the functioning of the entire complement cascade. Abnormality may be further investigated by measurement of individual complement components.

Immunodeficiency as a secondary disorder is suggested when signs of immune dysfunction are present in conjunction with

- concomitant or preceding viral infection
- certain malignancies, including chronic lymphoid leukemia, Hodgkin's, multiple myeloma
- immunosuppressive drug therapy
- history consistent with potential for HIV exposure

TABLE 18–8. Typical Patterns of Infectious Organisms in Immunodeficiency

Deficiency	Bacteria	Viruses	Fungi	Flagellate Parasites	Protozoa
B-cell	Hemophilus influenzae Streptococcus pneumoniae Staphylococcus aureus	Echoviruses		Giardia lamblia	
T-cell	Mycobacterium tuberculosis Mycobacterium avium	CMV Herpes zoster	Candida albicans		Pneumocystis carinii Toxoplasma gondii
Phagocytes	Staphylococcus aureus Staphylococcus epidermidis Pseudomonas aeruginosa Serratia marcescens Escherichia coli		Candida albicans Aspergillus flavus		
Complement: Classical pathway	Hemophilus influenzae Streptococcus pneumoniae Staphylococcus aureus				
Complement: Membrane attack pathway	Neisseria meningitidis Neisseria gonorrhoeae				

Adapted from Peakman M, Vergani D. *Basic and Clinical Immunology.* New York, Churchill Livingstone, 1997

TABLE 18–9. Clinical Symptoms Correlated with Type of Immunodeficiency and Laboratory Assays

Suspected Deficiency/Defect	Clinical Symptoms	Helpful Tests

T-Cell	Vaccination results in systemic illness
	Overwhelming infection with generally benign virus (varicella, CMV)
	Oral *Candida* not associated with antibiotics resists therapy or persists after age 6 months
	Candida moves from mucosal surfaces to contiguous cutaneous areas
	Patient has short limbed dwarfism
	Features of intrauterine graft vs host disease (scaling eryrodermia, alopecia, failure to thrive)
	Graft vs host disease follows transfusion of blood product
	Neonatal tetany
	Low lymphocyte count consistently < 1200/mm³
		T-cell count, CD3
		T-cell subset counts, esp:
		  CD4
		  CD8
		
		T-cell functional assessment:
		  PHA stimulation
		  antigen specific stimulation
		  IL-2 production

B-Cell	Recurrent infection with extracellular pyogenic organisms (*Hemophilus, Staph, Strep*—see Table 18–8)	B-cell count, CD20 Ig levels (IgG, IgA, IgM) IgG subclasses
Combined T- and B-cell	Features of Wiskott-Aldrich syndrome (draining ears, thrombocytopenia, eczema, esp in male) Features of ataxia-telangiectasia (telangiectasia of sclera, ears; facial expression is dull) Features listed above for T-cell deficiency and for B-cell deficiency are seen together	Tests listed for separate T-cell and B-cell deficiencies
Phagocytes	Recurrent, severe staph abscesses of skin (abscesses of deep organs occur less commonly) Chronic/recurrent osteomyelitis, draining lymph nodes (esp caused by *Klebsiella* or *Serratia* species)	Neutrophil count Neutrophil function test (nitroblue tetrazolium [NBT])

Symptoms are from Henry JB. *Clinical Diagnosis and Management by Laboratory Methods,* 19th ed. Philadelphia, Saunders, 1996; tests are from Peakman M, Vergani D. *Basic and Clinical Immunology.* New York, Churchill Livingstone, 1997

TABLE 18–10. Selected Immunodeficiencies

Disorder	Description
Severe combined immunodeficiency (SCID)	Congenital; rare; combined T- and B-cell deficiency; function severely impaired in any T- or B-cells present; serious recurrent infections, often fatal; bone marrow transplant is best treatment
DiGeorge anomaly	Congenital; rare; usually detected in newborn period as result of hypocalcemia and consequent tetany or cardiac defects; decreased T-lymphs, esp, CD4; reduced proliferative response; increased B-lymphs
X-linked agammaglobulinemia (Bruton syndrome)	Congenital; rare; usually becomes evident at 5 to 6 months of age (maternal antibody protection until this time) by recurrent infections; markedly decreased Ig levels; B-cells and plasma cells absent; normal T-cell function
Complement component deficiency	Deficiency/defect in one or more complement components; associated with increased risk of infection with pyogenic organisms; increased incidence of autoimmune disorder with classical pathway deficiency; alternate pathway deficiency associated with increased susceptibility to *Neisseria;* both seen with common pathway deficiency; C1 inhibitor most common deficiency
HIV/AIDS	Reduction in CD4 T-lymphs is most noteworthy finding and best monitor of disease progression; B-cell and macrophage immunity also compromised; see Chapter 14 for more info on HIV

Description summaries developed based on information from Henry, 1996; Peakman and Vergani, 1997; Ravel, 1995

18. SELF TEST

Choose the best response for each item. The answer key may be found in the appendices.

1. **Humoral immunity refers to**
    A. macrophage immune responses to foreign antigen
    B. T-lymphocyte immune responses to foreign antigen
    C. production of antibodies in response to foreign antigen

2. **_____ is the most abundant immunoglobulin and the antibody produced in the secondary immune response.**
    A. IgG
    B. IgA
    C. IgM

3. **Primary humoral responses involve this pentamer, consisting of five basic Ig molecules.**
    A. IgG
    B. IgA
    C. IgM

4. **After binding with an antigen, the antibody undergoes a conformational change that exposes a site that can bind with**
    A. the C5 complement component
    B. the C1q complement component
    C. antigenic sites other than the antigen stimulating antibody production
    D. phagocytic enzyme receptor sites on the surface of neutrophils

5. **Antigen-antibody complexes activate the _____ complement pathway.**
    A. classical
    B. alternate
    C. common

6. **The end result of activation of the complement cascade is**
   A. neutrophil depletion
   B. plasma cell formation
   C. lysis of the targeted cell

7. **Neutrophils are an important component of the cellular immune system involved in the**
   A. primary control of parasitic infection
   B. histamine production
   C. killing and removal of bacteria and fungi

8. **These cells serve as sophisticated phagocytes, release cytokines, and are involved in the processing and presentation of antigens to T-cells.**
   A. mononuclear phagocytes (MNPs)
   B. mast cells
   C. eosinophils
   D. neutrophilic phagocytes

9. **These cells are the tissue equivalent of the basophil.**
   A. mononuclear phagocytes (MNPs)
   B. mast cells
   C. eosinophils
   D. neutrophilic phagocytes

10. **Antibody producing plasma cells develop from**
    A. T-lymphocytes
    B. B-lymphocytes
    C. mononuclear phagocytes (MNPs)
    D. mast cells

11. **The T-lymphocyte subset that stimulates the production of antibody to processed antigens is called**
    A. T-suppressor (CD8) cells
    B. cytotoxic cells (T-killer cells)
    C. T-helper (CD4) cells

12. **This systemic autoimmune disease can affect virtually every organ, almost always produces an elevated ANA titer, and is associated with a characteristic "butterfly rash."**
    A. systemic lupus erythematosus
    B. systemic rheumatoid arthritis
    C. Sjögren's syndrome

13. **The rheumatoid factor is an antibody to**
    A. subcutaneous nodules
    B. Fc fragment of IgG antibody
    C. C-reactive protein molecules

14. **The autoantibody found in insulin resistant diabetes mellitus is directed at**
    A. islet cells
    B. glucose
    C. insulin receptors

15. **This organ-specific autoimmune disease targets the liver and is associated with ANA, smooth muscle, and mitochondrial autoantibodies.**
    A. autoimmune hepatitis
    B. primary biliary cirrhosis
    C. atrophic gastritis

16. **This rare congenital immunodeficiency results from a marked decrease in both T- and B-cells and is most successfully treated by bone marrow transplant.**
    A. DiGeorge anomaly
    B. SCID
    C. X-linked agammaglobulinemia

17. **The laboratory assay best suited for monitoring the disease progression in HIV infection is**
    A. B-cell count
    B. CD8 T-cell count
    C. CD4 T-cell count
    D. antibody to HIV

Appendix A

TESTING DURING PREGNANCY

Many advances have been made in laboratory methods for the detection of pregnancy, for assessment of fetal function and maturity, and for detection of some congenital anomalies. These tests are presented briefly in this appendix.

PREGNANCY TESTS

Most pregnancy tests are based on the placental secretion of the human chorionic gonadotropin (HCG) hormone. Tests may be either qualitative or quantitative and are performed on serum and/or urine. Serum levels of HCG reach about 25 mIU/mL 8 to 10 days after conception and then double every 1 to 3 days for the first 6 weeks of gestation. Serum concentrations are typically greater than urine concentrations until about 3 weeks, when the concentrations in both serum and urine are about the same. Urine concentrations are generally higher thereafter, but the amount recovered in testing is dependent on the method employed (Ravel, 1995). A rapid decline in serum and urine concentrations is seen late in the first trimester until levels stabilize at about 10,000 mIU/mL. Smaller changes may be seen in the third trimester (Figure A–1).

Human chorionic gonadotropin has two subunits, designated alpha and beta. The alpha-subunit is seen in other hormones, whereas the beta-subunit is different for each hormone. Today's test methods using antibodies to the HCG molecule or the beta-subunit of the molecule are far removed from earlier laboratory methods employing mice, rabbits, and frogs. Many methods are capable of detected pregnancy 1 to 2 weeks after conception and have sensitivity levels < 50 mIU/mL—most rapid, qualitative assays have sensitivities in the range of 25 to 50 mIU/mL; quantitative immunoassay tests may have sensitivities of ~ 2 to 3 mIU/mL. False positive results may be seen with some methods. Knowledge of the sensitivity of the method and whether the intact molecule or the beta-subunit is measured is important to the interpretation of test results. Home pregnancy tests are available that are similar to the rapid qualitative assays in clinical laboratories. With adequate sensitivity levels and strict adherence to the manufacturer's written procedure, results are generally valid. First morning urine specimens should be used for testing in all urine pregnancy tests. HCG assays may be used for purposes other than the early detection of normal pregnancy. These assays may be useful in ectopic pregnancy, spontaneous abortion, and the detection of HCG producing neoplasms. Other tests that may be performed during pregnancy are summarized in Table A–1.

TABLE A–1. Testing During Pregnancy

Purpose	Tests	Description
Congenital anomalies	Maternal serum alpha-fetoprotein (MSAFP)	Used for detection of neural tube defects and Down syndrome screening; AFP is produced initially by fetal yolk sac and then primarily by fetal liver—excreted into amniotic fluid (trisomy 21) and diffuses into maternal serum; maternal AFP defects ~ 85% to 90% of open neural tube detects
	Amniotic fluid alpha-fetoprotein	Amniotic fluid AFP levels performed if MSAFP elevation is detected and confirmed; AFP levels dependent on fetal age and variety of other factors
	Amniotic fluid acetylcholinesterase	Amniotic fluid acetylcholinesterase levels specific for neural tube defects and not as dependent on fetal age
		Table A–2 provides additional information on AFP levels; AFP in conjunction with HCG and unconjugated estriol (Triple screen/triple test) levels tested between 14 and 22 weeks' gestation provides improved accurcy in detecting Down syndrome (Fig. A–2)
	Amniotic fluid chromosome analysis	Used for detection/confirmation of specific conditions, including Down syndrome, Edward syndrome (trisomy 18), cystic fibrosis, X-linked muscular dystrophy, and fragile X syndrome
Fetal function	Urine estriol or total estrogens	Urinary excretion of estriol or estrogen generally correlates well with fetal health, but mild disorders may not be detected; dead/dying placenta or fetus indicated by failure of estriol level to continue rising or by sudden significant and sustained decreased in level; daily variation in levels and various maternal conditions, including hypertension, preeclampsia, and impaired renal function, affect results; serum unconjugated levels offer advantages over urine measurements and are generally used instead
Placental function	Serum unconjugated estriol	More specific for fetoplacental dysfunction than urinary excretion and less dependent on maternal renal function; single values may still be difficult to interpret because of day-to-day (and within day) variation in levels; used with AFP and HCG in maternal triple screen
	Serum placental lactogen	Placental lactogen produced only by placenta; levels indicative of placental function only; used particularly in third trimester; short half-life makes it a sensitive indicator of placental failure; estriol levels, assessing both placental and fetal funmction, are used more often
Fetal maturity	Lecithin/sphingomyelin (LS) ratio	Assessment of fetal lung maturity and likelihood of respiratory distress syndrome upon delivery; lecithin, major component of alveolar surfactant, is less than sphingomyelin until about 26 weeks' gestation; by about 35 to 36 weeks lecithin is twice sphingomyelin
	Phosphatidylglycerol	Also assesses fetal lung maturity; in minor component of alveolar surfactant, but produced almost entirely by mature alveoli—hence, provides good indicator of lung maturity

Table compiled with information from Henry, 1996; Jacobs, 1990; Ravel, 1995; SmithKline Beecham Test Information

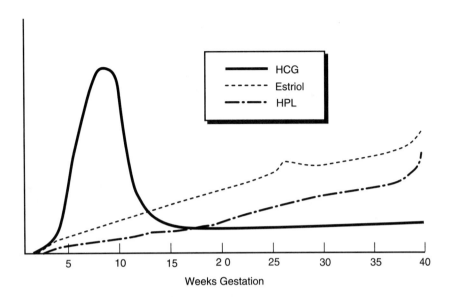

FIGURE A–1. HCG, estriol (total estrogens), and human placental lactogen (HPL) in normal pregnancy. (Adapted from Ravel R. *Clinical Laboratory Medicine: Clinical Application of Laboratory Data,* 6th ed. St Louis, Mosby, 1995, with permission)

TABLE A–2. Conditions Affecting MSAFP Levels

Decreased Levels	Increased Levels
Down syndrome	Open neural tube defects
Edward syndrome	Multiple pregnancy
Spontaneous, missed abortion	Underestimation of fetal age
Overestimation of fetal age	Hydrocephalus
Choriocarcinoma	Microcephalus
Molar pregnancy	Recent fetal death
Late fetal death	Fetal distress
	Congenital nephropathies and neoplasms
	Placental defects
	Abdominal pregnancy
	Growth retardation
	Cystic hygroma

Information from Ravel, 1995; Henry, 1996; SmithKline Beecham Test Information

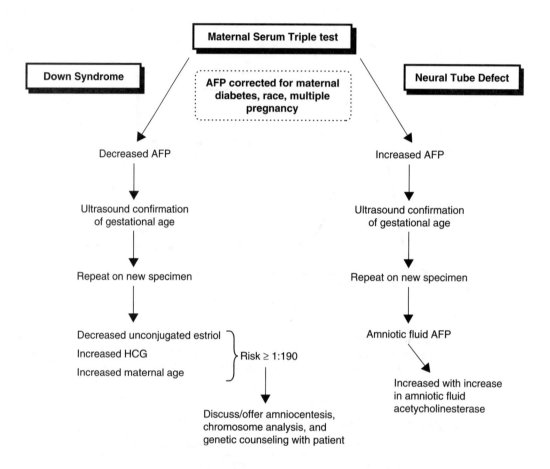

FIGURE A–2. Testing for Down syndrome and neural tube defects.

Appendix B
TUMOR MARKERS

Tumor markers are substances that do not normally appear in the circulation (or appear only in very small quantities) that are produced by neoplastic cells. The serum concentration of the marker can generally be correlated to changes in the mass of the primary tumor and its metastases and thus provides an efficient and effective means not only of detecting neoplasms, but also of monitoring disease progression and response to treatment. A variety of tumor markers are available, including specific enzyme markers, metabolic markers, tumor antigens, endocrine abnormalities, and gene alterations. In some instances the use of multiple markers can improve specificity and sensitivity. A few of the tumor markers that can be detected in serum are summarized in Table B–1.

Although not tested for in serum, progesterone and estrogen receptor assays and detection of human papillomavirus are described below.

- *Estrogen and Progesterone Receptor Assays* (ERA and PRA): useful in breast cancer as prognostic indicators and as an aid in selection of therapy; performed on tissue samples; immunoassay techniques estimate the number of binding sites (unoccupied or active, and inactive) for these hormones; 60% to 70% of patients with ERA positive tumors respond to hormonal manipulation; ERA negativity may indicate that chemotherapy is more likely to be effective; positive PRA in addition to positive ERA adds ~10% to 15% greater likelihood of response to hormonal manipulation (Ravel, 1995).
- *Human Papilloma Virus* (HPV): more than 50 types of HPV exist (Sacher and McPherson, 1991); some types are associated with common skin warts, others with venereal warts, and some types are associated with carcinoma of the cervix; specific types can be detected by DNA probe on cervical biopsy or smear material; type detected may also be indicative of the grade (low, intermediate, or high) of the malignancy.

TABLE B–1. Tumor Markers

Tumor Marker	Clinical Association
CEA	Carcinoembryonic antigen; elevations most frequently seen with colon cancer; also elevated in breast and lung cancer as well as other malignancies and in some benign conditions; smokers have slightly higher levels; major use is to follow therapy—baseline level drawn ≥ 4 weeks post-op with repeat levels every 2 months for 2 years (protocols vary); return of CEA to normal does not guarantee total elimination of tumor, but is good indicator that most is removed; subsequent elevations are suggestive of local recurrence of metastasis and may be seen several months prior to clinical evidence of recurrence
PSA	Prostatic specific antigen; more sensitive indicator of prostatic carcinoma than acid phosphatase levels (over detection rate 80 % to 90% [Ravel, 1995]); values in reference range seen in some patients with carcinoma; mild to moderate elevations suggest increased likelihood that prostatic carcinoma is present, but may be seen in benign prostatichyperplasia; values above 10 ng/mL are highly suggestive of carcinoma; especially useful for monitoring patients (in whom prostatic carcinoma has been proven) following therapy; may be useful in conjunction with PAP (see below)
PAP	Prostatic acid phosphatase; an isoenzyme of acid phosphatase that is distinctly different from the forms made in other cells (eg, platelets); may be used in conjunction with PSA to provide improved diagnostic sensitivity (more sensitive than either test used above); PSA is better test for monitoring disease progression and better indicator of prognosis
AFP	Alpha-fetoprotein; elevated in patients with primary hepatoma and some testicular tumors; most useful serum marker for hepatocellular carcinoma (Henry, 1996); may also be elevated in several benign liver conditions, including some cases of hepatitis
Beta-HCG	In addition to secretion in pregnancy, is secreted by choriocarcinomas and hyaditidiform moles in women and by germ line testicular carcinoma in men
CA-125	Antigenic determinant found in most ovarian carcinomas and detected using monoclonal antibody techniques; sensitivity in detection of ovarian cancer is ~75% to 80% (Ravel, 1995); elevations sometimes seen in other malignancies and in some benign conditions, including endometriosis, cirrhosis, and acute peritonitis
CA 19-9	Not a widely used marker, but is frequently significantly elevated in gastric and pancreatic carcinoma (Ravel, 1995); not highly specific; does not detect pancreatic carcinoma early enough to change prognosis; sensitivity improved when used in conjunction with CA-50 (Henry, 1996); has been used in conjunction with CEA to detect recurrence of colon cancer (Ravel, 1995); is related to Lewis A blood group antigen—persons negative for Lewis A antigen will not have elevation regardless of presence of carcinoma (Ravel, 1995)
CA 15-3	Antigen associated with breast cancer; more reliable in detecting and monitoring breast cancer than CEA (Henry, 1996); better correlation with tumor progression than with regression (Ravel, 1995); also may be elevated in other conditions, including some benign breast tumors, cirrhosis, and chronic hepatitis
CA 72-4	Moderate serum elevations seen with most carcinomas; despite poor sensitivity is currently considered best marker for managing patients with gastric carcinoma (Henry, 1996)
CA-549	Abnormal in 53% to 90% of patients with metastatic breast cancer (Ravel, 1995), but may also be elevated with other metastatic tumors and in some patients with benign breast tumors
CA-50	Differs only slightly from CA 19-9 and may be used in conjunction with this marker

Appendix C
THERAPEUTIC DRUG MONITORING

Laboratory assays are available for the quantitation of a number of drugs used for therapeutic purposes, including antibiotics, cardiac drugs, antiepileptics, psychiatric drugs, and others. Although the primary uses of therapeutic drug monitoring (TDM) are to ensure the patient is receiving sufficient medication to achieve the desired therapeutic effect and that the dosage is not large enough to produce toxic effects, TDM is used for a variety of reasons, including those summarized in Table C–1. A variety of methods are available for therapeutic drug assays, such as spectrophotometry, various chromatographic methods (thin layer chromatography [TLC]; gas chromatography [GC]; high performance liquid chromatography [HPLC]), radioimmunoassay (RIA), fluorescence-polarization immunoassay (FPIA), and enzyme multiplied immunoassay (EMIT). The development of immunoassay techniques that use antibodies reactive to a specific drug (and in some cases, metabolites of the drug) and are adaptable to automation has made it possible for most laboratories to offer at least some TDM. Other methods, still necessary in some instances, typically require highly specialized equipment and are generally available only through reference laboratories. Most assays measure the total amount of the drug present, including both the metabolically active unbound (or "free") portion and the protein bound portion.

A number of factors influence the blood level of therapeutic drugs, several of which are presented in Table C–2. An understanding of these factors is important in the evaluation of TDM test results and in ensuring appropriate specimen collection times. Levels may be requested as either peak or trough levels. When the drug is administered at regular intervals, serum levels go through a series of recurrent peak (highest) and trough (lowest) levels. Upon initiating the drug therapy, peak and trough levels gradually increase with each dose until a "steady state" is achieved. The steady state is a plateau at which peak concentrations are essentially the same from day to day as are trough levels. Serum drug concentrations are best measured at one (or both, in some instances) of these times (peak or trough) rather than at some random time between the two in order for results to be meaningful. Trough specimens are collected just prior to the next scheduled dose and peak levels are collected at a specified time (depending on route of administration and various characteristics of the drug itself, including rate of absorption) following administration. Table C–3 provides basic information about a number of therapeutic drugs.

TABLE C–1. Utilization of Therapeutic Drug Monitoring

Reason	Comments
To determine if therapeutic serum concentrations have been reached	Therapeutic effects may not be immediately evident, but determination of serum drug concentration assesses whether the level expected to produce the desired effects has been achieved
To avoid reaching toxic serum levels	Especially important when drugs have a narrow therapeutic window (ie, desired levels very close to toxic levels; narrow therapeutic range) and when the toxic effects of the drug are serious
Investigation of cases in which standard dose does not produce expected effect	Could be seen with low serum drug concentration, but could also occur in the presence of appropriate serum levels due to other factors, such as interference from other drugs
When patient has condition that is known to affect the achievement of desired levels (such as liver disease, kidney disorders, or altered digestive secretions)	Some conditions can interfere with the appropriate absorption of the drug, with adequate excretion of the drug and its metabolites, alter the protein binding of the drug, or interfere with or alter the metabolism of the drug
To assess patient compliance with prescribed regimen	Intentional or unintentional non-compliance by taking less than the prescribed amount, stopping medication altogether, taking more than the prescribed amount, taking medication at improper or irregular intervals

TABLE C–2. Factors Affecting Serum Levels of Therapeutic Drugs

Dosage and route of administration	IV, IM, or oral administration; peak levels achieved almost immediately with IV administration; achievement of peak level after oral administration is dependent on a number of factors, including absorption rate; influence of dosage is obvious
Drug transport and protein binding	Many drugs have large portions that are bound to proteins; protein bound molecules are not metabolically active; some conditions can alter the ratio of bound to unbound drug molecules (ratio generally relatively stable), making it possible to have a total serum concentration within therapeutic range with an unbound, metabolically active drug level that is toxic or to have a total serum drug level that is in the toxic range while the unbound drug level is in the therapeutic range; many assays measure total drug level only without distinction between bound and free; unbound or free drug assays are typically available from reference laboratories; significant alteration in binding proteins may also influence drug levels
Absorption of drug	May be altered by a number of factors, including alterations in gastric and pancreatic secretions, GI tract motility, malabsorption disorders, and in some instances, by interference from certain foods and drugs

(Cont.)

TABLE C–2. (*Cont.*)

Drug metabolism	Most therapeutic drugs are inactivated to some degree by the liver (digoxin and lithium are notable exceptions); rate of metabolism varies from drug to drug and among patients; liver damage can become a critical factor in the ability to metabolize a particular drug effectively; other drugs and substances, such as alcohol, can alter metabolism of some drugs
Half-life	The half-life of a drug is the time required for the body to reduce the drug concentration in the blood by 50%; an important factor in determining frequency of administration; depending on the type of drug and the patient's ability to metabolize and excrete the drug
Steady state	The steady state is when blood levels have reached equilibrium (the plateau at which peak values are relatively constant and trough levels do not vary significantly from one sampling to another); typically takes about five half-lives to achieve steady state (Ravel, 1995) unless loading doses are used
Uptake by target tissues and distribution space	Drugs typically act on tissues and often reach higher concentrations in tissues than in blood (blood levels are used for monitoring, however, because it is neither convenient nor feasible to perform routine monitoring on tissue samples; "distribution space" is the term used to refer to the relationship concentration in tissue and in blood; "larger distribution space" means that significantly more of the drug is in tissues than in blood; dependent on drug's chemical properties, including solubility characteristics; can be altered by conditions that affect tissue perfusion
Excretion	Most therapeutic drugs are excreted in large part by the kidney (a notable exception being theophylline [Ravel, 1995]); thus significantly impaired renal function impairs the ability to clear the drug and its metabolites from the blood
Interferences	Certain drugs and other substances can interfere with the absorption, metabolism, and other aspects of the therapeutic drug being measured; these substances may interfere with some laboratory assays
Patient factors	Any underlying condition such as liver or kidney disease that can influence one or more of the previously discussed factors
	Weight: weight based dosages may allow desirable blood levels to be achieved more readily than arbitrary standard doses
	Age: important dosage determinant, with children generally receiving twice the dose per unit of weight as adults, the elderly receiving less, and infants receiving about the same dose per unit of weight (Ravel, 1995)
	Compliance with prescribed drug regimen as discussed in Table C–1

TABLE C–3. Summary of Selected Therapeutic Drugs

Therapeutic Drug	Drug Class and Use	Collection	Peak Specimen Range	Therapeutic Half-Life	Serum Comments
Gentamicin	Aminoglycoside antibiotic; useful in infections with gram negative organisms, including *Pseudomonas aeruginosa*	30 min after IV administration 60 min after IM administration	Peak: 4 to 8 µg/mL; (Ravel, 1995)	2 to 3 h; variable	Both peak and trough levels usually monitored; peak values most useful for determination of effective dosage; trough levels correlate best with nephrotoxicity; excreted primarily through glomerular filtration; serum creatinine levels also used to aid dosage determinations; drug is also ototoxic; levels >10 µg/mL considered toxic (Ravel, 1995)
Vancomycin	Tricyclic glycopeptide antibiotic; useful for MRSA and *Clostridium difficile*	Recommendations vary from immediately to 15/30 min or 2 h after IV infusion; see comments	Peak: see comments Trough: 5 to 10 µg/mL (Henry, 1996)	4 to 8 h (adult) 2 to 3 h (child) (Ravel, 1995)	Serum levels fall quickly immediately after IV infusion, then more slowly; therapeutic range for peak level immediately after infusion is 30 to 40 mg/dL and at 15 min is 25 to 30 mg/dL (Ravel, 1995); only small amount absorbed from oral administration; this form used for GI tract organisms like *C difficile*; adverse effects include nephrotoxicity and ototoxicity; important to monitor renal function
Tobramycin	Aminoglycoside antibiotic; antibacterial action parallels that of gentamicin	30 min after IV infusion	Peak: 4 to 8 µg/mL Trough: 1 to 2 µg/mL (Henry, 1996)	2 to 3 h	Both peak and trough levels usually monitored; renal elimination; used in severe infections; adverse effects include ototoxicity and nephrotoxicity; renal function should be assessed
Phenytoin (Dilantin)	Anticonvulsant used in seizure disorders, tonic-clonic epilepsy, focal seizures, and acute state of uncontrolled seizures	Trough levels usually monitored 4 to 8 h (Ravel, 1995)	10 to 20 µg/mL	12 to 36 h (dose dependent) 4 to 11 h (children) (Sacher and McPherson, 1991)	Narrow therapeutic window with potential of toxicity > 20 µg/mL; 90% bound to serum proteins, primarily albumin; steady state usually 4 to 6 days (Ravel, 1995); most metabolized by liver; ~5% excreted unchanged in urine (Henry, 1996); levels may be increased in severe liverdisease; several drugs affect blood levels and may interfere with binding to albumin; assay available for free (unbound) phenytoin—therapeutic range 1 to 2 µg/mL (Sacher and McPherson, 1991); CNS symptoms in overdose—blurred double vision, drowsiness, nystagmus, muscular incoordination, and possible coma; long-term effects may include acne, gum hyperplasia, lymphoid hyperplasia, hirsutism, interference with vitamin D metabolism; phenobarbital affects phenytoin levels and conversely, phenytoin affects phenobarbital *(Cont.)*

TABLE C-3. (Cont.)

Therapeutic Drug	Drug Class and Use	Peak Specimen Collection	Therapeutic Range	Serum Half-Life	Comments
Valproic acid	Anticonvulsant; chemically unique; used for broad spectrum of seizures; also used in conjunction with antidepressant therapy in the treatment of bipolar disorder	Typically monitored by trough sample Peaks 1 to 3 h after oral dose	50 to 100 µg/mL (Sacher and McPherson, 1991)	15 to 20 h (Sacher and McPherson, 1991)	90% bound to proteins; well absorbed after oral administration; extensively metabolized by liver and excreted in urine; serum samples must remain tightly capped to avoid evaporation due to volatility; interacts with phenobarbital by inhibiting liver metabolism and with phenytoin by displacing plasma proteins (Sacher and McPherson, 1991); steady state reached in 2 to 3 days, but may take several weeks to see therapeutic effects (Ravel, 1995); although rare, may produce liver failure (potentially reversible) that progresses gradually several months into therapy (AST levels should be monitored) or more rarely, sudden and irreversible liver failure may occur soon after initiation of therapy (Ravel, 1995)
Carbamazepine (Tegretol)	Anticonvulsant used for grand mal and psychomotor epilepsy and in other seizures with pain component	Trough levels used to monitor. Peak occurs 6-8 hours after tablets	8-12 µg/mL (Sacher and McPherson, 1991) slightly lower if pt. is on another anticonvulsant	-35 hours (8-20 hours after 3-4 wks admin.)	Metabolized by liver—can speed its own metabolism; only ~1% excreted unchanged in urine (Ravel, 1995); steady state reached in about 2 weeks for initial therapy, shorter with subsequent doses (Ravel, 1995); clearance dependent on hepatic function and co-administration of other drugs (Sacher and McPherson, 1991) and in some instances protein binding (about 70% bound to protein); adverse effects include leukopenia (usually transient, but persists in some patients), rash, visual changes, ataxia, nausea, vomiting, thrombocytopenia (low incidence), hepatic failure or, rarely, aplastic anemia
Phenobarbital	Anticonvulsant barbiturate; used for tonic-clonic psychomotor, and focal epileptic seizures; not used for petit mal seizures	Trough levels used to monitor	20 to 40 µg/mL lower levels may be effective in children (Sacher and McPherson, 1991)	5 to 6 days (adults) 3-4 days (children)	Good absorption from stomach and small intestine; metabolized in liver with 10% to 30% excreted unchanged in urine (Ravel, 1995); increases degradation of the drugs metabolized by the hepatic microsomes; many potential interactions with other drugs; acidification of urine (such as occurs with valproic acid) delays clearance of phenobarbital (Sacher and McPherson, 1991); steady state reached in 2 to 3 weeks; acute alcoholism increases patient response and chronic alcoholism decreases patient response (Ravel, 1995); toxic effects include nausea, vomiting, vertigo, ataxia, respiratory depression

(Cont.)

TABLE C-3. (Cont.)

Therapeutic Drug	Drug Class and Use	Peak Specimen Collection	Therapeutic Range	Serum Half-Life	Comments
Theophylline	Antiasthmatic; used IV with acute exacerbation or orally for prevention of asthmatic episodes	Peak reached 30 min IV; 2 hrs oral; ~ 5 h with sustained release preparations	10 to 20 µg/mL (Henry, 1996; Sacher and McPherson, 1991)	8 to 9 Variable (shorter in smokers) 3 to 4 h children	Absorption is typically complete and occurs primarily in the small intestine for most preparations (Ravel, 1995); metabolized by liver with 10% to 15% excreted unchanged in urine (Ravel, 1995); serum levels are directly related to and predictive of bronchodilator effects (Sacher and McPherson, 1991); narrow therapeutic window; toxic symptoms of nausea and vomiting can occur > 20 µg/mL (Sacher and McPherson, 1991) and seizures, tachycardia, syncope, respiratory arrest, cardiac arrythmias or cardiac arrest > 30 µg/mL (Henry, 1996; Sacher and McPherson, 1991); blood level is best predictor of toxicity—not early symptoms
Digoxin	Cardiac drug used in congestive heart failure (increases force of myocardial contractions) and to control arrhythmias	Specimens for monitoring should be drawn at least 6 h after dose. Peaks 30 to 90 min after oral dose with plateau in 6 to 8 h	0.5 to 2.0 µg/mL	35 to 40 h, longer with decreased renal function	Only small amounts typically metabolized, with ~80% (Ravel, 1995) excreted unchanged in urine; narrow line between therapeutic and toxic levels; ≥ 2 µg/mL toxic; toxic levels can produce nausea, vomiting, headache, fatigue, disorientation, atria and ventricular arrhythmias, convulsions; steady state reached in about 7 days (Henry, 1996) with normal renal function and without loading dose; renal failure can increase half life to ~ 5 days (Ravel, 1995); variety of metabolic disorders and medications can alter serum levels; electrolyte abnormalities, hypothyroidism, and severe ischemic heart disease predispose to toxicity (Sacher, 1991)
Procainamide	Antiarrhythmic used to control ventricular and supraventricular arrhythmias	Trough specimen used for monitoring Peaks at 1.5 h (std preps (or 2 h (sustained release)	4 to 10 µg/mL (Henry, 1996) combined with NAPA 10 to 30 µg/mL (Ravel, 1995; Sacher and McPherson, 1991)	~ 3.5 h with normal renal function	Major metabolite is N-acetylprocainamide (NAPA) that has activity nearly equal to procainamide and has half-about twice that of procainamide; many investigators recommend measurement of both (Ravel, 1995; Sacher and McPherson, 1991); metabolized mainly by liver with 50% excreted unchanged in urine; steady state for standard preparations reached in ~ 18 h and for sustained release 24 to 30 h (Ravel, 1995); adverse effects include hypotension, bradycardia, irregular pulse, nausea, vomiting, malaise, confusion; long-term use can produce lupus erythematosus that is usually reversible (Henry, 1996; Sacher and McPherson, 1991)

Table compiled with data from Henry JB. *Clinical Diagnosis and Management by Laboratory Methods*, 19th ed. Philadelphia, Saunders, 1996; Jacobs DS, et al. *Laboratory Test Handbook*, 2nd ed. Cleveland, LexiComp Inc, 1990; Ravel R. *Clinical Laboratory Medicine: Clinical Application of Laboratory Data*, 6th ed. St Louis, Mosby, 1995; and Sacher RA, McPherson RA. *Widmann's Clinical Interpretation of Laboratory Tests*, 10th ed. Philadelphia, FA Davis, 1991

Appendix D

POINT OF CARE TESTING

In an effort to provide more "patient focused" care, many hospitals began efforts in the late 1980s and in the 1990s to design the delivery of health care services around the needs of patients. The belief was that providing services based on patient needs with less regard to organization of services around functional departments or professional groups would allow improvement in the quality of service, higher patient satisfaction levels, and cost reductions. Although numerous institutions embraced this philosophy, there are many variations in the extent to which the philosophy has been put into practice, the methods used to achieve the goals of patient focused care, and the degree to which implementation has been successful. Patient focused care typically involves at least some degree of cross training or multi-skilling, development of patient care teams assigned to particular patients who may be clustered according to clinical needs, and decentralization of ancillary services such as respiratory therapy, radiology services, physical therapy, and laboratory testing.

Testing performed at or near the patient's bedside is called *point of care testing* and is generally included (although to varying degrees) in efforts to reorganize the delivery of health care services around the patient's needs. When instituted after appropriate planning and evaluation and with the proper training, supervision, quality control, and quality assurance, point of care testing can provide significant benefits. Without the proper planning, training and understanding, quality control, and supervision, however, point of care testing has resulted in situations that not only horrify clinical laboratory scientists but produce outcomes in total opposition to the goals of improved quality and lowered cost and result in potentially catastrophic errors in treatment and diagnostic decisions. Quality point of care testing can provide more rapid access to test results (shorter turnaround time [TAT]), which allows medical intervention in a more timely manner and may reduce length of stay. Reduced TAT is of particular importance in settings where more critically ill patients are likely to be treated, such as the Emergency Department or Critical Care Unit. Other areas may also benefit from point of care testing. This appendix briefly summarizes the features of a good point of care testing program, factors to be weighed in deciding what testing is performed at the point of care and at which sites, and the issues to be addressed in implementing such testing. See Tables D–1 to D–4.

TABLE D–1. General Characteristics of a Good Point of Care Testing Program

No inappropriate duplication of resources

Test menu is appropriate for testing site

Responsibilities are clearly delineated for all aspects of the program, including testing, supervision, policy development, and program evaluation

Multidisciplinary involvement in planning, implementing, and evaluating the program (nursing and/or other non-laboratory testing personnel, laboratory staff, laboratory medical director)

Written quality control (QC) policies and procedures are developed, implemented, and adhered to

Appropriate follow-up is initiated and documented for all QC results out of the accepted range and is reviewed by supervisory staff

Quality control results are documented by testing personnel with regular monitoring and evaluation of results by individuals qualified to assess shifts, trends, and any statistically or medically significant QC results

Verification of instrument performance function (including precision, accuracy, and calibration verification or linearity) is conducted and documented initially and at regular intervals established by regulatory agencies and in accordance with regulatory standards with review by the medical director or designee

Well written, thorough testing procedures are readily available to and followed by testing personnel

Regular review of all policies and procedures is performed and documented and includes the approval of the laboratory medical director

Preventive maintenance procedures are performed and documented in accordance with manufacturer recommendations

A comprehensive training program is developed and implemented for testing personnel and includes test performance, limitations of the procedure, interfering substances, QC principles and procedures, calibration, basic troubleshooting, reporting of results, instrument maintenance, assessment of trainees' mastery of the material, and documentation of training

Competency assessment for testing personnel in accordance with regulatory agencies

Established mechanisms for follow-up of specified levels of low and high test results by confirmation testing in the central laboratory, including values outside the instrument's proven linearity range

Appropriate reference ranges specific for the methodology used have been developed or verified and are reported with test results

Established mechanisms for reporting all results and for those results that are critical

Regular evaluation of all aspects of the program (benefits, costs, compliance with regulatory agencies, necessary or desired changes, etc) that is documented along with any changes made in response to the results of the evaluation

Reagents are properly stored, prepared, and used in accordance with manufacturers' guidelines and are not used beyond stated expiration dates

---

TABLE D–2. Questions to Address in Point of Care Test and Test Site Selection

Which test results are likely to be needed on a stat basis?
   Are the results of the test often needed immediately in this patient care location?
   Would medical intervention be initiated immediately based upon test results?

How frequently is the test requested in this patient care area?
   Is the test often requested several times each day on a given patient? OR
   Is the test typically requested on most patients in this location?

Is suitable instrumentation available to perform this test at the point of care? (see also Table D–3)
Size of available instrumentation
   Instrument cost
   Ease of operation and instrument maintenance
   Whole blood vs serum or plasma samples
   Complexity of reagent preparation
   Reagent stability and storage requirements
   Validity of results

Will point of care testing at this site represent an unnecessary duplication of resources that is not outweighed by benefits gained?

Is the cost per reportable test acceptable based on the benefits to be achieved?

Does this patient care location have a sufficient number of staff members who are qualified (or can be trained) to perform this testing?

What is the CLIA designated test complexity level for the analytes under consideration? Can the regulations for this complexity level be reasonably met?

TABLE D–3. Desirable Features of Point of Care Testing Instrumentation

High level of accuracy
High level of precision
Easy to use with minimal operator intervention required
Good turnaround time
Sample factors:
  Small amount required for testing
  Whole blood used for testing (plasma or serum sample preparation requires additional time and equipment)
Portable or small in size
Minimal and easy to perform preventive maintenance procedures
Reporting format consistent with (or readily adaptable to) other laboratory methods
Ability to interface with laboratory information system
Good references from other users (preferably those using the instrument for at least 6 months)
Level of manufacturer support after purchase:
  Instrument set-up
  Performance or assistance with precision and accuracy studies, linearity studies, comparison to centralized laboratory method for same analyte(s)
  Warranty and service agreements
  Technical support
  Staff training
Detailed, easy to use operator's manual and procedural instructions
Use of one or more "built in" quality control features
Minimal or no reagent preparation requirements
Suitable length of reagent stability

TABLE D–4. Cost Factors Related to Point of Care Instrument Choice

Cost of instrument (outright purchase, title lease option, reagent rental agreement, etc)
Cost of consumable supplies required for testing
Preventive maintenance costs
Repair costs
Length of warranty
Service contract cost
Cost of interface to laboratory information system
Expected longevity of instrument
Cost of calibration standards and quality control (QC) materials
Frequency of required calibrations and QC testing
Reagent cost:
  Are there large volume purchase requirements that may result in expiration of unused quantities?
  Can a specific lot number be requested to reduce the frequency of additional testing required for new lot numbers?
  Reagent stability (unopened and opened)
Cost per reportable (or billable) test as opposed to cost per test; cost per reportable test includes all testing required to generate a valid patient result, including QC materials, consumables, calibration materials, etc. Cost per reportable or billable test is a more reliable indicator of operational costs than cost per test, which is often quoted by manufacturers' representatives if not clarified by the potential purchaser.

Although point of care testing can provide significant benefits, it is essential to ensure appropriate training, understanding of basic quality control principles, adequate supervision, assessment of testing personnel competencies, and other mechanisms to ensure that reliable data are provided by such testing. A failure to do so is to create an environment in which misdiagnoses and inappropriate treatment decisions can occur. A few examples of such problems from the author's experience and from those reported by the Joint Commission on Accreditation of Healthcare Organizations (JCAHO) are presented below.

- The nursing department with sole responsibility for point of care testing "...stopped running controls because the answers weren't coming out right." (Quote from *Point of Care Testing: The JCAHO Perspective*, by Anne C. Belanger, in MLO, June, 1994.)
- An Emergency Department physician who used an improperly stored, expired (1 year outdated) pregnancy test kit sent a pregnant woman for a radiologic procedure based on the negative test result obtained with invalid kit reagents. (*Point of Care Testing: The JCAHO Perspective*, by Anne C. Belanger, in MLO, June, 1994.)
- A medical assistant reported the presence of *Neisseria gonorrhea* in a vaginal specimen solely on the basis of a screening procedure intended only to rule out the presence of *N. gonorrhea* or to indicate the need for additional testing due to the possible presence of the organism. The error was detected by the supervising technologist during review of results the next day—after the physician had informed the patient of the erroneous results, treated the patient and her husband, and attempted to mediate a rather nasty marital spat. The patient actually had nothing more than a yeast infection. (Author's experience.)
- A certified physician's assistant performed a latex agglutination urine pregnancy test because the laboratorian for the clinic was not immediately available. Unfamiliar with the methodology employed (and failing to read procedural instructions for test interpretation), he interpreted the agglutination of the latex particles (which indicated an absence of HCG) as a positive test and informed the patient (who insisted it was impossible) that she was pregnant. His response to the laboratorian's query regarding his familiarity with the test was "Oh, yes. I'm sure it was positive. I've never seen one agglutinate that fast!" (Author's experience.)
- An Emergency Department physician, finding the developer reagent bottle empty, ran an occult blood slide under tap water instead. The same physician performed a Gram stain by decolorizing with safranin and counterstaining with crystal violet. (*Point of Care Testing: The JCAHO Perspective*, by Anne C. Belanger, in MLO, June, 1994.)
- Perhaps the most frightening example (and one that brings more than point of care protocols into question) is that of a resident in intensive care who informed a JCAHO surveyor that he "...had invented a new test for monitoring heparin therapy: monitor the patient's stool with an occult blood test. When the patient begins to bleed through the rectum, it's time to back off the heparin." (Quote from *Point of Care Testing: The JCAHO Perspective*, by Anne C. Belanger, in MLO, June, 1994.)

Appendix E

SAMPLE OF A MAXIMUM SURGICAL BLOOD ORDER SCHEDULE (MSBOS)

Procedure	# Units	Procedure	# Units	Procedure	# Units
GENERAL SURGERY		Small bowel resection	T/S	Esophageal reconstruction	T/S
Abdominal-perineal resection	2	Splenectomy	T/S	Esophagoscopy	0 or T/S
Amputations	T/S	Splenorenal artery bypass	3	Ethmoid artery ligation	4
Aneurysm, abdominal aortic	6	Sympathectomy	T/S	Ethmoidectomy	T/S
Aneurysm resection	4	Thrombectomy	T/S	Frontal sinus exploration	T/S
Aortobifemoral bypass	4	Thyroidectomy	T/S	Laryngectomy	1
Aortoiliac bypass	4	Total large colon resection	T/S	Laryngoscopy	0
Appendectomy	0	Tracheostomy	T/S	Maxillary fixation	T/S
Arterial bypass	1	Vein stripping	0	Maxillectomy	2
Biopsy	0	Whipple procedure	4	Myringotomy	0
Biopsy, node	0	**GYNECOLOGIC SURGERY**		Neck dissection	2
Bronchoscopy	0	Ap repair	1	Neurectomy	0 or T/S
Carotid artery exploration	1 or T/S	Cone biopsy (CO_2 laser)	0	Parotidectomy	0 or T/S
Cholecystojejunostomy	T/S	D & C	0 or T/S	Septoplasty	0 or T/S
Colon resection	2	Ectopic pregnancy	2	Sphenoidectomy	T/S
Colostomy closure	T/S	Endometrium ablation	0 or T/S	Thyroidectomy	T/S
Colostomy takedown	T/S	Exploratory laparotomy	T/S or 2	Tonsillectomy	0
Denver pertoneal shunt insertion	T/S	Exenteration procedure	4	Tracheoscopy	0
Denver shunt revision	T/S	Hysterectomy, total abdominal	T/S or 2	Tracheostomy	0 or T/S
Endarterectomy, carotid	1	Laparoscopy	0 or T/S	Tracheostomy (tube insertion)	0
Esophagogastrectomy	4	Laser vaporization	0	Tympanomastoidectomy	0 or T/S
Esophagectomy	4	Neosalpingostomy	T/S	Tympanoplasty	0
Exploratory laparotomy	T/S*	Ovarian wedge resection	T/S	**ORTHOPEDIC SURGERY**	
Femoral perineal bypass	2	Salpingo oophrectomy	0 or T/S	Amputation	T/S
Femoral popliteal bypass	1	Tubal ligation	0	Arthroscopy	0 or T/S
Gastric bypass	T/S	Tuboplasty	T/S	Arthroplasty	T/S
Gastrostomy	0 or T/S	Uterine suspension	0 or T/S	Carpal tunnel release	0
Hemicolectomy	T/S	Vaginectomy	T/S	Closed reduction	0
Hemorrhoidectomy	0 or T/S	Vulvectomy	T/S	Decompression laminectomy	1
Hepatic lobectomy	6	**VASCULAR SURGERY**		Discetomy	T/S
Hernia repair	0 or T/S	Aortofemoral/aortoiliac bypass	4	Fractures	0
Hickman catheter insert/remove	0 or T/S	Arterial bypass	2	Fusions, other	0 or T/S
Ileostomy	T/S	Carotid endarterectomy	T/S or 1	Hardware removal	0
Lumpectomy	0	Catheter insertion	T/S	Hip revisoin	3
Mastectomy	T/S	Femoral popliteal bypass	1	Hip screw and nailing	T/S
Mediastinoscopy	T/S	Iliac profunda bypass	1	Lumbar laminectomy	1
Oophorectomy	T/S	Renal artery repair	3	Meniscectomy	0
Pilonidal cyst	0	**OTOLARYNGOLOGIC (ENT) SURGERY**		Neuroma excision	0 or T/S
Portocaval shunt	4	Bronchoscopy	0 or T/S	Open reduction	T/S
Rib resection	0	Cochlear implant	0	Osteotomy	0 or T/S
Sigmoidectomy	T/S	Composite resection	4	Posterior rod fusion	2
Sigmoidoscopy	0 to T/S	Dissecting laryngoscopy	0	Rodding (Grosse and Kempf)	T/S

Procedure	# Units	Procedure	# Units	Procedure	# Units
Rotator cuff repair	T/S	Cystoscopy	0	Orchidopexy	0
Shoulder replacement	T/S	Cystotomy	0	Orchiectomy	0
Spinal fusions	1	Fulguration, bleeding bladder	0	Prostatectomy	2
Tendon repair	0	Hydrocelectomy	0	Pyelolithotomy	T/S
Total elbow	T/S	Ileal conduit	1	Reimplantation of ureter	T/S
Total hip	2	Lithotomy, utero	T/S	Tur	T/S
Total knee	T/S	Meatotomy	T/S	Ureterectomy	0
UROLOGIC SURGERY		Needle biopsy of prostate	0	Ureterolithotomy	T/S
Adrenalectomy	2	Nephrectomy, radical	2	Urethral fistulas, excision	T/S
Bladder resection	T/S	Nephrolithrotripsy	1	Vasectomy	0
Circumcision	0	Nephrostomy	T/S	Vasovasostomy	0
Cystectomy	2				

Courtesy of Ephraim McDowell Regional Medical Center Laboratory, WL Pesci, MD and RG Jackson MD, Medical Directors.

T/S, Type and Screen; 0, No Testing Required; *, Varies with Purpose.

Appendix F
CRITICAL VALUES

REFERENCE RANGE LISTS: Any list of reference ranges is not to be arbitrarily used in the evaluation of patient test results. Reference ranges vary (in some cases widely) among laboratories, by test methodology, and in regard to a variety of other factors including patient population. Each laboratory must provide a reference range specific to the test methodology used and the patient population served for use in interpreting patient data. Patient data must be evaluated by the clinician utilizing the reference range provided with the test report. It is important to note the units used in reporting test values and whether conventional or SI units are used. Common abbreviations employed in reporting units of measure for laboratory tests are provided in Table F-1. Representative ranges are provided in the text as appropriate to the discussion of particular tests. The reader is referred to Chapter 1 for information related to the determination of reference ranges.

CRITICAL VALUES: Critical values (also called panic values or alarm values) should also be established by each laboratory, ideally with input and approval by the medical staff routinely served by the testing facility. Critical values indicate the level at which immediate action is generally indicated and require immediate notification of the physician or other designated individual responsible for the care of the patient. Variation will be noted in published lists of critical values and in those values used by various laboratories with some following a more conservative approach. A typical listing of critical values is provided in Table F-2 as an example only. The values listed are for adults unless otherwise specified. Values for children, newborns, and in some instances, the elderly, may differ.

TABLE F-1. Common Abbreviations for Units of Measure and Prefixes

Abbreviation	Meaning	Prefix Abbreviation	Meaning	
L	liter	k	kilo	10^3
g	gram	d	deci	10^{-1}
mol	mole	m	milli	10^{-3}
m	meter	c	centi	10^{-2}
°C	degrees Celsius	μ	micro	10^{-6}
		n	nano	10^{-9}
		p	pico	10^{-12}

TABLE F-2. Representative List of Critical Values

Test	Critical Value	
	Above (High Level)	**Below (Low Level)**
Arterial blood gases: pH	7.5	7.3
pO_2		50 mm Hg
pCO_2	60mm Hg	20 mm Hg
BUN	100 mg/dL (indicates lower upper limit is critical in children)	uremia in adult;
Calcium	12.5 mg/dL	6.5 mg/dL
CK-MB	3.0%	
Creatinine	5.0 mg/dL	
Glucose	500 mg/dL	50 mg/dL
Hematocrit	60%	18% (higher for pre-op—30.0%)
Hemoglobin	20 g/dL (values may be critical in some disease states before this level is reached)	6.0 g/dL (higher for pre-op—10.0 g/dL)
Magnesium	5.0 mg/dL	1.0 mg/dL
Osmolality (serum)	325 mmol/kg	250 mmol/kg
Phosphorus	9.0 mg/dL	1.2 mg/dL
Platelet count	1,000,000/mm³ (10×10^9/L)	30,000/mm³ (3×10^9/L) assumes normal platelet function (higher for pre-op)
Potassium	6.2 mEq/L (7.0 mEq/L for newborn)	3.0 mEq/L
Prothrombin time	30 seconds (patient not anticoagulated)	
Sodium	160 mEq/L	120 mEq/L
WBC: peripheral blood	25,000/mm³ (on initial count)	2,500/mm³ (on initial count)
CSF	20 neutrophils	

Miscellaneous findings:
WBC differential: Peripheral blood—presence of blasts on initial examination; presence of sickled cells
Gram stain on cerebrospinal fluid: Organisms present
Blood culture: Organisms present
AFB stain or culture: Acid fast bacilli present
Stool culture: Enteric pathogen present
Transfusion service testing: Hemolytic transfusion reaction; inability to locate compatible donor units for crossmatch
Urinalysis: 3+ or 4+ ketones or glucose

Appendix G

ANSWER KEY FOR SELF TESTS

Question	CH. 1 (LAB)	CH. 2 (RENAL)	CH. 3 (CBC)	CH. 4 (LYMPHO/MYELO)	Question
1	C	B	D	A	1
2	B	A	A	C	2
3	D	C	B	B	3
4	A	A	C	C	4
5	D	D	B	B	5
6	B	C	D	A	6
7	C	B	B	C	7
8	B	A	C	B	8
9	D	D	A	D	9
10		B	B	C	10
11		A	C	A	11
12		D	A	B	12
13		C	D	C	13
14		C	B	A	14
15		B	C	C	15
16		A	B	C	16
17		C	D	A	17
18		D	C	C	18
19		B	A	D	19
20		A	C	D	20
21		D	B	C	21
22		D	B	C	22
23		C	C	A	23
24		A	A		24
25		D	D		25
26		B	B		26
27			A		27
28			C		28
29			B		29
30			D		30
31			A		31
32			C		32
33			A		33
34			B		34
35			C		35
36			D		36
37			B		37
38			B		38

Question	CH. 1 (LAB)	CH. 2 (RENAL)	CH. 3 (CBC)	CH. 4 (LYMPHO/MYELO)	Question
39			A		39
40			D		40
41			B		41
42			C		42
43			B		43
44			C		44
45			A		45
46			D		46
47			A		47

Question	CH. 5 (LIVER)	CH. 6 (GLUCOSE)	CH. 7 (LIPID)	CH. 8 (ELECTROLYTES)	Question
1	C	A	C	C	1
2	B	C	A	D	2
3	A	B	B	A	3
4	D	D	A	D	4
5	B	C	B	B	5
6	D	D	C	C	6
7	A	A	A	D	7
8	C	B	B	A	8
9	A	C	D	C	9
10	B	D	B	B	10
11	C	B	A	A	11
12	B	D	D	C	12
13	A	A	B	D	13
14	D		B	B	14
15	A		A	C	15
16	C		B	D	16
17	A			B	17
18	B			D	18
19	C			C	19
20				A	20
21				D	21
22					22
23					23
24					24
25					25

Question	CH. 9 (CHEM. PROF)	CH. 10 (PANCREATIC)	CH. 11 (ABGs)	CH. 12 (ACUTE MI)	Question
1	B	B	C	C	1
2	A	A	B	B	2
3	C	B	A	A	3
4	A	C	D	B	4
5	B	C	B	D	5
6	C	D	B	B	6
7	B	A	C	C	7

Question	CH. 9 (CHEM. PROF)	CH. 10 (PANCREATIC)	CH. 11 (ABGs)	CH. 12 (ACUTE MI)	Question
8	B	B	B	B	8
9	C	D	A	C	9
10	C	A	D	C	10
11	B	B	B	C	11
12	B		C		12
13	C		C		13
14	A		B		14
15	C		C		15
16	B		A		16
17	A		A		17
18	B				18

Question	CH. 13 (THYROID)	CH. 14 (ENDOCRINE)	CH. 15 (COAGULATION)	CH. 16 (TRANSF MED)	Question
1	C	A	A	B	1
2	A	C	C	C	2
3	B	D	C	D	3
4	C	B	D	A	4
5	D	C	B	B	5
6	C	A	D	C	6
7	C	D	C	D	7
8	B	B	A	C	8
9	A	A	D	C	9
10	B	C	D	B	10
11	C	D	C	D	11
12	A	B	A	D	12
13	C	B	C	C	13
14	D	A	B	A	14
15	B	D	C	B	15
16	C	D	A	D	16
17	A	C	D	D	17
18	B	A	B	B	18
19	E	B	D	C	19
20	D	D	C	A	20
21		C	C	D	21
22		A	D	B	22
23			B	B	23
24			A	B	24
25			C	A	25
26			A	A	26
27			B	C	27
28			C	C	28
29			C	C	29
30				A	30
31				B	31
32				C	32

Question	CH. 17 (MICRO)	CH. 18 (IMMUNE)	Question
1	B	C	1
2	B	A	2
3	C	C	3
4	C	B	4
5	C	A	5
6	B	C	6
7	D	C	7
8	C	A	8
9	B	B	9
10	D	B	10
11	C	C	11
12	B	A	12
13	A	B	13
14	D	A	14
15	B	A	15
16	D	B	16
17	C	C	17
18	D		18
19	A		19
20	C		20

REFERENCES

AABB Standards, 17th ed. 1996

AABB Technical Manual, 11th ed. 1993

American Diabetes Association. Clinical Practice Recommendations, volume 20, supplement 1, 1997

American Diabetes Association. Clinical Practice Recommendations, volume 21, supplement 1, 1998 (on-line, last revision 1-98)

Baskin LB, Morgan DL, Parupoa JY. A Rapid Immunoassay for Drugs of Abuse and Tricyclic Antidepressants. *Med Lab Obs,* 27:3, 1996

Belanger AC. Point of Care Testing: The JCAHO Perspective. *Med Lab Obs,* 26:6, 1994

Biggs R, Rizza CR, ed. *Human Blood Coagulation, Haemostasis and Thrombosis,* 3rd ed. Oxford, England, Blackwell Scientific Publications, 1984

Blaser MJ. Helicobacter Pylori and the Pathogenesis of Gastroduodenal Inflammation, *J Infec Dis,* University of Chicago, 1990

Cooney MM. A Collaborative Approach to Managing Risk. *Med Lab Obs,* Supplement, 24:9S, 1992

Corbett JV. *Laboratory Tests and Diagnostic Procedures with Nursing Diagnoses,* 3rd ed. Norwalk, CT, Appleton and Lange, 1992

Davis GL. Fibrinolysis Inhibitors. *Clin Lab Sci,* 10:4, 1997

Davis GL. Introduction to Hemostatic Inhibitors. *Clin Lab Sci,* 10:4, 1997

Endocrine Disorders Home Page [on-line], Endocrine Web, Inc., © 1997–1998

Forman DT. Controlling Error in Laboratory Testing. *Clin Lab Sci,* 10:4, 1997

Geyer SJ. Joining the Technological Evolution in Health Care. *Clin Lab Sci,* 10:4, 1997

Greenwood D, Slack R, Peutherer J. *Medical Microbiology: A Guide to Microbial Infections—Pathogenesis, Immunity, Laboratory Diagnosis and Control,* 15th ed. New York, Churchill Livingstone, 1997

Henry JB. *Clinical Diagnosis and Management by Laboratory Methods,* 19th ed. Philadelphia, Saunders, 1996

Hershman JM. *Hyperthyroidism: Diagnosis and Treatment. Thyroid Diagnosis and Management: A Technical Monograph.* National Health Laboratories Inc, La Jolla, CA

Hortin GL, Utz C, Gibson C. Managing Information from Bedside Testing, *Med Lab Obs,* 27:1, 1995

Jacobs DS, et al. *Laboratory Test Handbook,* 2nd ed. Cleveland, LexiComp Inc, 1990

Jensen R, Ens GE. Resistance to Activated Protein C: A Major Cause of Inherited Thrombophilia. *Clin Lab Sci,* 10:4, 1997

Kee, J LeF. *Laboratory and Diagnostic Tests with Nursing Implications,* 5th ed. Stamford, CT, Appleton and Lange, 1999

Kost GJ. The Hybrid Laboratory: Shifting the Focus to the Point of Care. *Clin Lab Sci,* 10:4, 1997

Lotspeich-Steininger C, Stiene-Martin A, Koepke J. *Clinical Hematology: Principles, Procedures, Correlations.* Philadelphia, Lippincott, 1992

Margulies P, MD. Medical Director, National Adrenal Disease Foundation, *Addison's Disease: The Facts You Need to Know,* (on-line, 1998)

Margulies P, MD. Medical Director, National Adrenal Disease Foundation, *Cushing's Syndrome: The Facts You Need to Know,* (on-line, 1998)

Mazzaferri EL. *Diagnosis and Management of Thyroid Nodules. Thyroid Diagnosis and Management: A Technical Monograph.* National Health Laboratories Inc, La Jolla, CA

Merck Manual (on-line), Section 8. Endocrine Disorders, Merck & Co, Inc, Whitehouse Station, NJ, © 1996–1997

Mollison PL, Engelfriet CP, Contreras M. *Blood Transfusion in Clinical Medicine,* 9th ed. Oxford, England, Blackwell Scientific Publications, 1993

Nardella A. Near-Patient Coag Testing, *Adv Adm Lab,* 2:6, 1998

Nicoloff JT. *Guide to Thyroid Function Testing for Laboratories and Physicians.* Abbott Diagnostics Educational Services, Abbott Diagnostics, Abbott Park, Illinois, 1991

NIH Publication No. 90-2964. *Recommendations for Improving Cholesterol Measurement: A Report from the Laboratory Standardization Panel of the National Cholesterol Education Program,* US Dept of Health and Human Services, Public Health Service, National Institutes of Health, February 1990

NIH Publication No. 96-3007. June, 1996 (on-line, 1998)

NIH Publication No. 90-3054. November, 1989, (on-line, 1998)

Ott D Trundle. Learn to Answer Troublesome Questions About Thyroid Tests. *Med Lab Obs,* 27:10, 1996

Paul SM, et al. One World One Hope: AIDS. *Med Lab Obs,* 28:10, 1996

Peakman, M, Vergani D. *Basic and Clinical Immunology.* New York, Churchill Livingstone, 1997

Phipps W, Long B, Woods N. *Medical-Surgical Nursing: Concepts and Clinical Practice,* 2nd ed. St Louis, Mosby, 1983

Popper C. Using Cost-Effectiveness Analysis to Weigh Testing Decisions. *Clin Lab Sci,* 10:4, 1997

Ravel, R. *Clinical Laboratory Medicine: Clinical Application of Laboratory Data,* 6th ed. St Louis, Mosby, 1995

Regulations and Point of Care Testing, Roundtable Discussion, *Med Lab Obs,* 28:8, 1997

Sacher RA, McPherson RA. *Widmann's Clinical Interpretation of Laboratory Tests,* 10th ed. Philadelphia, FA Davis, 1991

SmithKline Beecham. *Test Information: Helicobacter pylori Antibodies.* SmithKline Beecham Clinical Laboratories

SmithKline Beecham. *Test Information: Maternal Serum Alpha-Fetoprotein.* SmithKline Beecham Clinical Laboratories

SmithKline Beecham. *Test Information: The Triple Test: A Screening Test for Neural Tube Defects and Down Syndrome.* SmithKline Beecham Clinical Laboratories

Speiser PW, MD. *New Developments in the Treatment and Diagnosis of Congenital Adrenal Hyperplasia.* National Adrenal Disease Foundation, (on-line 1998)

Stein JH. *Internal Medicine: Diagnosis and Therapy,* 3rd ed. Norwalk, CT, Appleton and Lange, 1993

Surks MI. *Hypothyroidism: Diagnosis and Management. Thyroid Diagnosis and Management: A Technical Monograph.* National Health Laboratories Inc, La Jolla, CA

Travers EM, et al. Changing the Way Lab Medicine is Practiced at the Point of Care. *Med Lab Obs,* 26:7, 1994

Triple Screen "Major Advance" in Prenatal Dx of Retardation Causes, *Ob Gyn News,* 27:4, 1992

Triplett DA. Lupus Anticoagulants: Diagnostic Dilemma and Clinical Challenge. *Clin Lab Sci,* 10:4, 1997

Volpé R, *Autoimmune Thyroid Disease. Thyroid Diagnosis and Management: A Technical Monograph.* National Health Laboratories Inc, La Jolla, CA

Wartofsky L. *Altered Thyroid Function Tests in Patients with Systemic (Non-Thyroidal) Illness. Thyroid Diagnosis and Management: A Technical Monograph.* National Health Laboratories Inc, La Jolla, CA

Whalen F. An Outreach Program for Home Glucose Monitoring. *Med Lab Obs,* 26:7, 1994

Whitlock SA. *Immunohematology: Delmar's Clinical Laboratory Manual Series.* Albany, NY, Delmar Publishers, 1997

INDEX

Page numbers followed by *f* indicate illustrations and page numbers followed by *t* indicate table.